Anatomy and Physiology
For the MLA and Medical Exams

First and second edition authors
Michael Dykes
Phillip Ameerally

Third edition authors
Michael Dykes
Will Watson

Fourth edition author
Louise Stenhouse

Fifth edition authors
Samuel Hall
Jonny Stephens

6th Edition
CRASH COURSE

SERIES EDITOR

Philip Xiu

MA (Cantab), MB BChir, MRCP, MRCGP, MScClinEd, FHEA, MAcadMEd, RCPathME
Honorary Senior Lecturer
Leeds University School of Medicine
PCN Educational Lead
Medical Examiner
Leeds Teaching Hospital Trust
Leeds, UK

FACULTY ADVISOR

Claire F. Smith

BSc, PGCE, PhD, PFHEA, FAS, FLF, NTF, ACIEA, CATE
Professor of Anatomy
Deputy Pro Vice Chancellor Education and Innovation
Brighton and Sussex Medical School
Univeristy of Sussex
Brighton, UK

Anatomy and Physiology
For the MLA and Medical Exams

Jonny Stephens

BMBS, MMedSc, FRCA
Anaesthetic Registrar
London School of Anaesthesia
London, UK

Ross Munro

BMBS, BSc, MSc, FHEA, MAcadMEd
Resident Doctor/Anatomy Demonstrator
Brighton and Sussex Medical School
Univeristy of Sussex
Brighton, UK

Evelyn O'Rourke

BSc
Medical Student
Brighton and Sussex Medical School
University of Sussex
Brighton, UK

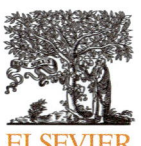

ELSEVIER

First edition 1998
Second edition 2002
Third edition 2007
Fourth edition 2012
Updated fourth edition 2015
Fifth edition 2019

Notice

Practitioners and researchers must always rely on their own experience and knowledge in evaluating and using any information, methods, compounds or experiments described herein. Because of rapid advances in the medical sciences, in particular, independent verification of diagnoses and drug dosages should be made. To the fullest extent of the law, no responsibility is assumed by Elsevier, authors, editors or contributors for any injury and/or damage to persons or property as a matter of products liability, negligence or otherwise, or from any use or operation of any methods, products, instructions, or ideas contained in the material herein.

ISBN: 978-0-443-24987-7

Content Strategist: **Trinity Hutton**
Content Project Manager: **Tapajyoti Chaudhuri**
Design: **Miles Hitchen**
Marketing Manager: **Deborah J. Watkins**

Printed in India

Last digit is the print number: 9 8 7 6 5 4 3 2 1

Working together to grow libraries in developing countries

www.elsevier.com • www.bookaid.org

Series editor's foreword

With great honour and pride, we present the latest edition of the Crash Course series. This series has traversed a journey of nearly a quarter century, stemming from the vision of Dr Dan Horton-Szar, and his legacy continues to walk with us on this pathway of knowledge.

The series has been popular with students worldwide, selling over **1 million copies** and being translated into more than **eight languages**, reinforcing our commitment to global learning. We remain extremely grateful for your unwavering trust. The series has once again been refreshed and fully upgraded in accordance with the rapidly changing medical guidelines, ensuring the content is comprehensive, accurate and fully up to date.

This latest series continues our tradition of integrating clinical practice with basic medical sciences, tailored meticulously for today's medical undergraduate curriculum. A central highlight of this instalment is our emphasis on high-yield examination content designed specifically for the Medical Licensing Assessment (MLA) curriculum.

Utilizing student feedback, we have strived to maintain the core principles of this series: delivering precise and readable text that brings together depth and clarity. The authors are experienced junior doctors who successfully navigated these examinations recently, ensuring practical and tested guidance. A team of expert faculty advisors from across the United Kingdom ensures the content's accuracy, making it resilient and reliable.

As we turn a new chapter with the latest edition, we honour the past, cherish the present and embrace the promise of the future. We wish you every success in your journey of learning and growth and hope that this series adds value to your life, both as students and as future medical professionals.

Philip Xiu

Authors

In essence, the anatomy and physiology of the human body encompasses the understanding of what things are and how they function, which is fundamental knowledge for all healthcare professionals. Only when you understand how the body functions normally can you understand how it fails in illness and what targets are available for treatment.

Anatomy and physiology are relevant to all specialities. Every medical practitioner will encounter these subjects daily, whether it be in the emergency department, on the ward, in a community clinic or at the surgical operating table. Once the fundamentals of anatomy and physiology are grasped, they will become far more enjoyable and also provide a solid foundation for your knowledge enabling development as you progress through your career. In addition, gaining knowledge in these topics will not only enhance individual capacity but also empower you to confidently and competently engage with and treat more effectively thousands of patients in your chosen career.

And if this is not enough to encourage you, you can be certain that anatomy and physiology will appear in examinations at every stage from medical school all the way through to speciality training exit examinations! We hope this book makes learning anatomy and physiology a more enjoyable and achievable experience.

Jonny, Ross and Evelyn

Faculty Advisor

The application of anatomy and physiology remains at the centre of safe clinical practice for doctors and allied healthcare professionals. To enable safe practice, understanding the structure and function of the body and how they present in health and disease is key.

I taught Samuel Hall, Jonny Stephens, Ross Munro and Evie O'Rourke at medical school. They know from recent first-hand experience how the anatomy and physiology they learned underpin their clinical work. I believe that learning is most productive when it is active and applied. One way to develop your knowledge beyond this book is to help teach others. This will really help you to cognitively process the information and truly learn it for understanding, not to just pass examinations. That is important too!

With so many resources available, it can be difficult to know which one to choose and whether it is at the correct level. This book gives you a concise review of the core anatomy and physiology that you simply cannot do without. We have worked to develop new diagrams, reflect diversity in the images and examples we use and add in updated clinical and anatomical information. As we learn anatomy and physiology, we not only gain an understanding of how to diagnose and treat patients, but we also understand more about our amazing own body. I hope you have a successful and interesting learning journey.

Claire F. Smith

Series editor's acknowledgements

We would like to express our sincere gratitude to those who have provided their support and expertise in preparing this sixth edition of the Crash Course series. Our junior doctor contributors' participation in crafting the manuscript has been indispensable. Their first-hand experience and current medical knowledge have infused realism and practicality into our content.

Our faculty editors deserve a special note of thanks. They have extensively validated the correctness of the information, ensuring that the content is not just accurate but also contemporaneous, credible and aligns with the latest medical standards.

We extend our heartfelt thanks to our publisher, Elsevier. Their staff have demonstrated an unwavering commitment to quality, maintaining the high standards since the first edition. Their insights have routinely enriched the content and process alike.

Our Commissioning Editor, Jeremy Bowes, deserves a special mention for his consistent support and guiding hand throughout the development process. His directions and advice have bettered this edition and spurred us on our quest for excellence.

We are greatly indebted to Alex Mortimer for her wisdom, practical insights and valuable guidance. A big thank you to our Content Strategists, Trinity Hutton and Jennifer Dooley, who need special acknowledgement for meticulously outlining the direction and scope of the content. They have managed to mix details with a strategic plan, keeping our readers in mind.

Lastly, much gratitude is owed to our Content Product Managers, Taranpreet Kaur, Ayan Dhar, Shivani Pal and Tapajyoti Chaudhuri, who have juggled their numerous day-to-day tasks with utmost dedication and perseverance. Despite the ever-approaching deadlines, they have shown remarkable patience and steadfast determination, ensuring that each step of the book's development was accomplished seamlessly.

In conclusion, we sincerely thank each of these wonderful people for their outstanding contributions and support, without which this work would not have been achieved. Their passion, commitment and collaborative effort have helped us bring this edition together.

Philip Xiu

Acknowledgements

Evie O'Rourke: I would like to thank the whole Elsevier team for their support and patience during this process. A big thank you to Claire F. Smith, Jonny Stephens and Ross Munro for all their guidance and putting up with my questions. Thank you to the Anatomy Team at BSMS for all your support and encouragement over the years. Thank you to my friends for providing levity and support over the years. Thank you to all my family, my many siblings, my dad Sean and stepmom Lou and to my grandparents John and Joyce for your constant support. Thank you to my sister Fi for being my role model and inspiration, always. The biggest thank you goes to my mum, Emily, for her unwavering love and belief, none of this would be possible without you.

Ross Munro: Thank you to my friends Evie O'Rourke, Jonny Stephens and Claire F. Smith for making the writing process fruitful, novel and enjoyable. Secondly, thanks to the Elsevier team for their guidance and assistance. Finally, I would like to thank my whole family for their steadfast love and support. To my parents Duncan and Lesley, my brother Scott and wife Elizabeth, thanks for everything!

Jonny Stephens: Thank you Evie O'Rourke, Ross Munro and Claire F. Smith for all of your hard work and for making the whole process a fulfilling and enjoyable one. I would like to thank my mum, Kim; dad, Bert; and sister, Daisy for being the best supporters from the very start. And my biggest thank you goes to my best friend and wife, Phoebe, for the sacrifices you make to allow me to do what I do, and to my little heroes, Hector and Xanthe, for always putting a smile on my face.

Claire F. Smith: I would like to express my heartfelt appreciation to Samuel Hall, Jonny Stephens, Ross Munro, and Evie O'Rourke for their outstanding writing contributions and thoughtful consideration of how this book can benefit students. I am truly grateful for the incredible support from the Elsevier team. I would also like to extend my deepest thanks to my husband, Trevor; my daughters Hermione and Elodie; my mother Susan; and in loving memory of my father Michael, for their unwavering love and support.

Special acknowledgements to digital artists

The anatomical illustrations in this work represent a significant step forward in addressing diversity within medical education, made possible through the expertise of two remarkable contributors.

Gusztav Velicsek, Director of 3D, and Dariusz Andrulonis, Digital Sculptor, brought exceptional skill and insight to this project. Their work with the anatomically precise illustrations that thoughtfully represent human diversity has enhanced the educational value of this book immeasurably.

I also want to thank the talented Joe Yapp who provided the illustration of the pre and post-operative transgender pelvis, which is the first to my knowledge in a medical anatomy textbook.

Combined with their understanding of the need for inclusive representation, has helped establish a new standard in anatomical visualisation. Their contributions will benefit students and healthcare professionals for years to come, providing a more comprehensive and representative foundation for anatomical study.

Philip Xiu

Contents

Contents

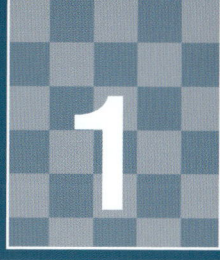
OVERVIEW OF THE BOOK

Anatomy and physiology are two essential sciences of medicine and healthcare. Anatomy is the understanding of the structure of organisms and their parts, from gross structures such as the bones of a limb to the microstructures of an individual cell. Physiology is the understanding of the normal functions of the human body, which healthcare providers must understand to treat the diseases that occur when these functions go wrong.

As you progress through this book and into your career, you will repeatedly find that structure is intrinsically related to function and vice versa. This book will progress from introducing the building blocks of life and key concepts required to understand anatomy and physiology, to describing the normal structure and function of the human body broken down into a regional approach. The aim of this book is to allow the readers to gain a good understanding of the concepts of anatomy and physiology that will be sufficient to pass medical and healthcare examinations.

CELL

The cell is the basic structural and functional unit of organisms and is responsible for carrying out essential processes that enable the organism to grow, develop and maintain homoeostasis. A cell comprises a membrane that acts as a barrier and regulates the movement of substances in and out of the cell. Inside the cell, the protoplasm has specific functions, such as energy production, and the nucleus acts as the control centre, storing and transmitting genetic information.

Microstructure of the cell

Protoplasm is the collective name given to the basic components and materials that make up the cell inside the cell membrane. The protoplasm therefore includes both the nucleus and cytoplasm. The protoplasm is formed of:

- Water – the major component of the cell, forming around 80% of the cell.
- Proteins – form around 15% of the cell. The two types are:
  - Structural proteins, forming the body of the cell.
  - Globular proteins that are mainly enzymes.

- Lipids – there are three main types of lipid in the cell:
  - Phospholipids – form the outer and intracellular membranous barriers.
  - Cholesterol – integrated into the outer and intracellular membranous barriers.
  - Triglycerides – an energy source of the cell.
- Carbohydrates – stored as glycogen and provide energy for the cell.
- Electrolytes – essential for cellular reactions (e.g. action potential): potassium ions (K^+), magnesium ions (Mg^{2+}), phosphate ions (PO_4^{3-}) and bicarbonate ions (HCO_3^-).

Organelles and their function

Within each cell are a number of highly organized physical structures – organelles – each with a specific function (Fig. 1.1).

Nucleus

The nucleus is present in almost all cells (mature red blood cells do not have a nucleus) and is the 'control centre' (Fig. 1.2). The nucleus stores and transmits information, in the form of DNA, to the next generation. The genes within the cell's nucleus determine the types of protein made by the cell during its lifetime.

Nuclear membrane and envelope

A nuclear membrane and envelope surround the nucleus, containing pores that regulate the entry and exit of molecules.

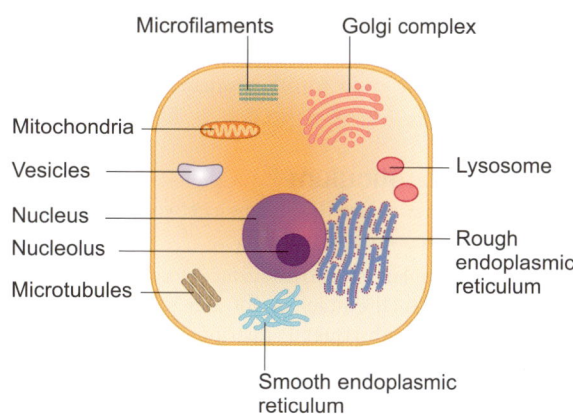

Fig. 1.1 Cell and organelles.

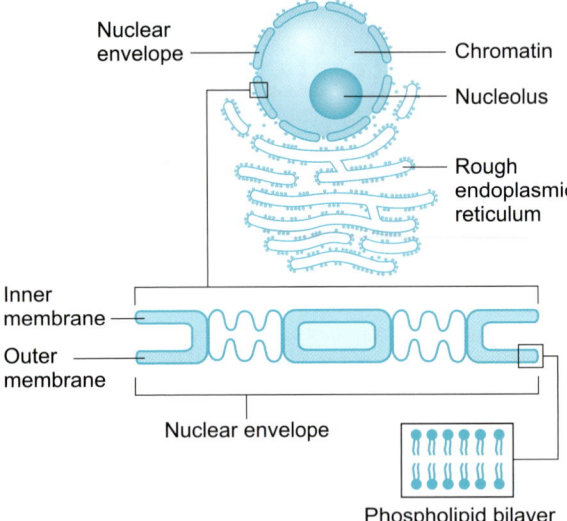

Fig. 1.2 The cell nucleus and nuclear membrane structure.

Nucleoli

The nucleoli are highly coiled structures within the nucleus of the cell. They contain ribonucleic acid (RNA) and protein components. The nucleoli are not enveloped by a nuclear membrane.

Ribosomes

Ribosomes are large organelles, composed of about 70 proteins and several RNA molecules, that serve as the site of protein synthesis. They include two subunits of different sizes, 30 s and 50 s, the former being smaller.

Proteins are synthesized from amino acid building blocks using a genetic template derived from DNA that is carried from the nucleus to the ribosomes as messenger RNA (mRNA). The proteins are then released into the cytosol (fluid part of the cell's cytoplasm) or transferred to other organelles via the Golgi apparatus.

Endoplasmic reticulum

The endoplasmic reticulum (ER) forms a network of membranes within the cell. There are two types:

1. Rough (or granular) ER carries surface ribosomes. Proteins are synthesized on the attached ribosomes, enter the lumen of the ER and are subsequently distributed within the cell or secreted to other cells.
2. Smooth (or agranular) ER does not have ribosomes on its surface. This type of ER synthesizes fatty acids and regulates cellular levels of calcium (Ca^{2+}), which controls many of the cell's activities.

Golgi apparatus

These membranous sacs sort and modify proteins arriving from the rough ER, packaging them into vesicles before sending them to other organelles within the cell or secreting them into the extracellular space.

Mitochondria

The mitochondria function to make energy available to cells in the form of adenosine triphosphate (ATP). Mitochondria are double-membraned, elongated structures with a smooth outer membrane and an inner membrane that is folded into tubes (cristae) designed to increase surface area. The cristae contain DNA for mitochondrial protein synthesis.

Lysosomes

Lysosomes are single-membraned organelles that contain highly acidic digestive enzymes that break down bacteria, cell debris and dead organelles.

Peroxisomes

Peroxisomes are single-membraned organelles that destroy the highly toxic compound hydrogen peroxide (H_2O_2), a by-product of certain cell reactions. Alternatively, the peroxisomes in the liver and kidney produce H_2O_2 and use it to detoxify various ingested molecules.

Filaments

A cell's shape is maintained by a cytoskeleton which is formed of protein filaments in the cytoplasm, which also act to aid cell movement.

Energy production in the cell

Cells use oxygen to break down macromolecules from food (carbohydrates to glucose, proteins to amino acids and fats to fatty acids) and form the compound ATP, the universal source of energy for all intracellular metabolic reactions.

Structure of adenosine triphosphate

ATP is a nucleotide containing the base adenine, the pentose sugar ribose and three phosphate molecules (Fig. 1.3). The two phosphate molecules at the end of ATP are connected by a high-energy bond. When broken, each liberates about 30.6 kJ/mol of energy, roughly the same as the energy in a single peanut. When the first covalent bond is hydrolyzed, adenosine diphosphate (ADP) is produced; the loss of another phosphate molecule forms adenosine monophosphate. Energy is released when each bond is hydrolyzed.

Formation of adenosine triphosphate

The majority (95%) of ATP is formed in the mitochondrial matrix. One molecule of glucose produces a net of 38 molecules of ATP during aerobic respiration. Other substrates can produce more ATP than carbohydrates. For example, 1 g of fat can produce twice as much ATP as 1 g of carbohydrate. Protein is used as a substrate only when all the carbohydrate and fat reserves have been utilized, that is, in a starvation state. There are four stages of ATP production:

Glycolysis
Glycolysis is the formation of pyruvic acid (PA). Glucose, fatty acids and amino acids enter the cell cytoplasm and are converted to PA, releasing energy for the formation of two molecules of ATP (Fig. 1.4).

Conversion of pyruvic acid to acetyl coenzyme A
PA enters the mitochondrial matrix, where the enzyme pyruvate dehydrogenase transforms it into acetyl coenzyme A (acetyl-CoA) (Fig. 1.4).

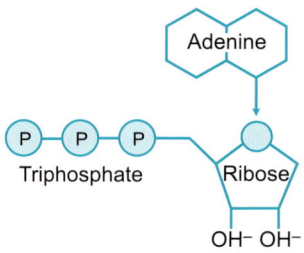

Fig. 1.3 Structure of adenosine triphosphate.

Citric acid/Krebs cycle
The citric acid cycle is also called the Krebs cycle or tricarboxylic acid cycle. Acetyl-CoA enters a series of chemical reactions in the mitochondrial matrix in which it is split into acetyl and CoA, as shown in Fig. 1.5. The acetyl portion enters the cycle, and the CoA is used in the formation of more acetyl-CoA. During the citric acid cycle, for every glucose molecule:

- Seven molecules of water are added.
- 16 hydrogen atoms and four molecules of carbon dioxide (CO_2) are released.
- Two molecules of ATP are formed.

The CO_2 diffuses out of the mitochondria and is expired as a waste gas from the lungs.

Oxidative phosphorylation (electron transport chain)
The largest amount of ATP formation occurs during oxidative phosphorylation (remember glycolysis and the citric acid/Krebs cycle only contribute 4 of the 38 ATP molecules produced) (Fig. 1.6). There are seven main steps:

1. Hydrogen is split into a hydrogen ion (H^+) and an electron.
2. The electron enters the electron transport chain on the inner mitochondrial membrane.

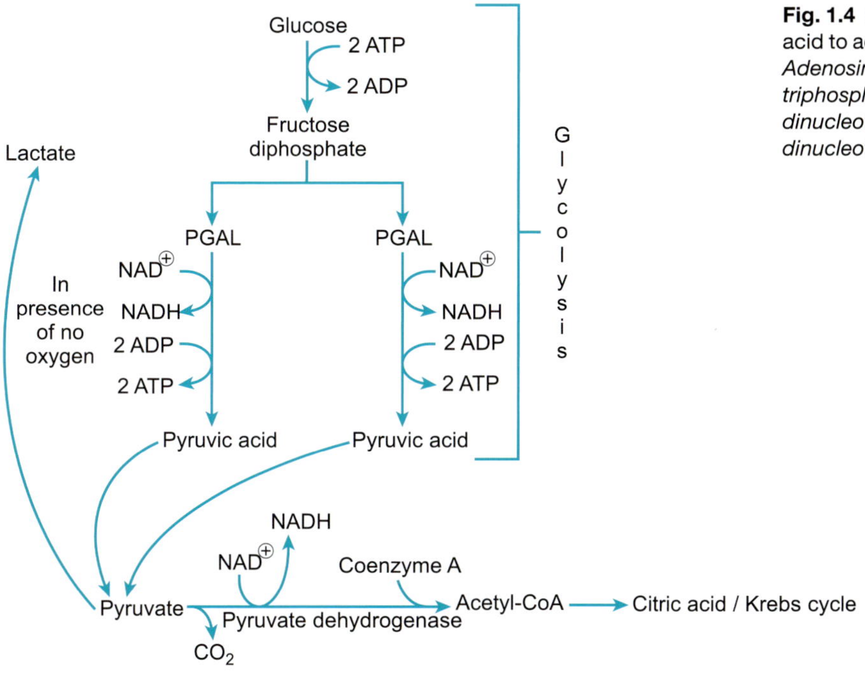

Fig. 1.4 Glycolysis and conversion of pyruvic acid to acetyl coenzyme (acetyl-CoA). ADP, *Adenosine diphosphate*; ATP, *adenosine triphosphate*; NAD, *nicotinamide adenine dinucleotide*; NADH, *nicotinamide adenine dinucleotide hydrogen* ; PGAL, *phosphoglycerate*.

3

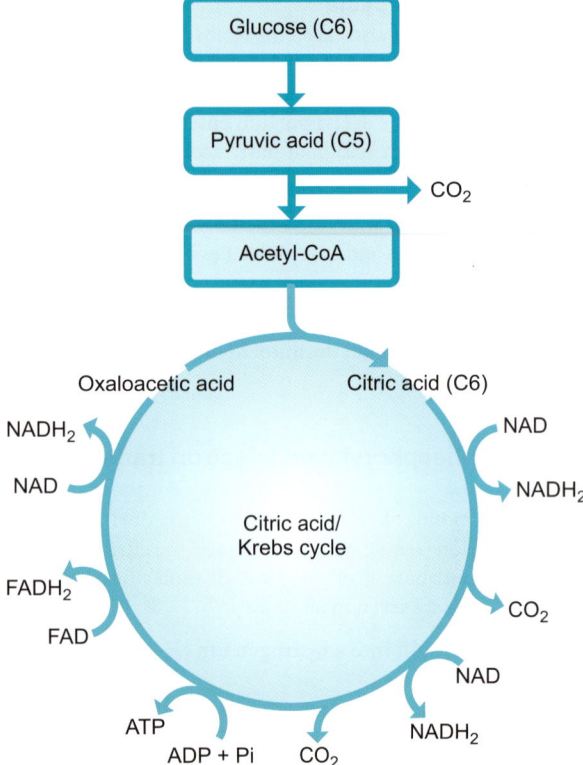

Fig. 1.5 Citric acid/Krebs cycle. ADP, *Adenosine diphosphate*; ATP, *adenosine triphosphate*; CoA, *coenzyme A*; FAD, *flavin adenine dinucleotide*; FADH$_2$, *flavin adenine dinucleotide–reduced form*; NAD, *nicotinamide adenine dinucleotide*; NADH, *nicotinamide adenine dinucleotide–reduced form*; Pi, *phosphate*.

3. The electron is transported from electron acceptor to electron acceptor (i.e. flavoproteins and cytochromes B, C and A) until it reaches cytochrome A3 (cytochrome oxidase).
4. Cytochrome oxidase helps form ionic oxygen, which combines with the H$^+$ to form water.
5. The large amounts of energy that are released during the electron transport chain happen because the electron transport pumps H$^+$ from the inner matrix of the mitochondrion to the space between the inner and outer membrane (outer chamber).
6. The high concentration of H$^+$ in the outer chamber flows over the enzyme ATPase, which is attached to the inner mitochondrial membrane. This energy from the H$^+$ flow is used by ATPase to convert ADP to ATP.
7. ATP is transferred by facilitated diffusion from the mitochondrion to the cell cytoplasm.

Anaerobic respiration

At times, tissues lack sufficient oxygen to undertake aerobic respiration (e.g. during intense muscle activity). The lack of oxygen means there is no terminal acceptor of H$^+$ at the end of the electron transport chain, leading to its termination with a subsequent reduction in glycolysis and the citric acid cycle. Therefore anaerobic respiration ensues, during which pyruvate, the product of glycolysis that normally enters the citric acid cycle under aerobic conditions, is converted to lactate facilitated by the enzyme lactate dehydrogenase.

This process generates the proton donor NAD$^+$ which can then be used for further glycolysis, which in turn generates a net production of 2 ATP molecules per cycle. This yield of ATP is significantly less than from aerobic respiration (38 molecules of ATP per molecule of glucose); however, anaerobic respiration is much faster and ensures that ATP continues to be formed in situations of high energy demand.

Lactate is highly acidic and must therefore be promptly removed from the tissues and blood. This can happen by one of two pathways:

- Cori cycle: occurs in the liver and describes the process of gluconeogenesis through the conversion of lactate into pyruvate and subsequently into glucose.
- Converted back to pyruvate in metabolically active tissues which can then be used by the citric acid cycle.

Functions of adenosine triphosphate

The functions of ATP are:

- To enable the transportation of molecules across cell membranes.
- To synthesize chemical compounds, for example protein synthesis on ribosomes, formation of cholesterol and phospholipids.
- To supply energy for mechanical work, for example muscle contraction and ciliary function.

Genetic control of the cell

Genes control cell function. Genes determine what proteins, both enzymes and structural proteins, are produced within the cell. Every gene is made of DNA, which regulates RNA to dictate the formation of particular proteins.

Deoxyribonucleic acid

DNA is a double helical chain composed of:

- Phosphoric acid, part of the backbone of the DNA molecule.
- A deoxyribose sugar, part of the backbone of the DNA molecule.
- Four nitrogenous bases:
  - Two purines: adenine (A) and guanine (G).
  - Two pyrimidines: thymine (T) and cytosine (C).

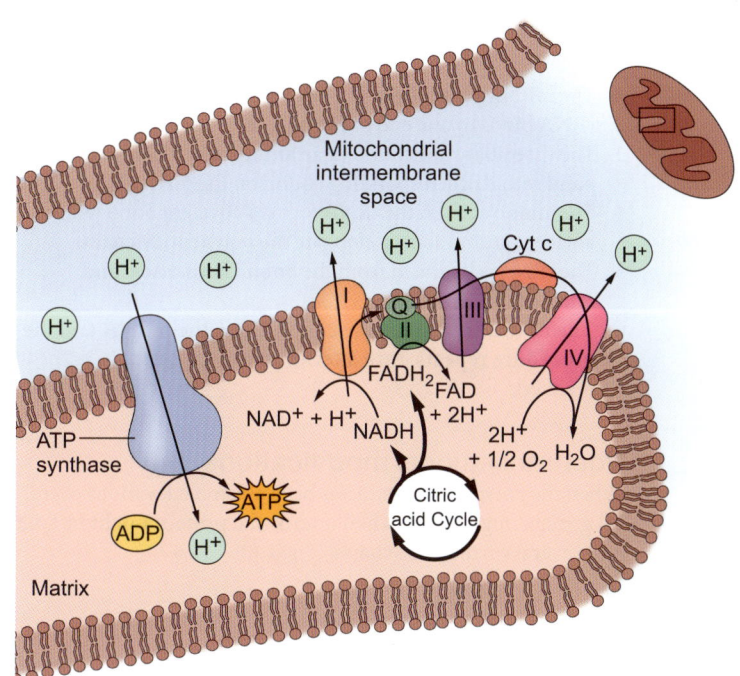

Fig. 1.6 Oxidative phosphorylation, the electron transfer chain and the citric acid chain. ADP, *Adenosine diphosphate*; ATP, *adenosine triphosphate*; Cyt c, *cytochrome C*; FAD, *flavin adenine dinucleotide*; FADH$_2$, *flavin adenine dinucleotide–reduced form*; NAD, *nicotinamide adenine dinucleotide*; NADH, *nicotinamide adenine dinucleotide–reduced form*. Ehem ocur.

The bases connect the two DNA strands, to form the double helical chain, via hydrogen bonds. Importantly:

- Adenine can bind only to thymine.
- Guanine can bind only to cytosine.

When DNA is split into its individual strands, the exposed bases provide the genetic code. Every three successive bases (triplet) code for one amino acid. Examples of each codon composition to form an amino acid can be found in the eBook version of this text. Chains of amino acids form proteins. The four bases can be arranged in 64 different three-letter combinations ($4 \times 4 \times 4 = 64$). As only 21 different amino acids are synthesized in the body, some amino acids are represented by more than one codon. There are also codons for start and stop signals, which indicate that the end of a genetic message has been reached. The remainder of the DNA that does not code for proteins has been classed as redundant DNA. However, new research is challenging this idea and hinting at the possibility that this 'noncoding DNA', previously known as 'junk DNA', has important functions, such as determining how and where new genes can evolve.

Super-coiling

DNA is a very long molecule and must be packaged very well to fit into a cell. The double helix gives it a natural twist, but further twisting packs it even tighter; this called is super-coiling.

Ribonucleic acid

For proteins to be produced, the DNA code must be transferred to an RNA code. As DNA is in the cell nucleus and the majority of cell function occurs in the cytoplasm, the RNA acts as an intermediary to these processes.

RNA is identical to DNA with two exceptions:

1. Deoxyribose is replaced with ribose.
2. Thymine is replaced by the pyrimidine uracil (which will only bind to adenine).

There are three types of RNA:

1. Messenger RNA (mRNA): carries the genetic code from the nucleus to the cytoplasm.
2. Transfer RNA (tRNA): transfers amino acids to the ribosomes to manufacture proteins.
3. Ribosomal RNA (rRNA): where the protein molecules are actually assembled.

HINTS AND TIPS

One amino acid is coded for by a sequence of three bases (a triplet).

HINTS AND TIPS

Remember that RNA is identical in structure to DNA apart from the fact that deoxyribose is replaced with ribose and thymine is replaced by uracil.

Protein synthesis

There are four key steps to protein production: transcription, splicing, translation and posttranslation modifications.

Transcription: messenger RNA synthesis

Transcription occurs following this sequence:

1. RNA polymerase attaches to the DNA promoter and moves along the helix (Fig. 1.7).
2. The DNA double helix unwinds and the strands separate.
3. RNA nucleotides attach – via hydrogen bonds – to the exposed bases on one DNA strand.
4. Covalent bonds are formed between the RNA nucleotide phosphate and ribose, producing mRNA.
5. When RNA polymerase comes across a DNA stop signal, it breaks away from the DNA strand. The stop signal indicates that the mRNA is complete.
6. The hydrogen bonds holding the mRNA to the DNA strand break, and the mRNA enters the nucleoplasm.

A three-base sequence in the mRNA transcript is known as a codon and is complementary to the three-base sequence in DNA (triplet).

Splicing

The primary mRNA transcript contains specific segments (exons) that code for amino acids; the remainder of the transcript does not code for any protein (introns). Splicing removes the introns and combines the remaining exons. This results in the final mRNA.

Translation

During translation:

1. The mRNA passes from the cell nucleus to the cytoplasm.
2. rRNA binds to one end of the mRNA.
3. The three-base anticodon in an amino acid–tRNA complex pairs with its corresponding codon on the mRNA.
4. The amino acid on the tRNA forms a covalent bond with the adjacent amino acid to elongate the polypeptide chain.
5. The tRNA is liberated from the bound amino acid and released.
6. The ribosome travels one codon along the mRNA and the procedure repeats until a termination sequence is reached.

Posttranslational modifications

When the polypeptide chain has been assembled, various chemical groups might be attached and/or the protein might be split into several smaller side chains (Fig. 1.8).

Cell movement

There are two types of cell movement:

1. **Amoeboid movement:** A protrusion from the cell – a pseudopodium – attaches to the substrate across which the cell is moving. The remainder of the cell body drags itself towards the pseudopodium (e.g. white blood cells through tissues). Amoeboid movement is initiated by chemical

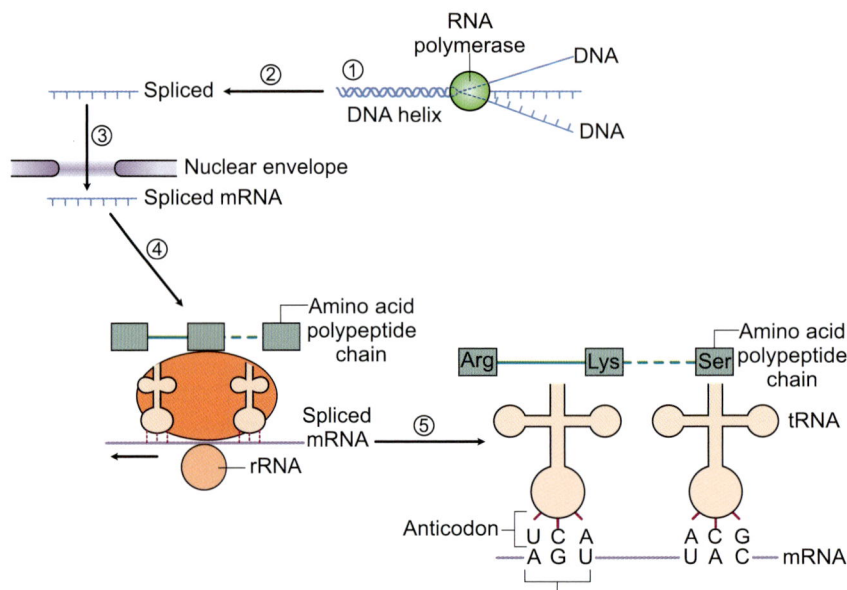

Fig. 1.7 DNA synthesis. mRNA, *Messenger ribonucleic acid*; RNA, *ribonucleic acid*.

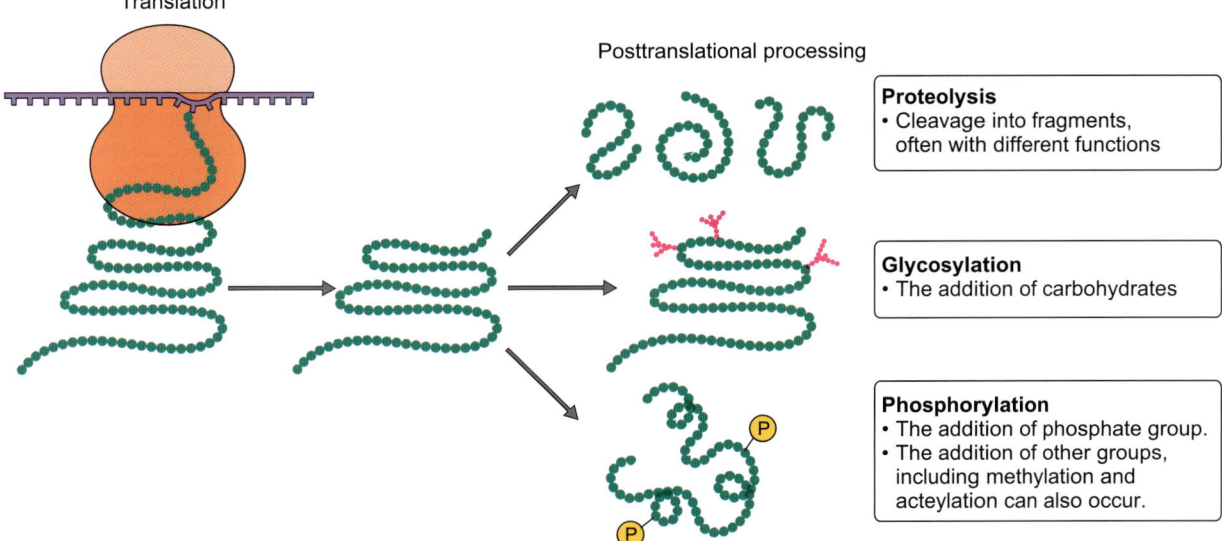

Fig. 1.8 Posttranslational modifications.

substances produced by the tissues (chemotaxis). The cells can move towards (positive chemotaxis) or away from (negative chemotaxis) an area of chemotactic substances.

2. **Ciliary movement:** Whip-like movements of cilia propel the cell. Such movement occurs on the inside surfaces of the respiratory airways and uterine tubes. In the respiratory airways, ciliary movements propel mucus towards the trachea; in the uterine tubes, they propel the ovum towards the uterine cavity.

Membrane physiology

The cell membrane consists of three components: lipids, proteins and carbohydrates (Fig. 1.9).

Cell membranes
Lipids
Phospholipid molecules form a lipid bilayer, which envelops the entire cell and organelle. One part of the phospholipid molecule is hydrophilic (water loving) and the other is hydrophobic (water hating). This results in the molecules lining up with the hydrophobic portions back to back, avoiding contact with water. Because there is no chemical bond linking the phospholipids to each other, they are free to move independently. This is sometimes termed 'the fluid mosaic model' and permits cells to change considerably without disruption to their structure.

The phospholipid bilayer regulates the movement of certain substances into and out of the cell. It prevents the entry of

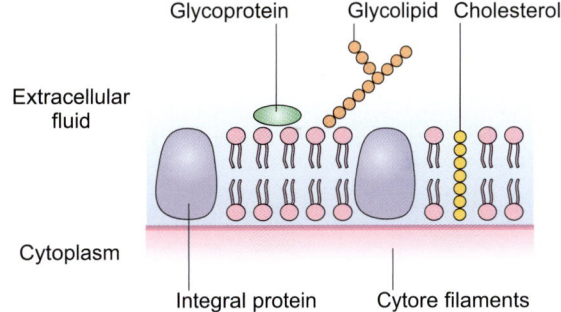

Fig. 1.9 Structure of cell membranes.

water-soluble substances (such as urea, glucose and ions) and allows the passage of fat-soluble substances (alcohol, oxygen and carbon dioxide).

Cholesterol, a steroid, inserts itself in the membrane with the same orientation as the phospholipid molecules. It functions to immobilize the first few hydrocarbon groups of the phospholipid molecules. If cholesterol was absent (as in a bacterium), a cell would need a cell wall. It also prevents the crystallization of hydrocarbons and the membrane from shifting.

Proteins
There are two types of protein in the cell membrane:
1. **Integral proteins:** These extend all the way through the bilayer (i.e. are transmembranous) and form structural channels through which ions and other water-soluble

substances can permeate. They also form receptors for enzyme binding.

2. **Peripheral proteins:** These are located on the inside of the membrane and form enzymes.

Carbohydrates (glycocalyx)

The carbohydrates in the cell membrane combine with proteins (to form glycoproteins) and lipids (to form glycolipids) that protrude outside the cell. They function to:

- Repel other negatively charged objects (because of their negative charge)
- Attach to other cells so they can identify them or be identified
- Provide binding sites for hormones

Cells involved in immunity use the glycocalyx for the recognition of host/foreign cells.

Membranous junctions

Adjacent cells can be joined together by different types of junction: tight junctions, gap junctions and spot desmosomes (Fig. 1.10).

Tight junctions

Tight junctions form an impermeable bond between adjacent cells. They direct the passage of substrates through the cells by preventing passage between them. They are found in the epithelial cell layer lining the small intestine and in the blood–brain barrier in the cerebral vessels.

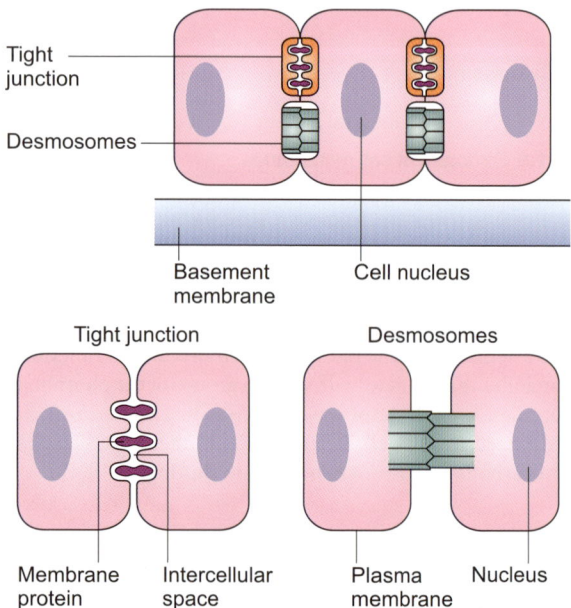

Fig. 1.10 Membranous junctions, showing a tight junction and desmosomes.

Gap junctions

Gap junctions are protein tunnels that form between adjacent cells. They allow for the passage of small molecules and/or ions between cells. Cells connected by gap junctions can work synchronously as a unit, instead of individually. In the heart, gap junctions allow a sequential and coordinated contraction of the atria and the ventricles.

Spot desmosomes

Spot desmosomes are large filamentous adhesions between nearby cells that serve as mechanical reinforcements. Tissues under stress, for example cardiac muscle, are connected by spot desmosomes.

Transport

The selective permeability properties of the cell membrane play an important role in cell function by controlling the entry into cells of small molecules and ions. Diffusion across biological membranes can be divided broadly into passive (diffusion) or active forms of transport.

Passive (diffusion)

The movement of small molecules and ions is dictated by their electrochemical concentration gradient. They move from high to low concentrations to neutralize a charge imbalance between two zones.

Size, electrical charge, shape and weight affect the rate of diffusion. If a substance is lipid soluble, diffusion across the cell membrane (which is a lipid bilayer) will occur more readily. However, with polar substances, diffusion rates through water-filled ion channels are greater.

If the solutions on either side of a membrane comprise only diffusible ions, diffusion occurs until equilibrium is reached and the ion distribution on each side is the same. At this point, this is the value of diffusible anions × diffusible cations.

There are several different types of diffusion (Fig. 1.11):

Simple diffusion. In simple diffusion, the movement of molecules occurs through a membrane opening. This opening either passes through the lipid bilayer (allowing the passage of lipid-soluble substances) or takes the form of protein channels, for example sodium and potassium (Na^+ and K^+) channels, through which water- and lipid-insoluble molecules pass. The protein channels regulate their permeability via a `gating' system.

Voltage gating. The electrical potential across the cell membrane influences the entry of certain substances. For example, during an action potential, an impulse passes down a neuron; the resulting reduction in the voltage causes sodium channels in the adjacent portion of the membrane to open. This allows the influx of sodium ions (Na^+) into the neuron by diffusion through the channel and hence the continuation of the nerve impulse.

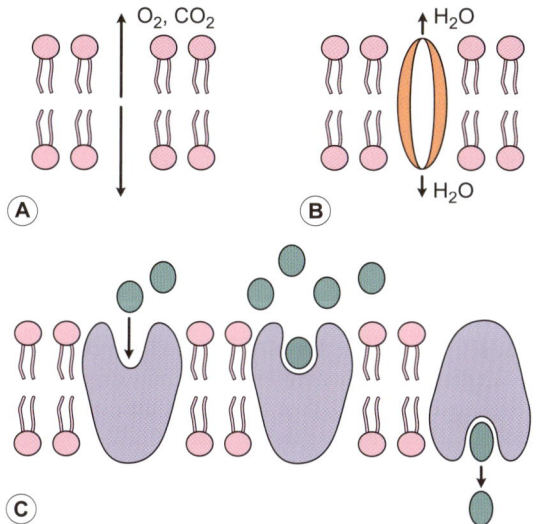

Fig. 1.11 Types of diffusion. (A) Simple diffusion. (B) Diffusion through channels: proteins and charged molecules are usually pulled through channels by water. (C) Facilitated diffusion: molecules (e.g. glucose) bind to protein, triggering a charge in protein shape. This transports the glucose molecules across the membrane.

Chemical gating. The binding of another molecule permits entry. For example, acetylcholine opens the acetylcholine channel, through which sodium ions (Na^+) diffuse, which allows nerve signals to propagate.

Facilitated diffusion. During facilitated diffusion, a carrier protein is required to transport a substance across the membrane. A good example is found in the liver cells, which help control the concentration of glucose in the blood. Liver cells store excess glucose as glycogen when blood sugar levels are high. The breakdown of glycogen is closely controlled by hormones. The breakdown products of glycogen are impermeable to the liver cell membrane, and so a transport protein, which functions by facilitated diffusion, allows the movement of glucose.

Nonionic diffusion. Although weak acids and bases cross cell membranes with difficulty in their ionic and dissociated forms, some have increased solubility in their undissociated form. Diffusion of such undissociated substances is called nonionic diffusion; it occurs in the kidneys and gastrointestinal tract.

Active transport

By using ATP, this energy-dependent system transports ions or molecules across a membrane against an electrochemical gradient. It can thus maintain the concentration of a substance against its natural diffusion gradient, for example the K^+ concentration is high intracellularly and low extracellularly.

Active transport depends on two types of transmembrane carrier protein, which derive their energy sources in different ways:

- **Primary transmembrane carrier proteins:** Receive their energy from ATP. They transport many different ions (e.g. Na^+, K^+, Ca^{2+} into and out of muscle cells; H^+ and K^+ into and out of the gastric glands). The most common type is the Na^+/K^+ pump system, hereafter referred to as Na^+/K^+-ATPase, which is present in all cells of the body. This pumps Na^+ out of the cell, K^+ into the cell and maintains the electrical potential across the cell membrane.
- **Secondary transmembrane carrier proteins:** Energy is generated from differences in ionic concentration between two sides of a membrane.

HINTS AND TIPS

As the result of the Na^+/K^+-ATPase, K^+ is predominantly intracellular and Na^+ is predominantly extracellular.

Cotransport

This term refers to transport across a cell membrane when a carrier is occupied by two substances simultaneously. There are two types:

- **Antiport:** A membrane carrier creates a gradient for the movement of one substance in one direction and another substance in the opposite direction.
- **Symport:** Two substances move in the same direction by means of a common carrier.

Osmosis

This is the diffusion of water across a semipermeable membrane (i.e. a membrane that allows only the passage of certain small molecules but prevents the passage of large molecules) (Fig. 1.12). Water molecules diffuse from a region of higher water concentration to a lower water concentration. The pressure at which water is drawn from the weak solution into the more concentrated solution is known as the osmotic pressure; the higher the solute concentration, the higher the osmotic pressure. *Note:* a low water concentration implies a high solute concentration.

Solute particles are seen as the osmotically active particles, the total concentration of which, regardless of exact composition, is referred to as *osmolarity*, which is expressed in osmoles (Osm):

$$1 \text{ Osm} = 1 \text{ mole } (6.02 \times 10^{23}) \text{ solute particles}$$

$$1 \text{ mOsm} = 1/1000 \text{ mole of solute particles}$$

The nature of the solute will dictate the osmolarity. Dissolving 1 mole of a nonionizing compound, such as glucose, in water will give a solution of 1 Osm. However, dissolving 1 mole of sodium chloride (NaCl), which dissociates into Na^+ and Cl^-, will give a solution of 2 Osm.

Osmolarity. Osmolarity (mOsm/L) is defined as the number of osmoles per unit volume.

This can be illustrated by putting x Osm of solute into a beaker, then adding water to make up 1 L of solution. Clearly, the water added would be less than 1 L.

Osmolality. Osmolality (mOsm/kg) is defined as the number of osmoles per unit weight.

Normally, osmolality is about the same as osmolarity. The normal osmolality value for plasma is 280 to 295 mOsm/kg.

At these normal plasma values, there is no net water movement. Lower or higher values will cause cell swelling (with danger of lysis/bursting) or shrinking, respectively.

The solutions inside and outside cells contain water; the cell wall is a semipermeable membrane. Thus osmosis applies to the movement of water molecules into and out of the cell.

- If the solution outside the cell contains a *higher* concentration of water molecules than the interior of the cell (i.e. the external solution is *hypertonic* for water), then water molecules will diffuse into the cell. This will cause the cell to swell and lyse (break).
- If the solution outside the cell contains a *lower* concentration of water molecules than the inside (i.e. the external solution is *hypotonic* for water), then water will diffuse out of the cell. This will cause the cell to shrink (crenate).
- If the concentrations of water molecules in the intracellular and extracellular concentrations are identical *(isotonic)*, there is no net movement of water.

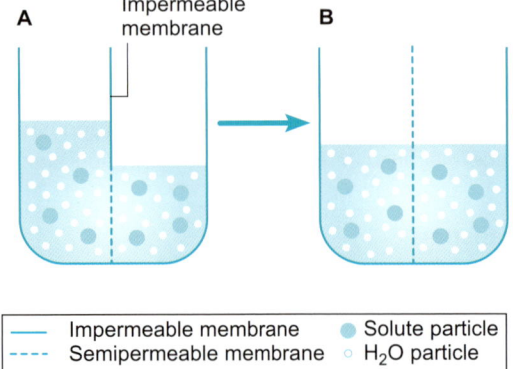

—— Impermeable membrane	● Solute particle
- - - Semipermeable membrane	○ H₂O particle

Fig. 1.12 Osmosis: flow of water across a semi-permeable membrane from a less concentrated (A) to a more concentrated solution resulting in (B).

LEVELS OF ORGANIZATION IN THE BODY

The human body, being a multicellular organism, has a wide variety of cell types. A group of similar cells that work together to perform a specific task is called a *tissue*, the largest of which is the skin. When two or more of these tissues are organized together to perform a particular function, they are referred to as an *organ*. Grouping of these organs related to function make up the different *organ systems* (Fig. 1.13).

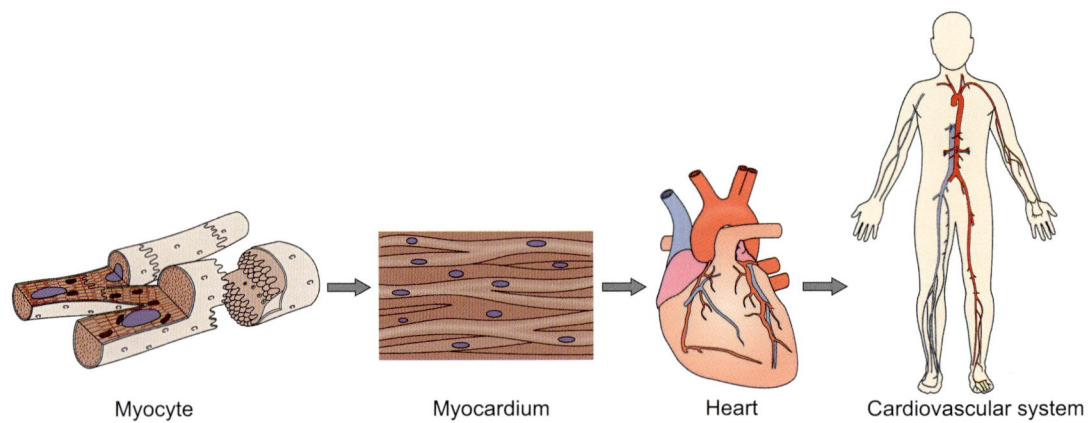

Myocyte   Myocardium   Heart   Cardiovascular system

Fig. 1.13 An example of levels of organization in the body.

Skin

The skin is the largest organ of the body and completely covers the body surface. The functions of the skin include:

- Protection from ultraviolet light, mechanical, chemical and thermal insults
- Sensation of pain, temperature, touch and pressure
- Thermoregulation
- Metabolic functions, for example vitamin D synthesis

The skin is composed of the following layers (Fig. 1.14):

- The epidermis is the outermost layer of the skin. It is stratified squamous keratinized epithelium, which forms a protective waterproof barrier. The epidermis is avascular and is continually shed and replaced.
- The dermis lies deep to and supports the epidermis. It is composed largely of interlacing collagen fibres, with some elastic fibres, giving the skin strength and elasticity. It also contains nerve endings (detecting pain, touch, pressure and temperature), blood vessels and glands. It contains mast cells, lymphocytes and macrophages that play a role in immunity.
- The hypodermis, or superficial fascia, lies deep to the dermis. It is composed of loose areolar tissue (subcutaneous fatty tissue), which provides thermal insulation and protection for underlying structures.

The skin appendages include:

- **Hair follicles (containing hair shafts)** – tubular invaginations of the epidermis into the dermis, lined by stratified squamous epithelium. At the base of each follicle, cell division, growth and maturation result in the formation of a column of dead, keratinized cells (hair shaft) that extrude from the follicle.

- **Sebaceous glands** – associated with the hair follicles. They produce sebum, which lubricates the skin and hair and creates a protective bactericidal layer.
- **Sweat glands** – produce sweat, which plays a role in thermoregulation.
- **Nails** – located at the distal end of the dorsal surface of each digit. They are composed of a nail plate and a nail bed. The nail plate is composed of tightly packed keratinized cells.

CLINICAL NOTES

MALIGNANT MELANOMA

Melanocytes are melanin-producing cells (melanin determines skin colour) located in the epidermis. A malignant melanoma is a tumour of the melanocytes. Most commonly, females develop melanoma of the lower limb, whereas males develop melanoma on the trunk. Early signs of melanoma can be summarized as follows:

Asymmetry
Border (irregular)
Colour (variegated)
Diameter (generally speaking, greater than 6 mm is more likely to be a melanoma)
Evolving/**E**nlarging – over time

Diagnosis is made by full-thickness excision (removal of the melanoma with a small margin of surrounding tissue) or by part removal of the lesion (biopsy) with subsequent histological examination. Melanoma metastasizes to nearby lymph nodes and then to distal organs, commonly the lungs, brain, bone and liver.

PHYSIOLOGY OF THE BLOOD AND BODY FLUIDS

Overview of body fluids and fluid compartments

The major component of the human body is water, which accounts for 63% of an adult male. In descending order of relative percentage composition, the remaining is composed of proteins and related substances, fat and minerals. An increased body fat content is associated with ageing, obesity and being female. Consequently, the percentage of water in females falls to 52%. Dissolved within this water are carbon dioxide (CO_2), nutrients, proteins and charged particles (ions).

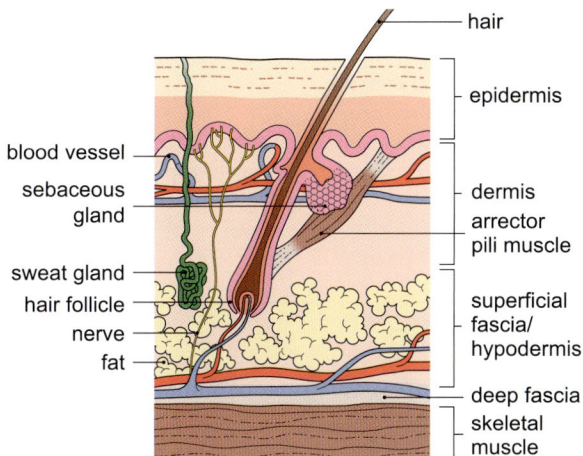

Fig. 1.14 Structure of skin and subcutaneous tissue.

(labels: hair, epidermis, blood vessel, sebaceous gland, dermis, arrector pili muscle, sweat gland, hair follicle, nerve, fat, superficial fascia/hypodermis, deep fascia, skeletal muscle)

Fluid in the body is distributed into different compartments (Fig. 1.15):

- **Intracellular fluid (ICF):** The fluid inside the cells (60%).
- **Extracellular fluid (ECF):** All fluids outside cells (40%), comprising:
  - **75% interstitial fluid (ISF):** The ECF that bathes the cells and lies outside the vascular system.
  - **25% plasma:** The noncellular part of the blood (within the vascular system).

Interstitial fluid and plasma are in a state of continual exchange via pores in the highly permeable capillary membrane. The two fluids therefore have a similar composition, with the exception of large proteins, which are trapped within the capillaries in the vascular system.

Transcellular fluid is another small compartment of body fluid and includes fluids such as cerebrospinal fluid and synovial fluid. Although it can be viewed as a specialized type of ECF, their compositions vary greatly.

Fluid movement between body compartments

The body's fluid compartments are normally in osmotic equilibrium, although they contain different amounts of various ions:

- ICF: K^+ contributes ~50% of osmolality.

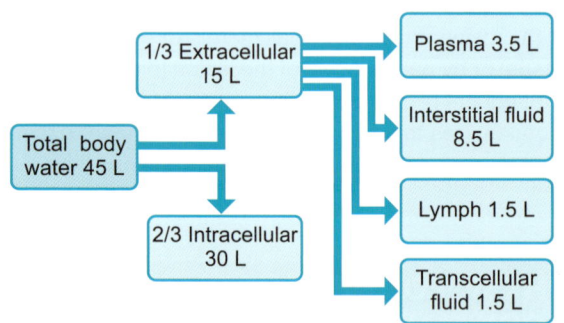

Fig. 1.15 Distribution of water in a 70-kg male.

- ISF and plasma: Na^+ and Cl^- are responsible for ~80% of osmolality.

Plasma and interstitial fluid exchange

The rate of filtration relies on Starling forces (Fig. 1.16), which are derived from two aspects of the ISF and capillary fluid:

- Oncotic pressure, which resists filtration
- Hydrostatic pressure, which favours filtration

In the capillaries, the osmolality of plasma is approximately 1 mOsm/L greater than the osmolality of ICF and ISF. Much of this is due to plasma proteins. This osmotic pressure draws fluid into the capillaries and is counterbalanced by the capillary hydrostatic pressure, which is 20 mm Hg greater than that of the ISF.

The exchange of water and ions occurs across the thin capillary wall, which is composed of endothelial cells. Substances can pass via:

- Vesicular transport (not discussed further but requires energy expenditure).
- Junctions between endothelial cells.
- Fenestrations (when present).

As well as this vesicular transport, simple diffusion and filtration are responsible for transport (see previously). Simple diffusion is responsible for 90% of exchange, relating mainly to net efflux of O_2 and glucose from plasma and influx of CO_2 into the plasma. Filtration is responsible for 10% of exchange.

Oncotic pressure
Oncotic pressure is the osmotic force produced by the proteins that are confined to a compartment/space by their relatively large size. Its value remains constant throughout the capillary. The effect of these proteins is to draw fluid into the compartment/space in which they are confined. In the plasma, oncotic pressure is 17 mm Hg, owing to imbalance of ions.

Hydrostatic pressure
The following determine vessel hydrostatic pressure:

- Arteriolar blood pressure.
- Venous blood pressure.
- Arteriolar resistance, on which depends the extent to which blood pressure is transferred along the capillary.

Fig. 1.16 Starling's law.

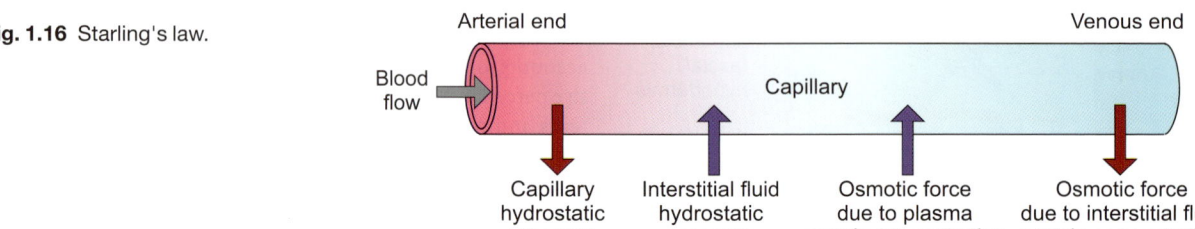

Hydrostatic pressure is maximal at the arteriolar end of the capillary (32 mm Hg), where it exceeds oncotic pressure (which is 25 mm Hg) and thus favours filtration. At the venous end, fluid re-entry into the capillary is favoured; hydrostatic pressure (12 mm Hg) is lower than oncotic pressure (25 mm Hg).

Exchange between interstitial fluid and the lymphatic vessels

The overall efflux of fluid from the capillaries would be expected to cause an increase in ISF hydrostatic pressure. However, this fluid, along with plasma proteins lost from the vascular space, enters a network of lymphatic channels, which is present in all organs and tissues. The fluid is returned to the circulatory system when the lymphatic system empties into the venous system via the thoracic duct in the neck. Normal lymph flow is 2 to 4 L/day.

Fluid and ion movement between the body and the external environment

A careful balancing of fluid intake against output maintains the composition of body fluids (Fig. 1.17). Daily water intake can be from two sources:

- Ingestion of fluid as liquids and as water in food: 2000 mL.
- Oxidative metabolism of food: 400 mL.

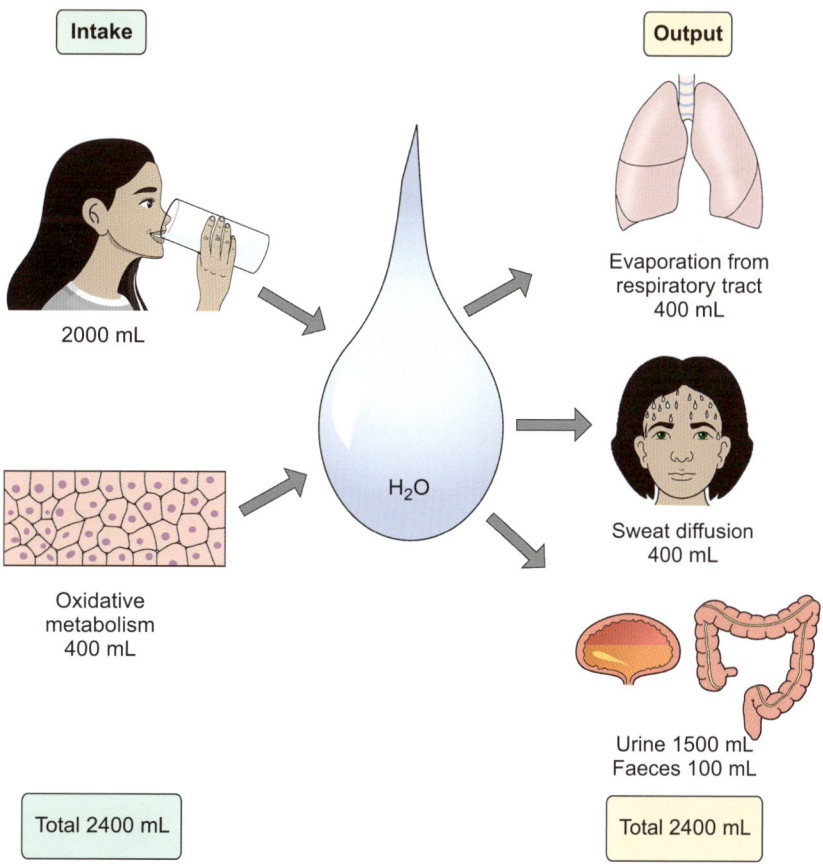

Fig. 1.17 Water balance.

Daily water loss occurs by several different mechanisms:

- **Urine/kidney** – the excretion of electrolytes and water by the kidney is the most important mechanism the body has to regulate fluid balance. The rate of water excretion is adjusted according to the body's needs and water intake. This occurs by filtration and reabsorption and can maintain body fluid volumes despite change in fluid intake or loss elsewhere, for example haemorrhage.
- **Lung** – water evaporates continuously from the respiratory tract. The amount varies with climate and humidity as well as respiratory physiology.
- **Skin** – diffusion through the skin occurs independent of sweating and is minimized by the cornified cholesterol-filled skin layer. Sweating can account for variable water loss. Values are normally 100 mL/day, although it can increase to 1 to 2 L/h, depending on weather and exercise.
- **Faeces** – water loss can be excessive with diarrhoea, compared with the small amount normally lost.

Blood physiology

Functions and components of the blood

Blood is the only liquid tissue. Blood volume can be estimated as approximately 70 mL/kg for adults and 80 mL/kg in children (roughly 5 L in a normal adult); this comprises approximately 8% of total body weight. The functions of blood relate to its composition:

- **Transport** – of gases, nutrients, waste products and hormones

- **Immunological** – defence against bacteria, viruses and foreign bodies by leucocytes
- **Homoeostatic** – temperature, pH, haemostasis and fluid exchange

There are two main components of blood (Fig. 1.18):

1. **Plasma (55%)** – a watery substance containing dissolved solutes and proteins in suspension.
2. **Cells and cellular fragments (45%):**
   - Erythrocytes (99%), also known as red blood cells (RBCs)
   - Platelets (<1%)
   - Leucocytes (<1%) or white blood cells (WBCs).

Plasma

Plasma comprises:

- **Water** – forms a medium for the suspension and transport of proteins, solutes and gases and so influences partial pressures and gas exchange. Water is important in temperature regulation because it releases heat. It also removes waste and breakdown products.
- **Solutes** – electrolytes in particular create osmotic pressure. Ions, for example HCO_3^-, are important in buffering pH change.
- **Proteins** – these are important transporters and buffers and also exert oncotic pressure. They include:
   - **Albumin** – particularly important for vascular oncotic pressure and fluid exchange. It also transports fatty acids, lipid-soluble hormones and some drugs.

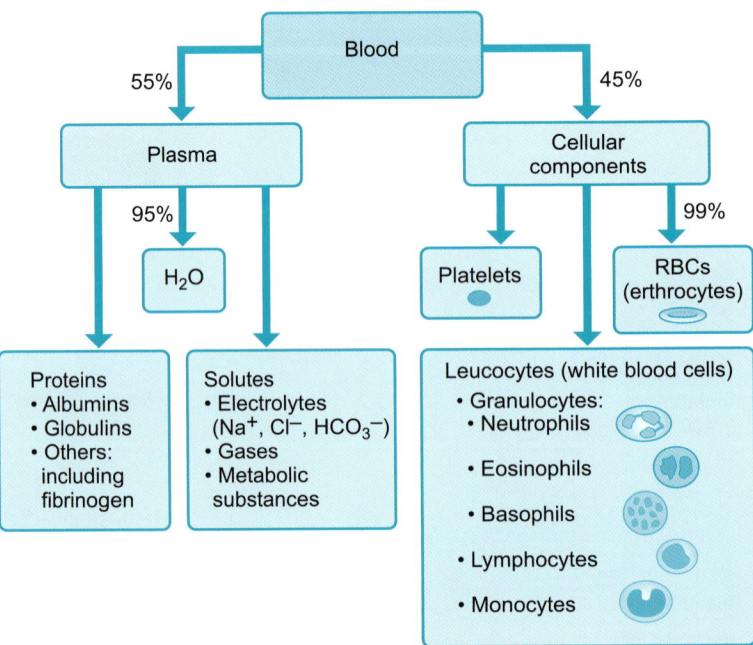

Fig. 1.18 Blood composition. RBCs, *Red blood cells*.

- **Globulins** – α- and β-globulins transport hormones and iron, respectively. γ-Globulins (antibodies) help defend against viruses and bacteria.
- **Other components** – for example fibrinogen is important in the process of blood clotting.

Cells

The types of cells found in blood are:

- **RBCs** – small, flexible, anucleate (nonnucleus) cells containing haemoglobin (~8 μm diameter). The biconcave shape suits their function in gas exchange and transport.
- **Platelets** – small cell fragments derived from megakaryocytes in the bone marrow. They initiate haemostasis and thrombus formation at injury sites (see later).
- **WBCs** – their numbers increase during infection, surgery or strenuous exercise and include:
    - **Neutrophils (60%)** – engulf and phagocytose bacteria and are also involved in inflammation. Numbers increase with bacterial infection, inflammation, burns and stress.
    - **Lymphocytes (20%)** – there are type B and type T cells, the immunological roles of which include generation of the specific immune response, including antigen–antibody reactions. Numbers increase in viral infections and some leukaemias.
    - **Monocytes (5%)** – phagocytose after transforming into macrophages. Numbers increase in viral or fungal infections, tuberculosis and some chronic diseases.
    - **Eosinophils (3%)** – destroy worm parasites. In allergic reactions, they combat histamine. Numbers increase in parasitic infections, allergic reactions and autoimmune diseases.
    - **Basophils (<1%)** – amplify the inflammatory response via the release of heparin and vasoactive substances. Numbers increase in allergic reactions, cancers and leukaemias.

CLINICAL NOTES

WHITE BLOOD CELL COUNT

White blood cell count, included on a full blood count, is often used to identify whether a patient has an infection. Trends in serial counts over several days are monitored to determine response to treatment.

Haemostasis

Haemostasis refers to the control of bleeding. Following injury to a blood vessel, responses occur in two phases:

1. **Rapid** – reactions of blood vessel and platelets:
    a. Slowing of blood flow.
    b. Aggregation of platelets to form a plug at the site of injury.
    c. Diffusion of tissue factors from the extravascular compartment, initiating the extrinsic coagulation pathway.
2. **Slow** – intrinsic coagulation pathway: formation of insoluble fibrin mesh that stabilizes the platelet plug.

Three mechanisms are involved with haemostasis:

1. Vasoconstriction.
2. Formation of a platelet plug.
3. Coagulation (formation of a blood clot) with eventual clot retraction.

Vasoconstriction

Immediately after an injury to a blood vessel, the smooth muscle in the vascular wall contracts, decreasing the vessel diameter and therefore blood loss. This occurs in response to:

- **Nervous reflexes** – as a result of pain and traumatized vessels causing release of catecholamines and vasopressin.
- Local myogenic spasm.
- Platelet thromboxane A_2 – this is more important in smaller than in larger vessels.

Formation of a platelet plug

The formation of a platelet plug is through platelet adhesion, activation and aggregation (Fig. 1.19).

Adhesion. Damage to the vascular endothelium exposes collagen and other connective tissue to which platelets adhere. This increases the concentration of platelets at the site of vascular injury.

Activation. During activation, platelets undergo:

- **Shape change** – they swell then extend many projections that facilitate greater contact with other platelets.
- **Granule release** – contractile proteins contract, causing a release of the following from granules:
    - **ADP and thromboxane A_2** – which activate and make platelets sticky.
    - **Serotonin and thromboxane A_2** – which cause vasoconstriction, so reducing blood loss.
- Expression of new receptors: glycoprotein (GP) IIb/IIIa.

Activated platelets recruit nearby platelets so that their effects are amplified.

Aggregation. The sticky, activated platelets attract one another and adhere, forming a loose clump. This platelet plug is effective at blocking small holes, and coagulation will not be necessary. However, injury to a blood vessel often requires coagulation.

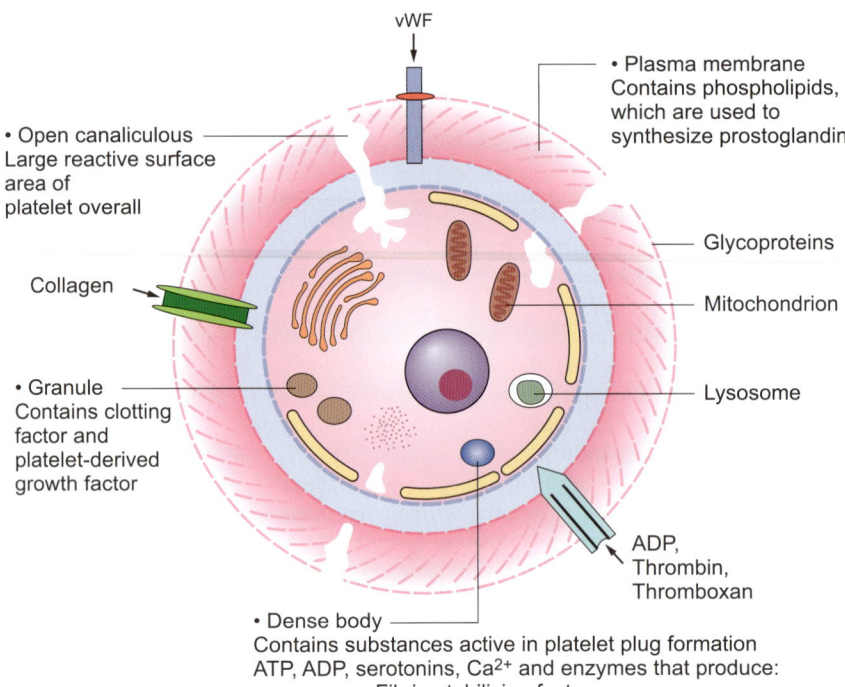

Fig. 1.19 Platelet structure. ADP, *Adenosine diphosphate*; ATP, *adenosine triphosphate*; vWF, *von Willebrand factor.*

vWF

- Plasma membrane
Contains phospholipids, which are used to synthesize prostoglandins

- Open canaliculous
Large reactive surface area of platelet overall

Collagen

Glycoproteins

Mitochondrion

- Granule
Contains clotting factor and platelet-derived growth factor

Lysosome

ADP, Thrombin, Thromboxan

- Dense body
Contains substances active in platelet plug formation ATP, ADP, serotonins, Ca^{2+} and enzymes that produce:
  - Fibrin-stabilizing factor
  - Thromboxane A_2

CLINICAL NOTES

ANTIPLATELET MEDICATIONS

Through inhibiting platelet activation and subsequently aggregation, antiplatelet drugs are commonly used in the primary and secondary prevention of conditions where ischaemia is caused through thrombotic events, for example cerebrovascular accidents (i.e. a stroke) or myocardial ischaemia. The primary mechanisms of action for two common drugs are:

- **Aspirin** – irreversibly blocks the formation of thromboxane A_2 by inactivating cyclooxygenase 1 and 2 enzymes.
- **Clopidogrel** – irreversibly inhibits the $P2Y_{12}$ subtype of ADP receptors.

Coagulation

Coagulation comprises a sequence of enzyme-catalyzed conversions of inactive factors to more active forms, culminating in the conversion of fluid blood into a solid clot.

Blood clot formation begins within seconds after trauma to the vascular wall and in minutes after injury to other areas of the body.

Two pathways are involved (Fig. 1.20):

1. The intrinsic pathway:
   - Is triggered by trauma to blood vessels and exposure to collagen.
   - Involves many enzyme-catalysed steps.
   - Is slow (minutes).
2. The extrinsic pathway:
   - Requires factors external to blood vessels, for example tissue factor (tissue thromboplastin).
   - Involves few enzymes and steps.
   - Is limited by the amount of tissue factor.
   - Is fast (seconds).

Both pathways produce prothrombinase (prothrombin activator), the formation of which appears to be the rate-limiting step in haemostasis. After this stage, pathways follow a common set of reactions, which is known as the final common pathway:

1. Prothrombinase and ionized Ca^{2+} cause prothrombin → thrombin (factor II).

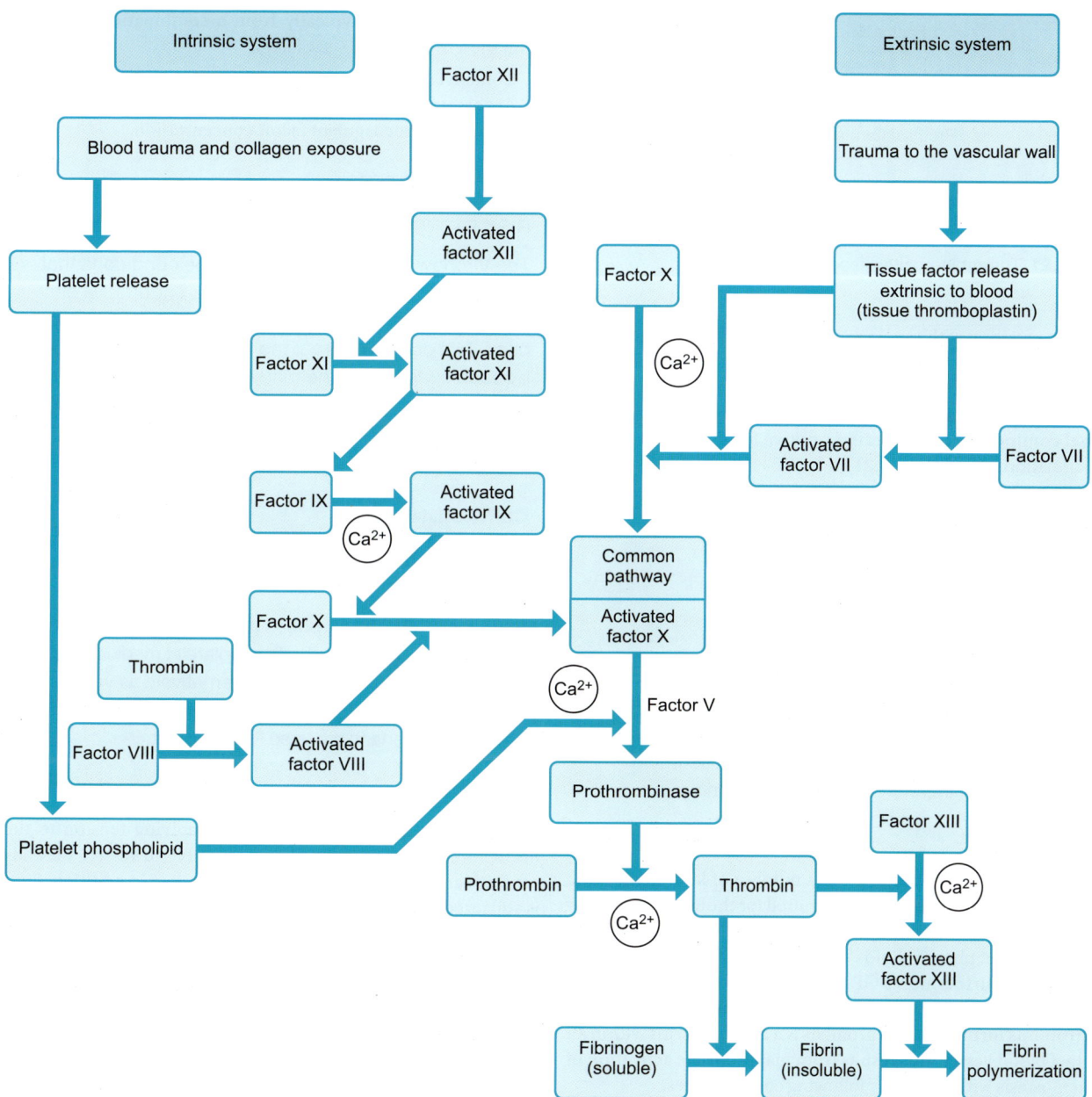

Fig. 1.20 Coagulation pathways.

2. 2a. Thrombin and ionized Ca^{2+} cause fibrinogen (soluble) → fibrin fibres (insoluble).
3. 2b. Thrombin activates fibrin-stabilizing factor (XIII), which cross-links the fibrin fibres.

The cross-linked fibrin strands mesh plasma, the platelet plug, plasmin and RBCs to form a blood clot. In clinical practice:

- The intrinsic pathway is monitored by partial or accelerated thromboplastin time.

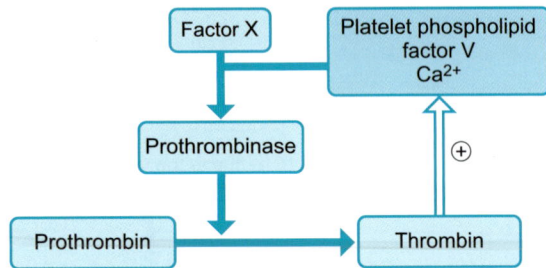

Fig. 1.21 Thrombin-positive feedback loop.

- The extrinsic pathway is monitored using the prothrombin time (PT). The PT forms the basis of the international normalized ratio.

Role of thrombin. Thrombin formed in the first stage of the final common pathway exerts a positive feedback effect on the coagulation cascade (Fig. 1.21):

- Acceleration of the formation of prothrombinase.
- Platelet activation.

> ### CLINICAL NOTES
>
> #### TRANEXAMIC ACID
>
> Tranexamic acid is an antifibrinolytic agent used to treat excessive blood loss after haemorrhage, especially in trauma or surgical patients. It reversibly binds to plasminogen or plasmin, preventing fibrin from becoming degraded and therefore stabilizing the fibrin mesh.

Role of platelets. Platelets serve a number of key haemostatic roles. Platelet phospholipids are required for the assembly of prothrombinase. Prothrombinase is produced following the interaction of platelet phospholipids with activated factors X and V and with Ca^{2+}. Furthermore, GP IIb/IIIa receptors bind to fibrin causing platelet aggregation with the fibrin glue.

Thrombus formation. A thrombus is a clot that forms within an intact blood vessel. This results from inappropriate activation of haemostasis with one of the following consequences:

- The thrombus dissolves spontaneously.
- The thrombus remains intact, with the risk of ischaemia and/or embolization.

Venous and arterial thrombi differ. Arterial thrombi (typically from rupture of atherosclerotic plaques):

- Contain large platelet and small fibrin components.
- Are associated with atheroma formation and turbulent blood flow.
- Have a rough endothelial surface that attracts the platelets.

Venous thrombi (typically from a combination of factors from the Virchow triad – see later):

- Contain large fibrin and large fibrin components.
- Are associated with slow blood flow, which causes a large increase in procoagulant factor concentration.

> ### CLINICAL NOTES
>
> #### RISK FACTORS FOR THROMBOSIS FORMATION
>
> The Virchow triad describes the three conditions that predispose to thrombosis formation: endothelial damage, stasis/turbulent flow of blood and hypercoagulability. To a certain degree, the thrombotic risk caused by each condition of the triad can be manipulated, that is stopping smoking or reducing blood pressure to limit damage of the blood vessel endothelium.

> ### CLINICAL NOTES
>
> #### PRIMARY AND SECONDARY PREVENTION OF THROMBOSIS
>
> Because arterial thromboses are mainly composed of platelets, they are treated with antiplatelet medications, for example aspirin or clopidogrel. Alternatively, as venous thrombosis is typically rich in fibrin, anticoagulants such as heparin and warfarin are used for treatment.

Clot retraction. Within a few minutes of its formation, a clot begins to contract owing to platelets applying tension to the fibrin fibres that are attached to damaged blood vessels, the ends of which are therefore brought closer together. In addition, fluid is squeezed out of the clot. Platelets are suited to clot retraction because they:

- Release factor XIII (fibrin-stabilizing factor), causing more cross-linking of fibrin and permitting further compression of the clot.
- Activate the self-contractile proteins thrombosthenin, actin and myosin; these allow the platelet to pull harder on the fibrin fibres.

Normal prevention of coagulation

The normal vascular system employs a number of mechanisms to keep haemostasis in check.

Prevention of activation of a haemostatic plug.

- Smooth endothelial cells discourage activation of the intrinsic pathway.
- The glycocalyx layer on the endothelium repels both platelets and clotting factors.

Fibrinolysis pathway

Fig. 1.22 Fibrinolysis pathway.

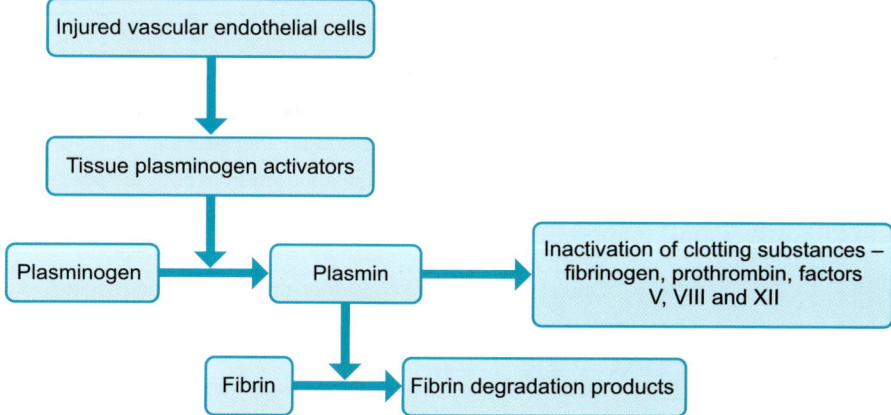

Inhibition of the coagulation cascade.

- **Endothelial-bound thrombomodulin** – binds thrombin and activates protein C, which is a plasma protein.
- **Protein C** – inactivates factors V and VIII.
- **Antithrombin III** (α-globulin and the most important circulating anticoagulant) – combines with thrombin, inactivating it for up to 20 minutes and blocking its effects on fibrinogen.
- **Heparin molecule** – is not active by itself but potentiates antithrombin III 100- to 1000-fold, with the added effect of removing activated factors XII, XI, X and IX.

Fibrinolysis. Plasmin is particularly important for removing inappropriately formed small blood clots; it acts to digest fibrin fibres and inactivate clotting substances: fibrinogen, prothrombin and factors V, VIII and XII (Fig. 1.22). Plasmin is formed from the inactive plasma enzyme plasminogen by:

- **Tissue plasminogen activator (t-PA)** – released by damaged endothelial cells at the periphery. It activates plasminogen in the presence of fibrin.
- **Clotting factors** – thrombin and activated factor XIII can activate plasminogen.

CLINICAL NOTES

THROMBOLYSIS

Certain acute thrombotic conditions, such as cerebro-vascular attack (i.e. stroke) or pulmonary embolism causing severe haemodynamic compromise, may be treated with thrombolytic drugs. Commonly, these drugs, such as alteplase, are recombinant tissue plasminogen activators, which aid in the formation of plasmin.

DESCRIPTIVE ANATOMICAL TERMS

The anatomical position

The anatomical position is a standard position used in both anatomy and clinical practice to allow an accurate and reproducible description of one body part in relation to another (Fig. 1.23).

- The head is directed forwards with the eyes looking into the distance.
- The body is upright, the legs together and the feet facing forwards.
- The arms are by the side of the body, with the palms facing forwards and the thumbs laterally.
- The penis and clitoris are considered in the erect position.

Anatomical planes

The anatomical planes are hypothetical planes used to transect the body (Fig. 1.23). They are useful when describing the location of structures in gross anatomy and the direction of movements. Cross-sectional imaging such as computed tomography (CT) or magnetic resonance imaging commonly produces images of the body in one or more of these planes.

- **The sagittal plane** – A vertical plane passing through the midline of the body from the head to the feet. Any plane parallel to this (i.e. to the left or right of the median sagittal plane) is termed paramedian or parasagittal.
- **The coronal plane** – These are vertical planes passing through the body from the head to the feet. They lie perpendicular to the sagittal planes.

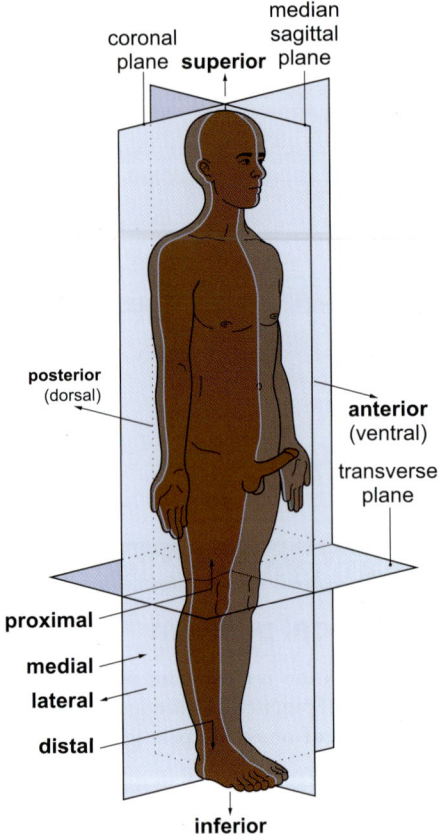

median sagittal plane
coronal plane **superior**

posterior (dorsal)

anterior (ventral)

transverse plane

proximal

medial

lateral

distal

inferior

Fig. 1.23 The anatomical position and the anatomical planes.

Table 1.1 Terms of position	
Position	**Description**
Anterior	In front of another structure
Posterior	Behind another structure
Superior	Above another structure
Inferior	Below another structure
Deep	Further away from body surface
Superficial	Closer to body surface
Medial	Closer to median sagittal plane
Lateral	Further away from median sagittal plane
Proximal	Closer to the trunk or origin
Distal	Further away from the trunk or origin
Ipsilateral	The same side of the body
Contralateral	The opposite side of the body

- **Transverse or axial horizontal plane** – These pass horizontally through the body from the front to the back. They lie at right angles to both the sagittal and coronal planes.
- **Oblique plane** – A plane that divides the body at an angle and is therefore not parallel to either of the former three.

Terms of position

The terms of position commonly used in anatomy and clinical practice are described in Table 1.1.

Terms of movement

The movements of the body are described as follows (Fig. 1.24):

- **Flexion** – a movement in the sagittal plane where there is a reduction in the angle between two parts of the body. There are exceptions to this, for example flexion at the glenohumeral joint increases the angle between the upper limb and the trunk.
- **Extension** – a backward movement in the sagittal plane where there is an increase in the angle between two body parts. Again, there are exceptions to this, for example at the knee joint, as a result of limb rotation during embryonic development.
- **Abduction** – movement away from the median sagittal plane.
- **Adduction** – movement towards the median sagittal plane.
- **Supination** – lateral rotation of the forearm causing the palm to face anteriorly, that is into the anatomical position.
- **Pronation** – median rotation of the forearm causing the palm to face posteriorly.
- **Eversion** – movement of the sole away from the median plane (turning the sole of the foot outwards).
- **Inversion** – movement of the sole towards the median plane (turning the sole of the foot inwards).
- **Rotation** – movement of part of the body around its long axis.
- **Circumduction** – a combination of flexion, extension, abduction and adduction.

The terms used to describe movements of the thumb refer to its being at a right angle to the movements of the fingers (see Video 1).

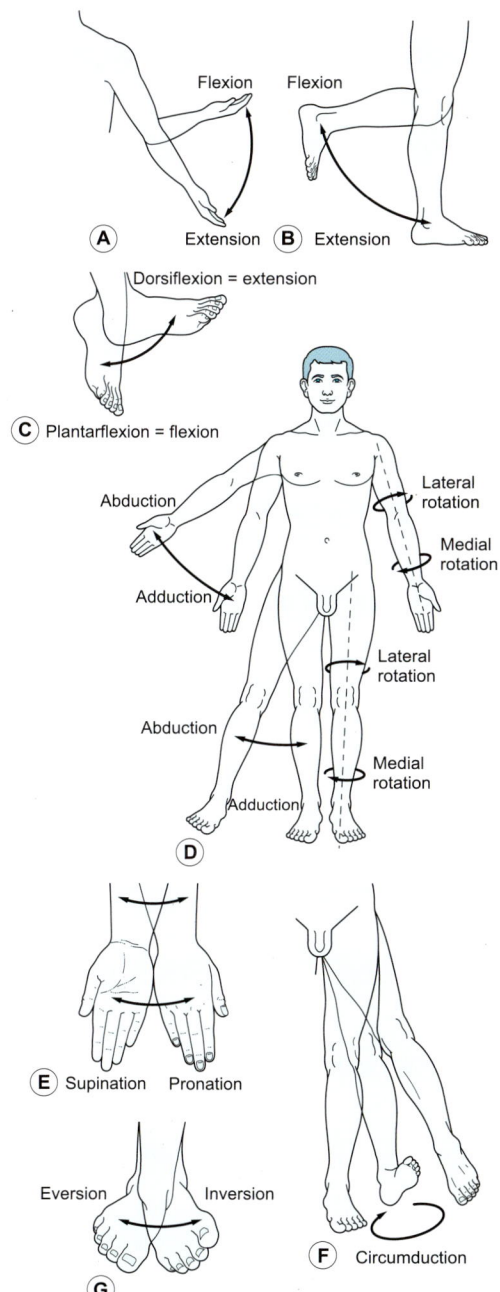

Natural variation of the body

There are many natural variations found within the body that may or may not relate to certain characteristics, for example sex. While aiming to present information in a concise format, it is important to be inclusive in understanding the body, and therefore, where known anatomical variation exists that is relevant to clinical practice, we have aimed to include it. Variations tend to be classified as accessory (e.g. an extra rib), lacking (e.g. absence of palmaris longus muscle) or varying (e.g. variation in the basilic vein).

HINTS AND TIPS

SKIN TONE AND EXAMINATION

Skin tone is influenced by the production, type, and distribution of melanin, a pigment produced by specialized skin cells called melanocytes. Darker skin contains more eumelanin, a type of melanin that provides a rich brown or black color.

When examining or assessing patients, be mindful that certain conditions may present differently on dark and light skin tones. For example:

- Rashes and Inflammation: Redness and erythema are often less visible on darker skin tones. Instead, look for swelling, warmth, or changes in texture.
- Bruising or Cyanosis: These may appear as a grayish or purple discoloration on darker skin, rather than the bluish tone commonly seen on lighter skin.
- Pallor (Paleness): In dark skin, pallor is better assessed in areas like the palms, soles, gums, or conjunctivae rather than relying on overall complexion.

Tip: Enhance your diagnostic skills by using resources that showcase conditions across a range of skin tones. Always ask the patient about changes they've noticed, as they may describe symptoms you cannot easily observe.

HINTS AND TIPS

UNDERSTANDING "DOUBLE-JOINTEDNESS"

Being "double-jointed" isn't about having extra joints—it's a common term for joint hypermobility, where a person's joints move beyond the typical range of motion.

While often harmless, hypermobility can sometimes be associated with joint pain, instability, or conditions like Ehlers-Danlos Syndrome (EDS).

Fig. 1.24 Terms of movement. (A) Flexion and extension of forearm at elbow joint. (B) Flexion and extension of leg at knee joint. (C) Dorsiflexion and plantarflexion of foot and ankle joint. (D) Abduction and adduction of right limbs and rotation of left limbs at shoulder and hip joints, respectively. (E) Pronation and supination of forearm at radioulnar joints. (F) Circumduction (circular movement) of lower limb at hip joint. (G) Inversion and eversion of foot at subtalar and transverse tarsal joints.

OVERVIEW OF THE HEAD AND NECK

Structure

The head in an adult comprises 22 bones: 8 cranial bones and 14 facial skeleton bones. The neck comprises seven cervical vertebrae. The brain is located within the skull and is supported by three layers (meninges). Leaving the brain are 12 cranial nerves (CNs) and the spinal cord. On the anterior aspect is the face with the key structures of the eyes, nose and mouth, with the ears located on the lateral aspect of the head. The neck connects the head to the thorax, enabling an extensive network of arteries and veins to be transported to the head, in addition to acting as conduit for the oesophagus and a location for the larynx.

Function

The head encases and protects the brain. The skull and facial skeleton provide attachments for muscles associated with facial expression and support of structures such as the tongue and larynx. The brain initiates and regulates a multitude of functions, including thought, memory, emotion, touch, motor skills, vision, breathing, temperature regulation, hunger and every physiological process within our body. Together, the brain and the connected spinal cord constitute the central nervous system (CNS).

Scalp

The scalp is the superficial covering of the skull and consists of five layers of tissue, the names of which form the acronym by which it is known: SCALP (skin, connective tissue, aponeurosis, loose connective tissue, periosteum). The layers have a rich blood supply and innervation (Fig. 2.1). The venous drainage mirrors the arterial supply and includes drainage through the emissary veins into the intracranial sinuses. These emissary veins are valveless and thus allow easy spread of infection from the scalp to the intracranial cavity.

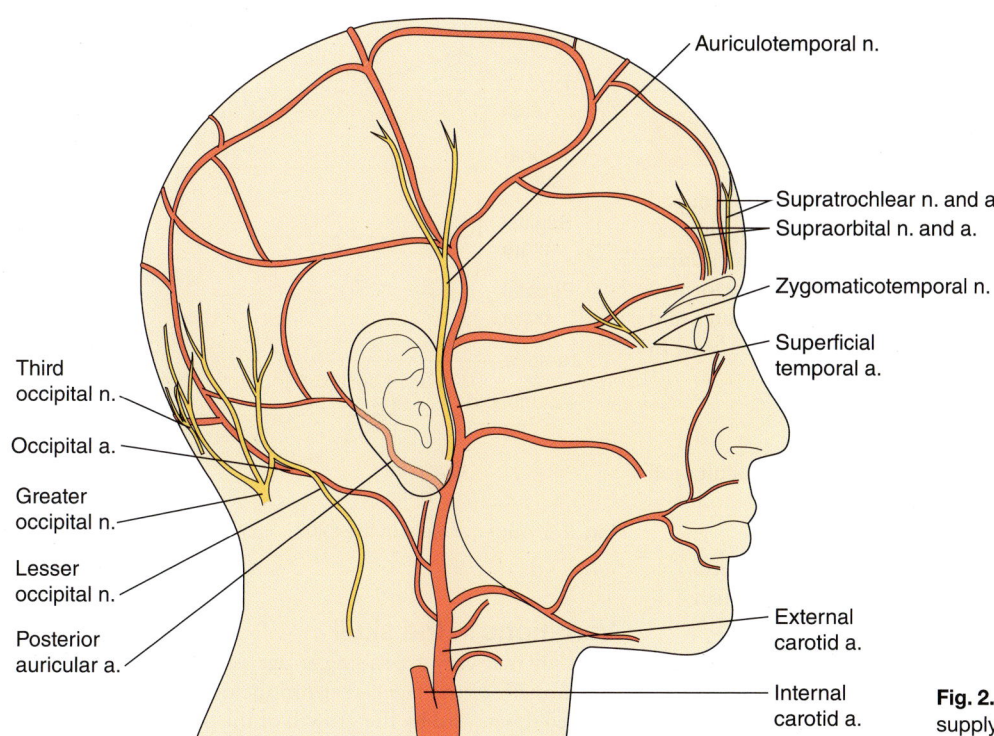

Auriculotemporal n.

Supratrochlear n. and a.
Supraorbital n. and a.

Zygomaticotemporal n.

Superficial temporal a.

Third occipital n.

Occipital a.

Greater occipital n.

Lesser occipital n.

Posterior auricular a.

External carotid a.

Internal carotid a.

Fig. 2.1 Arterial and nervous supply of the scalp. a, *artery*; n, *nerve*.

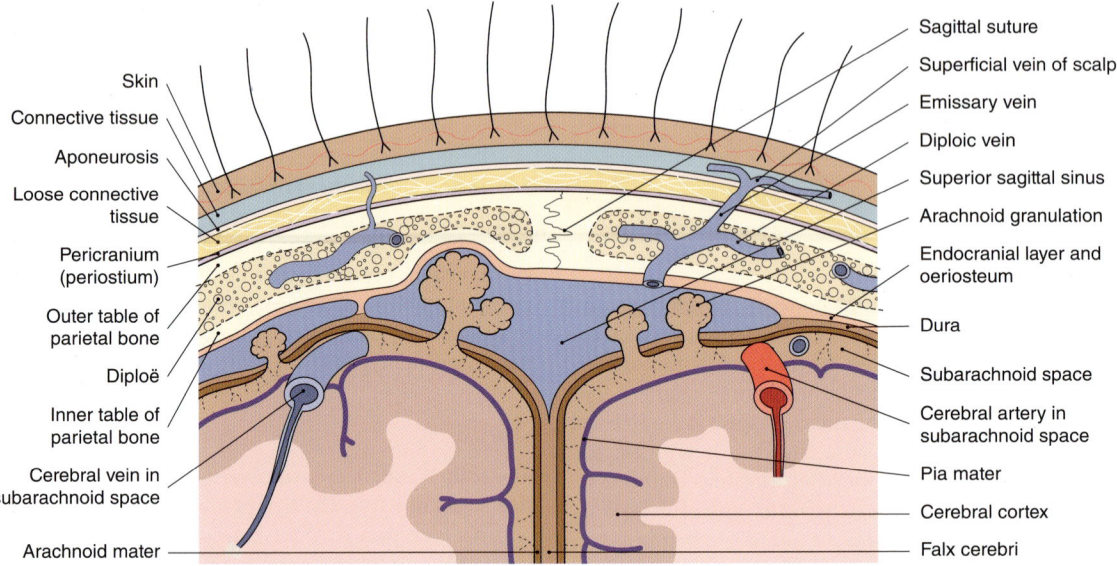

Fig. 2.2 A cross section through the scalp, cranium and meninges of the brain.

The cranial cavity

Beneath the scalp, the cranium protects the brain and its surrounding meninges. The cranial bones consist of outer and inner tables of compact bone, separated by porous cancellous bone containing red marrow throughout life (Fig. 2.2).

SKULL

The adult skull is composed of 22 bones, which can be grouped into the cranium and the facial skeleton (Figs 2.3–2.7). The cranium is subdivided into the upper part (the vault or calvarium) and the lower part (the skull base). The skull bones are formed from intramembranous ossification and create an outer and inner layer of cortical bone with a layer of cancellous bone in between.

The foetal skull

The foetal skull is not simply a smaller version of the adult skull and differs from the adult skull in the following ways:

- The facial skeleton is proportionally smaller.
- The alveolar and mastoid processes are underdeveloped.
- The frontal bone is divided by the metopic suture, which disappears by around 6 years of age.
- The skull has two main defects called the anterior and posterior fontanelles. The anterior fontanelle closes to form the bregma at 18 months, and the posterior fontanelle closes to form the lambda at 3 months.

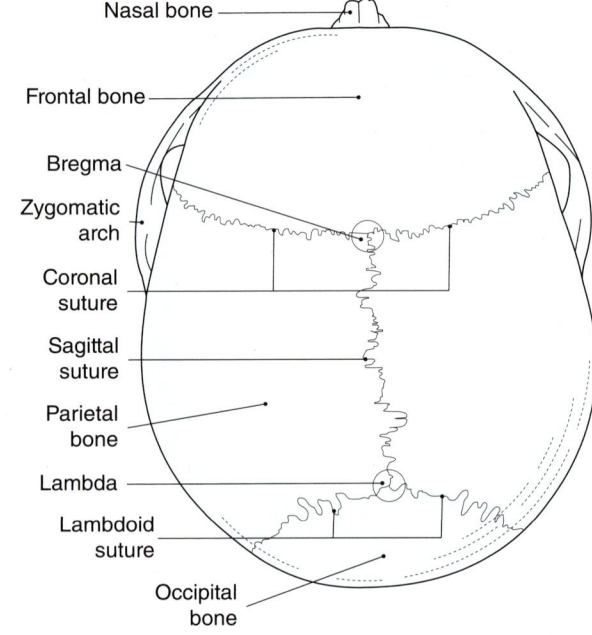

Fig. 2.3 Superior view of the skull.

Variations in the skull

The skull may vary depending on age, biological sex and ancestry. Growth of the facial skeleton includes the maxilla being carried downward by the growth of the orbits. The growth of the skull continues until puberty and reflects hormonal

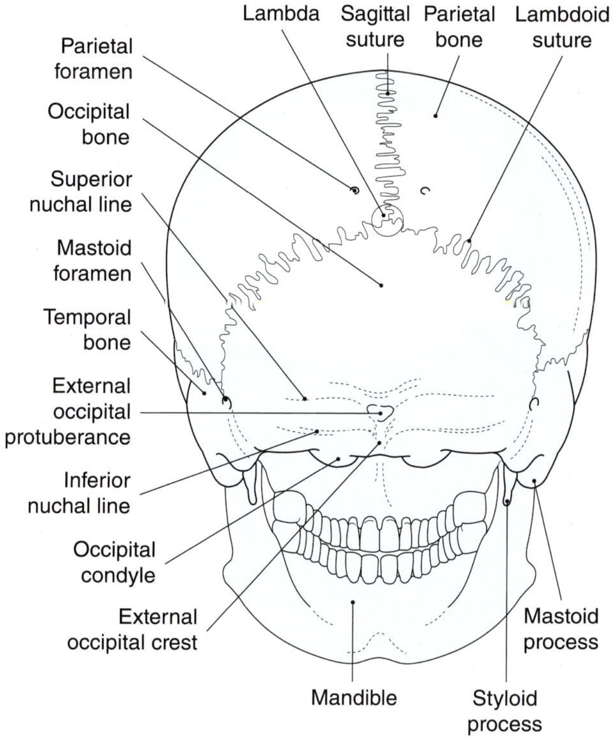

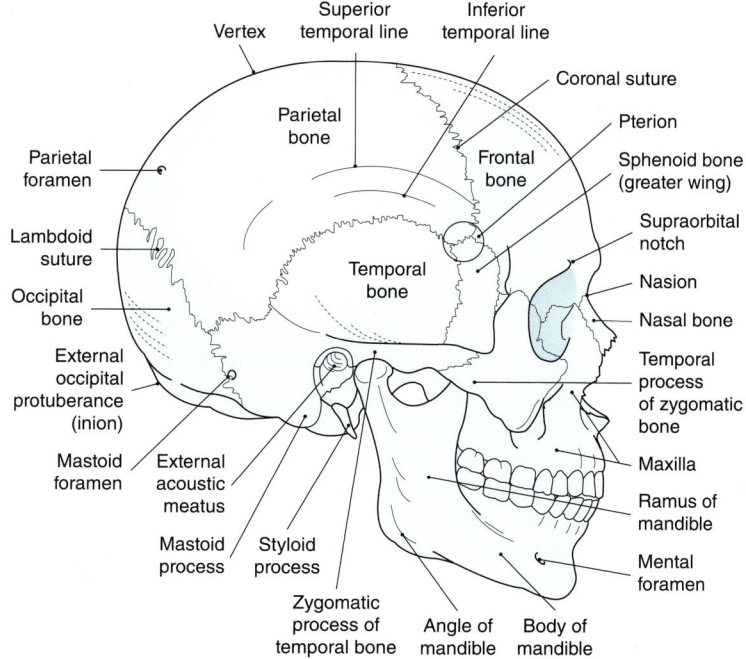

Lambda   Sagittal   Parietal   Lambdoid
            suture   bone   suture

Parietal
foramen

Occipital
bone

Superior
nuchal line

Mastoid
foramen

Temporal
bone

External
occipital
protuberance

Inferior
nuchal line

Occipital
condyle

External
occipital crest

Mandible   Styloid   Mastoid
            process   process

Fig. 2.4 Posterior view of the skull.

Nasal bone   Frontal bone

Supraorbital
notch (or
foramen)

Zygomatic
process of
frontal bone

Orbit

Zygomatic
bone

Frontal
process of
maxilla

Infraorbital
foramen

Nasal
aperture

Maxilla

Mandible   Mental
            foramen

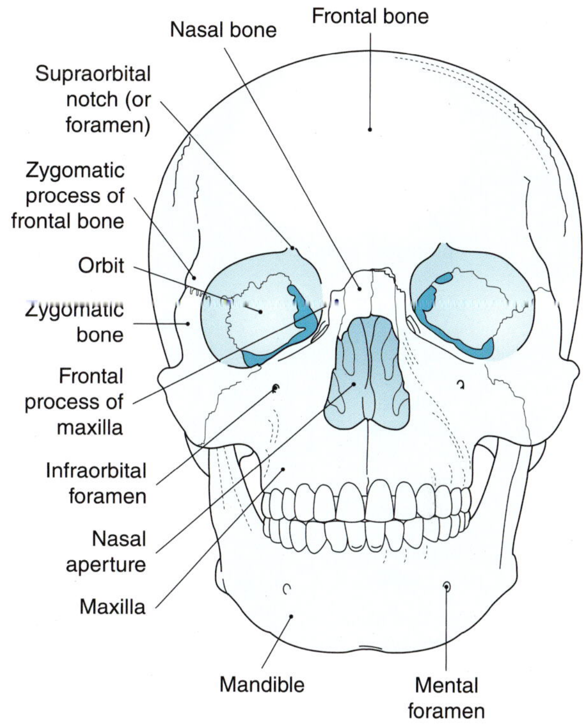

Fig. 2.5 Anterior view of the skull.

Superior   Inferior
            Vertex   temporal line   temporal line

                                    Coronal suture

Parietal
bone   Pterion

Parietal   Frontal   Sphenoid bone
foramen   bone   (greater wing)

                                    Supraorbital
Lambdoid   notch
suture
                        Temporal   Nasion
Occipital   bone
bone   Nasal bone

External   Temporal
occipital   process
protuberance   of zygomatic
(inion)   bone

Mastoid   External   Maxilla
foramen   acoustic
           meatus   Ramus of
                                    mandible
Mastoid   Styloid
process   process   Mental
                                    foramen
        Zygomatic
        process of   Angle of   Body of
        temporal bone mandible   mandible

Fig. 2.6 Lateral view of the skull.

25

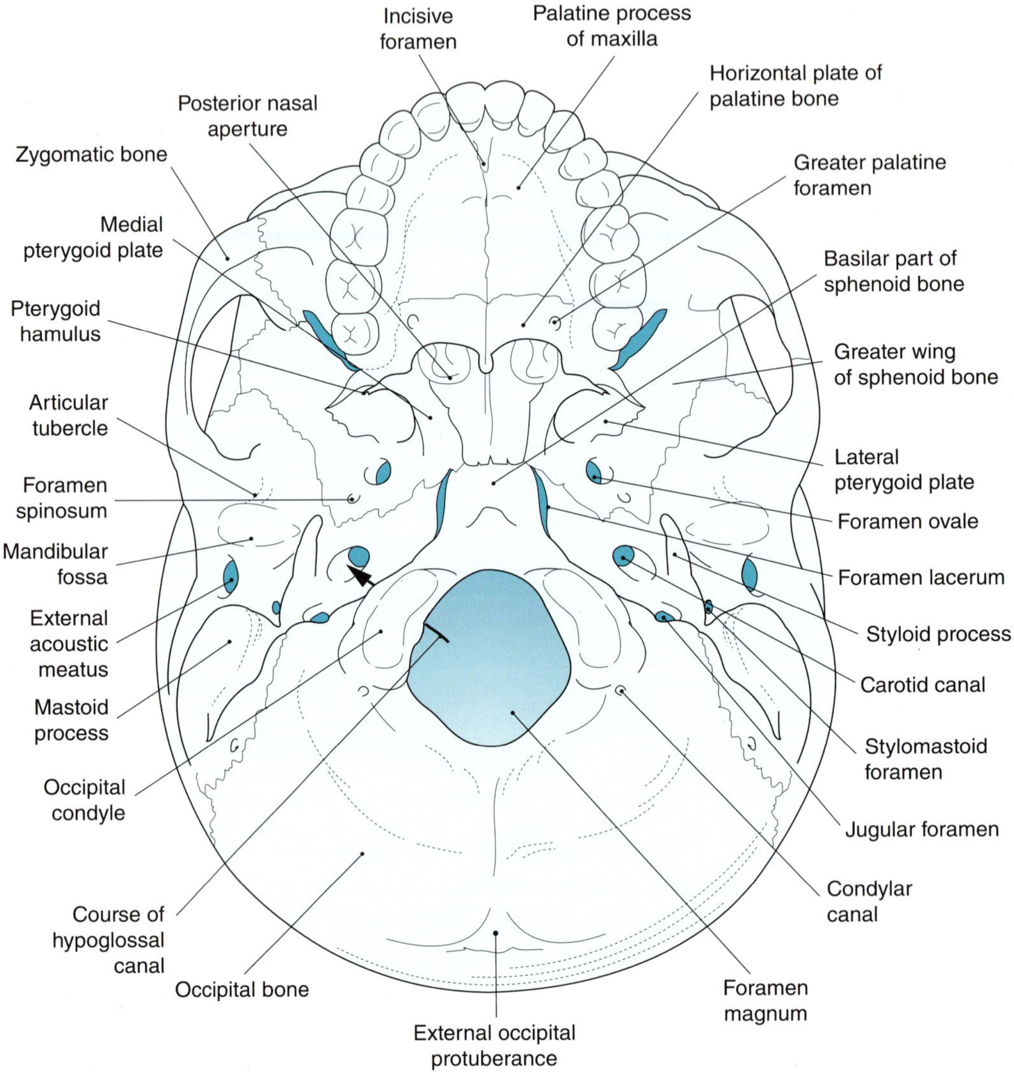

Fig. 2.7 Inferior view of the skull.

Labels (clockwise from top):
- Incisive foramen
- Palatine process of maxilla
- Horizontal plate of palatine bone
- Greater palatine foramen
- Basilar part of sphenoid bone
- Greater wing of sphenoid bone
- Lateral pterygoid plate
- Foramen ovale
- Foramen lacerum
- Styloid process
- Carotid canal
- Stylomastoid foramen
- Jugular foramen
- Condylar canal
- Foramen magnum
- External occipital protuberance
- Occipital bone
- Course of hypoglossal canal
- Occipital condyle
- Mastoid process
- External acoustic meatus
- Mandibular fossa
- Foramen spinosum
- Articular tubercle
- Pterygoid hamulus
- Medial pterygoid plate
- Zygomatic bone
- Posterior nasal aperture

influences. The final part of the skull to fuse is the jugular growth plate around age 20 to 30 years. Sutures over time fuse from around 30 years old. A male skull is generally considered to be more robust, with more pronounced supraorbital ridges, a larger mandible, well-defined glabella, larger mastoid process and external occipital protuberance. Female skulls are described as having a higher, more vertical and more rounded forehead than males. Genetic diversity does not easily align with ancestorial categories and may inadvertently reinforce stereotypes. Data that relate to population affinity are used by anthropologists to help understand features of the skull in human remains.

CLINICAL NOTES

ANTERIOR FONTANELLE

In babies, the anterior fontanelle can be used to crudely assess intracranial pressure as it bulges outwards when the pressure is raised, such as in patients with hydrocephalus.

Cranial fossae

The internal surface of the base of the skull is divided into anterior, middle and posterior cranial fossae (Fig. 2.8). The foramina

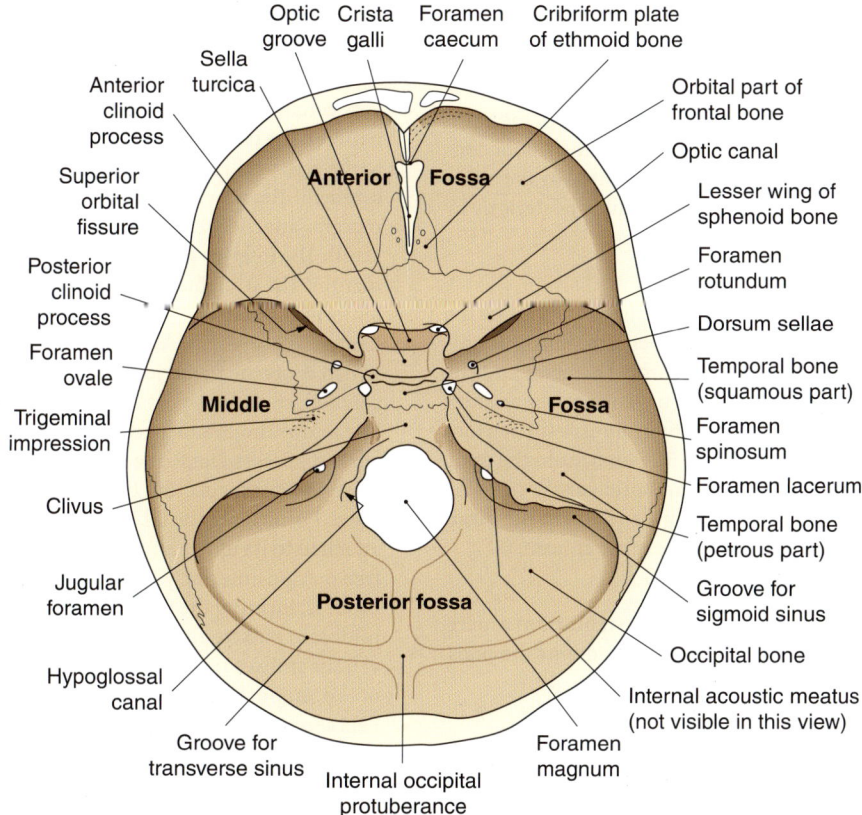

Fig. 2.8 Internal surfaces of the base of the skull, showing the cranial fossae.

Table 2.1 The key foramen in the skull and their contents

Opening in skull	Structures transmitted
Anterior cranial fossa	
Cribriform plate	Olfactory nerves
Middle cranial fossa	
Optic canal	Optic nerve, ophthalmic artery
Superior orbital fissure	V_1 (ophthalmic branch of trigeminal nerve); oculomotor, abducens and trochlear nerves; superior ophthalmic vein
Foramen rotundum	V_2 (maxillary division of trigeminal nerve)
Foramen ovale	V_3 (mandibular division of trigeminal nerve), lesser petrosal nerve
Foramen spinosum	Middle meningeal artery and vein
Posterior cranial fossa	
Internal acoustic meatus	Facial, vestibulocochlear nerves; labyrinthine artery
Jugular foramen	Glossopharyngeal, vagus, accessory nerves; sigmoid sinus becomes internal jugular vein
Hypoglossal canal	Hypoglossal nerve
Foramen magnum	Medulla oblongata, spinal part of accessory nerve, right and left vertebral arteries

of the cranial fossae and the structures passing through them are outlined in Table 2.1.

Anterior cranial fossa

The anterior cranial fossa contains the frontal lobes of the brain and the olfactory bulbs. The ethmoid bone of the fossa floor contains the thin cribriform plate, which is perforated by the olfactory nerve rootlets. The anterior fossa is bounded posteriorly by the sphenoid ridge.

Middle cranial fossa

The middle cranial fossa contains the temporal lobes of the cerebral hemispheres, the floor of the forebrain, the optic chiasm, the termination of the internal carotid arteries and the pituitary gland. A shallow depression (trigeminal impression) near the apex of the petrous temporal bone houses the sensory ganglion of the trigeminal nerve (CN 5). Superior to the optic groove sits the optic chiasm, with the optic canals running laterally from the groove. The pituitary gland lies in the pituitary fossa or sella turcica, inferior to the optic chiasm.

Posterior cranial fossa

The posterior cranial fossa is bordered by the tentorium superiorly and the occipital and petrous bones. It contains the pons, medulla, cerebellum and midbrain.

CLINICAL NOTES

PITUITARY TUMOURS

Tumours of the pituitary gland can compress the optic chiasm, which classically results in a bitemporal hemianopia caused by the decussation of the nasal fibres in the chiasm.

The meninges of the brain and spine

There are three meningeal layers surrounding the brain and spinal cord (Fig. 2.2).

Dura mater

The dura mater is composed of two layers. The outer layer is known as the endosteal layer and serves as the periosteum covering the inside of the skull. The inner layer is the meningeal layer—a dense fibrous layer covering the brain. The two layers are firmly adherent to each other throughout most of the skull, separating at intervals to form dural venous sinuses (described later). The dural sinuses drain cerebrospinal fluid and blood from the brain, into the internal jugular veins.

The dura is continuous with the dura mater of the spinal cord through the foramen magnum. Sleeves of dura surround the CNs, which fuse with the epineurium of the nerves outside the skull. The dura gives rise to the following septa that support the brain and restrict its movement (Fig. 2.9):

- Falx cerebri: A sickle C-shaped fold of dura which lies between the two cerebral hemispheres. It attaches anteriorly to the crista galli and blends posteriorly to the tentorium cerebelli. The superior sagittal sinus runs in its superior margin (attached to the endocranium on the vault of the skull). The inferior sagittal sinus runs in its free inferior margin. The straight sinus runs along its attachment to the tentorium cerebelli.
- Tentorium cerebelli: A crescent-shaped fold of dura mater which roofs the posterior cranial fossa. It covers the cerebellum and supports the occipital lobes of the brain. The tentorium is attached to either side of the posterior clinoid process, passes back along the petrous temporal bone and curves around the inner aspect of the occipital bone. Posteriorly, the falx cerebri and falx cerebelli are attached to its upper and lower surfaces, respectively. The free margin anteriorly is anchored to the anterior clinoid process, forming the tentorial notch through which the midbrain passes. The superior petrosal and transverse venous sinuses run along its attachment to the petrous part of the temporal bone and occipital bones, respectively.
- Falx cerebelli: Projects anteriorly between the two cerebellar hemispheres and is attached to the internal occipital crest. Its posterior margin contains the occipital sinus.
- Diaphragma sellae: In the middle cranial fossa is a small circular fold of dura forming the roof of the pituitary fossa.

Arachnoid mater

The arachnoid mater lies deep to the dura. It is separated from the pia mater by the subarachnoid space, containing cerebrospinal fluid (CSF). Where the arachnoid passes over the contours of the brain, the subarachnoid and pia mater are not closely apposed; the spaces formed in this way contain CSF. Some spaces are large and known as subarachnoid cisterns.

Pia mater

The innermost layer of the meninges is the pia mater, a thin, fibrous, water-impermeable tissue that invests the brain surface. The pia continues as a sheath around the small vessels entering the brain substance. The pia is translucent and therefore is the only meningeal layer that cannot be seen with the naked eye.

Blood and nerve supply of the meninges

The meninges are supplied by the middle meningeal artery and branches of the internal carotid, maxillary, ascending pharyngeal, occipital and vertebral arteries. Dura mater in the anterior and middle cranial fossae is innervated by the trigeminal nerve (CN 5). The dura of the posterior fossa is supplied by the upper three cervical nerves and meningeal branches from the vagus (CN10) and hypoglossal nerves (CN 12).

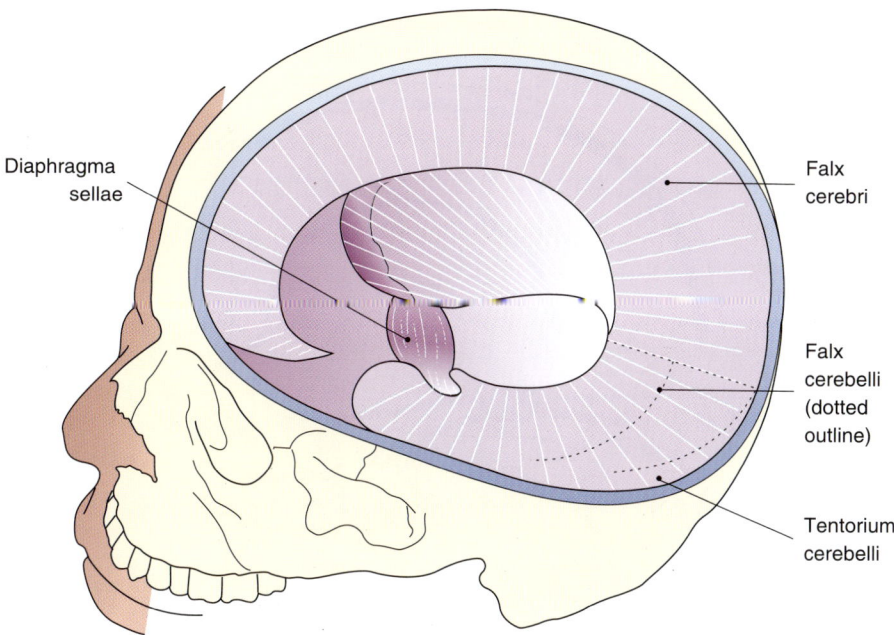

Diaphragma sellae

Falx cerebri

Falx cerebelli (dotted outline)

Tentorium cerebelli

Fig. 2.9 The falx cerebri, falx cerebelli, diaphragm sellae and tentorium cerebella.

CLINICAL NOTES

INTRACRANIAL HAEMORRHAGE

Bleeding within the cranium is typically classified ana-tomically and describes where the bleeding occurs in relation to the meningeal layers.

Extradural (epidural): Most often due to bleeding from the branches of the middle meningeal artery (e.g. caused by a fracture of the pterion) into the space between the periosteum and dura. A common presentation is brief unconsciousness following a trauma, followed by a lucid interval of several hours. Headaches, nausea/vomiting, focal neurological symptoms and ultimately death then develop as the intracranial pressure becomes raised.

Subdural: Sudden movements or trauma may shear the bridging veins leading from the brain to the dural venous sinuses. This results in bleeding between the dura and arachnoid mater. Subdural haemorrhages gen-erally develop more slowly compared with extradural haemorrhages, given that the bleeding site is venous compared with arterial. Brain atrophy in the elderly causes increased 'stretch' and, therefore, tension on these veins, making this patient group a high-risk group.

Subarachnoid: An artery in the subarachnoid space (e.g. a cerebral arterial circle aneurysm) ruptures causing bleeding into the cerebrospinal fluid. This results in a severe headache (classically described as a 'thunderclap' headache), loss of consciousness and, in some cases, death.

Dural venous sinuses

The dural venous sinuses lie between the two layers of the dura, are lined by endothelium and have no valves. Veins draining the brain, the diploë, the scalp, the orbit and the inner ear drain into the sinuses as described below and illustrated in Fig. 2.10

- Superior sagittal sinus: Runs in the upper border of the falx cerebri. It commences at the foramen caecum and passes posteriorly, grooving the vault of the skull. At the internal occipital protuberance, it forms the confluence of the sinuses and continues as a transverse sinus (usually the right). It receives numerous cerebral veins. CSF drains into the sinus via arachnoid granulations (Fig. 2.2).
- Inferior sagittal sinus: Lies in the free margin of the falx cerebri. It joins with the great cerebral vein to form the straight sinus. It drains cerebral veins from the medial side of the cerebral hemispheres.

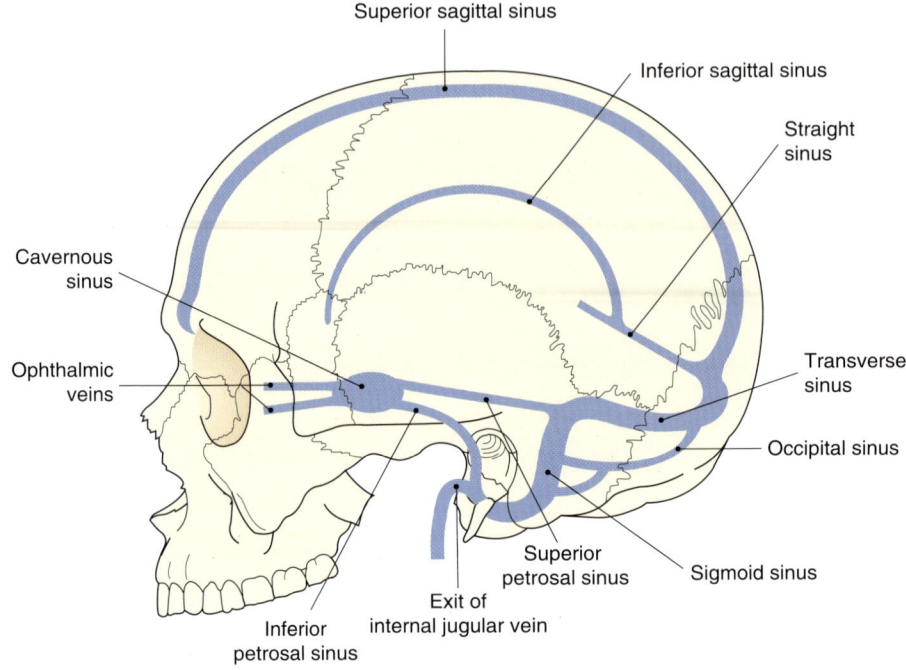

Fig. 2.10 The position of the cranial venous sinuses.

- Straight sinus: Lies between the falx cerebri and tentorium cerebelli and is formed by the junction of the inferior sagittal sinus and the great cerebral vein. It terminates by turning to form (usually the left) transverse sinus.
- Right and left transverse sinuses: These commence at the internal occipital protuberance and run in the attachment of the tentorium cerebelli. They end by turning inferiorly to form the sigmoid sinuses. They receive the superior petrosal sinuses and the inferior cerebral, cerebellar and diploic veins.
- Sigmoid sinuses: These turn inferiorly and medially to groove the mastoid process. They then turn downward through the posterior part of the jugular foramen to become continuous with the internal jugular vein.
- Occipital sinus: This lies in the attached margin of the falx cerebelli. It drains into the bases of the sigmoid sinuses.

Cavernous sinuses

Within the base of the skull, the cavernous sinuses lie in the middle cranial fossa on either side of the body of the sphenoid bone (Fig. 2.11); they extend from the superior orbital fissure anteriorly to the apex of the petrous temporal bone posteriorly. The cavernous sinuses receive:

- the superior and inferior ophthalmic veins.
- the cerebral veins.
- the sphenoparietal sinus.
- the central vein of the retina.

The cavernous sinuses drain posteriorly into the superior and inferior petrosal sinuses and inferiorly into the pterygoid venous plexus. The two sinuses communicate via anterior and posterior intercavernous sinuses.

The internal carotid artery, its sympathetic nerve plexus and the abducens nerve (CN 6) run through the sinus (Fig. 2.11). The oculomotor (CN 3) and trochlear (CN 4) nerves and the ophthalmic and maxillary divisions of the trigeminal nerve (CN 5) lie in the lateral wall of the sinus, between the endothelium and the dura.

Superior and inferior petrosal sinuses emerge from the cavernous sinus and lie at the superior and inferior borders of the petrous temporal bone, respectively. The superior sinus drains into the transverse sinus and the inferior sinus into the internal jugular vein.

CLINICAL NOTES

INFECTION

The central face drains to the cavernous sinus via the superior ophthalmic vein. This can serve as a route for infection to spread and cause meningitis or cavernous sinus thrombosis. Any infection in the 'danger area' of the face (a triangle with its base as the top lip and its apex at the bridge of the nose) should be treated aggressively.

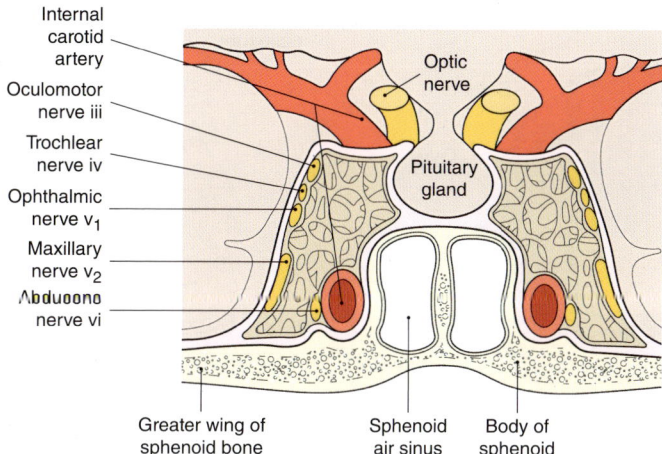

Internal
carotid
artery

Oculomotor
nerve iii

Trochlear
nerve iv

Ophthalmic
nerve v₁

Maxillary
nerve v₂

Abducens
nerve vi

Optic
nerve

Pituitary
gland

Greater wing of
sphenoid bone

Sphenoid
air sinus

Body of
sphenoid

Fig. 2.11 A coronal section of the cavernous sinus showing its relations.

Intracranial pressure

Within the cranium are three components: the brain (80%), blood (10%) and CSF (10%). In health, collectively these components occupy the average intracranial volume of 1700 mL at a pressure of 5 to 15 mm Hg, which is known as the intracranial pressure (ICP).

The Monro–Kellie doctrine dictates that because the skull is rigid and of a fixed size, any increase in the volume of either component will lead to an increase in ICP unless a reduction of another component occurs to maintain equilibrium. This compensation occurs primarily to prevent cerebral ischaemia and happens in a phased approach: first, there is a reduction in venous blood volume, then a reduction in CSF volume, finally followed by a reduction in arterial blood volume. If there is inadequate compensation for the increased intracranial volume, a sharp rise in ICP will follow, leading to global cerebral ischaemia (Fig. 2.12).

The next structure within the skull to consider is the brain, but before we do, it is helpful to explain the intersection of anatomy and physiology. The nervous system is divided into the CNS that involves the brain and spinal cord, and the peripheral nervous system (PNS) that involves the nerves connected to the CNS. Keeping within the skull, we will first explain the brain.

Brain

The CNS is composed of the brain and spinal cord. The brain is divided into two cerebral hemispheres, known collectively as the cerebrum, that are connected by the corpus callosum. Each cerebral hemisphere consists of four lobes: frontal, temporal,

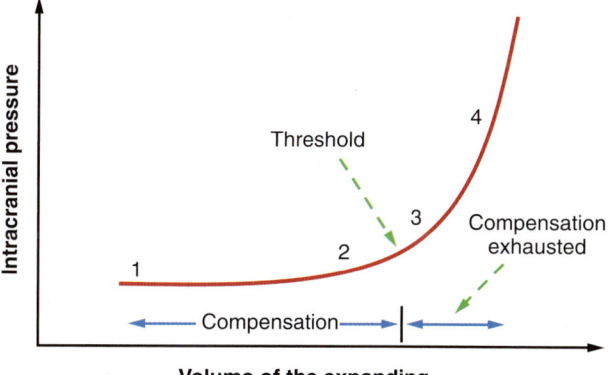

Intracranial pressure

Threshold

4

3

Compensation
exhausted

2

1

Compensation

**Volume of the expanding
intracranial content (one component)**

Fig. 2.12 Illustration of the effect of an expanding intracranial component on intracranial pressure (*ICP*). As the volume of an intracranial component increases from point 1 to point 2 on the curve, ICP remains relatively stable because of the compensatory mechanisms, including the translocation of cerebrospinal fluid from the intracranial space into the spinal subarachnoid space. Between points 1 and 2, the volumetric sum of all intracranial components remains relatively constant. Patients with intracranial tumours who are between point 1 and point 2 on the curve are unlikely to manifest clinical symptoms of increased ICP. The compensation ability is exhausted on the rising portion of the curve (point 3) when a small volumetric increase of the expanding intracranial component leads to a noticeable increase of ICP. Clinical signs and symptoms attributable to increased ICP are likely at this stage. Additional increases in intracranial volume at this point, as produced by increased cerebral blood flow secondary to hypercapnia or inhaled anaesthesia, can precipitate abrupt further increases in ICP (point 4).

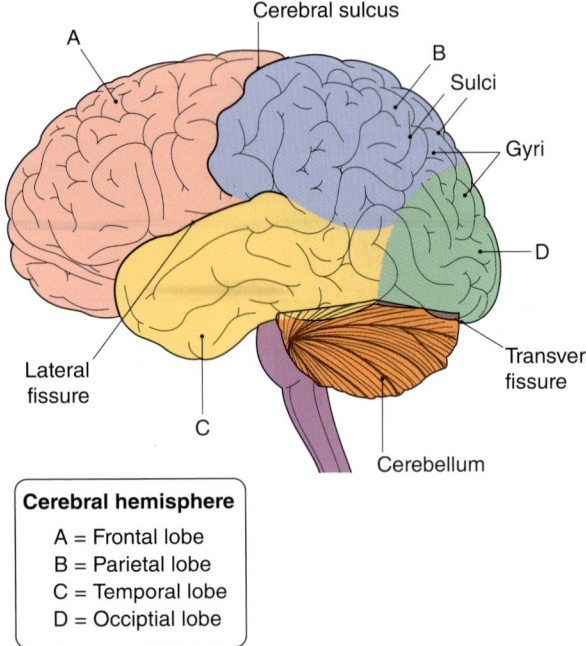

Fig. 2.13 Lateral view of the brain illustrating the major features.

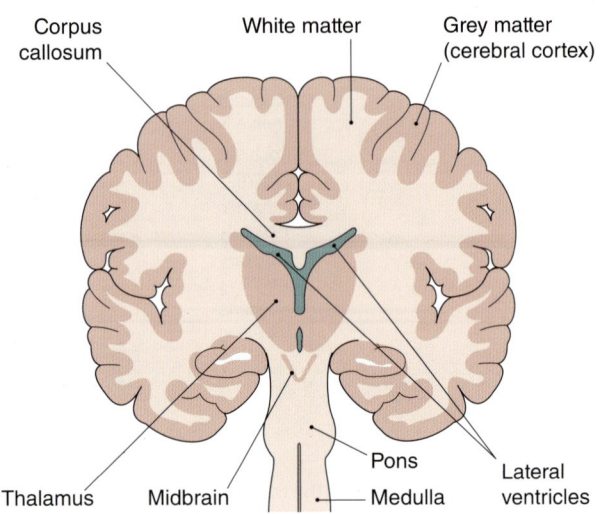

Fig. 2.14 Coronal section of the cerebrum illustrating grey and white matter.

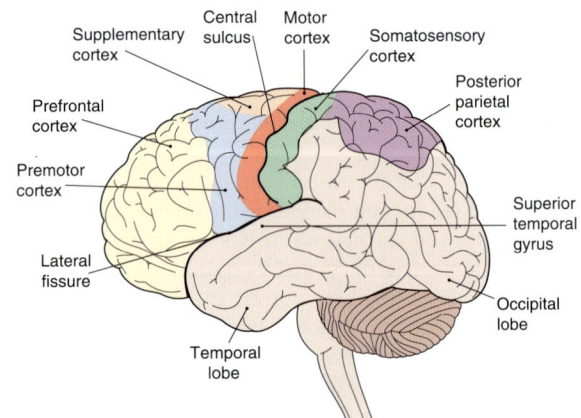

Fig. 2.15 Cortical representation including the motor cortex and associated areas.

parietal and occipital lobes. Ridges on the surface of the cerebrum are known as gyri. Grooves between the gyrus are known as sulci. The frontal and parietal lobes are separated by the central sulcus.

Deeper grooves are known as fissures, which divide the regions of the brain. The longitudinal fissure separates two cerebral hemispheres. The transverse fissure separates the cerebrum from the cerebellum. The lateral fissure (Sylvian fissure) separates the temporal lobe from the frontal and parietal lobes (Fig. 2.13).

The outer layer of the cerebrum is known as the cerebral cortex and is composed of grey matter (cell bodies). Deep to this lies white matter (myelinated axons) (Fig. 2.14). The cerebrum and a part of the brain known as the diencephalon together constitute the forebrain. Within the forebrain are areas of deep grey matter, known as the basal ganglia, which have a role in a number of neurological conditions (e.g. Parkinson disease).

The brainstem consists of the midbrain, pons and medulla oblongata (see Fig. 2.13). Within the brainstem, grey matter is arranged into distinct regions known as nuclei. These nuclei give rise to CNs 3 to 12.

Motor cortex

The primary motor cortex is the principal brain region that controls the planning, control and execution of voluntary movements

of the body, for example controlling the mouth when talking. The primary motor cortex lies in the posterior aspect of the frontal lobe, just anterior to the central sulcus (the prominent sulcus separating the frontal and parietal lobes). The motor cortex comprises the primary motor cortex, premotor cortex and supplementary cortex, all of which work in association (Fig. 2.15).

Primary motor cortex

The primary motor cortex is located on the precentral gyrus and is the primary generator of neural impulses that control the execution of movement. The cortex contains large neurones, known as Betz cells, that project their long axons down towards the spinal cord. The motor representation of the primary motor cortex controlling specific areas of the body is arranged in an orderly fashion. This somatotopic representation is termed the motor homunculus. The area of the primary motor cortex devoted to a specific part of the body is proportional and is determined by the relative density of motor receptors at the respective body part. Each hemisphere contains a primary motor cortex, which controls the contralateral side of the body (given the decussation (crossing) of the motor spinal tracts) (see 'Descending motor tracts' later).

Premotor cortex

The premotor cortex lies on the gyrus just anterior to the primary motor cortex (see Fig. 2.15). Although its exact function is not fully understood, it is considered to play a role in motor planning and the spatial guidance of movement, as well as the direct control of trunk muscles, given its projections to the spinal cord.

Supplementary cortex

The supplementary cortex lies in the medial aspect of the hemisphere on the gyrus just anterior to the primary motor cortex (Fig. 2.15). The functions of the supplementary cortex include planning complex movements and coordinating bilateral movements—both of which require information to be projected to the primary motor cortex and brainstem motor regions.

Basal ganglia

The basal ganglia are a collection of subcortical nuclei at the base of the forebrain; they are distinct areas of grey matter (Fig. 2.16). The basal ganglia have strong connections with the cortex, thalamus and brainstem and play a key role in the control of voluntary motor movements. The basal ganglia also have roles in procedural learning, eye movements, emotion and cognition.

On each side of the brain, the basal ganglia are divided broadly into four regions: the striatum, the globus pallidus, the substantia nigra and the subthalamic nucleus. Based on connections and function, the striatum is further divided into the ventral striatum (the nucleus accumbens and the olfactory tubercle) and the dorsal striatum (the caudate nucleus and the putamen). The globus pallidus is also divided into the globus pallidus interna and globus pallidus externa.

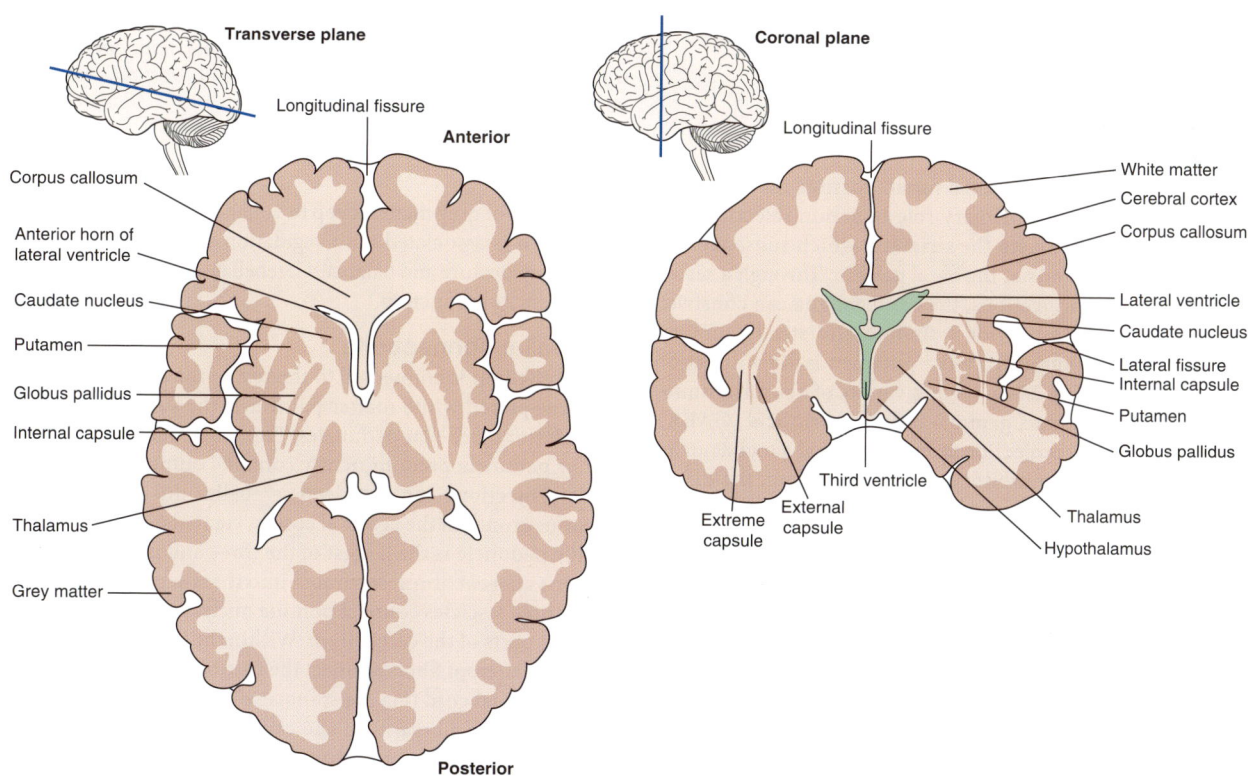

Fig. 2.16 Components of the basal ganglia.

CLINICAL NOTES

PARKINSON DISEASE

Parkinson disease (PD) is a progressive neurodegenerative disorder caused by the degeneration of the dopaminergic projections extending from the substantia nigra. It also affects neurones of the cholinergic and glutaminergic pathways. Although the pathophysiology is poorly understood, the inclusion of pathological Lewy bodies in the remaining cells of the substantia nigra is seen. The classical four symptoms of PD are movement-based findings of resting tremor, bradykinesia, rigidity and postural instability. However, nonmotor symptoms such as neuropsychiatric problems (mood, cognition, behaviour and thought alteration), autonomic dysfunction, sleep difficulties and sensory alterations can frequently cause as great or greater disability to the patient. Currently, there is no cure for the disease, and the mainstay of treatment is based around medications that increase dopamine levels within the brain. Novel interventions such as deep brain stimulation or ultrasound-based neuromodulation continue to be developed and may be considered for severe or drug-resistant PD.

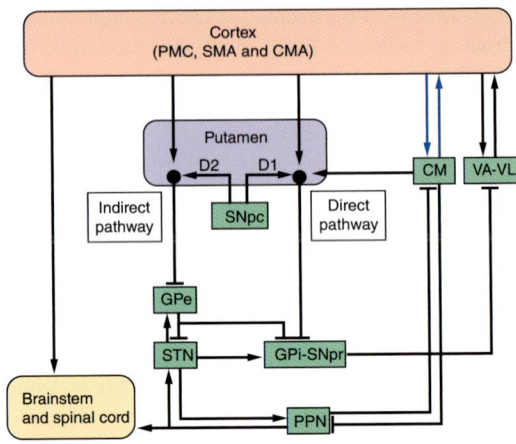

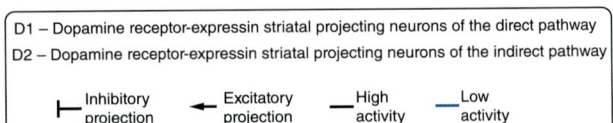

Fig. 2.17 Circuitry of the basal ganglia. CM, *Centromedian nucleus*; CMA, *cingulate motor area*; GPe, *globus pallidus external segment*; GPi-SNpr, *globus pallidus internal segment–substantia nigra pars compacta*; PMC, *primary motor cortex*; PPN, *pedunculopontine nucleus*; SMA, *supplementary motor area*; SNpc, *substantia nigra pars reticulata*; STN, *subthalamic nucleus*; VA-VL, *ventral anterior–ventral lateral nucleus*.

Circuits of the basal ganglia

The basal ganglia act as a funnel for all possible motor inputs and, in doing so, play a primary role in action selection. All cortical regions project via the striatum, which subsequently outputs to other regions of the basal ganglia. Through a series of interconnected projections, the basal ganglia can constrict motor movements to provide a smooth and steady, unitary stream of action. Output from the putamen is via a direct or indirect circuitry (Fig. 2.17). Using a variety of neurotransmitters including glutamate, gamma-aminobutyric acid (GABA) and dopamine, each projection around the basal ganglia nuclei may be excitatory or inhibitory. Broadly speaking, the direct pathway results in excitation of the thalamus, thereby facilitating movement. Conversely, the indirect pathway results in inhibition of the thalamus with subsequent inhibition of specific motor actions.

Cerebellum

The cerebellum is composed of two cerebellar hemispheres, the midline vermis and a flocculonodular lobe (consisting of the nodule and flocculus). The cerebellum sits in the posterior fossa beneath the tentorium cerebelli. Each hemisphere has a thin outer cortex of grey matter, deep to which lies white matter. The cerebellum is associated with regulation and coordination of movement, posture and balance. Cerebellar lesions result in ipsilateral deficits in function.

Cerebellar connections

The cerebellum is connected to the rest of the nervous system via three paired white matter pathways: the superior, middle and inferior cerebellar peduncles (Fig. 2.18). The superior cerebellar peduncle predominantly contains output projections. These projections connect deep cerebellar nuclei and upper motor neurones in the cerebral cortex, via thalamic nuclei. The middle peduncle is the largest of the three and predominantly contains afferent fibres, separated into three separate fascicles. These three fascicles connect pontine nuclei within the pons to different parts of the cerebellum. Within the inferior cerebellar peduncle, afferent fibres connect the vestibular nuclei, tegmentum and spinal cord (via the spinocerebellar tract) to the cerebellum. Output fibres from the cerebellum to the vestibular nuclei and reticular formation also connect via the inferior peduncle.

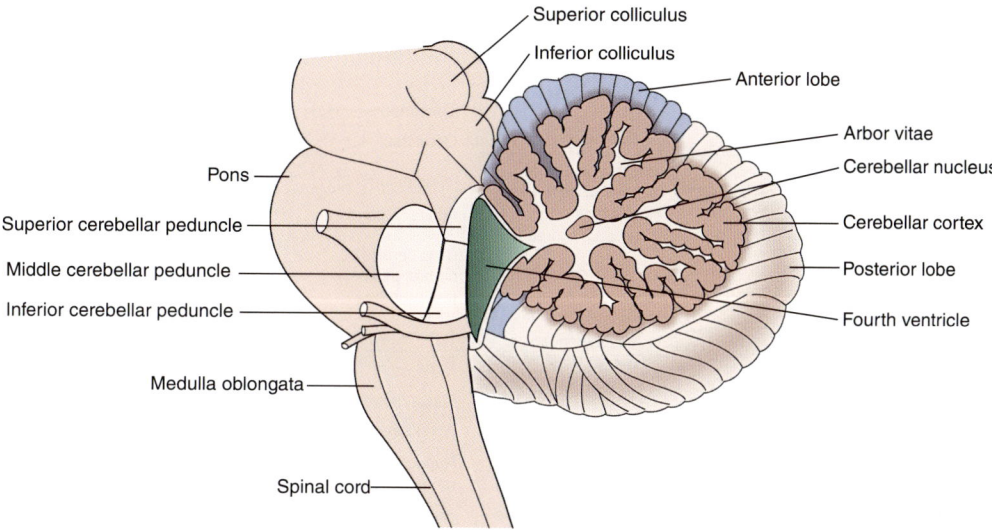

Fig. 2.18 Cerebellar peduncles.

Brainstem

The brainstem is sandwiched between the spinal cord and the diencephalon (Fig. 2.19). It consists of the midbrain, pons and medulla oblongata. It is here that the CNs and their respective nuclei originate.

Midbrain

The midbrain extends from the pons to the diencephalon and contains:

- Cerebral peduncles: These contain motor axons from the cerebrum to the spinal cord (corticospinal/pontine/bulbar) and sensory axons from the medulla to the thalamus.
- Colliculi: Four elevations in the posterior part of the midbrain:
  - Two superior colliculi: Some of the optic tracts enter here and regulate reflex eye movements, for example scanning, papillary reflex, accommodation reflex and the reflexes that occur with the eyes, head and neck regarding visual stimuli.
  - Two inferior colliculi: Conduit information from the auditory pathway to the thalamus.
- Nuclei substantia nigra: Darkly pigmented neurones extend from here to the basal ganglia, where they release dopamine and regulate subconscious muscle activities. The loss of these substantia nigra neurones can result in Parkinson disease.
- Red nucleus: Cerebellar and cerebral neurones synapse here and regulate muscular movements.
- CN nuclei 3 (oculomotor) and 4 (trochlear) are present here.

Pons

The word 'pons' means bridge. This 2.5-cm structure rests superior to the medulla and connects different parts of the brain via bundles of axons, which can be part of either the ascending or descending tract. The nuclei for CNs 5, 6, 7 and 8 (trigeminal, abducens, facial, vestibulocochlear) and the nerves that relay information from the cerebellum to the cerebral cortex are also present in the pons.

Medulla oblongata

The medulla oblongata contains three important functional regions:

- White matter: This contains all the sensory (ascending) and motor (descending) tracts. The pyramids are bulges of white matter consisting of large motor tracts; around 90% of these tracts decussate (cross over) to the opposite side of the body, which is the reason why the left brain controls the right side of the body and vice versa.
- Olives: Small olive-shaped structures, just lateral to the pyramids; proprioceptive impulses enter the medulla oblongata here and are then conducted to the cerebellum for processing.
- Nuclei: They are regions of grey matter where neurones synapse with each other. There are many different categories:
  - Gracile: Both the gracile and cuneate nuclei are implicated in sensations of touch and in consciousness.
  - Cuneate: Is also involved in proprioception, pressure and vibration.

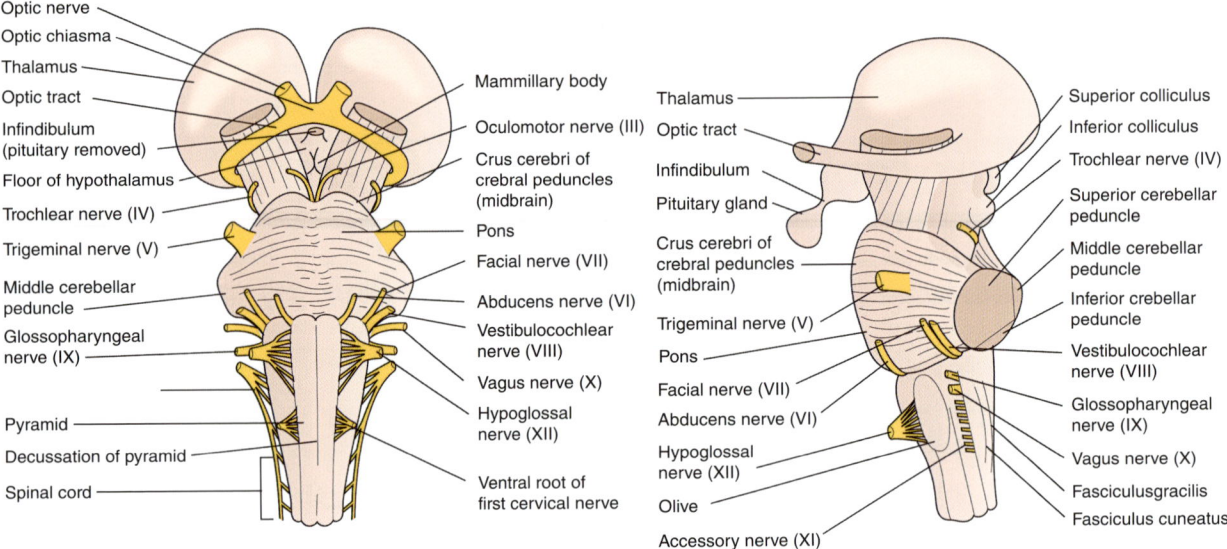

Fig. 2.19 The brainstem.

- ° Cranial nerve nuclei: There are between 8 and 12.
- ° Vital body function nuclei: Regulate the cardiovascular, respiratory, vomiting and coughing centres.

Reticular formation

The reticular formation is a loosely arranged network of white and grey matter in the brainstem. It has the following functions:

- Motor control: Via modulation of spinal interneurons and the transmission of information to the cerebellum.
- Sensory control: Exerts some control over activity in spinal reflex arcs. It is also important in the regulation of pain perception.
- Visceral control: Involved in the regulation of the respiratory and cardiovascular systems.
- Control of consciousness: A certain region of the sensory axons, which project to the cerebral cortex (reticular activating system), maintains consciousness. Damage to this region results in prolonged coma.

Cranial nerves

The CNs are 12 paired sets of nerves present on both sides of the body that emerge directly from the brain and brainstem. The CNs relay information between the brain and parts of the body; however, most nerves serve only the head and neck region. Table 2.2 summarizes all 12 cranial nerves. The detail of

their exact function is explained further when discussing the structures each nerve serves.

Ventricular system of the brain and cerebrospinal fluid

Four interconnected cavities (ventricles) exist within the brain that produce and circulate CSF throughout the brain and spinal cord.

Ventricles

There are four ventricles in the brain: two lateral ventricles (a left and a right), the third ventricle and the fourth ventricle (Fig. 2.20). The largest are the two lateral ventricles, which lie within the cerebrum and are separated in the midline by the septum pellucidum. The third ventricle lies between the right and left thalamus with the fourth ventricle lying posteriorly to the pons and upper half of the medulla.

Cerebrospinal fluid function

CSF is found between the pia mater and arachnoid mater throughout the brain and spinal cord; it helps protect the CNS from impact to the head as well as provides a degree of buoyancy and support against gravity. The CSF also supplies the brain with nutrients whilst providing chemical stability.

Cerebrospinal fluid production and reabsorption

Lining the whole ventricular system are ependymal cells, a specialized form of epithelium. As well as serving as a reservoir for

Table 2.2 Summary of cranial nerves

Nerve	Distribution and functions
Olfactory (CN 1)	Smell from nasal mucosa of roof of each nasal cavity
Optic (CN 2)	Vision from retina
Oculomotor (CN 3)	Motor to superior, medial and inferior oblique; parasympathetic innervation to sphincter pupillae and ciliary muscle (constricts pupil and accommodates lens of eye) carries sympathetic nerve fibres (from carotid plexus) to smooth muscle part of levator palpebrae superioris
Trochlear (CN 4)	Motor to superior oblique
Trigeminal (CN 5)—ophthalmic division (V_1)	Sensation from upper third of face, including cornea, scalp, eyelids, external nose and paranasal sinuses
Trigeminal (CN 5)—maxillary division (V_2)	Sensation from the middle third of face, including upper lip, maxillary teeth, mucosa of nose, maxillary sinuses and palate; supplies dura mater anteriorly
Trigeminal (CN 5)—mandibular division (V_3)	Motor to muscles of mastication, mylohyoid, anterior belly of digastric, tensor veli palatini and tensor tympani; sensation from lower third of face, including temporomandibular joint, and mucosa of mouth and anterior two-thirds of tongue; supplies dura mater anteriorly
Abducens (CN 6)	Motor to lateral rectus
Facial (CN 7)	Motor to muscles of facial expression and scalp, stapedius, stylohyoid and posterior belly of digastric; taste from anterior two-thirds of tongue, floor of mouth and palate; sensation from skin of external acoustic meatus; parasympathetic innervation to submandibular and sublingual salivary glands, lacrimal gland and glands of nose and palate
Vestibulocochlear (CN 8)	Vestibular sensation from semicircular ducts, utricle and saccule; hearing from the organ of Corti
Glossopharyngeal (CN 9)	Motor to stylopharyngeus, parasympathetic innervation to parotid gland; visceral sensation from parotid gland, carotid body and sinus, pharynx and middle ear; taste and general sensation from posterior third of tongue
Vagus (CN 10)	Motor to constrictor muscles of pharynx, intrinsic muscles of larynx and muscles of palate (except tensor veli palatini) and superior two-thirds of oesophagus; parasympathetic innervation to smooth muscle of trachea, bronchi, digestive tract and cardiac muscle of heart; visceral sensation from pharynx, larynx, trachea, bronchi and heart to the splenic flexure oesophagus, stomach and intestine; taste from epiglottis and palate; sensation from auricle, external acoustic meatus and dura mater of posterior cranial fossa
Accessory (CN 11) cranial root Spinal root	Motor to striated muscles of soft palate, pharynx and larynx via fibres that join the vagus nerve (CN10) in the jugular foramenMotor to sternocleidomastoid and trapezius
Hypoglossal (CN 12)	Sensory to dura mater, posteriorly; motor to intrinsic and extrinsic muscles of tongue (except palatoglossus)

neurodegeneration, the main function of these ependymal cells is to produce CSF. Each ventricle has a network of these cells, termed the choroid plexus. The greatest mass of choroid plexus sits within the lateral ventricles.

Within the venous sinuses lie small protrusions of arachnoid mater called arachnoid granulations. These granulations act like one-way valves to allow CSF to diffuse across the arachnoid into the venous circulation. The largest area of granulations lies along the superior sagittal sinus.

Cerebrospinal fluid flow

The majority of CSF is produced by the ependymal cells within the lateral ventricles. From here, it flows through the interventricular foramen (foramen of Munro) into the third ventricle, then through the cerebral aqueduct to the fourth ventricle. From the fourth ventricle, CSF flows to the central spinal canal and the median aperture or either of the two lateral apertures to enter the subarachnoid space, which surrounds the entire brain and spinal cord to the level of S1–S2. The CSF is then reabsorbed into the venous circulation via the arachnoid granulations. It is widely considered that CSF flows in a pulsatile manner, matching the pressure waves generated in blood vessels by the beating heart.

Blood supply and venous drainage to the brain and spinal cord

The brain is supplied by the two internal carotid arteries (ICAs) and the two vertebral arteries.

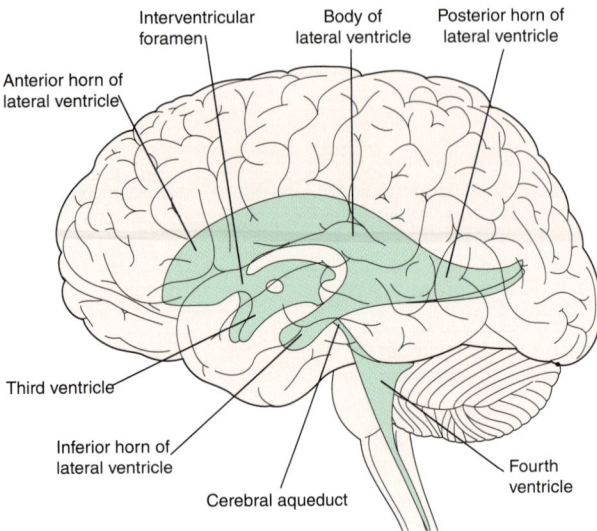

Fig. 2.20 The ventricles of the brain.

Internal carotid artery

The ICA is a terminal branch of the common carotid artery. On the left side of the body, the common carotid artery usually branches directly from the aortic arch. However, on the right side the brachiocephalic artery, a branch from the aortic arch, divides to become the subclavian artery and the right common carotid artery (Fig. 2.21). The ICA travels in the carotid sheath, enters the skull through the carotid canal and passes into the middle cranial fossa by traversing the foramen lacerum in the floor of the cavernous sinus. The artery runs forward in the cavernous sinus, turning superiorly to pierce the roof at the anterior end. It then enters the subarachnoid space and gives off the ophthalmic artery. Inferior to the anterior perforated substance of the brain, the ICA gives off the anterior cerebral and posterior communicating arteries, before continuing as the middle cerebral artery (Fig. 2.22). It is at this point where the ICA enters the cerebral arterial circle (circle of Willis).

Vertebral artery

The vertebral artery in the neck arises from the first part of the subclavian artery. It ascends in the foramina transversaria of the C6 to C1 vertebrae and enters the skull through the foramen magnum. The vertebral artery ascends superiorly on the surface of the medulla oblongata (Fig. 2.23) where the left and right vertebral arteries join to become the basilar artery in the midline.

Cranial branches of the vertebral artery include:

- the meningeal arteries.
- the anterior and posterior spinal arteries.

- the posterior inferior cerebellar artery.
- the medullary arteries.

Basilar artery

The basilar artery ascends on the anterior surface of the pons (Fig. 2.22), supplying the pons as it does so. At the upper border of the pons, it divides into the posterior cerebral arteries. Just before dividing, it gives off bilateral superior cerebellar arteries. The basilar artery also gives off branches to the inner ear via the anterior inferior cerebellar artery.

Cerebral arterial circle

The cerebral arterial circle is an anastomosis between branches of the ICAs and the vertebral arteries (Fig. 2.22), allowing blood entering either artery to flow to any part of either cerebral hemisphere. The cerebral arterial circle lies in the inferior surface of the brain, in the interpeduncular fossa beneath the forebrain. An anterior communicating artery connects the two anterior cerebral arteries, and posterior communicating arteries connect the internal carotid to the posterior cerebral artery.

CLINICAL NOTES

CEREBRAL AUTOREGULATION

The blood supply to the brain can autoregulate; that is when the perfusion pressure to the brain changes, the cerebral circulation can regulate itself to ensure that a relatively constant blood flow is maintained (Fig. 2.24). Several mediators and mechanisms are involved in cerebral autoregulation including oxygen (PaO_2), carbon dioxide ($PaCO_2$), H^+ and myogenic tone; conditions such as chronic arterial hypertension also affect cerebral autoregulation.

Cerebral perfusion

Cerebral perfusion pressure (CPP) is the principal determinant of cerebral blood flow, and therefore, an adequate CPP is crucial for oxygen and nutrient delivery to the brain. Normal CPP is 50 to 70 mm Hg and can be calculated as such:

$$CPP = MAP - (ICP \text{ or } CVP, \text{ whichever is highest})$$

Where

CPP = cerebral perfusion pressure
MAP = mean arterial pressure
ICP = intracranial pressure
CVP = central venous pressure

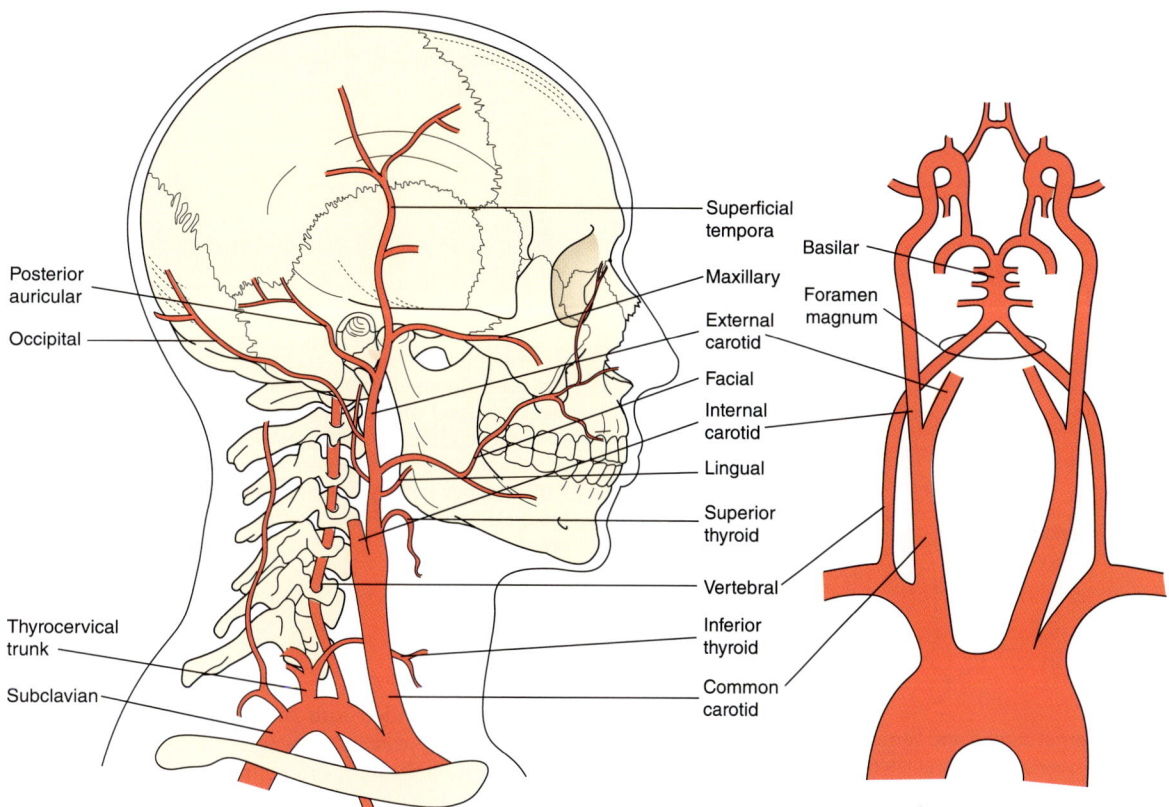

Fig. 2.21 Anatomy of the common carotid arteries.

If ICP rises significantly, CPP will thus be reduced, limiting the delivery of oxygenated blood to the brain and risking an ischaemic brain injury. This is one of the key reasons for preventing and/or treating a raised ICP.

Stroke (cerebrovascular accident)

A stroke is a loss of function of part(s) of the brain secondary to a disturbance in blood supply to the brain. Strokes can be classified as ischaemic (approximately 85% of all strokes) and haemorrhagic (approximately 15%). Ischaemic strokes occur due to thrombosis, emboli or hypoperfusion. Haemorrhagic strokes occur secondary to an aneurysm of arteriovenous malformation. The symptoms and signs of stroke depend on which part of the brain is affected. Patients commonly present with sudden onset of unilateral limb weakness, unilateral facial droop, speech disturbance or visual disturbance. Symptoms occur rapidly over minutes to hours. Typically, it is not possible to reverse the death of the brain tissue affected, although, with rapid restoration of blood supply to the area, a degree of reversibility can be achieved.

A transient ischaemic attack (TIA) produces symptoms often identical to those of stroke; however, the symptoms resolve in less than 24 hours and often last only for a few minutes. In these patients, the risk of a stroke is high, and they must undergo further investigations and receive prophylactic treatment.

Management of a severe traumatic brain injury

A patient with a severe traumatic brain injury requires urgent and specialist management to prevent any subsequent secondary brain injury. A key goal is to maintain an adequate CPP. If a patient is intubated and ventilated, controlling the PaO_2 and $PaCO_2$ of the patient, both of which have a significant effect on cerebral blood flow, is a cornerstone of management. For example if $PaCO_2$ is too high (e.g. >5.0 kPa), cerebral vasodilatation will occur, thus increasing the blood volume within the cranium. This will further increase ICP and reduce CPP.

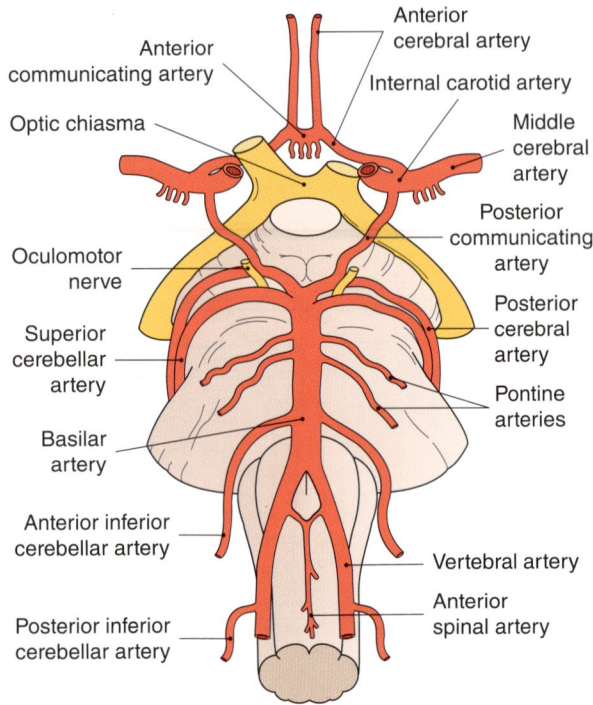

Fig. 2.22 Internal carotid and vertebral arteries and the cerebral arterial circle overlying the brainstem.

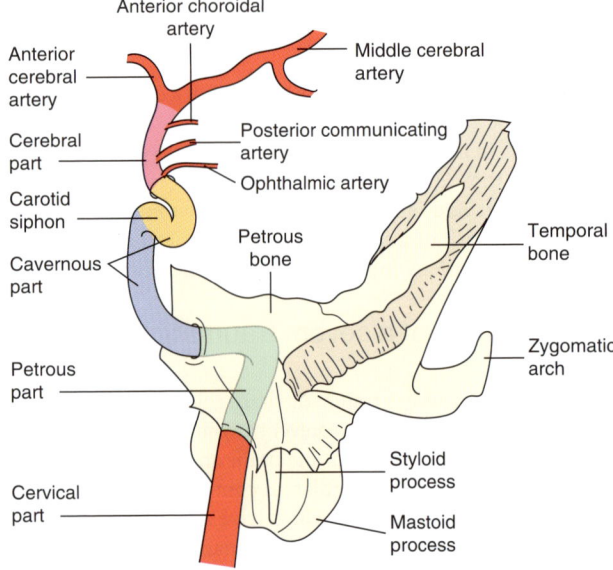

Fig. 2.23 Anatomy and course of the internal carotid artery.

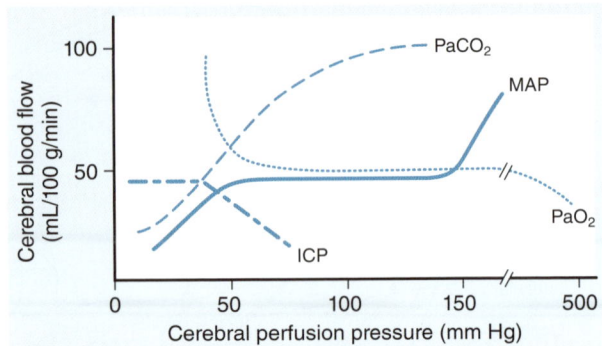

Fig. 2.24 Cerebral autoregulation and factors that affect cerebral blood flow (CBF). CBF is maintained steady at an average of 50 mL/min/100 g between the lower and upper limits of autoregulation. Below and beyond the limits of autoregulation, CBF changes linearly with systemic blood pressure. Other factors affecting CBF include $PaCO_2$, PaO_2 and intracranial pressure.

Peripheral nervous system

The PNS is divided into the somatic nervous system and the autonomic nervous system (sympathetic and parasympathetic). The PNS serves to connect the limbs and organs to the CNS.

Somatic nervous system

The somatic nervous system is composed of motor (efferent) and sensory (afferent) neurones. The efferent system carries impulses from the CNS to skeletal muscles. The afferent system carries sensory information to the CNS.

Autonomic nervous system

Autonomic nerves are either sympathetic or parasympathetic. They control involuntary visceral functions. The cell bodies of the preganglionic neurones of the sympathetic nervous system lie within the thoracic and first two lumbar segments of the spinal cord (T1–L2). The preganglionic axons exit via the anterior root of spinal nerves and synapse with postganglionic neurones in a ganglion of the sympathetic chain, which runs on either side of the vertebral column. The postganglionic axons then reenter the spinal nerve to supply the body wall and limbs. Some preganglionic axons do not synapse in the sympathetic chain. They can pass through the sympathetic ganglion and travel to autonomic plexuses in the thorax to supply thoracic viscera. Alternatively, they can pass through the ganglion to form the splanchnic nerves and synapse in a prevertebral ganglion, for example coeliac ganglion. Postganglionic axons supply abdominal viscera.

The cell bodies of the parasympathetic preganglionic neurones lie in the nuclei of CN 3, 7, 9 and 10 and in the grey matter of the spinal cord between S2 and S4. Their axons travel in cranial nerves (CN 3, 7, 9, 10) and sacral nerves (S2–S4). They synapse in ganglia, which lie within, or in proximity to, the viscera they supply.

HINTS AND TIPS

SYMPATHETIC VERSUS PARASYMPATHETIC NERVOUS SYSTEMS

The activity of the sympathetic and parasympathetic nervous systems can be remembered by the following: the sympathetic nervous system controls 'flight-or-fight' reactions (e.g. dilation of the pupils, increase in heart rate and decrease in activity of the gut). The parasympathetic nervous system is concerned with 'rest and digest' (increases activity of the gut, etc.).

Sensation, perception and pain

Sensation

Sensation is the conscious or subconscious awareness of external/internal stimuli. The reaction to the sensation is dependent on the CNS target of the impulses. For example touching a hot oven will elicit the spinal reflex arc, which results in the rapid removal of the hand from heat.

Sensory modalities

The term 'modalities' describes the different types of sensation, of which there are two:

General
- Somatic: Provides information from sensory receptors in the skin and mucous membranes and includes:
  - tactile, for example touch, vibration and pressure.
  - pain.
  - thermal.
  - proprioception, which tells the brain the relative positions of the body in space.
  - visceral: provides information about the internal organs.

Special—These include smell, vision, hearing and balance. These are all discussed later.

Sensory receptors

The different types of sensory receptors monitor stimuli and can be classified functionally or structurally (Table 2.3).

Table 2.3 Types of sensory receptor

Functional attributes of receptors		
Type	**Stimulus**	**Where present**
Mechanoreceptor	Mechanical pressure	Skin
Thermoreceptor	Temperature changes	Skin
Nociceptor	Pain	Skin, eyes, muscles
Osmoreceptor	Osmotic pressure of body fluids	Hypothalamus—detect osmolality of body fluids and result in ADH regulation
Chemoreceptor	Chemical changes	Mouth (taste), nose (smell)
Photoreceptor	Light changes	Retina
Structural attributes of receptors		
Type	**Description**	**Associated with**
Free nerve endings	The dendrites are not covered in myelin	Pain, tickling, touch
Encapsulated nerve endings	These dendrites are surrounded by a connective tissue substance	Touch, e.g. Pacinian corpuscles
Separate cells	These synapse with other neurones to detect sensation	Taste, e.g. gustatory receptors in the taste buds

ADH, *Antidiuretic hormone.*

The mechanism of sensation—The mechanism of sensation is demonstrated below using the increase in external temperature as an example:

1. The receptor is stimulated, for example the increase in temperature stimulates the skin thermoreceptors.
2. The receptor converts this into a graded potential in the neurone.
3. When this reaches a threshold, it triggers an action potential (AP).
4. The AP propagates towards the CNS via afferent fibres; for example temperature signals travel through the spinothalamic tract.
5. Certain regions of the cerebral cortexes, for example the hypothalamus, process the information.
6. The cerebral cortex sends signals via the efferent fibres to particular regions of the body to respond to the stimulus; for

example if the body is too hot, then the sympathetic tone is reduced and the blood vessels dilate passively.

Adaption—During a continued stimulus, the generator potential decreases in amplitude causing fewer and fewer APs. Consequently, the perception of sensation declines. An example is when you go into your flatmate's room and it has a pungent smell (!). After a while, you get used to it and cannot smell it anymore. This is not because the smell has gone away but because your olfactory system has adapted.

Somatic sensations

These arise from stimulation of sensory reception in the skin and mucous membranes.

Tactile receptors—Tactile sensation includes touch, pressure, vibration, itching and tickling. It is sensed by a combination of the following receptors (the first three activate encapsulated large-diameter myelinated A fibres):

- Meissner corpuscles: Comprising free nerve endings. These are egg-shaped masses in the skin dermal papillae. They sense fine touch and predominate in the fingertips, lips, nipples, clitoris and glans penis.
- Mechanoreceptors: For example Merkel discs, flattened free nerve endings in the stratum basal of skin, for fine touch sensation.
- Ruffini corpuscles: Stretch receptors present deep in the dermis, ligaments and tendons.
- Hair root plexus: Found in hairy skin; detects movements of hair.
- Pacinian corpuscles: Large, multilayered connective tissue capsules. They are found in the dermis and subcutaneous layer, where they detect pressure.
- Free nerve endings: Small-diameter, unmyelinated C fibres stimulated by chemicals, such as bradykinin, for tickle and itch sensation.

Thermal receptors—These are free nerve endings, specifically:

- Cold receptors: Found in the stratum basal where they mainly attach to mediu m-diameter myelinated A fibres.
- Warmth receptors: Present in the dermis. They are attached to small-diameter, unmyelinated C fibres.

Photoreceptors—Photoreceptors are light-sensitive proteins involved in the function of photoreceptor cells. An example is the rhodopsin in the retina.

Chemoreceptors—A chemoreceptor is a cell, or a group of cells, that transduces a chemical signal into an AP. There are two types: distance and direct. An example of a distance chemoreceptor is the olfactory receptor neurones in the olfactory system. Examples of direct chemoreceptors include taste buds in the gustatory system and carotid bodies that detect changes in pH inside the body.

Perception

Perception describes the conscious awareness and interpretation of the sensations. One example is the awareness of extremes of temperature.

Pain

Pain describes the unpleasant sensory and emotional experience associated with actual or potential tissue damage. Pain can therefore play a vital protective function by alerting the body to tissue injury. Nociceptors are the receptors for pain and are found almost everywhere. Nociceptors are activated by thermal, mechanical or chemical stimuli, stimuli that are transformed into electrical signals and conducted to the CNS. An understanding of the mechanisms of pain and pain regulation will allow you to be able to provide adequate analgesia (pain relief medications) to your patients—a central pillar of medicine.

There are two types of pain:

Fast—occurs within 0.1 second of application of the stimulus and is:

- conducted along medium-diameter myelinated Aδ fibres.
- very well localized.

An example is a finger on a sharp object.

Slow—occurs 1 to 2 seconds after application of the stimulus and persists. It is:

- conducted along small-diameter, unmyelinated C fibres.
- localized and diffuse.

An example is renal colic.

Pain can be superficial somatic (in the skin), deep somatic (in deeper structures like muscles, joints and tendons) or visceral organ pain, which can occur away from the organ that is damaged, that is referred pain. This is due to the damaged visceral organ and the referred region being innervated by the same spinal cord segment; for example irritation of the diaphragm can refer pain to the shoulder tip. In this example, the irritated diaphragm (causes of which include liver damage, intraabdominal bleeding or free air within the abdomen after abdominal surgery) is innervated by C3, C4 and C5 nerve branches, which also supply sensation to the shoulder tip.

Regulation of pain

The body has a variety of mechanisms to regulate the degree of pain experienced. This regulation can happen peripherally and/or centrally:

- Peripheral regulation: activity in the low-threshold mechanoreceptors can inhibit the spinothalamic nerve impulses, for example rubbing the area of pain.

- Central regulation (Fig. 2.25). The CNS has its own pain control areas:
  ○ Periaqueductal grey areas of the midbrain and pons.
  ○ Raphe magnus nucleus—located in the lower region of the pons and superior medulla.
  ○ Reticular formation regions in the dorsal horn—nucleus reticularis paragigantocellularis and locus coeruleus. Stimulation of opiate and 5-HT (5-hydroxytryptamine, i.e. serotonin) receptors in these areas can inhibit the pain pathway and cause analgesia.

Analgesia

Several classes of analgesic medications exist. Selecting the most appropriate agent will depend on a variety of factors including the source, nature and severity of the pain and, crucially, the side effect profile of the analgesic (Fig. 2.26).

Paracetamol—Paracetamol is the most common analgesic agent used worldwide, typically useful for mild to moderate pain; it is also used as an antipyretic. Although its mechanism of action is not entirely understood, paracetamol has been found to reduce the activity of cyclooxygenase, which may account for its pain- and fever-reducing properties.

Nonsteroidal antiinflammatory drugs—Nonsteroidal antiinflammatory drugs decrease the sensitization of nociceptors that occurs in inflammation by inhibiting the formation of inflammatory mediators.

Opiates—Throughout the CNS, there are three classes of opioid receptors that act to modulate pain:

1. Mu (μ).
2. Delta (δ).
3. Kappa (κ).

These receptors can be activated by endogenous opiate-like peptides derived from three large molecules: proenkephalin, proopiomelanocortin and prodynorphin. They act on the μ and δ (mu and delta) opioid receptors in the spinal cord, brainstem and hypothalamus to block pain signals.

Opioid receptors can also be stimulated exogenously by opiates (naturally occurring molecules, e.g. morphine) or opioid drugs (synthetic agents that stimulate opioid receptors, e.g. fentanyl).

Each drug will stimulate different opioid receptors to varying degrees. For example morphine stimulates the μ-receptors, resulting in nonendogenous analgesia, euphoria, sedation and respiratory depression. However, all opioids have a range of side effects (Table 2.4):

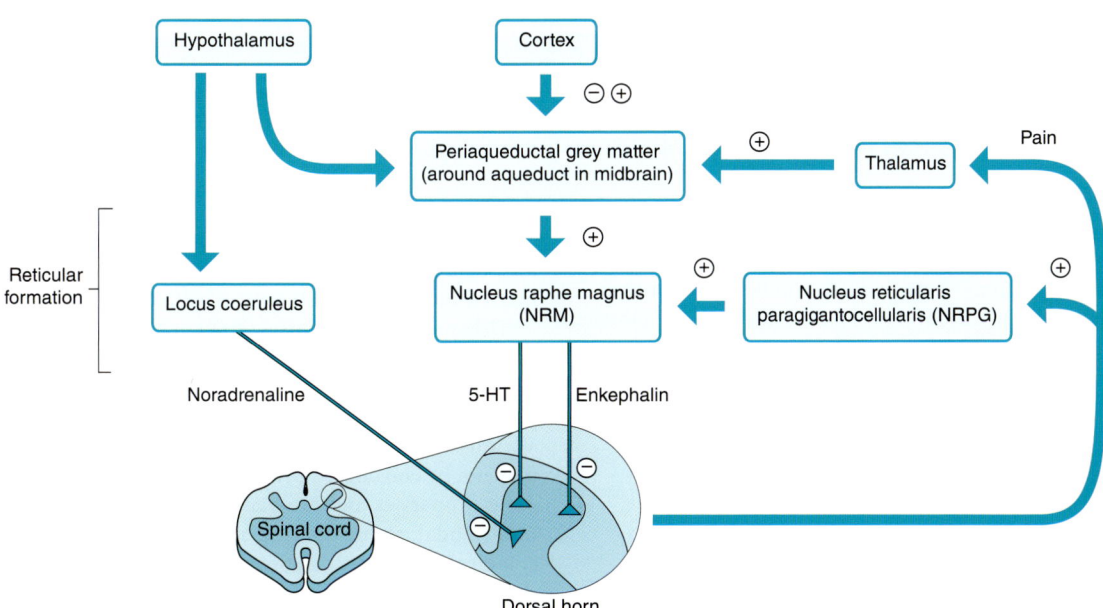

Fig. 2.25 Central pain regulation.

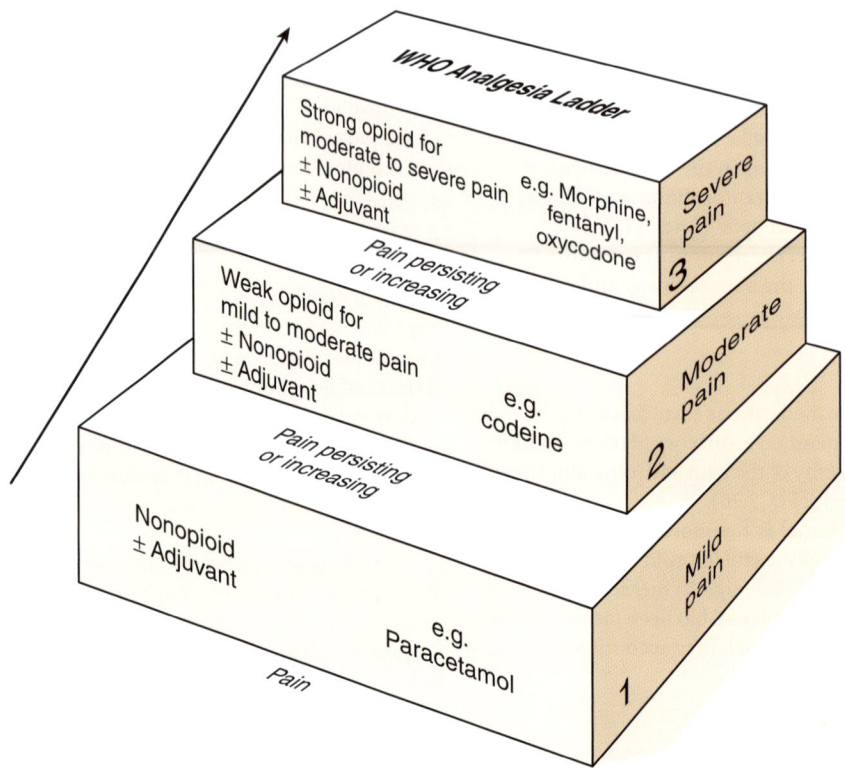

Adjuvants include NSAIDs such as ibuprofen or naproxen (if no contraindications), TENS machine

Fig. 2.26 The World Health Organization (WHO) analgesic ladder. Originally designed for cancer-related pain, the principles of the model are translated to most analgesic regimes. NSAIDs, *Nonsteroidal antiinflammatory drugs*; TENS, *transcutaneous electrical nerve stimulation*. (Adapted from WHO guidelines for the pharmacological and radiotherapeutic management of cancer pain in adults and adolescents. Geneva: World Health Organization; 2018. Available at https://iris.who.int/bitstream/handle/10665/279700/9789241550390-eng.pdf. Accessed 19 May 2025. WHO is not responsible for the content or accuracy of this adaptation.)

- Respiratory depression, reducing the sensitivity of the brainstem to arterial PCO_2 ($PaCO_2$).
- Nausea/vomiting: Opiates/opioids stimulate the chemical trigger zone (CTZ) within the fourth ventricle, which then stimulates the vomiting centre of the medulla. Stimulation of the CTZ can be inhibited by antiemetic drugs such as ondansetron.
- Constipation: Caused by reduced motility of the gastrointestinal tract.

Repeated administration of morphine causes:

- Tolerance: Decreased responsiveness to the drug so that more must be taken to achieve the same effect.
- Dependence: Not physical (where a withdrawal causes physical symptoms, e.g. nausea, muscle cramping) and psychological (drug-seeking behaviour, anxiety).

Overdose with opiates can result in pinpoint pupils, respiratory depression and a comatose patient. Treatment includes intravenous μ-antagonists such as naloxone.

Other analgesic agents—Other analgesic agents exist such as ketamine, gabapentin and amitriptyline. Their mechanism of action is varied, with some used to target specific types of pain; for example gabapentin is useful for neuropathic pain. Various other medications such as magnesium and clonidine may not be considered primarily as analgesics but have analgesic properties and are becoming increasingly popular in multimodal, opiate-sparing analgesic regimes. Nonpharmacological techniques can be used to supplement/replace medications and include transcutaneous electrical nerve stimulation (TENS) and acupuncture. Typically, the side effect profile of nonpharmacological techniques is more

Table 2.4 Opioid drugs and their pharmacology

μ-Agonist	Bioavailability and administration	Metabolism	Potency and length of action	Clinical use	Notes
Morphine	Poor availability when given orally due to high rate of first-pass metabolism. Intravenous administration provides reliable dosing	Active metabolite morphine-6-glucuronide	$t_{1/2}$ 3 h	Acute and chronic pain	Cannot be given in labour as foetal liver cannot conjugate
Diamorphine (heroin)	More lipid soluble. Given orally or by intramuscular, intravenous or subcutaneous injection	Partly to morphine	Very potent, rapid onset, $t_{1/2}$ 2 h	Acute and chronic pain	
Codeine	High oral bioavailability	To other opioids including morphine	One-sixth potency of morphine	Mild pain, headache, dental pain	Potent antitussive, low side effect profile
Pethidine	High lipid solubility. Given orally and by intramuscular injection	Metabolite norpethidine interacts with MAOIs	One-tenth potency of morphine	Acute pain, labour	Does not cause miosis
Fentanyl	High lipid solubility. Given intravenously, epidurally, transdermally.		Very potent, short acting	Intraoperative pain	Intraoperative analgesia
Buprenorphine	Increase first-pass metabolism. Given sublingually, intrathecally		$t_{1/2}$ 12 h, slow onset	Acute and chronic pain	Partial agonist and difficult to reverse effects in overdose
Methadone	Given orally or by injection		$t_{1/2}$ >24 h, very slow onset	Maintenance of drug addicts	Does not produce euphoria

MAOIs, *Monoamine oxidase inhibitors*; $t_{1/2}$, *half-life*.

favourable than drugs and should therefore be considered where possible.

CELLULAR PHYSIOLOGY OF THE NERVOUS SYSTEM

Neurones: structure and function

The conducting cells of the nervous system are termed neurones. A typical motor neurone consists of a cell body (containing a nucleus), which gives rise to a single axon (nerve fibre) and numerous dendrites (Fig. 2.27). The cell bodies of most neurones are located within the CNS. Aggregations of cell bodies in the CNS and PNS are known as nuclei and ganglia, respectively. Axons conduct electrical impulses (APs) away from the cell body. They communicate with other neurones at synapses (via neurotransmitter release) with target organs or glands. Axons of a neurone may be wrapped in a myelin sheath (myelinated) or not (unmyelinated). Myelinated fibres conduct impulses faster than unmyelinated fibres. Dendrites extend outward from the cell body. Dendrites receive signals from other neurones and transmit them to the cell body.

Classification of neurones
Projection neurones: Golgi type 1
These neurones influence cells located in different parts of the nervous system. This function is helped by the fact that the cells have long neurones (known as axons) and sometimes produce collateral branches.

Interneurones: Golgi type 2
These neurones influence cells located in close proximity. They have shorter axons than the projection neurons, although they

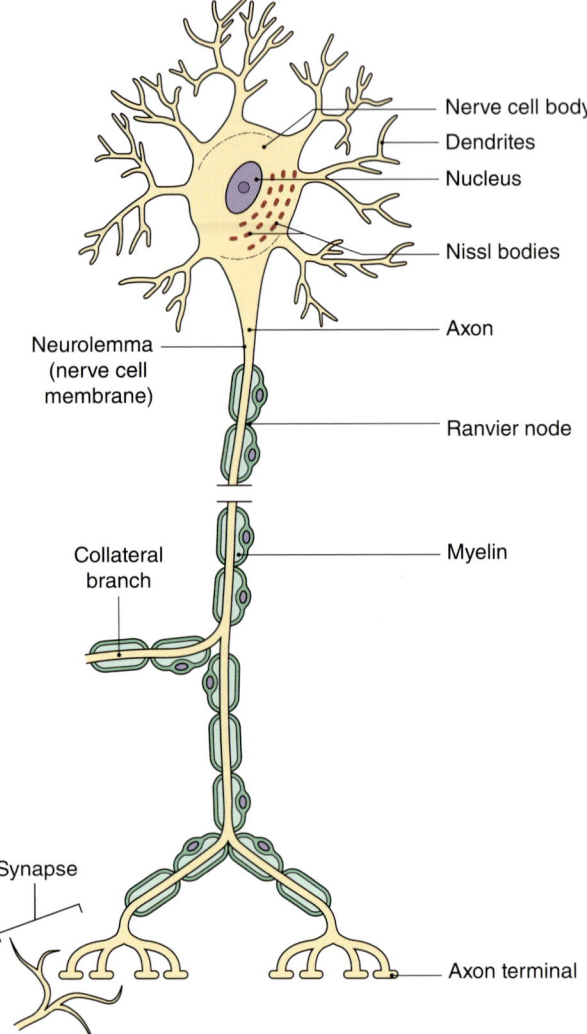

Nerve cell body

Dendrites

Nucleus

Nissl bodies

Axon

Neurolemma
(nerve cell
membrane)

Ranvier node

Collateral
branch

Myelin

Synapse

Axon terminal

Fig. 2.27 Structure of a typical motor neurone.

too sometimes produce collateral branches, which increase their ability to relay information.

Neuronal excitation and inhibition

An electrical potential gradient exists across the nerve cell membrane. This gradient is caused by the relative permeability of the cell membrane to sodium ions (Na^+) in the extracellular fluid and potassium (K^+) in the intracellular fluid. The value of this potential determines whether an AP is generated.

Resting potential

There is a potential difference of $-70\,mV$ across the membrane of a resting neurone, the outside being positive relative to the inside. This is due to a greater concentration of K^+ ions inside the cell, which results in a negative inside and positive outside and hence a potential difference (diffusional potential).

Diffusion takes place until an equilibrium state is reached. This is where the electrical force attracting the positive K^+ into the cells is equal to the chemical force of the concentration gradient. The electrical potential is also affected by the diffusion of ions, such as Na^+ moving across the cell membrane in the opposite direction to the K^+.

There is always a degree of unregulated leakage of Na^+ into the cell and K^+ out of the cell: down the concentration gradient. However, this is counteracted by an energy-dependent Na^+/K^+-adenosine triphosphatase (ATPase) exchange pump that stabilizes the resting membrane potential. The pump ejects three Na^+ in exchange for every two K^+ transports into the cell.

Action potentials

An AP is the feature of muscle and nerve cells that results in self-propagating membrane depolarization. When a nerve cell is stimulated, the electrical potential across the membrane changes. If the stimulus is strong enough and reaches a certain value (threshold potential), an AP is generated. APs have three distinct properties:

1. They are all or nothing: this means that an AP will occur when the threshold potential has been exceeded. Increasing the stimulus further does not change the shape or size of the AP.
2. They have a refractory period: during an AP, it is either impossible or very difficult to stimulate a second AP. There are two types of refractory period:
   a. Absolute: In the early part of the AP, no further stimulus is possible.
   b. Relative: A further AP is possible, but a larger-than-normal stimulus is required.
3. They are self-propagating: Once the AP has been initiated, it spreads throughout the excitable tissue.

Ionic mechanism of an action potential

The propagation of a nerve impulse along an axon begins when synapses on a neurone receive neurotransmitters from adjacent nerve endings. This causes the electrical potential across the cell membrane to change, setting off a chain of events that results in the AP.

There are three stages to the generation of an AP (Fig. 2.28):

1. The threshold: To initiate an AP, the stimulus must increase the membrane potential to about $20\,mV$ above the resting potential of $-70\,mV$. When this happens, Na^+ enters the neurone via voltage-gated Na^+ channels.

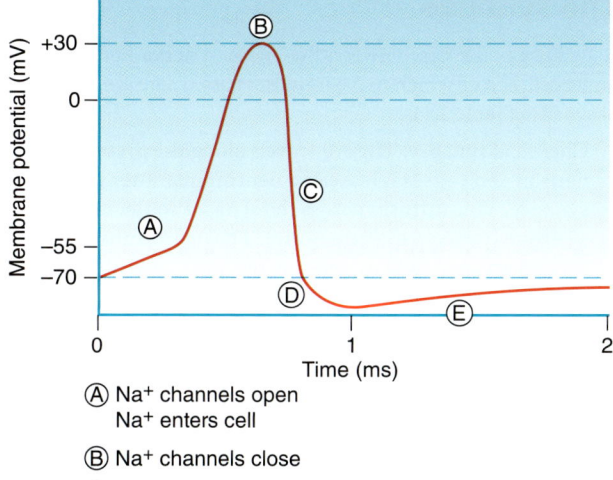

A Na⁺ channels open
  Na⁺ enters cell

B Na⁺ channels close

C K⁺ channels open
  K⁺ leaves cell

D K⁺ channels close

E Refractory period

Fig. 2.28 Mechanism of an action potential.

2. Depolarization (upstroke) (A): If the threshold is reached, more voltage-gated Na^+ channels open and further depolarization takes place (positive feedback). The membrane potential rises towards 0 mV and then overshoots to +30 mV (B).
3. Repolarization (downstroke) (C): Once 0 mV is passed, the positive intracellular charge resists further Na^+ entry and slow-inactivation gates begin to close. The slow voltage-gated K^+ channels are fully open at +30 mV, K^+ leaves the cell and the internal negativity of the membrane is returned. There is a period of hyperpolarization when the voltage-gated K^+ channels are not fully closed, permitting additional K^+ to leave—the absolute refractory period (D). Restoration of the resting membrane potential occurs when voltage-gated Na^+ and K^+ channels are closed (E). The Na^+/K^+-ATPase continues to actively pump Na^+ out of, and K^+ into, the cell throughout the AP.

After potentials

Sometimes the Na^+ and K^+ channels do not return to their previous states. This causes either an over- or undershoot, leading to hyper- or hypopolarization, respectively.

Myelinated and unmyelinated fibres

Myelin comprises proteins and lipids that form a sheath around some nerves (Fig. 2.29) and increases the speed of impulse

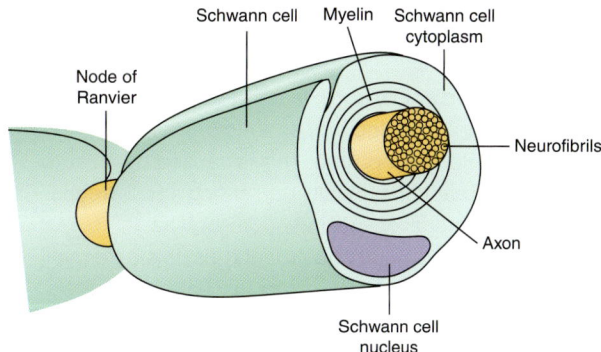

Fig. 2.29 Myelinated fibre.

transmission. There are roughly twice as many myelinated fibres as unmyelinated. Examples of where nerves are myelinated include the brachial plexus and the radial nerve in the upper limb.

Myelin sheath in the PNS is formed by Schwann cells (also known as neurolemmocytes), which envelop the naked axon and produce a cellular membrane containing the lipid substance sphingomyelin. This insulates the axon, decreases the ion flow through the membrane and consequently reduces its capacitance.

Between every two Schwann cells there is a small, exposed area of axon where ions can still flow between the axon and extracellular fluids; these are the nodes of Ranvier. APs jump from node to node by saltatory conduction where sodium rushing into the node creates an electrical force, thus 'pushing on' the ions already inside the axon (Fig. 2.30). The importance of saltatory conduction is twofold:

1. The conduction velocity of APs is increased as the depolarization jumps from node to node.
2. As only the nodes depolarize, less adenosine triphosphate (ATP) is required and energy is conserved.

CLINICAL NOTES

DEMYELINATING DISEASES

Lack of myelin can cause a number of diseases, of which the two most common are:
- Multiple sclerosis: This disease of unknown aetiology is characterized by multiple plaques of demyelination and inflammation within the neurones of the CNS. Specifically, it causes a loss of oligodendrocytes—the cells responsible for creating and maintaining the myelin sheath. It most commonly affects the white matter in the optic nerve, brainstem, basal

(Continued)

ganglia and spinal cord, leading to optic neuropathy, diplopia, vertigo and spastic paraparesis.

- Guillain-Barré syndrome: This is caused by an autoimmune reaction typically presenting 1 to 3 weeks after a bacterial or viral infection such as *Campylobacter jejuni* gastroenteritis. It is a demyelinating neuropathy that results in weakness in the distal muscle progressing proximally with time. It can sometimes lead to respiratory failure.

Speed of conduction

The speed of conduction of an AP depends on:

- Myelinated versus unmyelinated fibres—see later.
- Fibre diameter: The thicker the fibre, the faster the speed of conductance.

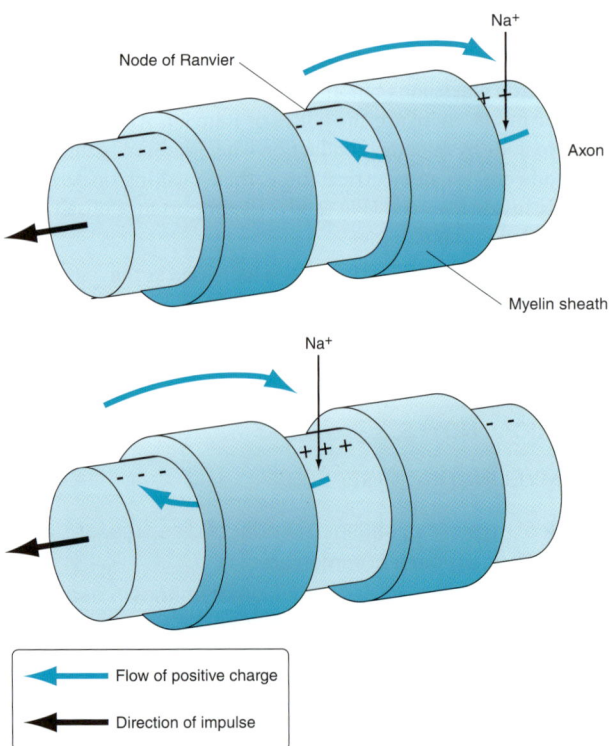

Fig. 2.30 Saltatory conduction.

The synapse

A synapse is the gap between the end of a nerve fibre and the target cell, across which nerve impulses pass. There are two types of synapse (Table 2.5):

1. Chemical synapse: The AP travels along the presynaptic neuron and causes release of a neurotransmitter into the synapse. This diffuses across the synapse to the next neurone (postsynaptic neurone). The neurotransmitter acts on postsynaptic membrane receptors, causing either excitation or inhibition of the neurone. An example of a chemical synapse is the neuromuscular junction, the connection between motor neurones and muscle fibres.
2. Electrical synapse: These have direct channels (usually gap junctions) that conduct ions (electricity) from one cell to another.

THE PROCESS OF NERVOUS TRANSMISSION

Nervous transmission describes the domino-like process of a neurone receiving an impulse and transmitting it along the neurone from one end to another before passing it on to the next neurone. There are two types of transmission:

1. Chemical
2. Via a second messenger

Chemical transmission

The process of chemical transmission is displayed in (Fig. 2.31) and detailed below:

1. When the AP spreads over the presynaptic terminal, the depolarization causes the opening of voltage-gated calcium channels within the membrane.
2. This causes a large influx of Ca^{2+} ions into the terminal boutons of the presynaptic membrane.
3. As a result of the Ca^{2+} ion influx, neurotransmitter-containing vesicles migrate towards the end of the presynaptic terminal, using an actin cytoskeleton. Using proteins, including the soluble NSF attachment protein receptor (SNARE) complex, the vesicles dock and then fuse with the presynaptic membrane. When they reach the synapse, they exocytose and release their contents into the synaptic cleft.
4. The postsynaptic neuronal membrane contains large numbers of receptor proteins. The neurotransmitter diffuses across the cleft and binds to these receptors.

Table 2.5 Comparison of electrical and chemical synapses

Feature	Electrical	Chemical
Cytoplasmic continuity	Yes	No
Delay	None	0.8–1.5 ms
Agent	Ion	Neurotransmitter
Space between cells	2 nm	30–50 nm
Direction of signal	One way or both ways	One way
Variation in function	Either on or off	Modifiable activity levels

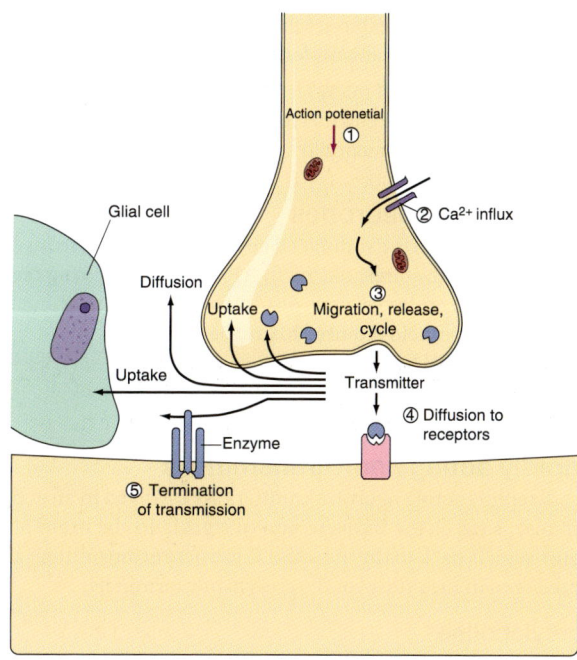

Fig. 2.31 Synaptic transmission. AP, *Action potential*.

Once bound, the neurotransmitter causes a change in postsynaptic membrane potential and can activate either ionotropic receptors or second-messenger systems.

5. The transmitter is cleared from the synaptic cleft via several different mechanisms, rendering the transmitter unable to cause further postsynaptic activation.

Ionotropic receptors are coupled with an ion channel and can either inhibit or stimulate the postsynaptic neurone. There are two types:

- Cation/excitatory postsynaptic potential (EPSP) ionotropic receptors: These allow Na^+ to pass into the postsynaptic neurone, causing excitations and propagation of the AP down the postsynaptic neurone.
- Anion/inhibitory postsynaptic potential ionotropic receptors: These allow Cl^- to enter, which inhibits the postsynaptic neurone.

Second-messenger transmission

Ion channels close within milliseconds and so do not permit prolonged postsynaptic neural changes as is required in memory formation. The second-messenger system allows a prolonged response via second messengers such as cyclic adenosine monophosphate or calmodulin.

Removal of the transmitted substance

To prevent continued action, the neurotransmitter must be removed from the synapse. This is done by:

- Active reuptake of the neurotransmitter into the presynaptic terminal.

Diffusion of transmitter out of a synaptic cleft into the extracellular fluid.

- Enzyme degradation; for example acetylcholine (ACh) is broken down by acetylcholinesterase.
- Active uptake of the neurotransmitter by glial cells.

CLINICAL NOTES

MYASTHENIA GRAVIS

Myasthenia gravis is an autoimmune neuromuscular disease that leads to varying degrees of muscle weakness. It is caused by the antibodies that destroy or block the nicotinic ACh receptors on the postsynaptic neurone at the neuromuscular junction. This results in the prevention of synaptic transmission. Treatment of this condition is generally by acetylcholinesterase inhibitors (such as pyridostigmine), which inhibits the breakdown of ACh in the synapse, increasing the concentration of ACh at the neuromuscular junction.

Summation

The excitation of a single presynaptic terminal on the surface of a neurone will rarely cause an AP. This is because even though an EPSP might be generated, on its own, it is insufficient to pass the threshold. Many EPSPs need to summate (the cumulative effect of several input impulses) to reach the threshold and produce an AP. There are two mechanisms for this:

- Spatial: Activation of many terminals near each other.
- Temporal: The same channel reopens continuously so more EPSPs can occur sequentially.

Facilitation of neurones

Facilitation is when the summated effects of the ESPS are insufficient to exceed the threshold for an AP to occur, requiring excitation signals from other neutrons to facilitate the neurone in reaching the threshold required to fire the AP.

Neurotransmitters

Rapidly acting neurotransmitters

Small, rapidly acting neurotransmitters are involved in an acute response, such as the transmission of signals to the brain and motor signals back to the muscles. These neurotransmitters are synthesized in the cytosol of the presynaptic terminals.

Acetylcholine

ACh is secreted in the motor cortex, basal ganglia, motor neurones innervating skeletal muscle, preganglionic neurones of the autonomic nervous system and postganglionic neurones of both the sympathetic and parasympathetic nervous systems. It can have both inhibitory and excitatory effects. Reduced ACh concentrations in certain parts of the brain are associated with Alzheimer disease. ACh is the primary neurotransmitter of the autonomic nervous system and will act on a variety of postsynaptic receptors, depending on its function (Fig. 2.32).

Noradrenaline (norepinephrine)

Noradrenaline is the main neurotransmitter of ganglion cells in the sympathetic nervous system, which excite some organs (e.g. myocardium to contract stronger) and inhibit others (e.g. lung bronchial muscle to dilate). Noradrenaline also causes constriction of peripheral blood vessels (see Fig. 2.32). Secretion of noradrenaline by the locus coeruleus in the pons is a key component in the control of sleep. Blockage of its removal at synapse is the mode of action of tricyclic antidepressants.

Amino acids

There are two types of amino acid neurotransmitter:

- Excitatory, for example glutamate and aspartate. Glutamate is the most common amino acid and stimulates two receptors: N-methyl-D-aspartate (NMDA) and α-amino-3-hydroxy-5-methyl-4-isoxazolepropionic acid (AMPA). The former is thought to be involved in the formation of memory.
- Inhibitory, for example GABA and glycine. GABA is secreted by nerve terminals present in the basal ganglia, cerebellum

and spinal cord. Glycine is mainly present in the spinal cord, particularly in the interneurons.

Slow-acting neuropeptide transmitters

These are larger in size than the rapidly acting transmitters and cause prolonged responses (e.g. long-term changes in the numbers of receptors and synapses). They are manufactured in the neuronal cell body and have a broad range of functions (e.g. pain modulation by opioids).

ORBIT

Eyelids

The external surface of the eyelids is covered by skin and the internal surface is covered by mucosa—the conjunctiva, which reflects at the superior and inferior fornices onto the eyeball. The space between the eyeball and eyelid is the conjunctival sac (Fig. 2.33). The space between the eyelids is the palpebral fissure. The fibrous framework of the eyelids is the orbital septum (Fig. 2.34; see also Fig. 2.33), which is thickened at the lid margins to form the tarsal plates and for the attachment of the medial and lateral palpebral ligaments. The levator palpebrae superioris muscle is attached to the superior tarsal plate.

The lacrimal gland lies at the superolateral aspect of the orbit and is wrapped around the tendon of levator palpebrae superioris. Its ducts open into the conjunctival sac, and it receives parasympathetic supply from the facial nerve (CN 7) via the greater petrosal nerve, which synapses on the pterygopalatine ganglion. Postganglionic fibres to the lacrimal gland hitchhike along the maxillary nerve and pass into the zygomaticotemporal nerve before innervating the gland.

The tears produced by the lacrimal gland are spread over the conjunctiva by blinking to stop it dehydrating. The tears are then drained through the lacrimal punctum, which drains via the nasolacrimal duct, which in turn opens below the inferior meatus of the nasal cavity.

Osteology of the orbit

The bony orbit is formed by (Fig. 2.35):

- Superiorly: frontal bone and lesser wing of the sphenoid
- Medially: axilla, lacrimal, ethmoid and body of the sphenoid
- Inferiorly: axillary, zygomatic, palatine
- Laterally: ygomatic and greater wing of the sphenoid

Muscles of the orbit

The muscles of the orbit are summarized in Table 2.6 and demonstrated in Fig. 2.36.

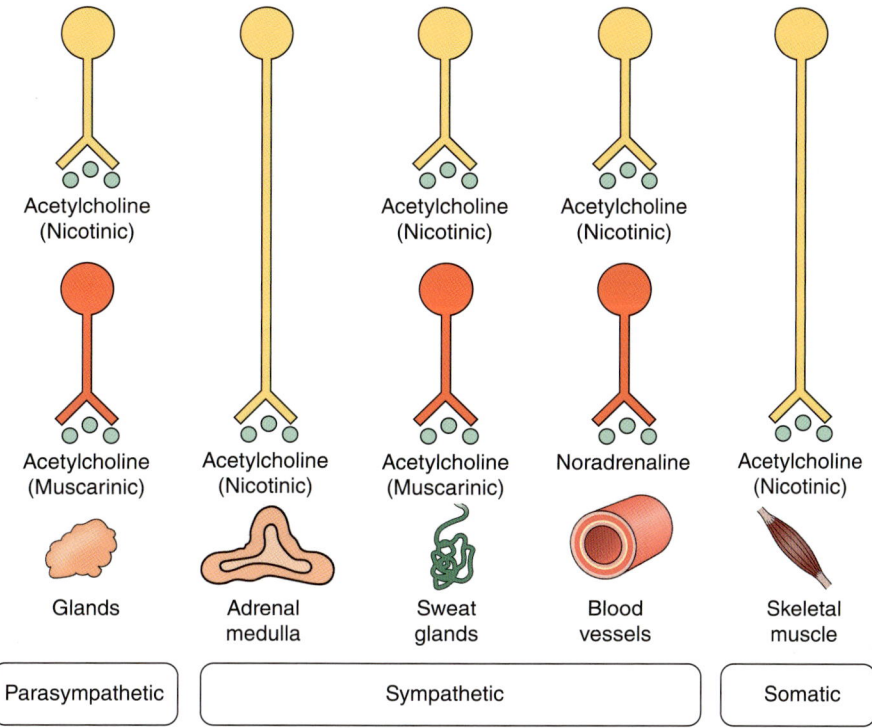

Fig. 2.32 Neurotransmitters of the autonomic nervous system.

Vessels of the orbit

The arterial supply is via the ophthalmic artery (branch of the internal carotid), which courses with the optic nerve. The venous drainage is through the superior ophthalmic vein, which communicates anteriorly with the facial vein and posteriorly with the cavernous sinus, and the inferior ophthalmic vein, which runs through the inferior orbital fissure to drain into the pterygoid venous plexus.

Nerves of the orbit

Optic nerve (CN 2)

The optic nerve is surrounded by a dural sheath which fuses with the sclera on entering the globe. The optic nerve carries afferent impulses from the retina to the visual cortex.

CLINICAL NOTES

PAPILLOEDEMA

The dural/meningeal sheath of the optic nerve is in continuity with the subarachnoid space, so any increase in intracranial pressure will cause swelling of the optic nerve head and swelling of the optic disc (where the nerve enters the globe), which can be visualized on fundoscopy.

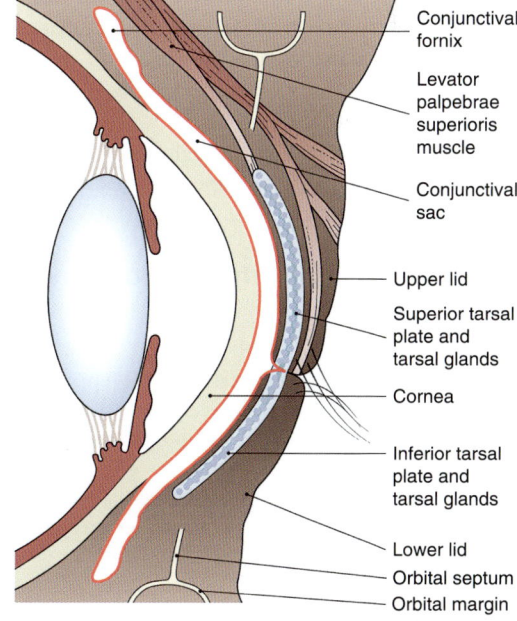

Fig. 2.33 Cross section of the eyeball, conjunctival sac and eyelids.

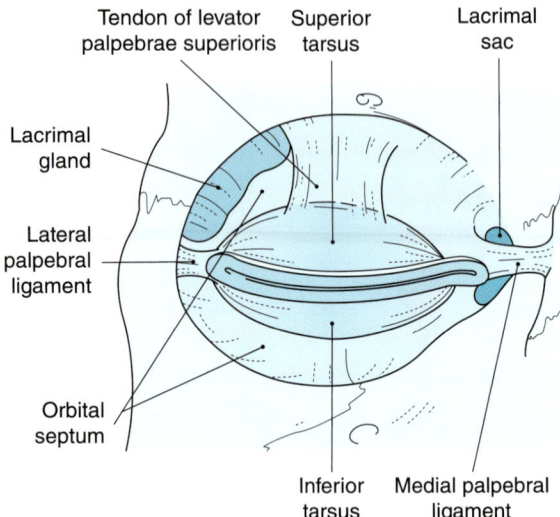

Fig. 2.34 Orbital septum and palpebral ligaments.

Oculomotor nerve (CN 3)

Upon entering the orbit, the oculomotor nerve (CN 3) divides into a superior branch and a larger inferior branch.

- Superior division: Supplies the superior rectus and levator palpebrae superioris muscles.
- Inferior division: Supplies the inferior and medial recti and the inferior oblique muscles. The nerve to the inferior oblique sends parasympathetic branches to the ciliary ganglion to cause constriction of the pupil.

Trochlear nerve (CN 4)

The trochlear nerve (CN 4) runs through the orbit and crosses the origin of the levator palpebrae superioris medially to supply the superior oblique muscle.

Ophthalmic division of the trigeminal nerve (CN 5, V$_1$)

This gives off three branches in the orbit:

- Frontal nerve: The main continuation of V$_1$. It passes outside the annulus of Zinn and runs between the levator palpebrae superioris and the bone. It branches into the supraorbital and supratrochlear nerve.
- Lacrimal nerve: Passes along the lateral rectus muscle to supply the skin and conjunctiva of the upper eyelid and is joined by the parasympathetic fibres from the zygomaticotemporal nerve.
- Nasociliary nerve: Runs on the medial wall of the orbit above the medial rectus muscle before branching into the infratrochlear and anterior ethmoidal branches (Table 2.7).

Abducens nerve (CN 6)

The abducens nerve (CN 6) supplies the lateral rectus muscle.

The visual system

The visual system comprises the eye, with its photoreceptive cells transducing light rays into receptor potentials. These are transmitted via the optic nerve (CN 2) to the CNS, where the collection of electrical potentials is combined to produce a perceived image.

Anatomy of the eye

A cross-sectional diagram and frontal image of the eye are shown in Figs 2.37 and 2.38. The definitions for the main structures of the eye are as follows:

- Anterior chamber: The space between the cornea and the iris, which is filled with aqueous humour.
- Choroid: The vascular portion of the posterior segment of the eye; this provides nutrition to the retina.
- Ciliary body: Aqueous fluid is produced here.
- Ciliary muscles: These smooth muscles attach the ciliary body to the lens via the zonular ligaments.
- Conjunctiva: This lines the inner surface of the eyelids.
- Cornea: The clear tissue in front of the eye. It has an epithelial surface layer, a stroma that comprises most of the corneal tissue, a tough layer called Descemet membrane and an endothelium on the inner surface.
- Iris: The coloured part of the eye. It consists of dilator and constrictor muscles and vascular tissue. The pupil is the opening in the centre of the iris. Dilation and constriction of the iris alter the size of the pupil, increasing or decreasing the amount of light able to pass into the eye, respectively.
- Lacrimal apparatus: A group of structures that produce and drain lacrimal fluid (tears). The lacrimal glands secrete

lacrimal fluid, which drains into the lacrimal ducts. It then enters the nasolacrimal duct and finally drains away into the basal cavity.

- Lens capsule: A fibrous capsule over the lens.
- Lens: A ball-like structure that changes shape to focus the image on the retina.

- Lids: Provide protection for the eye and the glands within the eyelid.
- Limbus: Where the cornea meets the sclera.
- Tarsal glands (Meibomian glands): Secrete an oily substance that helps stabilise the tear film.

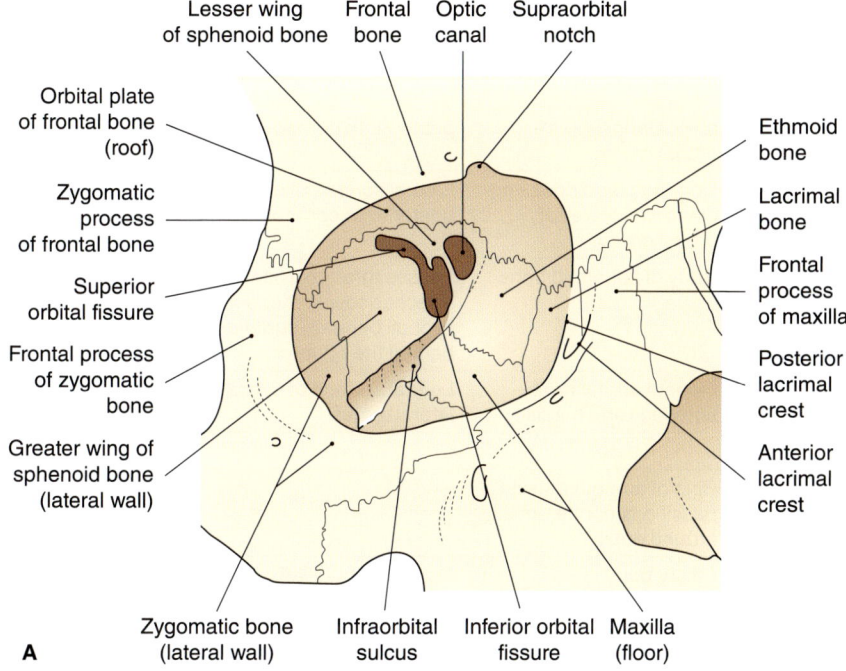

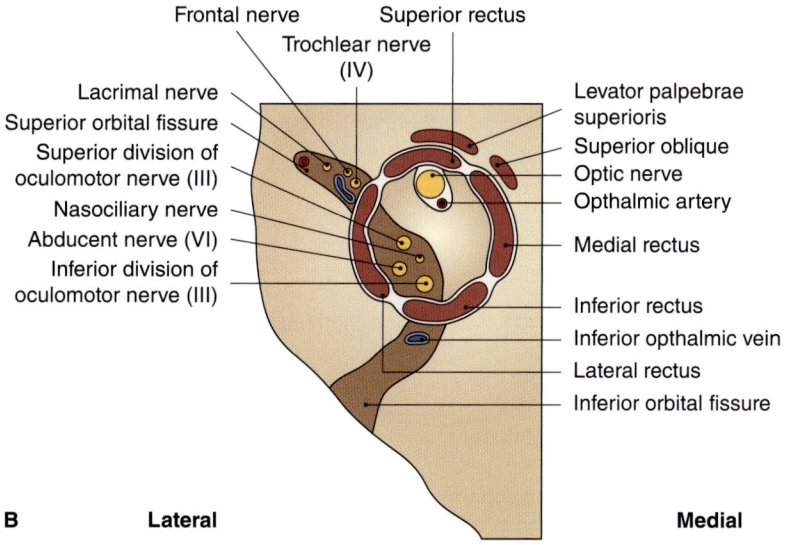

Fig. 2.35 Bones (A) and contents (B) of the bony orbit.

Table 2.6 Muscles of the orbit

Name of muscle (nerve supply)	Origin	Insertion	Action
Extrinsic muscles of eyeball (striated skeletal muscle)			
Superior rectus (CN 3)	Common tendinous ring on posterior wall of orbital cavity	Superior surface of eyeball just posterior to corneoscleral junction	Moves eye upward and medially
Inferior rectus (CN 3)	Common tendinous ring on posterior wall of orbital cavity	Inferior surface of eyeball just posterior to corneoscleral junction	Moves eye downward and medially
Medial rectus (CN 3)	Common tendinous ring on posterior wall of orbital cavity	Medial surface of eyeball just posterior to corneoscleral junction	Moves eye medially
Lateral rectus (CN 6)	Common tendinous ring on posterior wall of orbital cavity	Lateral surface of eyeball just posterior to corneoscleral junction	Moves eye laterally
Superior oblique (CN 4)	Body of sphenoid bone	Passes through trochlea and is attached to superior surface of eyeball beneath superior rectus, behind the equator	Moves eye downward and laterally
Inferior oblique (CN 3)	Floor of orbital cavity, anteriorly and medially	Lateral surface of eyeball deep to lateral rectus	Moves eye upward and laterally
Intrinsic muscles of eyeball (smooth muscle)			
Sphincter pupillae of iris (parasympathetic via CN 3)	Ring of smooth muscle passing circumferentially around pupil	—	Constricts pupil
Dilator pupillae of iris (sympathetic)	Ciliary body	Sphincter pupillae	Dilates pupil
Ciliary muscle (parasympathetic via CN 3)	Corneoscleral junction	Ciliary body	Controls shape of lens; in accommodation, makes lens more globular
Muscles of eyelids			
Orbicularis oculi (CN 7)	Medial palpebral ligament, lacrimal bone	Skin around orbit, tarsal plates	Closes eyelids (helps spread tears across conjunctiva)
Levator palpebrae superioris (striated muscle: CN 3 nerve; smooth muscle: sympathetic)	Lesser wing of sphenoid bone	Superior tarsal plate	Raises upper lid

- Optic disc: The part of the fundus where all the nerve fibres from the retina meet to form the optic canal.
- Optic nerve (CN 2): A sensory nerve that runs from the retina to various parts of the brain.
- Posterior chamber: The space between the iris and the lens, filled with aqueous fluids.
- Retina: Nervous tissue that lines the posterior three-quarters of the eyeball. Photoreceptive cells in the retina convert the light image into a bioelectrical signal for the brain to understand (see below).
- Sclera—the fibrous shell of the eye.
- Vitreous: A jelly-like material that fills the posterior segment of the eye.
- Zonular ligaments: The ligaments connecting the ciliary muscle to the perimeter of the lens, stabilizing the position of the lens.

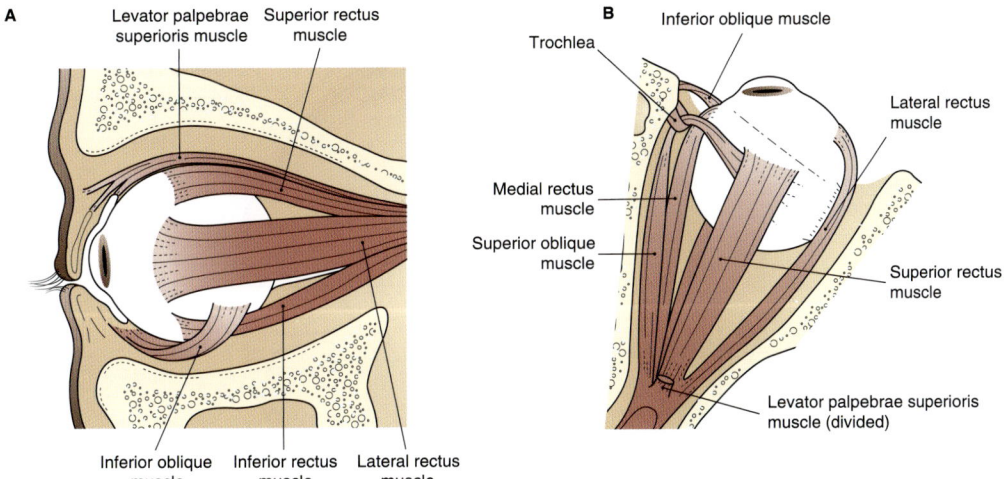

Fig. 2.36 Muscles of the orbit: (A) lateral view, (B) superior view.

Table 2.7 Branches of the nasociliary nerve

Branch	Action
Communicating branch	Communicates with the ciliary ganglion—general sensory fibres from the eyeball pass to the ciliary ganglion via the short ciliary nerves and then to the nasociliary nerve via the communicating branch
Long ciliary nerve	Two or three branches containing sympathetic fibres for the dilator pupillae—runs with the short ciliary nerves and pierces the sclera to reach the iris
Posterior ethmoidal nerve	Exits through the posterior ethmoidal foramen to supply the ethmoidal and sphenoidal air sinuses
Infratrochlear nerve	Passes below the trochlea to supply the skin over the upper eyelid
Anterior ethmoidal nerve	Exits via the anterior ethmoidal foramen and enters the anterior cranial fossa on the cribriform plate of the ethmoid; then enters the nasal cavity via an opening opposite the crista galli to supply the mucosa of the nose; then supplies the skin of the nose as the external nasal nerve

CLINICAL NOTES

LACRIMATION

The function of lacrimation is to moisten the surface of the cornea and remove waste. Lacrimation is stimulated by many things, including emotion. You may have wondered before why you get a 'runny nose' when you cry. This is due to the increased amount of lacrimal fluid, that is tears, draining through the nasolacrimal duct into the nasal cavity.

Aqueous humour production and flow

Aqueous humour, the transparent liquid located within the anterior and posterior chambers of the eye that maintains intraocular pressure at roughly 10 to 20 mm Hg and gives the eyeball its roughly spherical shape, is produced by the ciliary body in the posterior chamber of the eye. From here, aqueous humour flows between the lens and the iris in the posterior chamber and through the pupil to enter the anterior chamber. Within the anterior chamber, aqueous humour leaves the eye via the trabecular meshwork to enter Schlemm's canal before returning into the venous circulation. Aqueous humour is constantly being produced and must therefore be drained by the trabecular meshwork at the same rate; otherwise, intraocular pressure will rise significantly (Fig. 2.39).

Glaucoma

Glaucoma is defined by damage to the optic nerve (CN 2) typically as a result of raised intraocular pressure. It is broadly divided into two categories:

Open-angle glaucoma: Caused by a reduction in the outflow of aqueous humour through the trabecular meshwork. This is a chronic disease with a gradual reduction in peripheral vision.

Closed-angle glaucoma: An ophthalmic emergency caused by the iris being forced against the trabecular meshwork inhibiting the drainage of aqueous humour. Irreversible damage to the optic nerve (CN 2) and subsequent blindness can occur rapidly unless treated.

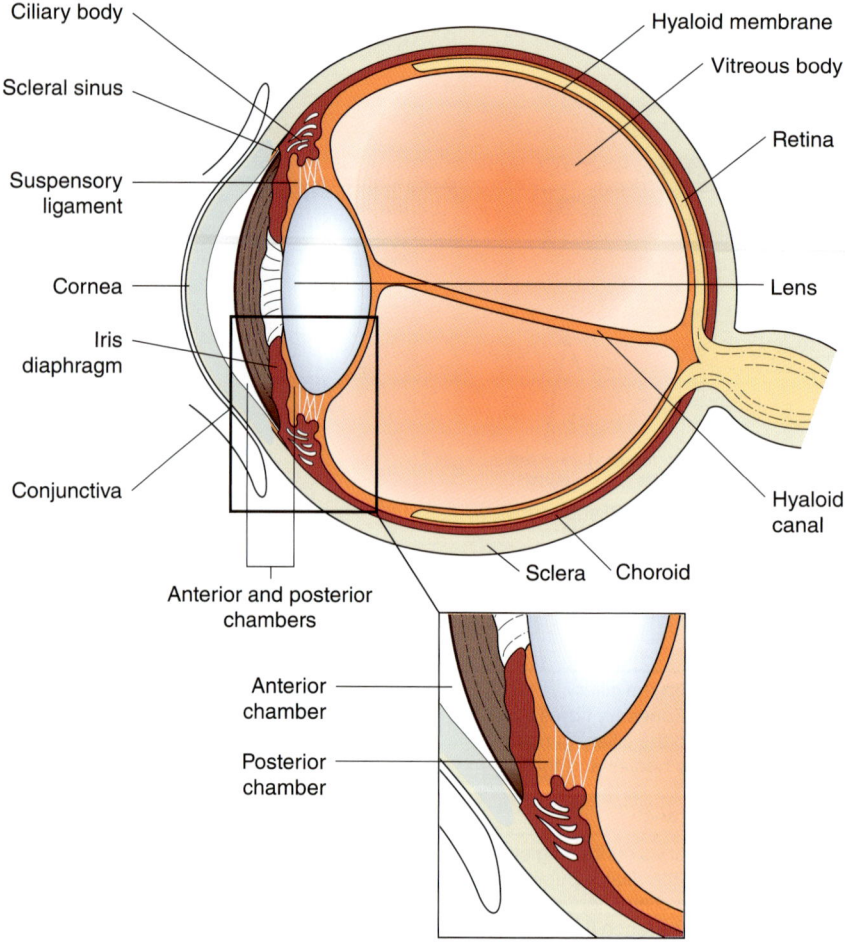

Fig. 2.37 Cross section through the eye showing the main structures.

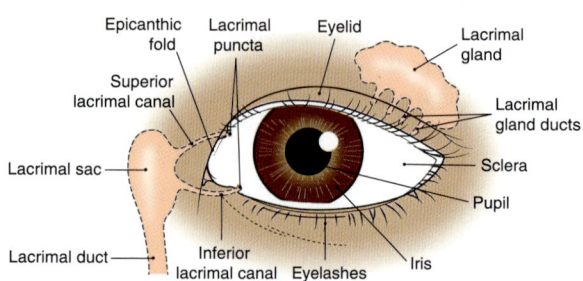

Fig. 2.38 Anatomy of the eye from a frontal view.

Anatomy of the retina

The retina forms the inner surface of the eyeball. It has two layers:

- Deep pigmented layer: This melanin-coated epithelial sheet prevents the scattering of light rays and focuses them on the retina.

- Superficial neural layer: Processes the incoming light source and sends information to the optic nerve. This information is analyzed in the brain and an image is formed. The neural layer is divided into three cell levels: photoreceptive cells, bipolar cells and ganglion cells.

These two levels (Fig. 2.40) are separated by two synaptic cell layers where synaptic contacts are made. Two other types of cells are present: horizontal and amacrine cells. These alter the signals from the photoreceptive, bipolar and ganglion cells.

Photoreceptive cells—Two cell types transduce light rays into receptor potentials:

- Rods: It contain the blue-green light-absorbing photopigment rhodopsin. Dim light stimulates the rods, enabling vision with minimal light, but not in colour.

- Cones: React to bright light and produce colour vision. The cones contain three different types of photopigment, which absorb blue, green and yellow-orange light. These

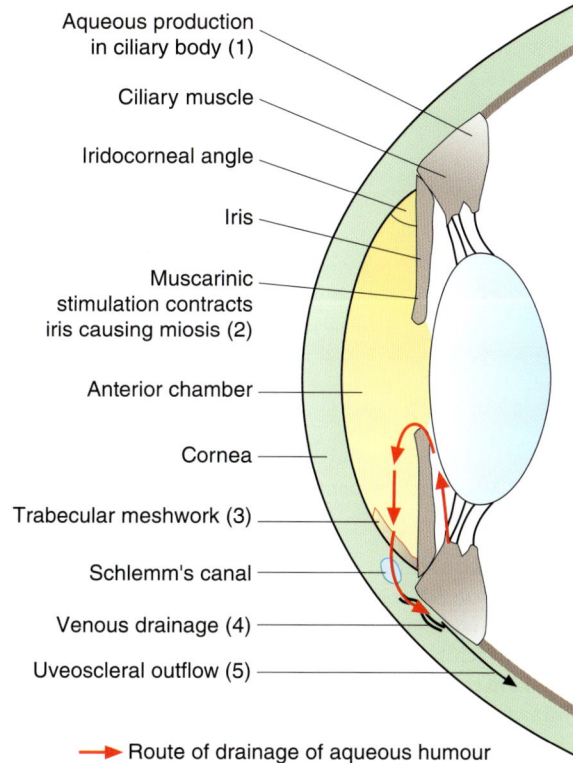

Aqueous production in ciliary body (1)

Ciliary muscle

Iridocorneal angle

Iris

Muscarinic stimulation contracts iris causing miosis (2)

Anterior chamber

Cornea

Trabecular meshwork (3)

Schlemm's canal

Venous drainage (4)

Uveoscleral outflow (5)

→ Route of drainage of aqueous humour

Fig. 2.39 The route of drainage of aqueous humour from the eye and the sites of action of drugs used in the treatment of glaucoma. The mechanisms by which some drugs benefit glaucoma are still uncertain but are thought to include the following: (a) in angle-closure glaucoma, muscarinic agonists (e.g. pilocarpine) facilitate aqueous humour drainage (3, 4) by constricting the iris (2), which widens the iridocorneal angle; (b) carbonic anhydrase inhibitors (e.g. acetazolamide) decrease aqueous humour production (1); (c) β-adrenoceptor antagonists (e.g. timolol) reduce aqueous humour production (1) and increase drainage (3); (d) selective α_2-adrenoceptor agonists (e.g. brimonidine) decrease aqueous humour production (1); (e) prostaglandin F2α analogues (e.g. latanoprost) enhance aqueous humour outflow (3, 4, 5) and may improve ocular blood flow.

photopigments are composed of two parts: opsin (glycoprotein) and retinol (a vitamin A derivative). Each photopigment contains a different variant of opsin, which permits the absorption of different wavelengths of light and hence the ability to see different colours.

Processing visual stimuli—Light enters the eye through the pupil and strikes the photopigment in the retina. This results in:

- Isomerization: A change in the conformation of retinol from the *cis*- to the *trans*- form.
- Bleaching: Transretinol separates from opsin. It appears colourless.

Reconversion—When no light is present, the enzyme retinol isomerase converts *trans*-retinol back to *cis*-retinol.

Regeneration—The *cis*-retinol then binds to opsin and the pigment resynthesizes.

Optics

The light that enters the eye is refracted by the cornea—to a lesser degree by the lens—so that it is focused exactly on the retina (convergence). If the rays do not meet at the same retinal point, the image produced is unfocused (Fig. 2.41). A person for whom images of nearby objects fall on the retina, but images of far objects do not, is considered to be short/near-sighted (myopic). Conversely, a person is considered long/far-sighted (hypermetropic) if images of far objects focus on the retina but images of near objects do not.

Accommodation—Light that reflects off objects that are very close to the eye hits the cornea at a greater angle and requires greater refraction to meet at the retina. The lens is responsible for this extra refraction. The ciliary muscles contract, causing the zonular fibres to relax and thus easing the tension on the lens, making it shorter and broader in shape. This refracts the light rays so they meet at the same point in the retina.

The accommodation reflex of the eye involves the optic nerve (CN 2) as the afferent component and the oculomotor nerve (CN 3) and its parasympathetic component, via the Edinger–Westphal nucleus, as the efferent component.

CLINICAL NOTES

VISUAL ACUITY

Visual acuity describes how precisely an image is seen: the greater the precision, the higher the acuity. The area of greatest acuity in the retina is the central fovea, which contains only cones. Clinically, visual acuity is tested by using a Snellen chart. This contains rows of letters in decreasing size. Patients stand 6 m away from the chart and are required to read the smallest sized letter possible. They are then given a score, expressed as a fraction, corresponding to the smallest number row they can read at that distance. In modern practice, the ability to read the row labelled 6 from 6 m is considered 'normal visual acuity' and is the equivalent of the old-style score of 20 at 20 ft, that is 20/20 vision.

However, many patients do not have normal visual acuity. After testing, they will be given a score expressed as a fraction of the test distance (6 m is standard) over the smallest letter size achieved. Therefore patients with poorer visual acuity will only be able to accurately read larger letter sizes and therefore will be given a higher number. This means a score of 6/24 would equate to worse visual acuity than 6/6.

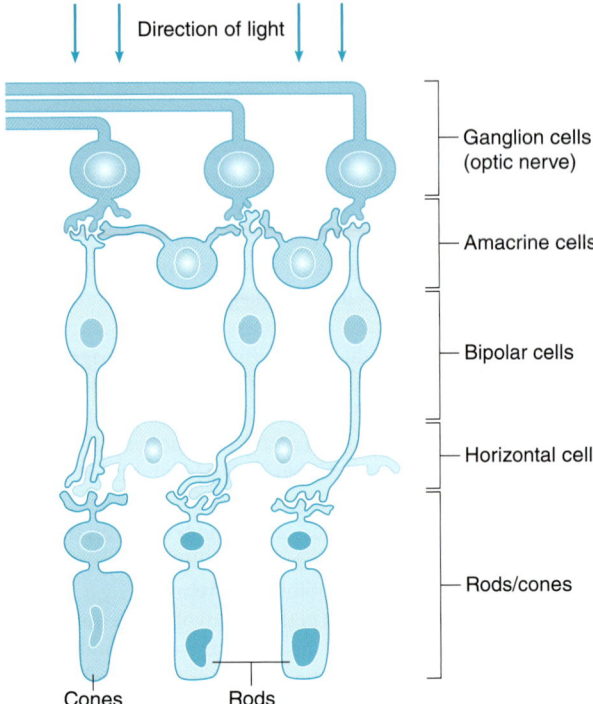

Fig. 2.40 Layers of the retina.

Dark and light adaption—After a person has been sitting in a bright room for a while, much of the photochemical in the rods and cones will have been converted to retinol (which is subsequently converted to vitamin A) and opsins. This reduction in the amount of photoreceptive chemical reduces the sensitivity of the eye to light even further.

Conversely, sitting in a dark room for a while results in the photochemical being converted back into light-sensitive pigments, so much dimmer levels of light can be detected.

Central visual processing

After leaving the eyes, the optic nerves pass through the optic chiasma, where some nerve fibres (temporal retinal fibres receiving light from the nasal visual field) cross and travel to the opposite side of the brain from which the visual stimuli came (Fig. 2.42). After the chiasma, the axons become the optic tract, which ends in one of the following locations:

- Lateral geniculate nucleus (LGN): The retinal fibres terminate in six discrete layers of the LGN of the thalamus. A given area of the retina projects to a certain level in the LGN. This organization is preserved all the way to the visual cortex.
- Pretectal nuclei and superior colliculus in the midbrain: Activate the pupillary pathway light reflex and govern rapid directional eye movements.
- The suprachiasmatic nucleus in the hypothalamus: Involved with the control of circadian rhythms.

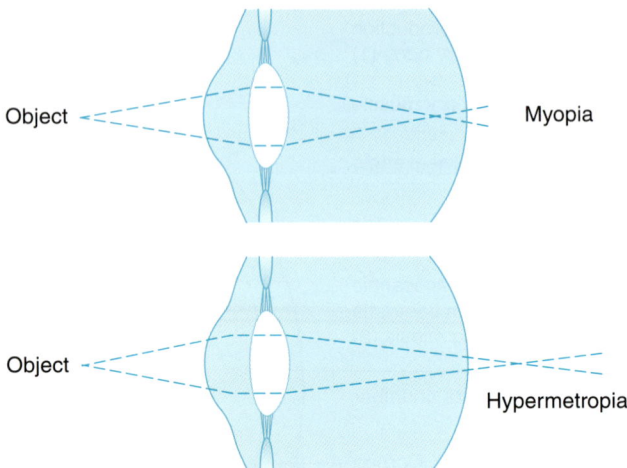

Fig. 2.41 Myopia and hypermetropia.

The visual cortex

The primary visual cortex lies in the medial occipital cortex and contains six layers of cells arranged in millions of vertical hypercolumns, each representing a different function. For example orientation columns enable lines to be discriminated and ocular dominance columns enable the perception of the depth of an object. There are also colour-detecting regions. All this information is processed individually and then brought together to form an image. Although it is unclear precisely how these cells interact to form an image, the process no doubt involves excitatory and inhibitory interplay between the cells.

NOSE

The nose consists of:

- An external nose of nasal bones and the cartilaginous process separated by the nasal septum.
- The nasal cavity.

Nasal cavity

The walls of the nasal cavity are listed in Table 2.8. The mucosa of the nasal cavity is ciliated columnar epithelium, which contains numerous serous and mucous glands. Hairs in the mucosa trap inspired particles. The rich vascular plexus of the mucosa also warms the inspired air. The roof and superior lateral wall contain specialized olfactory epithelium. The blood and nerve supply to the nasal cavity are shown in Fig. 2.43.

Physiology of smell

The nose contains specialized olfactory epithelium, within the olfactory region (superior aspect) of the nose. This epithelium

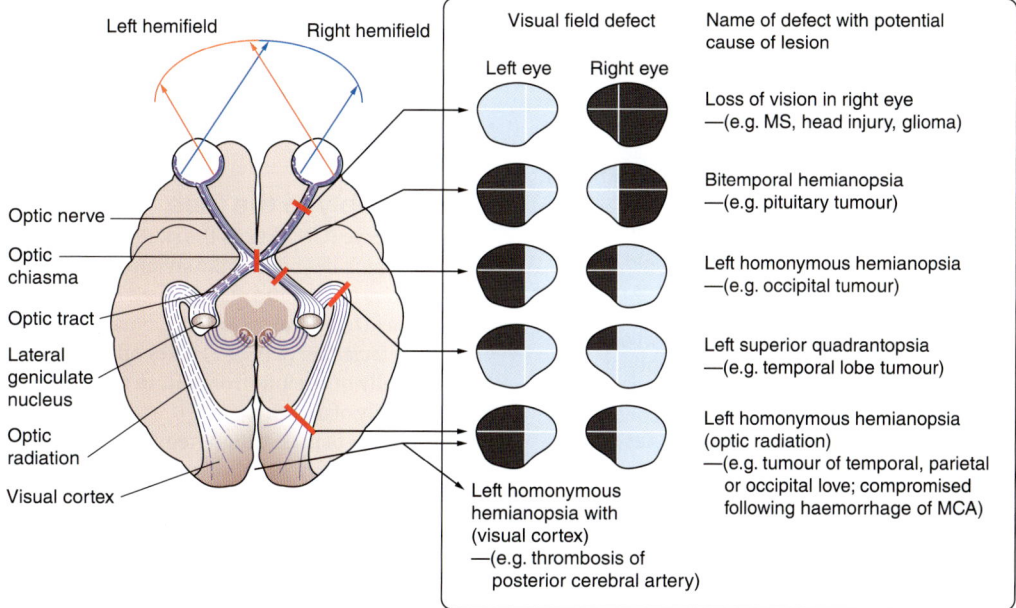

Fig. 2.42 Pathway of visual processing. MCA, *Middle cerebral artery*; MS, *multiple sclerosis*.

has abundant chemoreceptors known as olfactory receptors that convert chemical signals into nervous impulses that are subsequently carried via fibres of the olfactory nerve (CN 1) through the cribriform plate and into the olfactory bulb which lies on the superior surface of the cribriform plate. The olfactory nerve (CN 1) then transmits this information for central processing. Disruption of this process at any point can lead to anosmia, the loss of the sense of smell, for example head trauma leading to a skull base fracture that disrupts the cribriform plate, severing fibres of the olfactory nerve (CN 1).

Paranasal sinuses

The paranasal sinuses lie in the skull and facial bone surrounding the nasal cavity. The paranasal sinuses create spaces within the bones that help lighten the skull and assist in voice resonance. The paranasal sinuses are as follows:

- Maxillary: In the maxilla bones.
- Ethmoidal: Medial and superior in the nasal cavity within the ethmoid bone.
- Frontal: Behind the brow ridge in the frontal bone.
- Sphenoidal: posterior and superior within the sphenoid bone, immediately anterior to the pituitary fossa.

FACE

Sensation of the face

The sensation to the face is via the trigeminal nerve (CN 5), which is divided into three sections. The terminal branches of these divisions, which supply the skin, can be seen in Fig. 2.44.

Muscles of facial expression

The muscles of facial expression (Fig. 2.45) are supplied by the facial nerve (CN 7). The four muscles of facial expression that are tested clinically are:

- Occipitofrontalis: Formed by a frontal and occipital belly connected by an aponeurosis. Its function is to raise the eyebrows.
- Orbicularis oculi: Consists of an orbital and a palpebral part that screws the eyes shut and closes the eyelids, respectively. Orbicularis oculi is connected to the scalp at

Table 2.8 Walls of the nasal cavity

Surface	Components
Floor	Palatine process of maxilla, horizontal process of palatine bone, i.e. the hard palate
Roof	Nasal, frontal, sphenoid and ethmoid bones; above lies the anterior cranial fossa and the sphenoidal sinus
Lateral wall	Maxillary, palatine, sphenoid, lacrimal and ethmoid bones and the inferior concha; the superior and middle conchae are projections of the ethmoid bone; the superior, middle and inferior meatus lie beneath their respective conchae; sphenoethmoidal recess lies above the superior concha
Medial wall (nasal septum)	The perpendicular plate of the ethmoid, the vomer and the septal cartilage

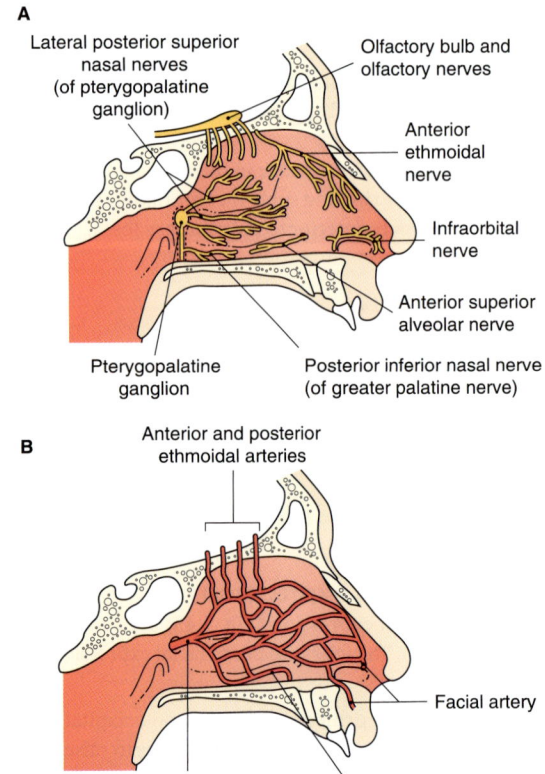

Fig. 2.43 Nerves (A) and arteries (B) of the nasal cavity.

the medial angle of the eye by the medial palpebral ligament.
- Buccinator: Inserts into the angle of the mouth; acts to expel food from the cheeks and pulls the mouth into a smile.
- Orbicularis oris: Narrows the opening of the mouth.

Motor supply to the face

The facial nerve (CN 7) exits the skull through the stylomastoid foramen, which lies behind the styloid process. The facial nerve (CN 7) enters the parotid gland where it divides into five terminal branches (temporal, zygomatic, buccal, mandibular and cervical). The facial nerve (CN 7) gives off smaller branches to the occipital belly of occipitofrontalis, to the stylohyoid and to the posterior belly of digastric.

The muscles of mastication (temporalis, masseter, medial and lateral pterygoid) are supplied by the mandibular branch (V_3) of the trigeminal nerve (CN 5).

Vessels of the face

The face receives its blood supply from the superficial temporal and facial arteries, both of which are branches of the external carotid.

- The facial artery ascends medial to the mandible and in the face gives off the inferior labial, superior labial and lateral nasal branches before terminating as the angular artery at the medial canthus of the eye.
- The superficial temporal artery is a terminal branch of the external carotid and begins in the parotid gland. It ascends superficial to the zygomatic process before dividing into frontal and parietal branches. The superficial temporal artery pulse can be felt anterior to the tragus of the ear.
- The remaining blood supply to the face comes from the supraorbital and supratrochlear arteries, which are terminal branches of the ophthalmic artery.

The veins drain the face following a similar course as the arteries as described below:

- The supraorbital and supratrochlear veins unite to form the facial vein that descends in the face and receives tributaries from the branches corresponding to the facial artery.
- The superficial and maxillary veins join to form the retromandibular vein in the parotid gland.
- The posterior auricular and posterior division of the retromandibular vein form the external jugular vein.
- The facial vein and the anterior division of the retromandibular vein drain into the internal jugular vein.

Lymphatics of the face drain to the deep cervical lymph nodes (see Fig. 2.57).

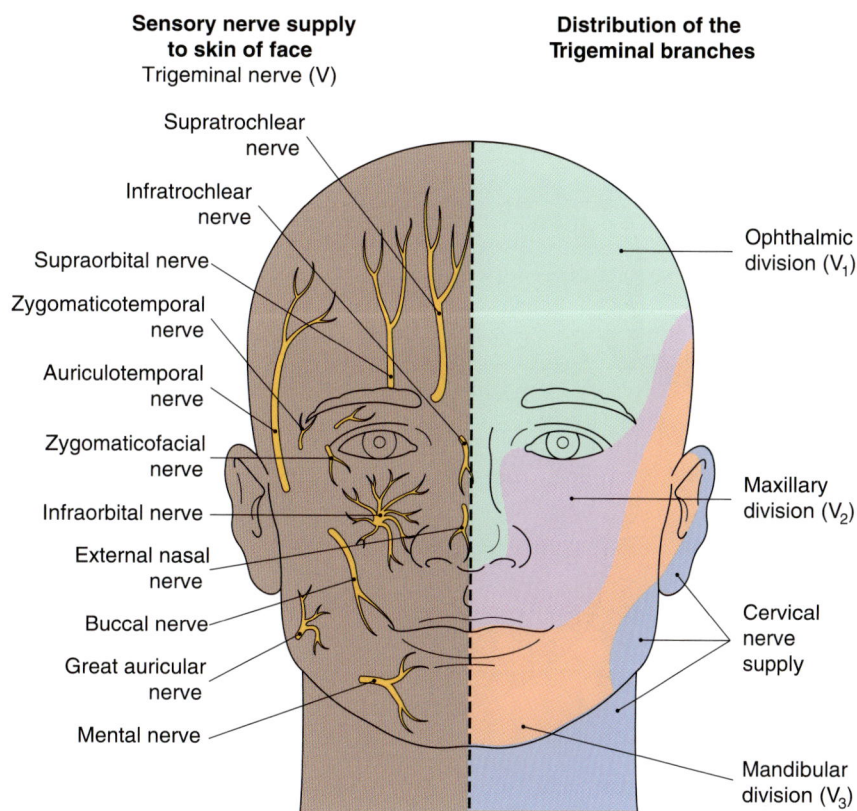

Sensory nerve supply
to skin of face
Trigeminal nerve (V)

Distribution of the
Trigeminal branches

Supratrochlear nerve

Infratrochlear nerve

Supraorbital nerve

Zygomaticotemporal nerve

Auriculotemporal nerve

Zygomaticofacial nerve

Infraorbital nerve

External nasal nerve

Buccal nerve

Great auricular nerve

Mental nerve

Ophthalmic division (V₁)

Maxillary division (V₂)

Cervical nerve supply

Mandibular division (V₃)

Fig. 2.44 Distribution of the trigeminal divisions and terminal sensory branches.

PAROTID REGION

Parotid gland

The parotid gland is the largest salivary gland and lies between the ramus of the mandible and the sternocleidomastoid muscle (Fig. 2.46). The gland is surrounded by a capsule that is derived from the investing fascia of the neck. The free edge of the fascia becomes the stylomandibular ligament. The parotid duct (Stenson duct) passes over the masseter muscle, pierces the buccinator and opens in the oral cavity opposite the upper second molar tooth.

Structures within the parotid gland

The structures from superficial to deep are (Fig. 2.47):
- Facial nerve (CN 7): Divides into its five terminal branches within the parotid gland. The facial nerve (CN 7) separates the superficial from the deep part of the gland.
- Retromandibular vein: Formed by the union of the superficial temporal and maxillary veins. It divides into

an anterior and posterior portion; the former drains via the facial vein into the internal jugular vein, and the latter joins the posterior auricular vein to form the external jugular vein.
- External carotid artery: Divides into its two terminal branches (superficial temporal and maxillary) within the gland.

Blood supply, innervation and lymphatic drainage

The arterial supply to the parotid gland is from the external carotid artery.

The parasympathetic fibres that stimulate salivation from the parotid gland originate in the glossopharyngeal nerve and then pass to the otic ganglion via the lesser petrosal nerve. The postganglionic fibres reach the parotid via the auriculotemporal nerve (a branch of CN 5 V₃). General sensation of the parotid gland is carried by the auriculotemporal nerve, and sensation of the capsule is via the greater auricular nerve.

The lymphatics drain into the deep cervical lymph nodes.

61

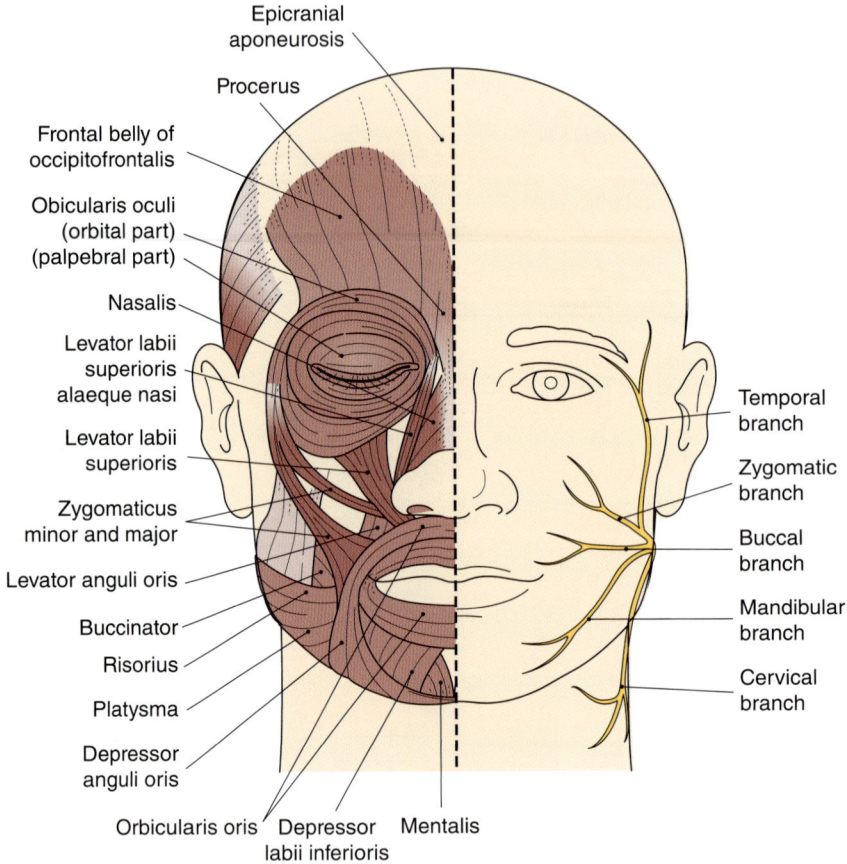

Epicranial aponeurosis

Procerus

Frontal belly of occipitofrontalis

Obicularis oculi (orbital part) (palpebral part)

Nasalis

Levator labii superioris alaeque nasi

Levator labii superioris

Zygomaticus minor and major

Levator anguli oris

Buccinator

Risorius

Platysma

Depressor anguli oris

Orbicularis oris   Depressor   Mentalis
                    labii inferioris

Temporal branch

Zygomatic branch

Buccal branch

Mandibular branch

Cervical branch

Fig. 2.45 Main muscles of the face and the motor branches of the facial nerve.

TEMPORAL AND INFRATEMPORAL FOSSA

Temporal fossa

The temporal fossa lies on the lateral aspect of the skull and is bordered superiorly by the superior temporal line, anteriorly by the lateral orbital rim and inferiorly by the zygomatic arch. It contains the temporalis muscle and the overlying temporalis fascia, which inserts onto the zygomatic arch of the zygoma. The deep temporal nerves (branches of V_3) and vessels (maxillary) emerge from the border of the lateral pterygoid to supply the temporalis muscle. The auriculotemporal nerve also emerges from behind the temporomandibular joint (TMJ) and crosses the zygomatic arch into the temporal fossa to supply the scalp in this region.

Infratemporal fossa

The infratemporal fossa lies in the space between the ramus of the mandible and the pharynx; its boundaries can be seen in

Fig. 2.48. It communicates with the temporal fossa above through the zygomatic arch. The key contents of the infratemporal fossa include the medial and lateral pterygoid muscles, the mandibular nerve, the otic ganglion, the chorda tympani nerve and the maxillary artery (Fig. 2.49).

Mandible

The mandible comprises a body, angle and ramus. The two halves are joined in the midline by the symphysis menti; on either side of this symphysis lies the mental foramen through which the terminal branches of the inferior alveolar nerve pass (Table 2.9). The muscle attachments on the mandible are shown in Fig. 2.49.

The temporomandibular joint

The TMJ is a synovial joint through which the mandible articulates with the mandibular fossa of the temporal bone.

The TMJ is separated into an upper and lower part by a disc which attaches the joint capsule and the lateral pterygoid

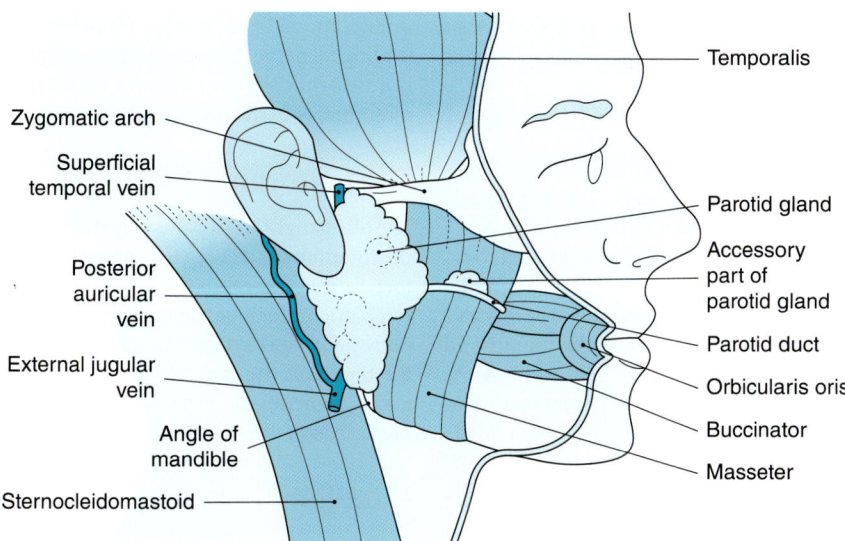

Fig. 2.46 The parotid gland. (Adapted from Snell, R. S. (1992). *Clinical anatomy for medical students* (4th ed.). Little Brown & Co. Reproduced with the permission of Lippincott Williams and Wilkins. http://lww.com.)

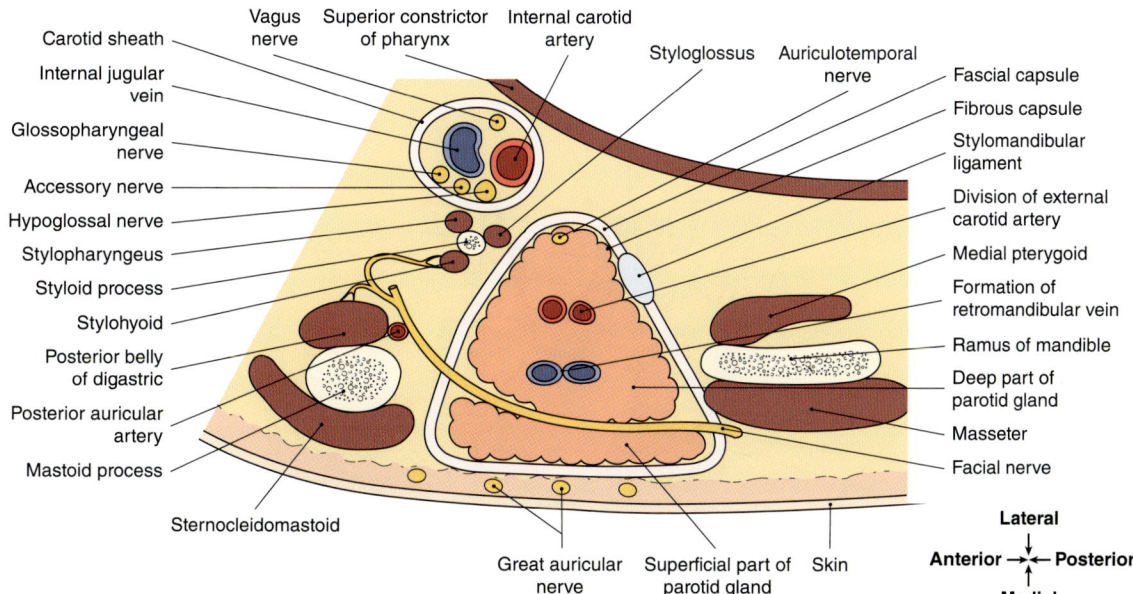

Fig. 2.47 Transverse section through the parotid region. (Adapted from Snell, R. S. (1992). *Clinical anatomy for medical students* (4th ed.). Little Brown & Co. Reproduced with the permission of Lippincott Williams and Wilkins. http://lww.com.)

(Fig. 2.50). The hinge-like movements (elevation and depression) of the jaw take place in the lower compartment, and protraction of the jaw by the medial pterygoids takes place in the upper compartment.

Mandibular nerve

The mandibular nerve is the third division (V_3) of the trigeminal nerve (CN 5), which enters the infratemporal fossa through the foramen ovale. The nerve lies deep to the lateral pterygoid muscle and is separated from the pharynx by the tensor veli palatine muscle. The mandibular nerve divides into two main branches—the lingual nerve to the tongue and the inferior alveolar nerve, which runs in the body of the mandible. The lingual nerve supplies sensory information to the anterior two-thirds of the tongue, joined by the chorda tympani which carries taste to the anterior two-thirds of the tongue. Other branches of the mandibular can be seen in Table 2.10.

Chorda tympani

The chorda tympani is the final branch of the facial nerve (CN 7) in the temporal bone (after the greater superficial petrosal nerve and the nerve to the stapedius). Chorda tympani enters the infratemporal fossa through the petrotympanic fissure and joins the lingual nerve. Chorda tympani carries taste fibres to the anterior two-thirds of the tongue as well as parasympathetic secretomotor fibres to the submandibular ganglion.

Otic ganglion

The otic ganglion is a parasympathetic ganglion lying inferior to the foramen ovale. Preganglionic fibres from the inferior salivatory nucleus travel in the glossopharyngeal nerve, then in the tympanic branch of the tympanic plexus and finally the lesser petrosal nerve to reach the otic ganglion. Postganglionic fibres hitchhike on the auriculotemporal nerve to enter the parotid gland. Sympathetic and sensory fibres to the parotid gland also pass through the ganglion without synapsing.

Maxillary artery

The maxillary artery is the larger of the terminal branches of the external carotid artery and begins behind the neck of the mandible. It then passes between the heads of the lateral pterygoid to enter the pterygopalatine fossa. The branches of the maxillary artery are shown in Table 2.11.

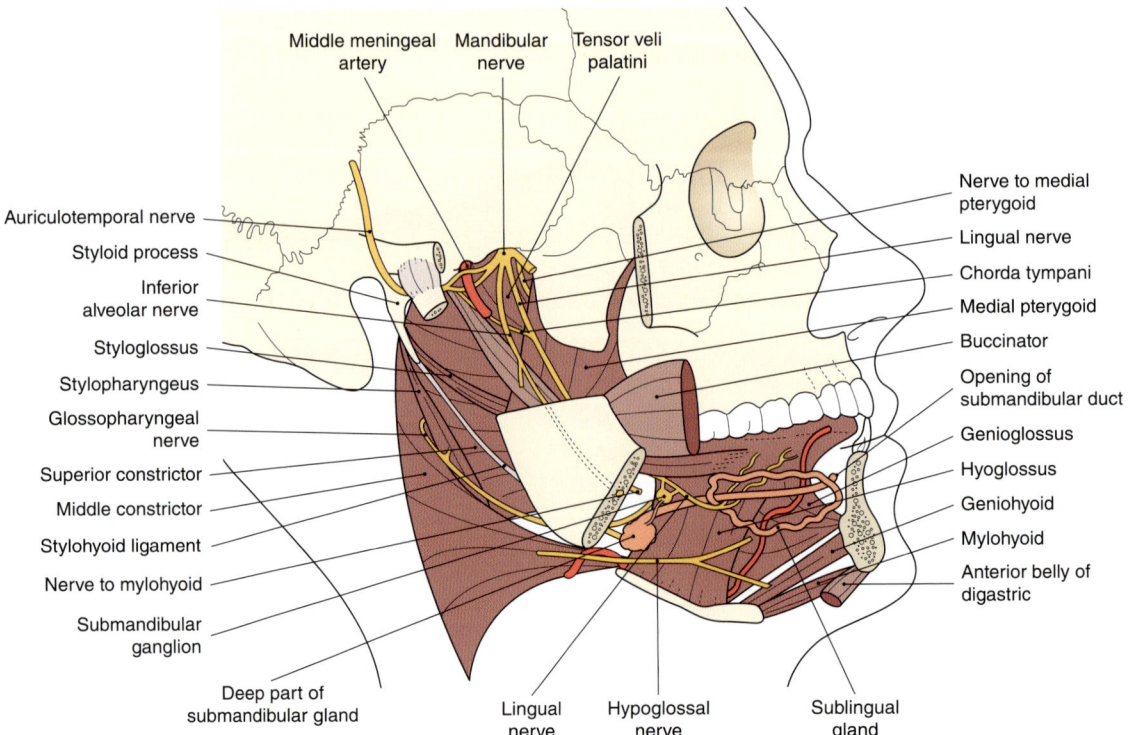

Fig. 2.48 The contents of the infratemporal fossa.

Medial aspect (left side)

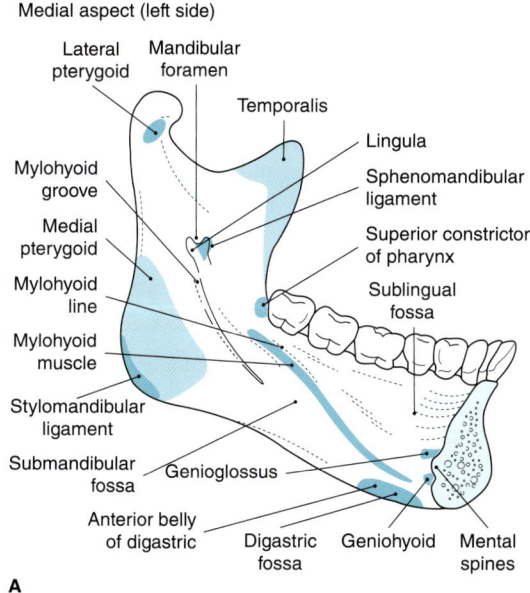

Lateral aspect (right side)

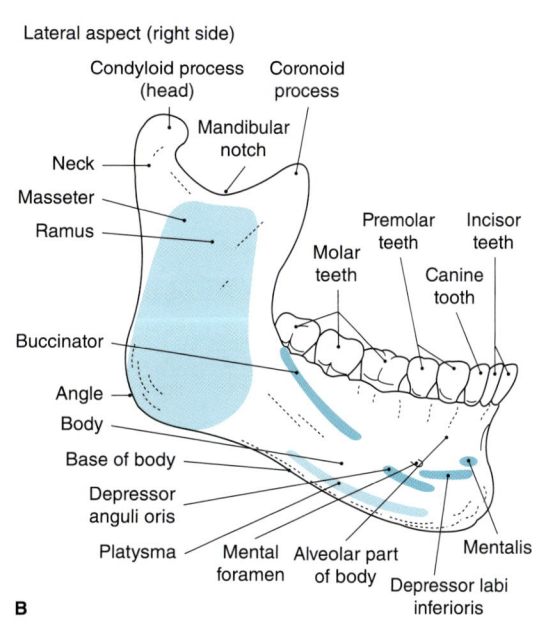

Fig. 2.49 The mandible: (A) medial view, (B) lateral view.

Table 2.9 The muscles of mastication

Muscle	Origin	Insertion	Action
Temporalis (V_3 nerve)	Temporal fossa floor up to inferior temporal line	Coronoid process	Elevates mandible; posterior fibres retract a protruded mandible
Masseter	Lower border and deep surface of zygomatic arch	Lateral surface of ramus of mandible	Elevates and protrudes mandible
Lateral pterygoid—superior head	Infratemporal surface of sphenoid bone	Neck of the mandible	Acting together, they protrude the mandible and pull the articular disc anteriorly; acting alone on one side produces deviation of mandible to contralateral side
Lateral pterygoid—inferior head	Lateral surface of lateral pterygoid plate	Articular disc	
Medial pterygoid—superficial head	Tuberosity of maxilla	Medial surface of ramus and angle of the mandible	Acting together, they elevate the mandible; acting alone on one side produces deviation of mandible to contralateral side
Medial pterygoid—deep head	Medial surface of lateral pterygoid plate		

Pterygopalatine (sphenopalatine) fossa

The pterygopalatine fossa is a medial extension of the infratemporal fossa, which is connected via the pterygomaxillary fissure. It is a small pyramidal space below the apex of the orbit that lies behind the maxilla and in front of the pterygoid process of the sphenoid bone. It contains the terminal maxillary artery, the maxillary nerve, the nerve of the pterygoid canal and the pterygopalatine ganglion.

CLINICAL NOTES

DISLOCATION OF THE TEMPOROMANDIBULAR JOINT

When yawning, if the lateral pterygoid contracts too much, the mandibular head can pass anteriorly to the articular tubercle and the mouth will no longer close. It can be reduced by applying downward pressure on the molars whilst pulling up on the chin.

A

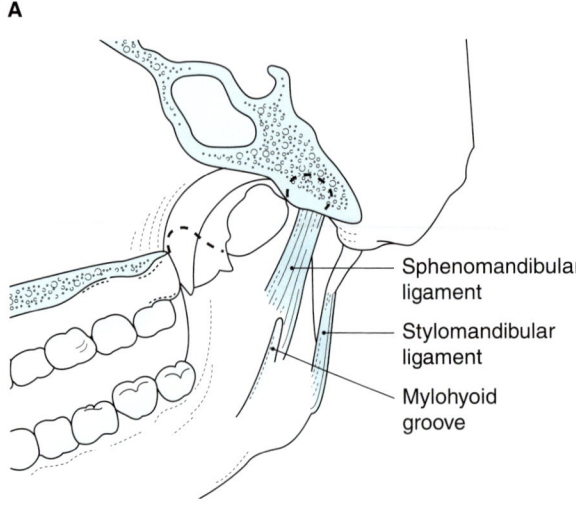

Sphenomandibular ligament

Stylomandibular ligament

Mylohyoid groove

B

Mandibular fossa   Articular disc   Articular tubercle

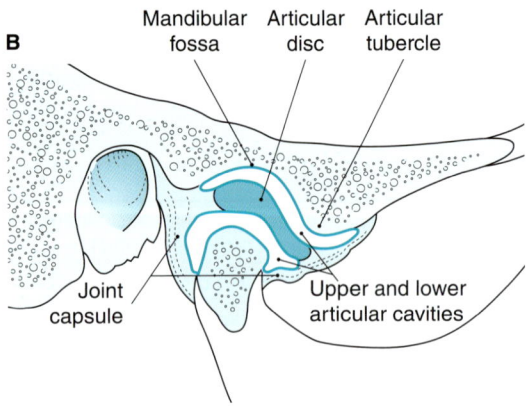

Joint capsule

Upper and lower articular cavities

Fig. 2.50 The temporomandibular joint viewed (A) medially and (B) laterally.

Pterygopalatine ganglion

The pterygopalatine ganglion is a parasympathetic ganglion lateral to the sphenopalatine foramen and suspended from the maxillary nerve. The preganglionic fibres begin in the superior salivatory nucleus of the brainstem and travel in the facial nerve (CN 7). The fibres leave the facial nerve (CN 7) as the greater superior petrosal nerve, which is joined by sympathetic fibres (from the carotid plexus) to form the nerve of the pterygoid canal. The nerve of the pterygoid canal then supplies the pterygopalatine ganglion whose postganglionic fibres then supply the lacrimal gland. The ganglion also receives ganglionic branches from the maxillary nerve.

Branches of the pterygopalatine ganglion are shown in Table 2.12.

Branches of the maxillary nerve in the pterygopalatine fossa

- Infraorbital nerve: Sensation of the medial cheek, nose and lips.
- Zygomatic nerve: Divides into the zygomaticotemporal (sensation to the temple) and zygomaticofacial branches (sensation to the malar region of the cheek).

EAR AND VESTIBULAR APPARATUS

The ear is divided into the external, middle and inner ear.

External ear

The external ear is composed of the auricle and the external auditory meatus and canal with the tympanic membrane at the end. The surface anatomy landmarks of the external ear are shown in Fig. 2.52.

Auricle

The auricle is a cartilaginous structure which captures sound and directs it towards the tympanic membrane. The sensory innervation of the ear is shown in Fig. 2.51.

External auditory canal (ear canal)

This extends from the auricle to the tympanic membrane. The lateral third is cartilaginous, and the medial two-thirds are the petrous bone. It is layered with skin and sebaceous glands, which produce cerumen (earwax).

Tympanic membrane

The thin membrane is covered by skin externally and mucous membrane internally, the concave surface of which points outward (Fig. 2.52). The membrane moves in response to sound waves, and this vibration is transmitted to the three bones of the middle ear. The external membrane has sensory innervations from the auriculotemporal nerve and the inner surface from the glossopharyngeal nerve.

Middle ear

The middle ear lies in the petrous bone and comprises the tympanic cavity and the epitympanic recess. The middle ear is connected to the pharynx by the Eustachian tube and the mastoid air cells via the aditus. The middle ear contains the ossicles, the stapedius and tensor tympani muscles and the chorda tympani. Table 2.13 describes the boundaries of the middle ear.

Table 2.10 The branches of the mandibular nerve

Branch	Area supplied
Main trunk	
Meningeal branch	Reenters cranial cavity via foramen spinosum
Nerve to medial pterygoid	Medial pterygoid and a branch that passes through otic ganglion to supply tensor tympani and tensor veli palatini
Anterior division (motor except the buccal nerve)	
Deep temporal nerves	Two or three nerves emerge from the upper border of lateral pterygoid—enter and supply temporalis
Masseteric nerve	Passes through mandibular notch to supply masseter muscle
Nerve to lateral pterygoid	Enters deep surface of lateral pterygoid and supplies it
Buccal nerve	Passes anteriorly between heads of lateral pterygoid to appear at anterior border of masseter; is sensory to skin of cheek and underlying buccal mucosa and gingiva
Posterior division (mainly sensory)	
Lingual nerve	Appears at lower border of lateral pterygoid and runs over superior surface of medial pterygoid to lie just beneath mucosa lining inner aspect of mandible adjacent to third molar tooth (its subsequent course is described with the mouth); deep to lateral pterygoid, the nerve receives the chorda tympani
Inferior alveolar nerve	Runs parallel with lingual nerve over medial pterygoid; enters mandibular foramen and supplies teeth of lower jaw; at mental foramen, a branch of the nerve, the mental nerve, exits mandible to supply lower lip and chin region; mylohyoid nerve arises from inferior alveolar nerve just above mandibular foramen to supply mylohyoid and anterior belly of digastric
Auriculotemporal nerve	Emerges from behind the temporomandibular joint, crosses the root of the zygomatic arch behind the superficial temporal artery; supplies the skin of the auricle, the external auditory meatus and scalp over the temporal region

Table 2.11 Branches of the maxillary artery

Branch	Site of origin	Area supplied
Middle meningeal artery	Infratemporal fossa	Enters cranial cavity via foramen spinosum to supply meninges
Inferior alveolar artery	Infratemporal fossa	Follows inferior alveolar nerve into mandibular canal and supplies lower jaw and teeth, and surrounding mucosa
Deep temporal arteries Masseteric artery Pterygoid branches	Infratemporal fossa	Muscles of mastication
Posterior superior alveolar artery	Pterygopalatine fossa	Enters posterior aspect of maxilla to supply molar and premolar teeth of maxilla
Anterior superior alveolar artery	Infraorbital canal	Incisor and canine teeth

Table 2.12 Branches of the pterygopalatine ganglion

Branch	Course and distribution
Nasopalatine nerve	Passes through the sphenopalatine foramen to supply the nasal septum and incisive gum of the hard palate
Lateral posterior superior nasal nerve	Exits via the sphenopalatine foramen to supply the lateral wall of the nose
Greater palatine nerve	Passes through the greater palatine canal and foramen to supply the mucosa of the palate and the lateral wall of the nose
Lesser palatine nerve	Exits through the lesser palatine foramina to supply the soft palate and the mucosa over the palatine tonsil
Pharyngeal nerve	Passes via the palatovaginal canal to supply the nasopharynx
Lacrimal fibres	Parasympathetic fibres to the lacrimal gland join the zygomaticotemporal nerve of V_2 then the lacrimal nerve before supplying the gland

Auditory tube

The auditory tube (Eustachian tube) connects the middle ear to the nasopharynx. The posterior one-third is bony and the remainder is cartilaginous. The mucosa is continuous with the nasopharynx and the middle ear. The Eustachian tube allows the pressure in the middle ear to equilibrate with the environment during swallowing, chewing and Valsalva.

Ossicles

The three ossicles are the bones of the internal ear and are the malleus, incus and stapes, which form a chain between the tympanic membrane and the oval window. The vibrations of the ossicles are dampened during loud noise by two muscles—the tensor tympani connects to the tympanic membrane and the stapedius muscle connects to the stapes.

Inner ear

The inner ear lies in the petrous bone and is the site of sound amplification and conversion of sound into electrical impulses (Fig. 2.53). The inner ear is formed by a bony labyrinth that is lined by a membranous labyrinth. The space between the bony and membranous labyrinths is filled with perilymph.

The bony labyrinth has three parts, the vestibule (utricle and saccule), the cochlea and the semicircular canals, each of which is lined with membranous labyrinth.

The vestibule is the organ of balance and is continuous anteriorly with the cochlea and posteriorly with the semicircular canals. The membranous vestibule has receptors that respond to vertical and horizontal acceleration.

The cochlear is responsible for hearing and has a membranous cochlear duct that makes 2.5 turns around a central bony core called the modiolus. The cochlear duct has the scala tympani above and the scala vestibuli below it, which also contain perilymph and are continuous at the tip of the cochlear duct. The duct itself contains the organ of Corti, which has the nerve endings responsible for hearing.

The three membranous semicircular canals are orientated in all three axes so that they can detect rotational changes in any direction.

Cranial nerves in the temporal bone

Facial nerve (CN 7)

The facial nerve (CN 7) begins as two roots (the motor root and the sensory nervus intermedius), which then fuse in the internal acoustic meatus before reaching the medial wall of the middle ear. In the middle ear, it turns posteriorly above the promontory (the geniculate

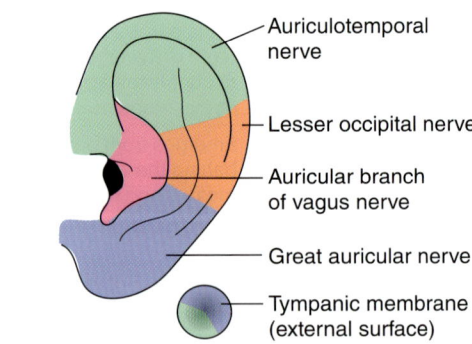

Auriculotemporal nerve

Lesser occipital nerve

Auricular branch of vagus nerve

Great auricular nerve

Tympanic membrane (external surface)

Fig. 2.51 Sensory innervations of the external ear.

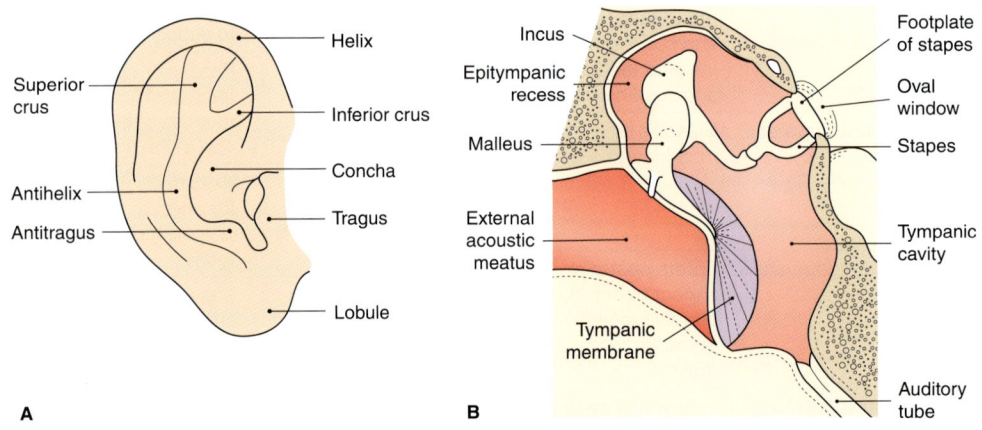

Fig. 2.52 (A) External ear and (B) tympanic membrane.

A

Helix

Superior crus

Inferior crus

Concha

Antihelix

Tragus

Antitragus

Lobule

B

Incus

Epitympanic recess

Malleus

External acoustic meatus

Tympanic membrane

Footplate of stapes

Oval window

Stapes

Tympanic cavity

Auditory tube

ganglion lies at the sharp posterior bend). It then turns inferiorly to exit the bone through the stylomastoid foramen (Fig. 2.54).

The branches of the facial nerve (CN 7) in the petrosal temporal bone are as follows:

- Greater superior petrosal nerve: Branches at the geniculate ganglion and is joined by the deep petrosal nerve to form the nerve of the pterygoid canal.
- Nerve to the stapedius.

- Chorda tympani: Branches just before the stylomastoid foramen and crosses the tympanic membrane before entering a canal for the petrotympanic fissure.

Vestibulocochlear nerve (CN 8)

This nerve has two components, a cochlear and vestibular nerve. The vestibular nerve forms the vestibular ganglion and its fibres supply the utricle, saccule and semicircular canals. The cochlear nerve forms the spiral ganglion before becoming the organ of Corti.

ORAL CAVITY

The oral cavity is divided into two parts:

- The vestibule is located between the cheeks/lips and the teeth.
- The oral cavity proper, bound within the teeth and the hard palate. The floor is formed of the tongue and glossal muscles and has a fold of mucosa called the frenulum, which can be seen when lifting the tongue.

The sensation of the mouth arises from:

- The roof: greater and lesser palatine, and nasopalatine nerves.
- The floor: lingual nerve.
- The cheek: buccal nerve (from CN 5 V_3).

The salivary glands (parotid, submandibular and sublingual) drain into the oral cavity.

Table 2.13 The boundaries of the middle ear

Wall	Components
Roof (tegmental wall)	Tegmen tympani (thin plate of bone): separates cavity from dura in floor of middle cranial fossa
Floor (jugular wall)	A layer of bone separates tympanic cavity from superior bulb of internal jugular vein
Lateral wall (membranous)	Tympanic membrane with epitympanic recess superiorly
Medial wall (labyrinthine)	Separates tympanic cavity from inner ear
Anterior wall (carotid)	Separates tympanic cavity from carotid canal; superiorly lies opening of auditory tube and canal for tensor tympani
Posterior wall	Connected by aditus to mastoid antrum and air cells

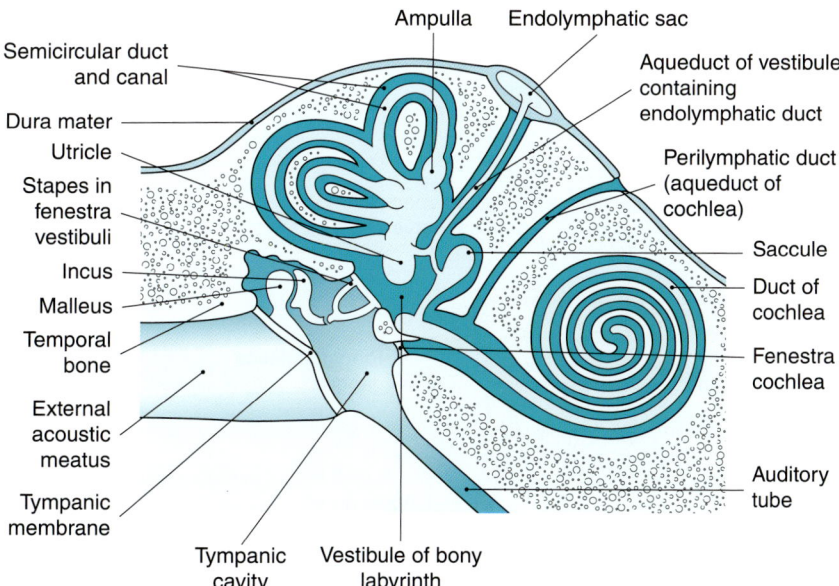

Fig. 2.53 The inner ear.

Lips

The lips function to seal the oral cavity and aid in speech. They are covered by mucosa internally and skin externally. The orbicularis oris muscle, superior and inferior labial vessels and nerves all lie in the lips.

Tongue

The tongue is a muscular structure which has its anterior two-thirds in the oral cavity and posterior third in the oropharynx. The sulcus terminalis is a V-shaped line that separates the anterior two-thirds from the posterior third and is a remnant of the embryonic thyroglossal duct. Just anterior to the sulcus are 10 to 12 vallate papillae—nipple-like structures that increase the surface area of the tongue and aid in the manipulation of food.

The anterior two-thirds of the tongue are relatively smooth but covered with numerous filiform and fungiform papillae. The under surface has lateral folds called the plica fimbriata.

The blood supply to the tongue is via the lingual arteries and veins. The innervation is shown in Table 2.14. Lymphatic drainage is to the deep cervical, submental and submandibular nodes.

The features of the tongue are shown in Fig. 2.55 and the muscles of the tongue are listed in Table 2.15.

HINTS AND TIPS

The hypoglossal nerve (CN 12) supplies all of the muscles in the tongue except for palatoglossus, which is supplied by the pharyngeal plexus.

Submandibular region

This is the region between the mandible and the hyoid bone. The submandibular region contains:

- Muscles: digastric, mylohyoid, hyoglossus, genioglossus, geniohyoid and styloglossus.
- Salivary glands: submandibular and sublingual.
- Nerves: lingual, glossopharyngeal and hypoglossal.
- Vessels: facial and lingual.

Lingual nerve

The lingual nerve branches from the mandibular nerve deep to the lateral pterygoid and is joined by the chorda tympani. The lingual nerve passes between the medial pterygoid and the ramus of the mandible and then between the hyoglossus muscle and the submandibular gland to supply the taste and somatic sensation to the anterior two-thirds of the tongue.

Hypoglossal nerve

Behind the angle of the ramus of the mandible, the hypoglossal emerges from deep to the digastric and then runs deep to the hyoglossus, styloglossus and genioglossus. It supplies all the muscles of the tongue except for the palatoglossus, which is supplied by the vagus nerve (CN 10).

Submandibular gland

The submandibular gland is responsible for the production of the majority of saliva in the unstimulated (resting) mouth; the saliva helps keep the mouth moist. Upon stimulation, the parotid gland takes over and produces saliva to aid digestion. The submandibular gland has a partly superficial section and a small deep part that are continuous around the border of the

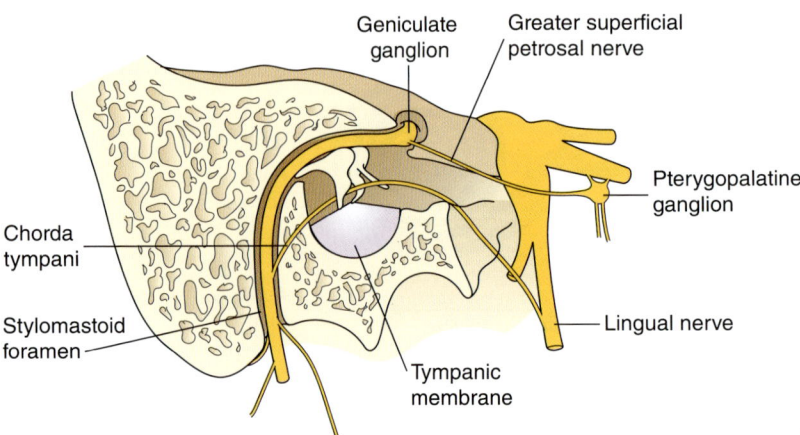

Fig. 2.54 The facial nerve in the petrous bone.

Table 2.14 Nerve supply to the tongue

	Anterior two-thirds	**Posterior one-third**
General sensory	Lingual nerve (V$_3$)	Glossopharyngeal nerve (CN 9)
Taste	Chorda tympani (CN 7) (via the lingual nerve)	Glossopharyngeal nerve (CN 9) (also vallate papillae)

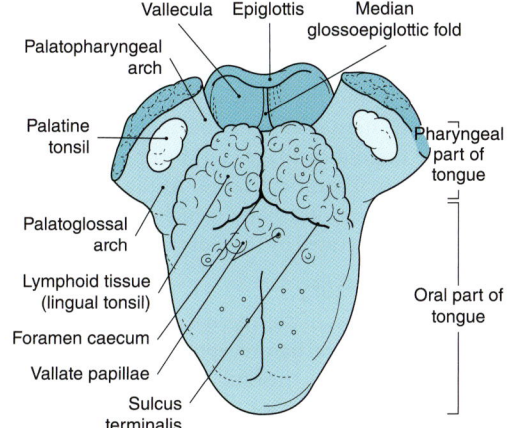

Fig. 2.55 The tongue.

mylohyoid muscle. Its arterial supply is from the facial and lingual vessels. Its parasympathetic supply is from the submandibular ganglion, with the sympathetic supply coming from fibres travelling with the facial artery.

Palate and tonsils

The palate is the roof of the mouth and the floor of the nasal cavity. It has two parts:

- The hard palate is made of the maxilla and palatine bone.
- The soft palate is a mobile fibromuscular fold lying posterior to the hard palate. It is composed of muscles (Table 2.16) and the palatine aponeurosis, which is the expanded aponeurosis of the tensor veli palatine.

Blood supply to the palate is from the greater and lesser palatine arteries, which are terminal branches of the maxillary artery. The greater and lesser palatine nerves arise from the pterygopalatine ganglion.

The palatine tonsils are lymphoid masses lying between the palatoglossal and palatopharyngeal arches.

NECK

The neck connects the head and the torso, enabling key structures to pass between them. The neck is supported by the seven cervical vertebrae and contains the larynx, pharynx and thyroid gland. The vertebrae and muscles of the neck enable it to be a

Table 2.15 Muscles of the tongue

Name of muscle (nerve supply)	Origin	Insertion	Action
Intrinsic muscles			
Longitudinal (CN 12)	Mucous membrane	Mucous membrane	Shortens tongue
Transverse (CN 12)	Mucous membrane and median septum	Mucous membrane	Narrows tongue
Vertical (CN 12)	Mucous membrane	Mucous membrane	Lowers tongue
Extrinsic muscles			
Palatoglossus (pharyngeal plexus)	Palatine aponeurosis	Lateral aspect of tongue	Pulls tongue upward and backward and narrows oropharyngeal isthmus
Genioglossus (CN 12)	Superior mental spine (genial tubercle) of mandible	Merges with other tongue muscles	Draws tongue forward and pulls tip backward
Hyoglossus (CN 12)	Body and greater cornu of hyoid bone	Merges with other tongue muscles	Depresses tongue
Styloglossus (CN 12)	Styloid process of temporal bone	Merges with other tongue muscles	Draws tongue upward and backward

mobile structure to assist the senses of the eyes and ear in inter-acting with the external environment.

Soft tissues in the neck

Fascia (Fig. 2.56)

Superficial fascia

This is a thin layer that encloses the platysma muscle.

Deep fascia

- Investing fascia: Completely encircles the neck and divides to enclose the trapezius and sternocleidomastoid muscles. The fascia attaches superiorly on the mandible and the zygomatic arch (enclosing the parotid in the process), and it attaches inferiorly to the clavicle, manubrium and acromion.
- Pretracheal fascia: Encloses the thyroid and parathyroid gland. The pretracheal fascia lies deep to the infrahyoid muscles and is attached superiorly to the thyroid and cricoid cartilages. Inferiorly, the fascia enters the thorax and blends with the fibrous pericardium.
- Prevertebral fascia: Encloses the vertebra and associated muscles. Superiorly, the fascia attaches to the skull base and inferiorly it blends with the anterior longitudinal ligament. Anterior to this fascia is the retropharyngeal space.
- Carotid sheath: Encloses the carotid artery, jugular vein and vagus nerve.

Triangles of the neck

The anterior triangle of the neck is bounded posteriorly by the anterior border of the sternocleidomastoid muscle and anteriorly by the midline. The anterior triangle is further subdivided into the submental, submandibular, carotid and muscular triangles (Fig. 2.57). The contents of the anterior triangle are shown in Table 2.17 and Fig. 2.57.

The posterior triangle is bordered by the trapezius, the posterior border of sternocleidomastoid and the middle third of the clavicle. The posterior triangle can be further subdivided into the occipital and subclavian triangles by the posterior belly of omohyoid. The contents of the posterior triangle can be seen in Fig. 2.58 and Table 2.18.

Vessels of the neck

Carotid artery

The common carotid artery arises from the brachiocephalic trunk on the right and the aortic arch on the left. They both course deep to the sternocleidomastoid in the carotid sheath to the level of the thyroid cartilage (C3) before dividing into the external and internal carotid arteries. At the common carotid bifurcation lies the carotid body, which contains peripheral chemoreceptors innervated by the glossopharyngeal nerve.

Internal carotid artery

The first few centimetres of the internal carotid are dilated as the carotid sinus, a peripheral baroreceptor used to measure blood pressure. It passes through the skull base in the carotid canal. It has no branches in the neck.

External carotid artery

This ascends to enter the parotid gland and terminates as the superficial temporal and maxillary arteries. The branches of the external carotid are shown in Fig. 2.59.

Table 2.16 Muscles of the soft palate

Name of muscle (nerve supply)	Origin	Insertion	Action
Tensor veli palatini (nerve to medial pterygoid V$_3$)	Spine of sphenoid, auditory tube, scaphoid fossa of pterygoid process	With muscle of other side, forms palatine aponeurosis	Tenses soft palate
Levator veli palatini (pharyngeal plexus)	Petrous part of temporal bone, auditory tube	Palatine aponeurosis	Elevates soft palate
Musculus uvulae (pharyngeal plexus)	Posterior border of hard palate	Mucous membrane of uvula	Elevates uvula
Palatopharyngeus (pharyngeal plexus)	Palatine aponeurosis horizontal plate of palatine bone	Posterior border of thyroid cartilage	Elevates pharyngeal wall and pulls palatopharyngeal folds medially and depresses soft palate
Palatoglossus (pharyngeal plexus)	Palatine aponeurosis	Lateral aspect of tongue	Pulls tongue upward and backward and narrows oropharyngeal isthmus and depresses soft palate

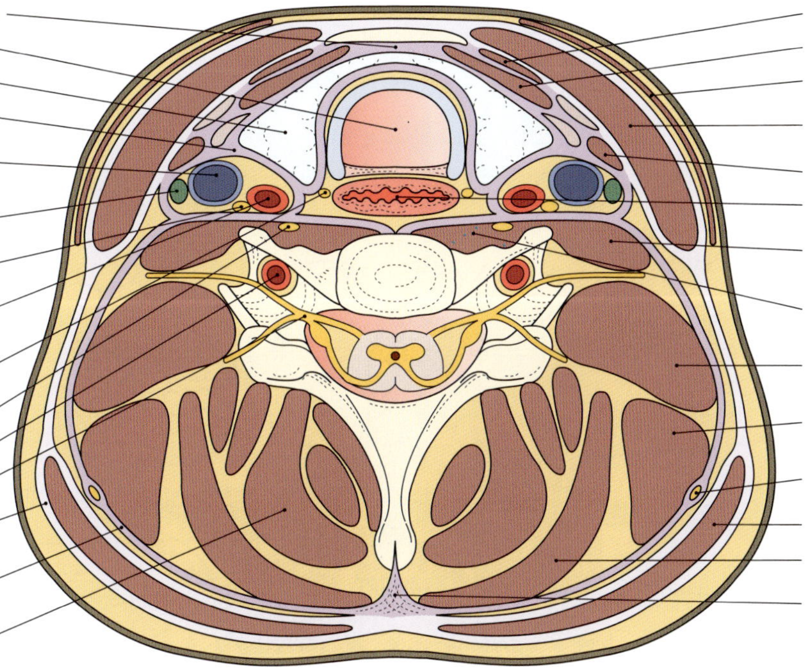

Pretracheal fascia
Trachea
Thyroid gland
Carotid sheath
Internal jugular vein
Deep cervical lymph node
Vagus nerve
Common carotid artery
Recurrent laryngeal nerve
Sympathetic trunk
Vertebral artery
Spinal nerve
Investing layer of fascia
Prevertebral layer of fascia
Semispinalis capitis
Sternohyoid muscle
Sternothyroid muscle
Platysma
Sternocleidomastoid muscle
Omohyoid muscle
Oesophagus
Scalenus anterior muscle
Longus colli cervicis muscle
Scalenus medius muscle
Levator scapulae muscle
Spinal part of accessory nerve
Trapezius
Splenius capitis
Ligamentum nuchae

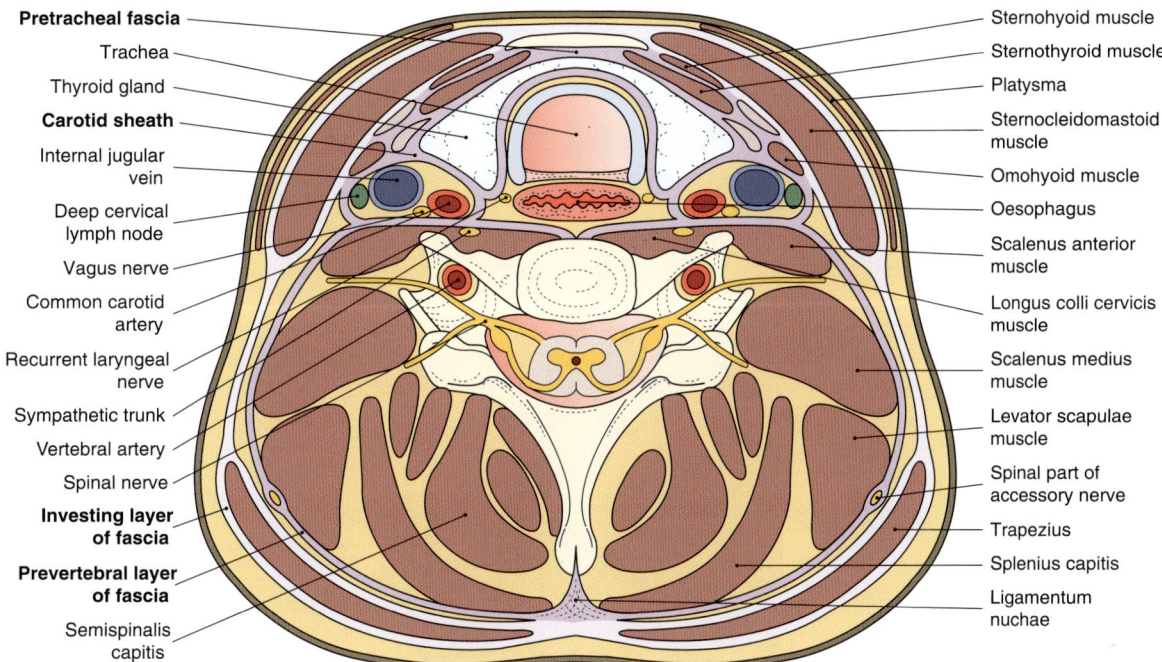

Fig. 2.56 The deep fascia of the neck.

Jugular veins

Internal jugular vein

The internal jugular vein commences at the sigmoid sinus and leaves the skull through the jugular foramen. The internal jugular vein descends through the carotid sheath, initially posterior to and then lateral to the carotid artery. It unites with the subclavian vein to form the brachiocephalic vein.

External jugular vein

The external jugular vein is formed from the posterior auricular and retromandibular vein behind the angle of the mandible. It runs over the sternocleidomastoid, pierces the investing fascia in the subclavian triangle and drains into the subclavian vein.

Muscles of the neck

The major lateral muscles of the neck are listed in Table 2.19. The supra- and infrahyoid muscles are shown in Table 2.20.

Nerves of the neck

Glossopharyngeal nerve (CN 9)

This nerve emerges through the jugular foramen and passes between the internal and external carotid arteries. The glossopharyngeal nerve gives a branch to the carotid body and then passes between the superior and middle pharyngeal constrictor muscles to supply sensation and taste to the posterior third of the tongue and the oropharynx.

Vagus nerve (CN 10)

The vagus exits through the jugular foramen and descends in the carotid sheath. It passes anterior to the subclavian artery and then into the thorax. The vagus nerve has a recurrent laryngeal branch which supplies the muscles of the larynx.

Spinal accessory nerve (CN 11)

The accessory nerve forms from C1 to C6 roots in the cervical spine, enters the skull through the foramen magnum and then immediately leaves through the jugular foramen. The spinal accessory nerve supplies the sternocleidomastoid and trapezius muscles.

HINTS AND TIPS

The left accessory nerve and thus the left sternocleidomastoid muscle rotate the head to the right.

Hypoglossal nerve (CN 12)

This emerges from the hypoglossal canal and passes between the internal jugular and internal carotid vessels. At the angle of the

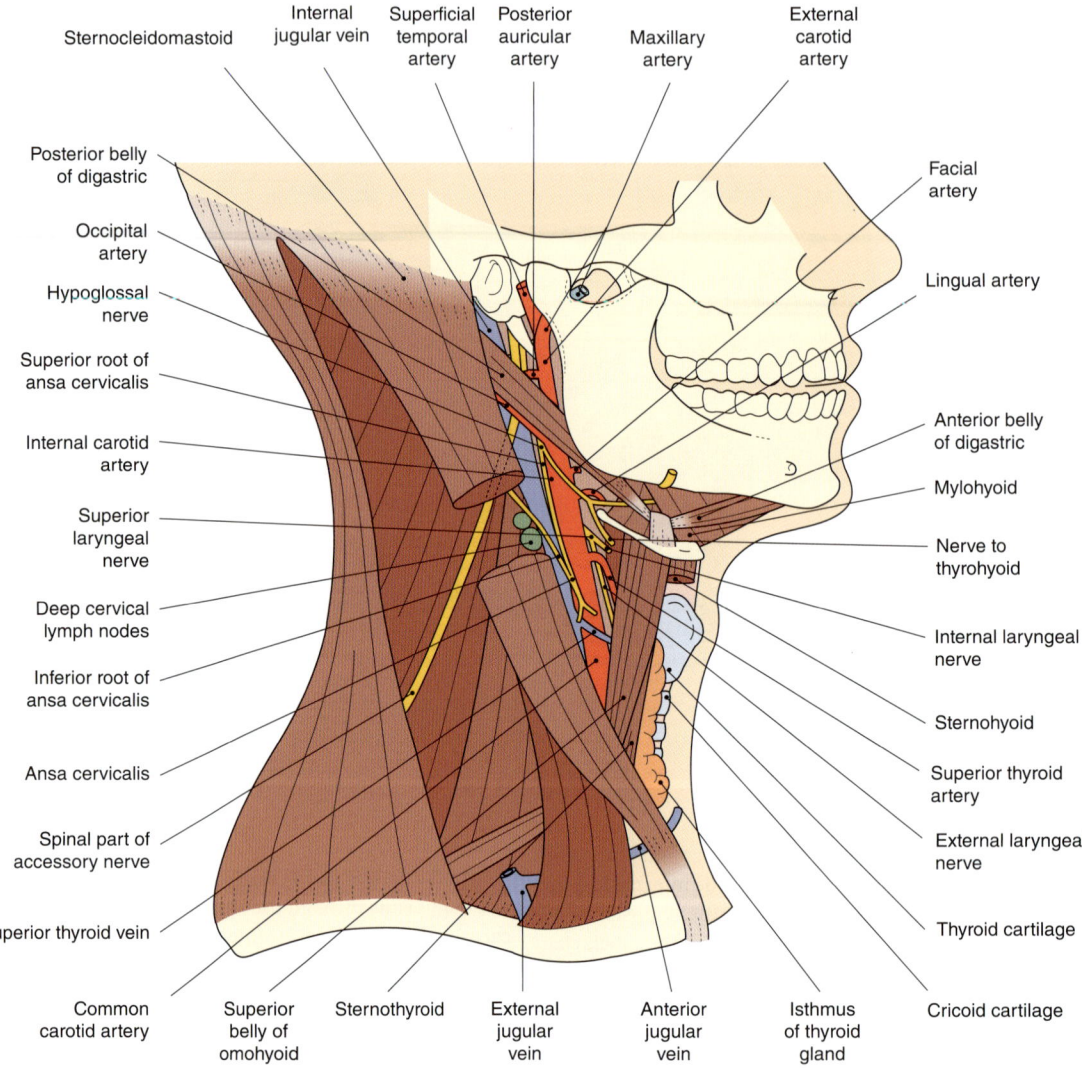

Fig. 2.57 The anterior triangle of the neck.

Table 2.17 The contents of the anterior triangle of the neck

Triangle	Main contents
Carotid	External carotid artery; larynx and pharynx, and internal and external laryngeal nerves
Muscular	Sternothyroid and sternohyoid muscles, superior belly of omohyoid; thyroid gland, trachea and oesophagus
Digastric (sub-mandibular)	Submandibular gland and lymph nodes; facial artery and vein; external carotid artery; internal carotid artery, internal jugular vein, glossopharyngeal (CN 9), vagus (CN 10) and hypoglossal (CN 12) nerves
Submental	Submental lymph nodes

mandible, it passes outwards from the lower border of the posterior digastric. It loops around the occipital artery and enters the submandibular region to supply the muscles of the tongue.

Ansa cervicalis

This nerve loop is formed from the C1 to C3 nerve roots and supplies the omohyoid, sternohyoid and sternothyroid.

Sympathetic chain

The sympathetic chain lies between the carotid sheath and the prevertebral fascia. It has a superior, middle and inferior ganglion; the latter fuses with the first thoracic ganglion to form the stellate ganglion. The postganglionic fibres follow the arteries into the head.

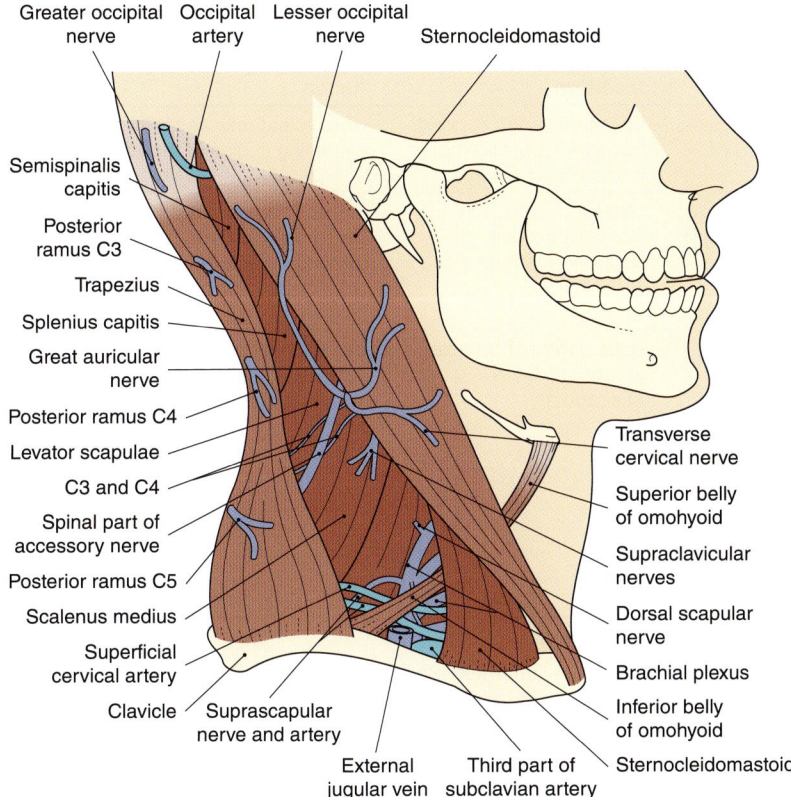

Greater occipital nerve · Occipital artery · Lesser occipital nerve · Sternocleidomastoid

Semispinalis capitis
Posterior ramus C3
Trapezius
Splenius capitis
Great auricular nerve
Posterior ramus C4
Levator scapulae
C3 and C4
Spinal part of accessory nerve
Posterior ramus C5
Scalenus medius
Superficial cervical artery
Clavicle · Suprascapular nerve and artery
External jugular vein · Third part of subclavian artery

Transverse cervical nerve
Superior belly of omohyoid
Supraclavicular nerves
Dorsal scapular nerve
Brachial plexus
Inferior belly of omohyoid
Sternocleidomastoid

Fig. 2.58 The posterior triangle of the neck.

Table 2.18 The contents of the posterior triangle	
Structure	**Origin**
Third part of subclavian artery	Enters anterior inferior angle of triangle
Superficial cervical artery	Branch of thyrocervical trunk of subclavian artery
Suprascapular artery	Branch of thyrocervical trunk
Brachial plexus	Roots of plexus enter posterior triangle by emerging between scalenus anterior and medius; trunks and divisions also lie in posterior triangle before entering the axilla
Accessory nerve	Spinal part of accessory nerve enters posterior triangle by emerging from deep to posterior border of sternocleidomastoid
Cervical plexus	The four cutaneous branches emerge from posterior border of sternocleidomastoid

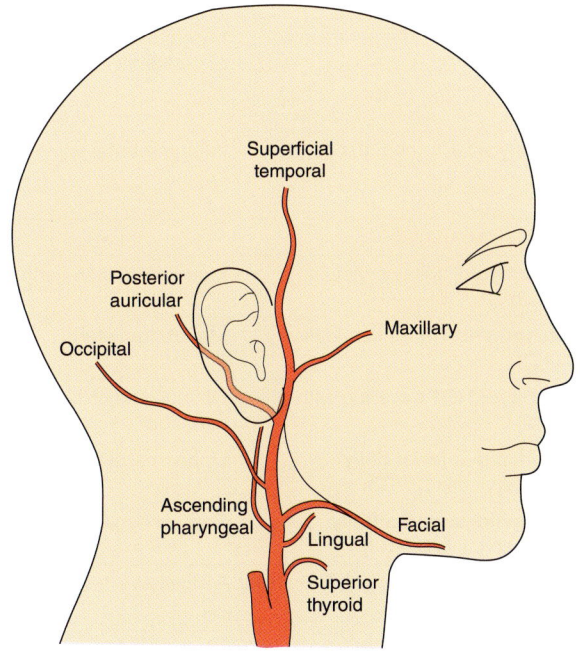

Superficial temporal
Posterior auricular
Occipital
Maxillary
Ascending pharyngeal
Lingual
Facial
Superior thyroid

Fig. 2.59 Branches of the external carotid artery.

Table 2.19 Lateral muscles of the neck

Name of muscle (nerve supply)	Origin	Insertion	Action
Platysma (CN 7 nerve)	Inferior border of mandible; skin and subcutaneous tissues of lower part of the face	Fascia covering superior parts of pectoralis major and deltoid muscles	Used to express sadness and fright by pulling angles of mouth down
Sternocleidomastoid (CN 11 (spinal part), C2, C3)	Anterior surface of manubrium of sternum; medial third of clavicle	Mastoid process of temporal bone and superior nuchal line	Individually, each muscle laterally flexes neck and rotates it so face is turned upwards toward opposite side; both muscles act together to flex neck
Trapezius (CN 11 (spinal part), C2, C3)	Superior nuchal line; external occipital protuberance; ligamentum nuchae; spinous processes of C7–T12 vertebrae	Lateral third of clavicle; acromion; spine of scapula	Elevates, retracts and rotates scapula laterally so that the glenoid 'looks upwards'

Table 2.20 Suprahyoid and infrahyoid muscles

Name of muscle (nerve supply)	Origin	Insertion	Action
Suprahyoid muscles			
Posterior belly of digastric (CN 7)	Mastoid process	Intermediate tendon bound to hyoid bone	Depresses mandible and elevates hyoid bone
Anterior belly of digastric (CN 5 inferior alveolar V_3 nerve)	Lower border of mandible near midline	Intermediate tendon bound to hyoid bone	Depresses mandible and elevates hyoid bone
Stylohyoid (CN 7)	Styloid process of temporal bone	Body of hyoid bone	Elevates hyoid bone
Mylohyoid (CN5 inferior alveolar V_3 nerve)	Mylohyoid line on medial surface of mandible	Body of hyoid bone and mylohyoid raphe	Elevates floor of mouth and hyoid bone, and depresses mandible
Geniohyoid (C1 through CN 12 nerve)	Inferior mental spine	Body of hyoid bone	Elevates hyoid bone and depresses mandible
Infrahyoid muscles			
Sternohyoid (ansa cervicalis C1–C3)	Manubrium sterni and clavicle	Body of hyoid bone	Depresses hyoid bone
Sternothyroid (ansa cervicalis C1–C3)	Manubrium sterni	Oblique line on lamina of thyroid cartilage	Depresses larynx
Thyrohyoid (C1 travelling with CN 12)	Oblique line on lamina of thyroid cartilage	Body of hyoid bone	Depresses hyoid bone and elevates larynx
Omohyoid–inferior belly (ansa cervicalis C1–C3)	Upper margin of scapula	Intermediate tendon bound to clavicle and first rib	Depresses hyoid bone
Omohyoid–superior belly (ansa cervicalis C1–C3)	Body of hyoid bone	Intermediate tendon bound to clavicle and first rib	Depresses hyoid bone

Adapted from Hall-Craggs, E. C. B. (1995). Anatomy as a basis for clinical medicine. Williams & Wilkins.

MIDLINE STRUCTURES OF THE NECK

Pharynx

The pharynx is a tube lying poster to the nasal cavity (nasopharynx), the oral cavity (oropharynx) and the larynx (laryngopharynx). It extends to the cricoid cartilage at the level of C6, where it is continuous with the oesophagus.

The layers of the pharynx are the mucosa, the pharyngobasilar fascia (which is continuous with the skull base periosteum) and the muscular layer of pharyngeal constrictors (Fig. 2.60; Table 2.21). The arterial supply to the pharynx is via the ascending pharyngeal, ascending palatine, facial, maxillary and lingual arteries. The venous drainage is via the pharyngeal venous plexus draining into the internal jugular vein.

The nerve supply to the pharynx is as follows:

- Nasopharynx: maxillary nerve (V_2).
- Oropharynx: glossopharyngeal nerve.
- Laryngopharynx: internal laryngeal nerve (branch of the vagus nerve).

Nasopharynx

The nasopharynx is posterior to the nasal cavity, with continuity with one another through the posterior nasal apertures. The role of the nasopharynx is to transmit inspired air. The nasopharynx contains the openings to the Eustachian tube and the adenoid on the posterior wall. During swallowing, the soft palate moves upwards and the posterior wall comes forward to occlude the nasopharynx and prevent the entry of food into the nasal cavity. The muscles of the pharynx are described in Table 2.21.

Oropharynx

The oropharynx extends from the soft palate to the epiglottis. The palatine tonsils lie in the lateral walls. The anterior wall of the oropharynx is made of the posterior third of the tongue with its underlying lingual tonsil. The mucosa of the oropharynx is reflected from the base of the tongue to form one medial and two lateral glossopharyngeal folds with two pouches (valleculae) between them.

Laryngopharynx

The laryngopharynx lies posterior to the larynx. The piriform fossae are grooves on either side of the laryngeal inlet that guide food away from the laryngeal opening.

HINTS AND TIPS

The four sets of tonsils (tubal, pharyngeal, lingual and palatine) form a ring of lymphoid tissue around the oropharynx called Waldeyer ring.

Larynx

The larynx is continuous with the laryngopharynx above and the trachea below. It is responsible for protecting the airways from food and for phonation. The laryngeal cartilages and the laryngeal membranes that link these cartilages are shown in Fig. 2.61 and Table 2.22.

Laryngeal cavity

The laryngeal inlet is demarcated by the epiglottis, aryepiglottic and interarytenoid folds (Fig. 2.62). The laryngeal inlet leads to the vestibule, which extends as far as the vestibular folds. The vestibular ligament/fold forms the false cord, which is superior to the vocal/true cords. The rima glottis is the space between the folds, and the infraglottic cavity lies below the folds.

The mucosa above the vocal fold is supplied by the superior laryngeal artery and the internal laryngeal nerve. The mucosa below the fold is supplied by the inferior laryngeal artery and the recurrent laryngeal nerve.

Intrinsic muscles of the larynx

The intrinsic muscles of the larynx are described in Table 2.23. They are all paired except for the transverse arytenoids muscle. They serve to alter the length and tension of the folds and rima glottis for speech production.

HINTS AND TIPS

The intrinsic muscles of the larynx are supplied by the recurrent laryngeal nerve except for the cricothyroid, which is supplied by the external (superior) laryngeal nerve.

Joints of the larynx

There are two pairs of synovial joints in larynx:

- Cricothyroid joint: Between the inferior cornu of the thyroid cartilage and the facet of the cricoid cartilage.
- Cricoarytenoid joint: Allows the arytenoids to rotate and glide on the cricoid cartilage.

CLINICAL NOTES

TRACHEOSTOMY AND CRICOTHYROIDOTOMY

During a tracheostomy, the skin of the neck is incised, the strap muscles moved to one side and the thyroid isthmus moved inferiorly or clamped and divided if necessary. An incision is then made through the second to fourth tracheal cartilages and a tracheostomy tube inserted.

A cricothyroidotomy (a short-term, emergency procedure) is performed by passing a needle through the cricothyroid membrane directly below the thyroid prominence. This is useful when there is a blockage at the rima glottides, as the needle passes below this level.

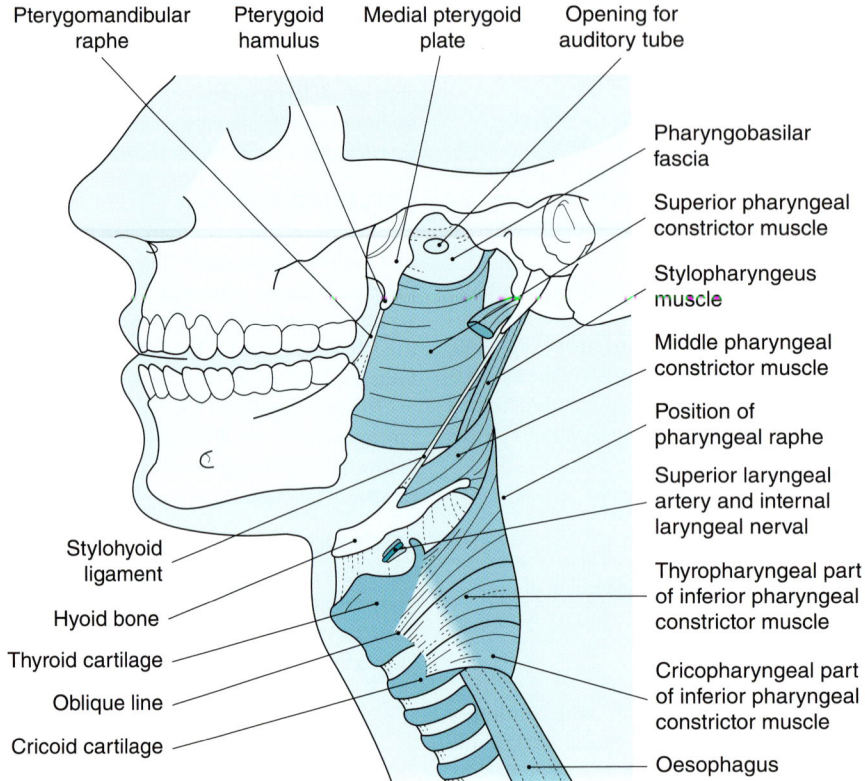

Fig. 2.60 Muscles of the pharynx.

Table 2.21 Muscles of the pharynx

Name of muscle (nerve supply)	Origin	Insertion	Action
Superior constrictor (pharyngeal plexus)	Medial pterygoid plate, pterygoid hamulus, pterygomandibular raphe, mylohyoid line of mandible	Pharyngeal tubercle of occipital bone, midline pharyngeal raphe	Assists in separating oro- and nasopharynx and propels food bolus downward
Middle constrictor (pharyngeal plexus)	Stylohyoid ligament, lesser and greater cornua of hyoid bone	Pharyngeal raphe	Propels food bolus downward
Inferior constrictor (pharyngeal plexus)			
Thyropharyngeus	Lamina of thyroid cartilage	Pharyngeal raphe	Propels food bolus downward
Cricopharyngeus	Cricoid cartilage	Contralateral cricopharyngeus	Upper oesophageal sphincter
Palatopharyngeus (pharyngeal plexus)	Palatine aponeurosis Horizontal plate of palatine bone	Thyroid cartilage	Elevates pharyngeal wall and pulls palatopharyngeal folds medially
Salpingopharyngeus (pharyngeal plexus)	Auditory tube	Merges with palatopharyngeus	Elevates pharynx and larynx
Stylopharyngeus (CN 9)	Styloid process of temporal bone	Thyroid cartilage	Elevates larynx during swallowing

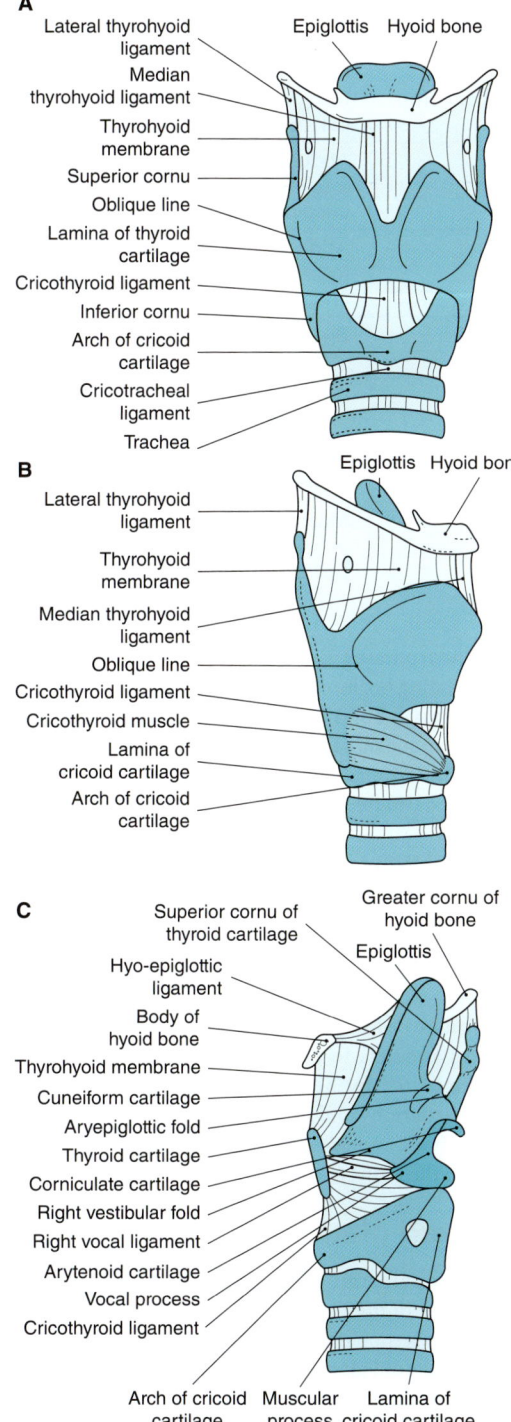

Fig. 2.61 Laryngeal cartilages from the (A) front, (B) right hand side and (C) left hand side without the left lamina of the thyroid cartilage.

Table 2.22 Laryngeal membranes

Membrane	Attachments
Thyrohyoid	Runs between the thyroid cartilage and hyoid bone; has a midline thickening and two lateral thickenings, the median thyrohyoid ligament and lateral thyrohyoid ligaments, respectively
Quadrangular	Runs between the epiglottis and the arytenoid cartilage; its lower free border is the vestibular ligament
Cricothyroid	Joins the cricoid, thyroid and arytenoid cartilages; its upper free border is the vocal ligament; there is also a midline thickening, the median cricothyroid ligament
Cricotracheal	Runs from the cricoid cartilage to the trachea

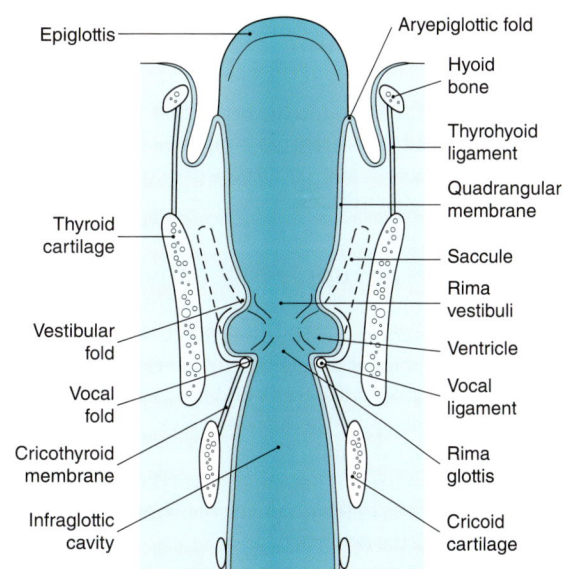

Fig. 2.62 Coronal section of the larynx. (Adapted from Williams, P. (Ed.). (1995). *Gray's anatomy* (38th ed.). Churchill Livingstone.)

Trachea

The trachea begins at the level of C6 and is continuous with the larynx above and ends at its bifurcation into the main bronchi at the level of the sternal angle (T4). Its walls are reinforced by the C-shaped cartilaginous rings that stop it from collapsing during ventilation.

Table 2.23 Intrinsic muscles of the larynx

Muscle (nerve supply)	Origin	Insertion	Action
Cricothyroid (external laryngeal nerve)	Cricoid cartilage arch	Inferior border of thyroid cartilage and inferior cornu	Lengthens and tenses vocal cords by tilting cricoid and thus arytenoid cartilages
Posterior cricoarytenoid (recurrent laryngeal nerve)	Cricoid cartilage lamina	Muscular process of arytenoid cartilage	Abducts vocal cords by laterally rotating arytenoid cartilages on cricoid cartilage
Lateral cricoarytenoid (recurrent laryngeal nerve)	Cricoid cartilage arch	Muscular process of arytenoid cartilage	Adducts vocal cords by medially rotating arytenoid cartilages on cricoid cartilage
Thyroarytenoid (recurrent laryngeal nerve)	Posterior surface of thyroid cartilage	Muscular process of arytenoid cartilage	Shortens vocal cord
Transverse arytenoid (recurrent laryngeal nerve)	Body of arytenoid cartilage	Body of contralateral arytenoid cartilage	Closes rima glottis by adducting arytenoid cartilages
Oblique arytenoid (recurrent laryngeal nerve)	Muscular process of arytenoid cartilage	Apex of contralateral arytenoid cartilage	Closes rima glottis by drawing arytenoid cartilages together
Vocalis (recurrent laryngeal nerve)	Vocal process of arytenoid cartilage	Vocal ligament	Maintains/increases tension in anterior part of vocal ligament; relaxes posterior part of vocal ligament

Thyroid gland

The thyroid gland is an endocrine organ that lies between the trachea behind and the infrahyoid strap muscles in front. It is covered by the capsule and the pretracheal fascia. It has two lobes, connected by an isthmus.

Blood and nerve supply to the thyroid

The superior thyroid artery (the first branch of the external carotid artery) is accompanied by the external laryngeal nerve to supply the upper poles of the gland. The inferior thyroid artery arises from the thyrocervical trunk and runs with the recurrent laryngeal nerve to supply the inferior poles. All four arteries anastomose behind the gland.

The thyroid ima artery is present in 3% of the population and arises from either the brachiocephalic trunk or the aortic arch and enters through the isthmus.

Venous drainage is through the superior and middle thyroid veins, which drain into the internal jugular vein and the inferior thyroid vein, which drains into the brachiocephalic vein (Fig. 2.63).

Thyroid hormones

The thyroid hormones are triiodothyronine (T3) and thyroxine (T4), which are tyrosine-based hormones produced by the follicular cells. The production of thyroid hormones begins with thyroglobulin, which is produced by the follicular cells and iodinated by the thyroperoxidase enzyme. Lysosomal enzymes in colloid are incorporated through endocytosis in response to thyroid-stimulating hormone, and the lysosomal enzymes cleave T4 from the thyroglobulin.

Thyroid hormones are transported in the blood bound to proteins (thyroxine-binding globulin and albumin) with only a small fraction (<1%) free in the plasma and able to produce metabolic effects.

The effects of thyroid hormones are to increase cardiac output, blood pressure and basal metabolic rate. They also potentiate the effects of catecholamines.

Calcitonin

This is a hormone produced by the C-cells (parafollicular) of the thyroid gland and acts to reduce the serum calcium level. Its release is stimulated by high serum calcium and gastrin. Its actions oppose parathyroid hormone by inhibiting osteoclastic activity in the bone and preventing calcium reabsorption in the tubular cells of the kidney.

Parathyroid glands

The parathyroids are four small glands (6 × 4 × 2 mm) on the posterior surface of the thyroid glands. They produce parathyroid hormone in response to low serum calcium. Both the upper and lower parathyroid glands are supplied by the inferior thyroid artery. They are at risk of damage during thyroidectomy, which causes severe postoperative hypocalcaemia.

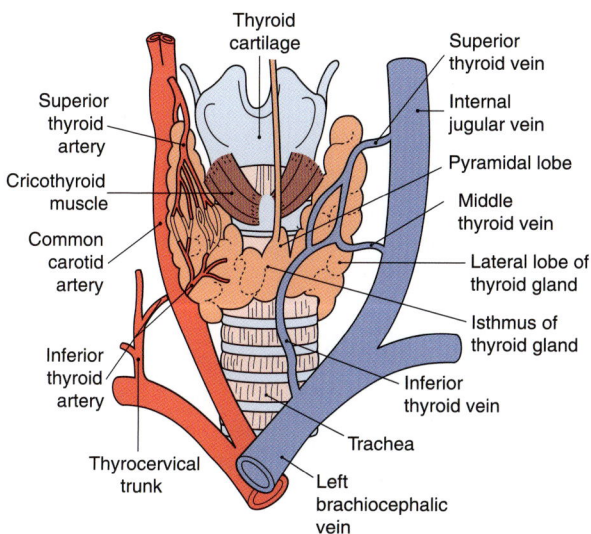

Fig. 2.63 Blood supply of the thyroid gland.

HINTS AND TIPS

The term somatic refers to 'the body' and allows controls of conscious activities and also feeds back information to the brain. By contrast, the autonomic system mediates unconscious activities.

CLINICAL NOTES

THYROGLOSSAL CYSTS, GOITRE AND THYROIDECTOMY

The thyroid gland develops as a down growth from the back of the tongue—attached to it by the thyroglossal duct. This duct usually disappears; however, remnants may persist. A cyst may form in these remnants. These can be distinguished from a midline sebaceous cyst (or a goitre) by asking a patient to swallow or stick out the tongue, which will pull the thyroglossal cyst upwards. An enlargement of the thyroid is referred to as a goitre and may compress structures adjacent to the thyroid. A thyroidectomy (removal of the thyroid) may be total (e.g. for carcinoma) or subtotal (e.g. in the treatment of hyperthyroidism), where part of the gland is preserved. Owing to the close relationship between the inferior thyroid arteries and the recurrent laryngeal nerve, these are tied rather than cut during a thyroidectomy, as damage to the nerve results in hoarseness.

OVERVIEW OF THE THORAX

This chapter will cover the anatomy of the thorax and the organs within it and explore the fundamental physiology of both the cardiovascular and respiratory systems.

Structure of the thorax

The thorax is delineated by the sternum anteriorly, 12 ribs bilaterally and 12 central thoracic vertebrae posteriorly. Inferiorly, the diaphragm, a dome-shaped muscle, separates the thoracic and abdominal cavities. The thoracic framework supports and protects the crucial organs within it. The mediastinum houses the heart, a muscular organ central to circulatory function. The pericardium envelops and protects the heart, comprising visceral and parietal layers. Within pleural cavities, the lungs perform respiratory functions with bronchi that branch from the bifurcation of the trachea, the carina. Vascular structures intricately traverse throughout the thorax, including the great vessels, the aorta, vena cava and pulmonary vessels.

Functions of the respiratory system

The primary purpose of the respiratory system is gaseous exchange; however, it has many other roles crucial for homoeostasis. It actively regulates the acid–base equilibrium, responding to CO_2 and H^+ concentrations as impaired gas exchange in respiratory diseases can lead to acidosis or alkalosis. Metabolically, the system facilitates the uptake of vascular substances, including prostaglandins, noradrenaline and leukotrienes, and produces functional substances such as surfactants, enzymes and immunologically active material. It also secretes hormones, responsible for converting angiotensin 1 to angiotensin 2 and releasing prostaglandin I_2 to prevent platelet aggregation.

In addition, the lung's capillary bed acts as a filter to trap blood clots, emboli and cancer cells, subsequently cleared by macrophages and lymphatic drainage. Serving as a 500-mL volume reservoir, the respiratory circulation ensures constant blood flow to the left ventricle. Additionally, the lungs excrete volatile drugs and contribute to phonation, controlling laryngeal muscles for speech and singing. Overall, the respiratory system is a complex body system that is responsible for many aspects of homoeostasis, but its predominant role is gaseous exchange.

Functions of the cardiovascular system

The cardiovascular system consists of the heart, blood vessels and lymphatics. Primarily, it acts as a pump resulting in the circulation of blood and lymph. The cardiovascular system has a number of additional transport and homoeostatic functions, outlined in Fig. 3.1. The heart is a hollow, muscular organ that beats, on average, 72 times per minute. The right side of the heart receives deoxygenated blood from the systemic venous circulation and pumps it to the lungs. The left side of the heart receives oxygenated blood from the lungs and pumps it throughout the remaining parts of the body.

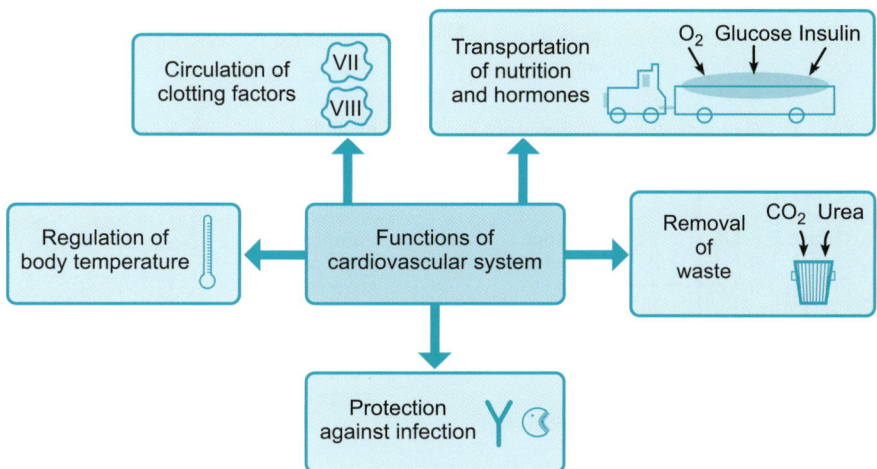

Fig. 3.1 Functions of the cardiovascular system.

SURFACE ANATOMY OF THE THORAX

Bony landmarks

The bony landmarks are illustrated in Fig. 3.2. There are many imaginary vertical lines used clinically to describe locations in the thorax:

- *Midsternal line:* The sagittal midline of the body.
- *Midclavicular line:* Halfway between the tip of the acromion and the midsternal line.
- *Anterior axillary line:* Corresponds to the anterior axillary fold/lateral edge of pectoralis major.
- *Posterior axillary line:* Corresponds to the posterior axillary fold/lateral edge of latissimus dorsi.
- *Midscapular line:* Passes through the inferior angle of the scapula.

The key transverse line/plane is between the manubrium and the body of the sternum at the level of T4 to T5. This is known as the sternal angle (angle of Louis) and is the landmark for several key thoracic structures:

- Divides the mediastinum into superior and inferior regions.
- Level of the second costal cartilage.
- The beginning and end of the aortic arch.
- Bifurcation of the trachea (the carina).
- Superior border of the pericardium.
- The point where the thoracic duct crosses to the left-hand side of the thorax.

- Entry of the azygos vein into the superior vena cava (SVC) (note that while anatomical variations exist, drainage into the SVC is the normal configuration).

Note: Natural variation has been shown to affect the position of the structures listed above.

CLINICAL NOTES

CHEST DRAIN LANDMARKS

The midclavicular line is used as a landmark for emergency needle decompression to treat tension pneumothorax. The needle is inserted on the midclavicular line in the second intercostal space. Chest drains are inserted in the 'triangle of safety', which is bordered by the anterior and posterior axillary line, and the fifth intercostal space. Inserting the drain slightly anterior to the midaxillary line avoids injury to the long thoracic nerve.

Trachea, lungs and pleura

The larynx can be palpated in the midline of the neck with its thyroid cartilage (Adam's apple) at the level of C5. Just below this is the cricoid cartilage at C6, which forms the first cartilaginous ring of the trachea. The level of the trachea bifurcation is marked externally by the angle of the sternum.

Superiorly, the pleura and lungs extend 2 cm above the clavicles. The pleurae extend to T12 posteriorly and follow the costal margin around to the sternum (Fig. 3.3).

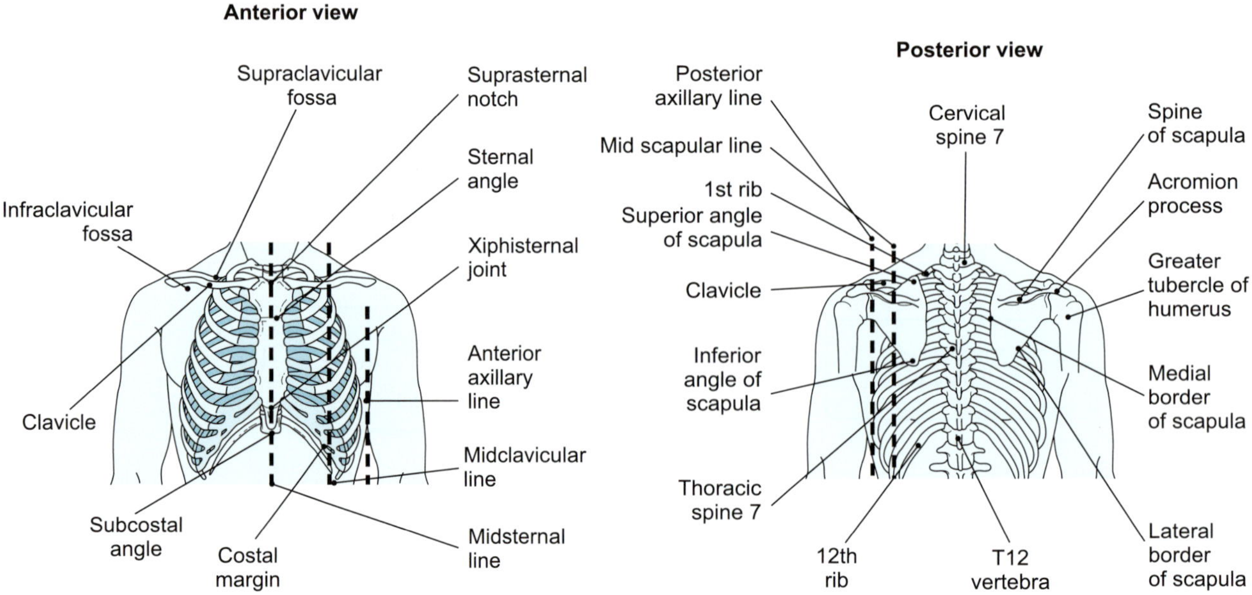

Anterior view

Supraclavicular fossa
Suprasternal notch
Sternal angle
Xiphisternal joint
Infraclavicular fossa
Anterior axillary line
Clavicle
Midclavicular line
Subcostal angle
Costal margin
Midsternal line

Posterior view

Posterior axillary line
Mid scapular line
1st rib
Superior angle of scapula
Clavicle
Inferior angle of scapula
Thoracic spine 7
12th rib
T12 vertebra
Cervical spine 7
Spine of scapula
Acromion process
Greater tubercle of humerus
Medial border of scapula
Lateral border of scapula

Fig. 3.2 Surface markings of the anterior and posterior thoracic walls.

Ribs and costal cartilages

There are 12 pairs of ribs that articulate with the vertebral column posteriorly. Anteriorly, ribs 1 to 7 articulate directly with the sternum (true ribs) and ribs 8 to 10 articulate with the costal cartilage of the rib above (false ribs). Ribs 11 and 12 do not articulate anteriorly and are known as floating ribs.

Typical ribs

A typical rib has the following features (Fig. 3.4):

- A head with two demifacets to articulate with its own vertebrae and the vertebra above.
- The neck between the head and the tubercle.
- The tubercle articulates with the transverse process of its own vertebrae.

CLINICAL NOTES

THORACIC OUTLET OBSTRUCTION

Cervical ribs are found in 1% of patients and can range from small stubs to fully formed ribs. They are a known cause of thoracic outlet obstruction.

Atypical ribs

The first rib has many features not seen in the other ribs. It is shorter, broader and more sharply curved. The scalene tubercle lies on the inner border and is the attachment of the anterior scalene muscle. The subclavian artery and vein pass posteriorly and anteriorly to this tubercle, respectively. The artery forms the subclavian groove in the rib's surface.

Intercostal spaces

There are 11 paired intercostal spaces and each one contains a neurovascular bundle and three muscle layers (Fig. 3.4). The three muscles are the external, internal and innermost intercostal muscles. The innermost muscle is lined with endothoracic fascia and the parietal pleura.

Intercostal nerves and vessels

The intercostal nerves are formed from the anterior rami of the corresponding spinal nerves T1 to T11. The anterior rami of T12 runs inferior to the 12th rib and is known as the subcostal nerve. Each intercostal nerve initially runs between the parietal pleura and the posterior intercostal membrane; then at the angle of the rib, the nerve comes to lie in the costal groove of the corresponding rib between the internal and innermost muscle.

Each intercostal nerve has several branches:

- Rami communicantes branch to the sympathetic trunk.
- A collateral branch at the angle of the rib, which then runs superior to the rib.

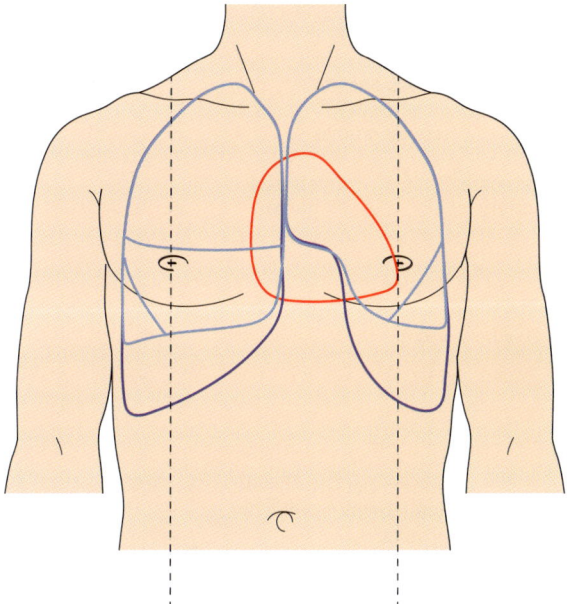

Fig. 3.3 Anterior view of the surface anatomy of the thorax: lungs at expiration *(light blue)* and full inspiration *(dark blue)*. (Adapted from Standring, S. (Ed.). (2016). *Gray's anatomy* (41st ed.). Elsevier.)

THORACIC WALL

The bony structure of the thoracic wall is composed of the sternum, the ribs and the vertebrae.

Sternum

The sternum has three components:

1. *The manubrium:* Articulates with the first and second rib. The sternal notch (jugular notch) is palpable at the superior border of the manubrium.
2. *Body of sternum:* Forms the main part of the sternum and articulates with ribs 2 to 7.
3. *Xiphisternum:* The most inferior part of the sternum. It can be palpated at the junction of the sternum and the epigastrium.

HINTS AND TIPS

The sternal angle (also known as the angle of Louis) sits at the level of T4, between the manubrium and the body of the sternum, and articulates with the second ribs laterally. During examination, the sternal angle is used as a surface landmark to identify thoracic structures during clinical examination, including auscultation of the heart and lungs.

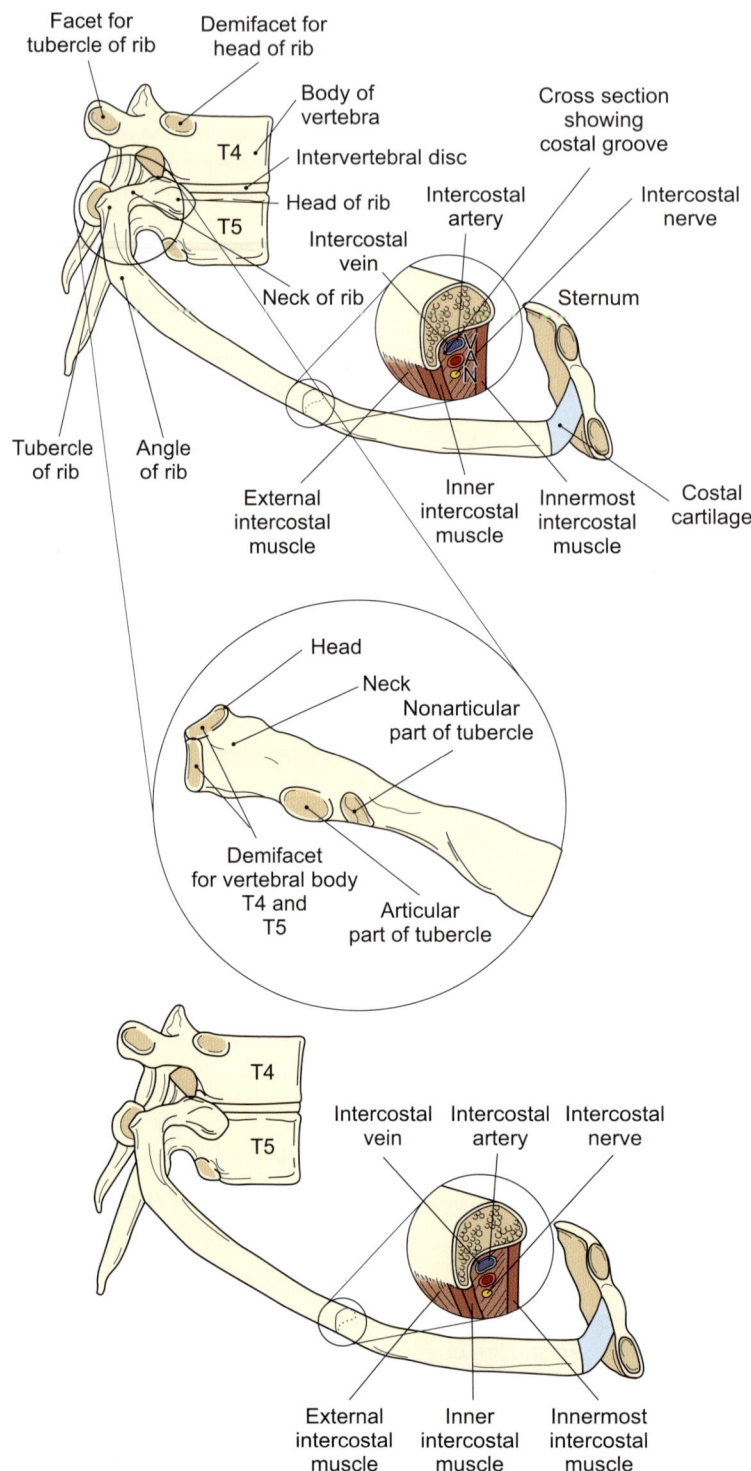

Fig. 3.4 Right fifth rib with the inset showing the posterior surface of the rib. A typical rib including the intercostal muscles and neurovascular bundle.

- Lateral cutaneous branch, which divides into an anterior and posterior branch to supply the skin.
- Terminal branch: the anterior cutaneous branch further divides into medial and lateral branches.

The first intercostal nerve divides into a superior and inferior branch, the former joining the brachial plexus and the latter passing beneath the first rib and running in the first intercostal space. The 7th to 11th intercostal nerves pass from the intercostal space to lie between the anterior abdominal wall muscles at the costal margin to supply the skin of the anterior abdominal wall.

HINTS AND TIPS

The neurovascular bundle runs in a groove at the inferior border of each rib. The order of structures from superior to inferior can be remembered with the acronym 'VAN' (*v*ein, *a*rtery, *n*erve).

Openings into the thorax

Thoracic inlet (superior thoracic aperture)

The thoracic inlet allows communication between the neck and the thoracic cavity. It is bounded posteriorly by the T1 vertebrae, laterally by the first rib and anteriorly by the superior border of the manubrium of the sternum. The thoracic inlet transmits the oesophagus, trachea, lung apices and the major vessels and nerves.

Thoracic outlet (inferior thoracic aperture)

The thoracic outlet lies between the thorax above and the abdominal cavity below. It is bound by the T12 vertebrae, the 12th ribs and the xiphisternum. The thoracic outlet is filled by the diaphragm. Fig. 3.5 shows the structures that pass through the diaphragm. Table 3.1 shows the arterial supply to the thoracic wall.

Diaphragm

The diaphragm is the primary muscle of respiration and consists of a central tendon and peripheral muscular segments (costal section). The costal segment inserts onto the sternum and the lower six ribs. The diaphragm has a left and right dome, with the right being higher owing to the presence of the liver below it. The crural region of the diaphragm has two crura that pass on either side of the oesophagus and insert onto the vertebrae (right onto L1–L3 and left onto L1–L2). During inspiration, the diaphragm contracts downwards to increase thoracic volume. The blood and nerve supply of the diaphragm are shown in Table 3.2.

THORACIC CAVITY

The thoracic cavity contains the pleural cavity and lungs laterally and the mediastinum centrally.

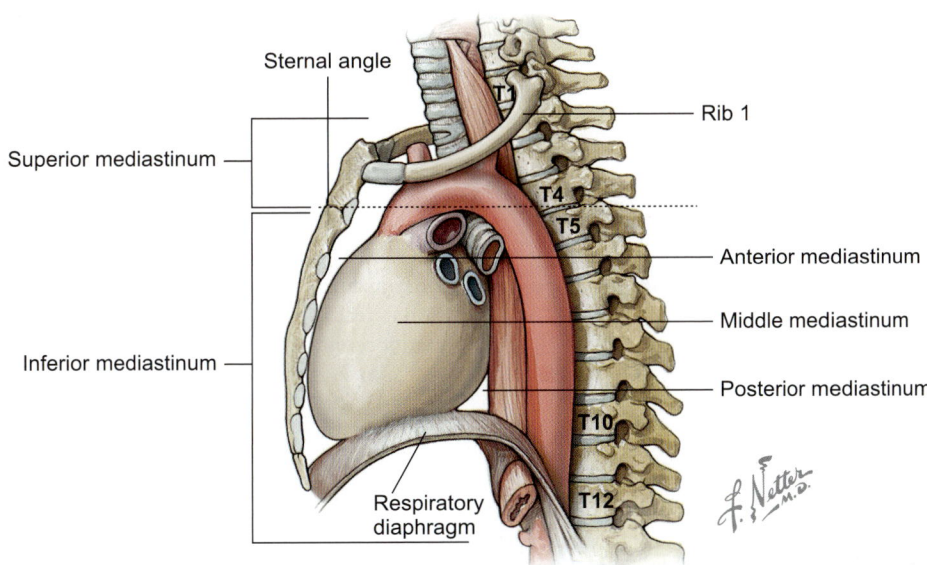

Fig. 3.5 Lateral view of the mediastinum. (From Hansen, J. (2023). *Netter's clinical anatomy* (5th ed.). Elsevier Inc.)

Table 3.1 Arterial supply to the thoracic wall

Artery	Origin	Distribution
Anterior intercostal (spaces 1–6)	Internal thoracic artery	Intercostal spaces and parietal pleura
Anterior intercostal (spaces 7–9)	Musculophrenic artery	
Posterior intercostal (spaces 1–2)	Superior intercostal artery (from costocervical trunk of subclavian artery)	
Posterior intercostal (all other spaces)	Thoracic aorta	
Internal thoracic	Subclavian artery	Runs inferiorly, posterior to the costal cartilages and lateral to the sternum, terminating by dividing into the superior epigastric and musculophrenic arteries
Subcostal	Thoracic aorta	Abdominal wall

Table 3.2 Nerves and vessels of the diaphragm

Innervation	Motor supply: phrenic nerves (C3–C5) Sensory supply: centrally by phrenic nerves (C3–C5), peripherally by intercostal nerves (T5–T11) and subcostal nerve (T12)
Arterial supply	Superior phrenic arteries; musculophrenic arteries; pericardiacophrenic arteries; inferior phrenic arteries
Venous drainage	Musculophrenic and pericardiacophrenic veins drain into internal thoracic vein; superior and inferior phrenic veins
Lymphatic drainage	Diaphragmatic lymph nodes drain to posterior mediastinal nodes, eventually to the superior lumbar lymph nodes; lymphatic plexuses on superior and inferior surfaces communicate freely

Mediastinum

The mediastinum is divided into superior and inferior regions by the angle of Louis. The superior mediastinum is bordered by the manubrium and the T1 to T4 vertebrae. It contains the thymus (in adults), the aortic arch (with its branches), the SVC (and brachiocephalic veins), the trachea and oesophagus and the phrenic and vagus nerves.

The inferior mediastinum is divided into anterior, middle and posterior sections.

- Anterior: Between the sternum and pericardium. It contains fat, lymph nodes and, in children, the thymus.
- Middle: Contains the pericardium, heart, ascending aorta and pulmonary trunk.
- Posterior: Between the pericardium and the thoracic vertebra. It contains the thoracic descending aorta, oesophagus, azygos veins and sympathetic trunks. Note that the posterior mediastinum extends from T4 to T12 owing to the long posterior surface of the diaphragm dome.

Nerves of the thorax

The phrenic nerves originate from spinal nerves C3 to C5. The right nerve runs lateral to the SVC, anterior to the hilum of the lung, and continues lateral to the inferior vena cava (IVC) before piercing the diaphragm. The left phrenic nerve also passes anterior to the hilum and along the pericardium overlying the left ventricle. The phrenic nerves provide both motor supply to the diaphragm and sensory information from the central tendon, with the sensation of the lateral diaphragm supplied by the intercostal nerves.

The vagus nerves originate in the brainstem and exit the skull through the jugular foramen to run in the carotid sheath. The right vagus nerve runs anterior to the subclavian artery (where it gives off the right recurrent laryngeal branch) and behind the brachiocephalic vein until it lies on the lateral surface of the trachea. Unlike the phrenic nerve, the vagus nerves run posterior to the lung hila. In the superior mediastinum, the vagus nerve (cranial nerve 10) gives off cardiac branches before reforming along the oesophagus, which it follows into the abdomen. The left vagus nerve takes the same course as the right except that it gives off its recurrent laryngeal branch as it passes over the aortic arch.

HINTS AND TIPS

'C3, C4, C5 keeps the diaphragm alive.' – Phrenic nerve

Thoracic sympathetic trunk

The sympathetic trunks lie over the heads of the ribs. There is a ganglion for each spinal nerve except for T1, which merges with the inferior cervical ganglion to form the stellate ganglion. White and grey rami communicantes connect the sympathetic trunk to the spinal nerves. Branches from the T1 to T6 ganglia innervate the thorax and heart. Ganglia from T7 to T12 innervate the abdominal cavity via the greater (T7–T9), lesser (T10–T11) and least (T12) splanchnic nerves, which pass posterior to the diaphragm.

Trachea

The trachea begins at the level of C6 at the lower border of the cricoid cartilage. It runs in the superior mediastinum anterior to

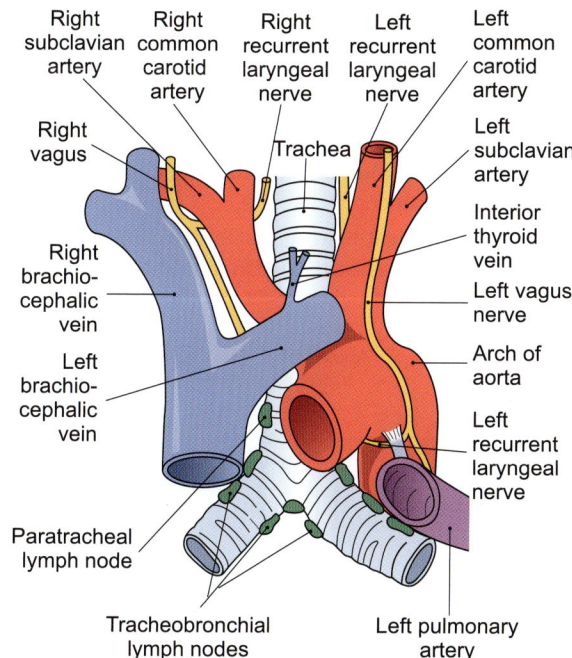

Fig. 3.6 Trachea and its main relations anteriorly and laterally.

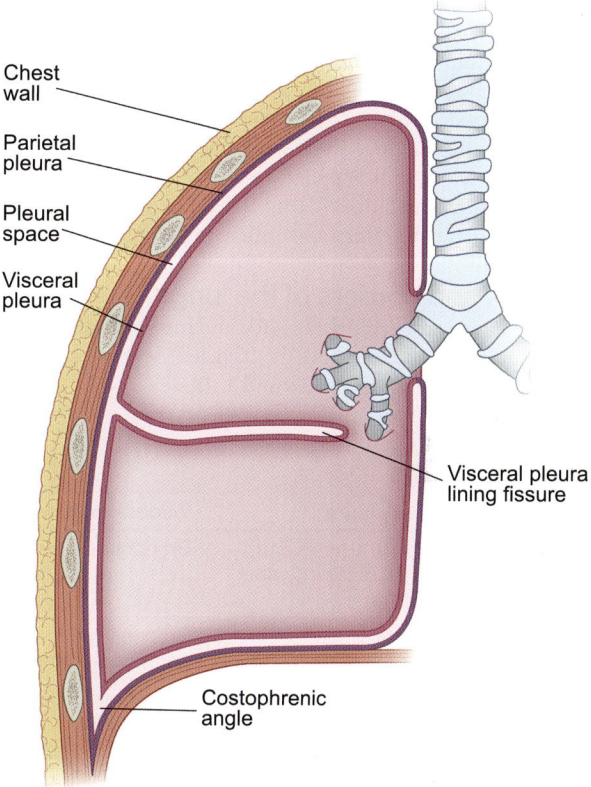

Fig. 3.7 The visceral and parietal pleurae with the pleural space in between.

the oesophagus (Fig. 3.6). At the sternal angle (T4), the trachea bifurcates into the right and left main bronchi. This bifurcation is called the carina. The right main bronchus is wider, straighter and shorter than the left, which is why it is the usual location for lodged aspirated material or foreign bodies. The trachea is supported by C-shaped cartilaginous rings in its wall that help maintain its shape and stop it from collapsing during respiration.

PLEURAE AND LUNGS

Pleurae

Each pleural cavity is lined by the pleural membrane. The membrane covering the internal surface of the thoracic wall is the parietal pleura, and the lining covering the lung is the visceral pleura. The two pleurae are continuous at the hilum of the lung. The parietal pleura is named after the surface that it covers (costal, mediastinal and diaphragmatic). The visceral pleura invaginates into the fissures of the lungs. The parietal and visceral pleurae with the pleural space in between are seen in Fig. 3.7.

At the inferior hilum, a double fold of pleura hangs down (the pulmonary ligament), which allows space for the hilum to descend during inspiration.

The pleural space between the two layers of pleura contains 4 mL of pleural fluid that acts as a lubricant to allow the lung to move freely. Certain medical conditions cause an increase in the volume of pleural fluid, called a pleural effusion.

The arterial supply and venous and lymphatic drainage of the pleura are described in Table 3.3.

CLINICAL NOTES

PLEURAL DISEASES

Many respiratory pathologies impact the pleura and pleural space. Inflammation of the pleura is called pleuritis and causes a localised sharp pain that is worse on inspiration. If any substance enters the pleural space, it can collapse the lung and cause difficulty breathing. The name of the pathology depends on the substance within the pleural space:

- Air: pneumothorax
- Fluid: pleural effusion
- Blood: haemothorax
- Pus: empyema

Lungs

The lungs are light, spongy organs responsible for gas exchange. Their gross colour is pink, but this darkens with age due to breathing atmospheric pollution. The right lung comprises three lobes (further divided into 10 bronchopulmonary segments), and the left lung comprises two (with nine bronchopulmonary segments). Each lung is supplied by a main bronchus, which divides into segmental bronchi (Fig. 3.8). When the airways no longer contain cartilage, they are termed bronchioles.

Surfaces and borders of the lungs

The lungs have a costal, diaphragmatic and mediastinal surface, and the apices extend 2 cm above the clavicle. The gross structure of the lungs can be seen in Figs 3.9 and 3.10.

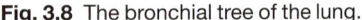

Table 3.3 Arterial supply, venous drainage and lymphatic drainage of the pleura		
	Parietal pleura	**Visceral pleura**
Arterial supply	Intercostal arteries and branches of the internal thoracic artery	Bronchial arteries
Venous drainage	Intercostal veins	Bronchial and pulmonary veins
Lymphatic drainage	Intercostal, internal thoracic (parasternal), posterior mediastinal and diaphragmatic nodes	Bronchopulmonary (hilar) nodes

Blood supply of the lungs

The lungs have a dual blood supply:

1. *Bronchial arteries from the aorta:* Supply the walls of the bronchi and bronchial tree down to the level of the terminal bronchioles.
2. *Pulmonary arteries:* Receive the entire cardiac output from the right ventricle and supply the blood undergoing gas exchange (pulmonary circulation).

The pulmonary circulation begins at the pulmonary artery, containing partially deoxygenated blood from the right ventricle. This then splits into the right and left main branches, which go to their

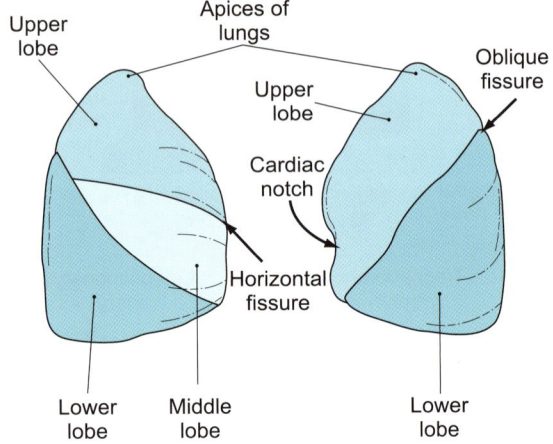

Fig. 3.9 Surface of the lungs (anterior view).

Fig. 3.8 The bronchial tree of the lung.

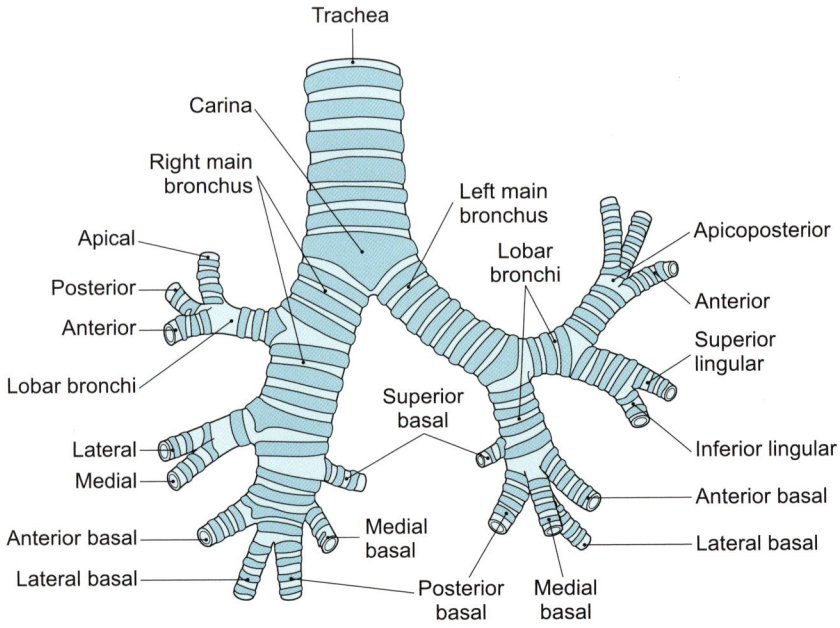

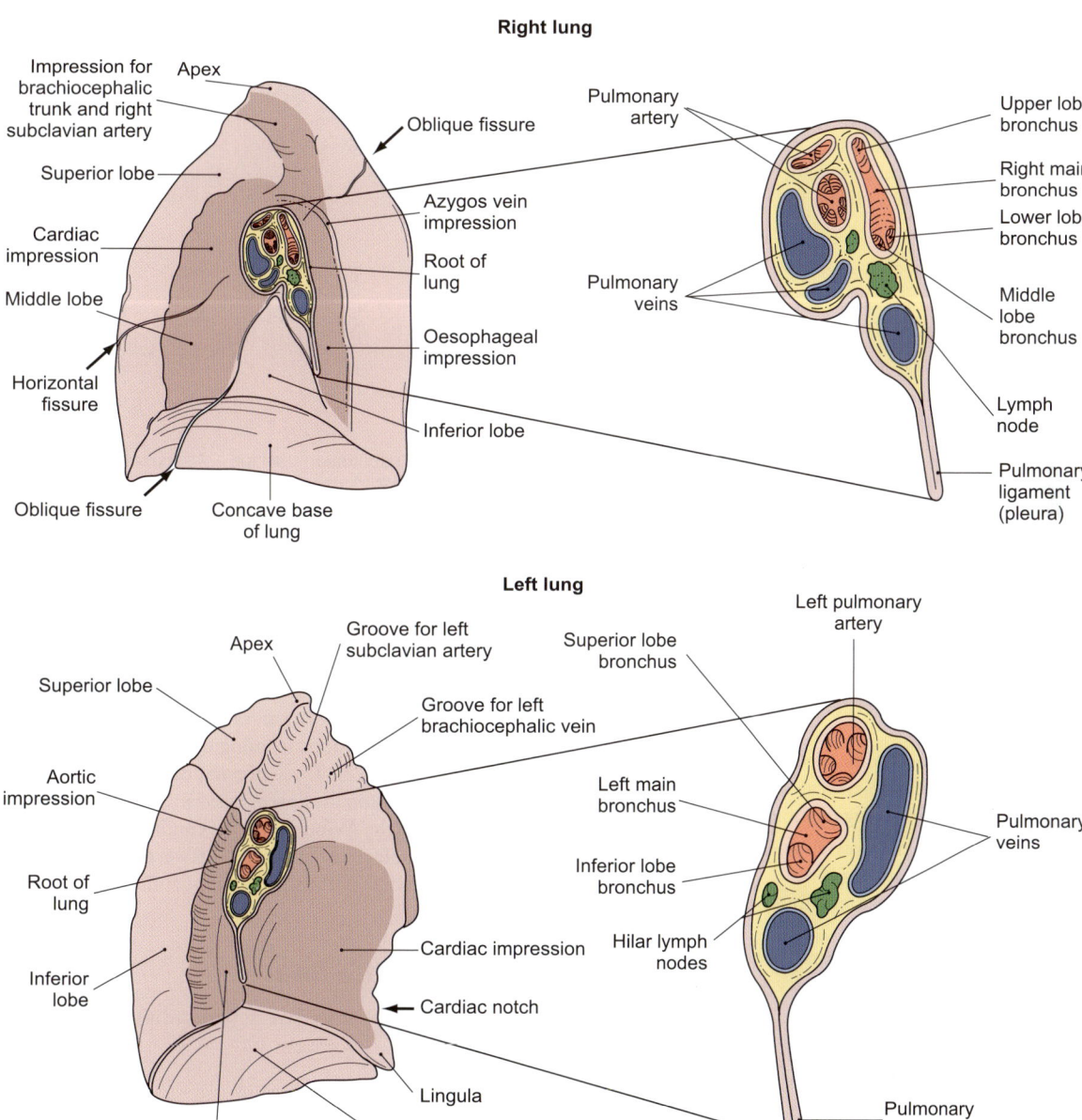

Fig. 3.10 Medial aspect of the right and left lungs and contents of their roots. Impressions are only seen in fixed lungs.

respective lungs. These main arteries branch successively, closely following the airways. Beyond the terminal bronchioles, the vessels form the capillary bed starting with smaller arterioles that function as capillaries, as gaseous exchange starts at this level. The capillary bed forms a dense network in the walls of the 300 million alveoli; this bed is made up of approximately 280 billion capillaries. Hence, a rich mesh structure, likened to a flowing blood sheet, produces a huge surface area for gaseous exchange; the area is estimated at 50 to 100 m². As the average pulmonary capillary diameter is 6 mm, erythrocytes with a diameter of 8 mm have to squeeze through, thereby reducing the diffusion distance and facilitating efficient gaseous exchange. Oxygenated blood then flows into the pulmonary veins, which pass between lung lobules. These are also short and unite to form four large veins that empty into the left atrium.

The pulmonary circulatory vessels differ from their systemic counterparts in the following ways:

- Thinner walls.
- Less vascular smooth muscle.
- No particular muscular vessels.
- Greater distensibility and compliance.
- Terminal branches have a greater internal diameter.
- Rapid subdivision.

CLINICAL NOTES

PULMONARY EMBOLUS

Venous thrombosis in the deep veins of the legs can embolize, travel through the right side of the heart and lodge in the pulmonary circulation. This impairs blood flow and thus blood oxygenation, resulting in hypoxia. This is called a pulmonary embolus. Severe impairment of blood flow can cause circulatory collapse.

Nerve supply of the lungs

The nerves are supplied by the sympathetic and parasympathetic system via the nerve plexus at the hilum.

Position of the heart

The heart is located in the middle mediastinum, which is the central compartment of the thorax, located between the two pleural sacs. The heart has the following relations:

- *Superior to the heart:* great vessels and bronchi.
- *Inferior to the heart:* diaphragm.
- *Lateral to the heart:* pleurae and lungs.
- *Anterior to the heart:* thymus.
- *Posterior to the heart:* oesophagus.

CLINICAL NOTES

APEX BEAT

The apex of the heart (the most inferior and lateral point of the heart) is normally located at the fifth intercostal space in the midclavicular line. Displacement of the apex can signify pathology. For example, the apex beat may move inferior and laterally with heart failure. Palpation and auscultation over the apex beat, therefore, form part of a routine cardiovascular system examination. Fig. 3.11 shows the normal physiological position of the heart within the thorax and identifies where a stethoscope should be placed during auscultation of the heart.

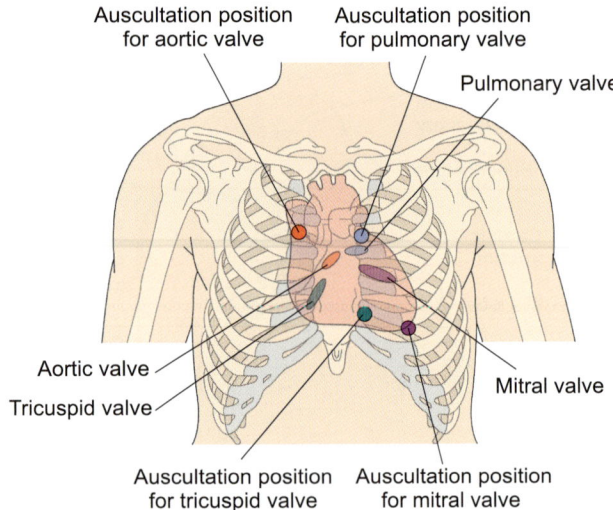

Fig. 3.11 Surface anatomy of the heart.

Skeleton of the heart

The cardiac skeleton consists of four bands of dense collagenous tissue, known as fibrous rings. The muscle fibres of the atria and ventricles are attached to a pair of fibrous rings around the atrio-ventricular (AV) orifices, forming the bases of the cusps of the AV valves (Fig. 3.12). These prevent distension during cardiac contraction and stop the flow of nerve impulses between the atria and ventricles (the AV bundle of the conducting system provides the only physiological connection between the atria and ventricles). Two further fibrous rings support the aortic and pulmonary valves.

Layers of the heart

The heart wall has three layers: pericardium, myocardium and endocardium.

Pericardium

The pericardium is a fibroserous sac enclosing the heart and the roots of the great vessels. It is composed of two layers. The strong outer layer, the fibrous pericardium, limits the movement of the heart and is attached inferiorly to the central tendon of the diaphragm, anteriorly to the sternum (via the sternopericardial ligaments) and superiorly to the tunica adventitia of the great vessels. The inner layer is known as the serous pericardium and is itself divided into two layers—the parietal pericardium, which is firmly adherent to the fibrous pericardium, and the visceral pericardium, a serous layer that reflects onto the great vessels and surface of the heart. The visceral pericardium also forms the outer layer

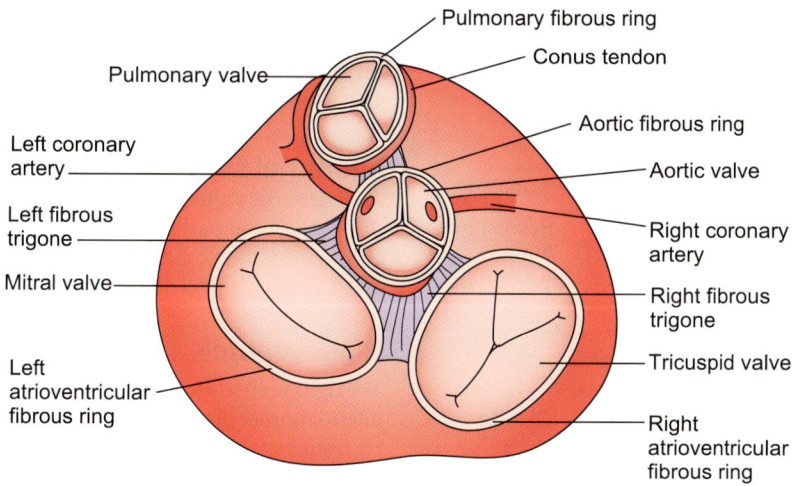

Fig. 3.12 Skeleton of the heart.

of the heart, known as the epicardium. There is a potential space between the parietal and visceral pericardial layers, which is normally filled with a thin layer of serous fluid (approximately 50 mL), allowing the heart to move smoothly within the pericardium. The main arterial supply to the pericardium is via the pericardiacophrenic artery (a branch of the internal thoracic artery). Venous drainage is via the pericardiacophrenic veins and the azygos veins. The phrenic nerve (C3–C5) provides sensory innervation to the fibrous and parietal layers of the pericardium. This can result in referred pain to the skin above the clavicle within the C3–C5 dermatomes. The visceral layer has no somatic innervation and so is insensitive to pain.

CLINICAL NOTES

PERICARDIAL DISEASES

Pericarditis (inflammation of the pericardium) occurs secondary to many causes, including bacterial or viral infection. It results in central chest pain that is worse on inspiration and is relieved by sitting forward. A pericardial rub may be heard on auscultation, caused by inflammation of the opposing pericardial surfaces. Blood (haemopericardium) or fluid (pericardial effusion) in the pericardium may result in cardiac tamponade (compression of the heart) due to the indistensible nature of the fibrous pericardium. The result is a heart that cannot contract fully, leading to falling cardiac output and death if untreated.

Pericardial sinuses

Pericardial sinuses are spaces within the pericardial sac. The two main pericardial sinuses are the oblique sinus and transverse sinus:

- The reflection of the serous pericardium around the pulmonary veins forms a recess posterior to the left atrium known as the oblique sinus. The oesophagus lies immediately posterior to the oblique sinus.
- The transverse sinus is formed from a reflection of the serous pericardium around the aorta and the pulmonary trunk anteriorly, and around the SVC and pulmonary veins posteriorly. The transverse sinus separates the arterial outflow and venous inflow of the heart (Fig. 3.13).

Myocardium

This makes up the majority of the heart and consists of cardiac muscle cells (myocytes) that are responsible for its contractility. Myocytes have the following features:

- A striated and branched network.
- They are 50 to 100 μm in length and 10 to 20 μm in diameter.
- A single nucleus is (usually) present.
- A dense mitochondrial network.

The myocytes are connected by intercalated discs that help the cells adhere at desmosomes (proteoglycan bridges that glue cells together). Between these are gap junctions made of connexin proteins. These pores allow electrical conductivity through the myocardium.

Like skeletal muscle, the myocytes contain actin and myosin filaments—the contractile components of the heart. The actin and myosin form a similar network to that in skeletal muscle (see Chapter 9), with M and Z lines and A, H and I bands. At the Z

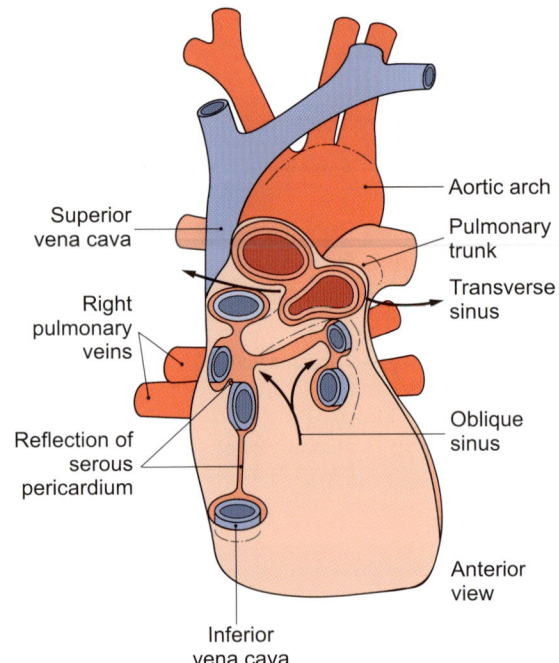

Superior
vena cava

Right
pulmonary
veins

Reflection of
serous
pericardium

Inferior
vena cava

Aortic arch

Pulmonary
trunk

Transverse
sinus

Oblique
sinus

Anterior
view

Fig. 3.13 Pericardial sinuses. (Adapted from Williams, P. (Ed.). (1995). *Gray's anatomy* (38th ed.). Churchill Livingstone.)

line, the sarcolemma forms the transverse tubular structure, which enables rapid electrical conduction by activating the whole contractile apparatus. The sarcoplasmic reticulum stores the calcium required for muscle contraction.

Endocardium

The endocardium has three layers and is continuous with the endothelial lining of the large blood vessels attached to the heart:

- Outermost connective tissue layer containing nerves, veins and Purkinje fibres (specialized conducting fibres).
- Middle layer of connective tissue.
- Inner layer of endothelial cells.

Chambers of the heart

The heart has four chambers of varying size and wall thickness dependent on function. The right and left sides of the heart are separated by the interatrial and interventricular septa. The atrium and ventricles are separated by the AV septum.

Right atrium

The right atrium forms the right border of the heart. It consists of the right atrium proper and an atrial appendage, the right auricle. The ridged anterior wall of the atrium (composed of pectinate muscles) and the smooth posterior wall are separated by a ridge known as the crista terminals, and externally by a groove known as the sulcus terminalis. The right atrium receives blood from the SVC, the IVC and the coronary sinus.

Interatrial septum

The interatrial septum separates the left and right atria. A depression in the lower part of the septum, known as the fossa ovalis, is a remnant of the closed foramen ovale of the foetal heart. Failure of this closure after birth results in an ASD.

Right ventricle

The right ventricle forms the majority of the anterior surface and inferior border of the heart. Its internal surface has several notable features:

- *Trabeculae carneae:* Irregular muscular bundles that line the wall of the ventricle.
- *The moderator band:* Runs from the interventricular septum to the anterior wall of the ventricle and transmits part of the conducting system of the heart.
- *Chordae tendineae:* Fibrous cords attached to both the free edges of the tricuspid valve and to the papillary muscles within the wall of the ventricle.
- *The infundibulum:* The outflow tract of the right ventricle.

Left atrium

The left atrium forms most of the base of the heart. It consists of the left atrium proper and the left auricle. The interior of the atrium is smooth, while the auricle is ridged due to the presence of pectinate muscles. Four pulmonary veins open into the posterior wall of the atrium delivering oxygenated blood from the pulmonary circulation.

Left ventricle

The left ventricle forms the apex and left border of the heart. It supplies blood to the entire body, with the exception of the lungs. Its wall is three times thicker than that of the right ventricle, and pressures within it are up to six times greater. Its internal surface has several notable features, some of which are similar to those of the right ventricle:

- Well-developed trabeculae carneae.
- Chordae tendineae between the free edges of the aortic valve and the papillary muscles.
- The aortic vestibule: the outflow tract of the left ventricle.

The interventricular septum is of equal thickness to the rest of the left ventricle, and consequently, it bulges into the right ventricle. It is composed of a superior membranous region and an inferior muscular region and transmits the AV bundle of the conduction system.

CLINICAL NOTES

CONGENITAL HEART DEFECTS

Failure of the foramen ovale to close results in an atrial septal defect (ASD). This allows oxygenated blood to pass from the left atrium into the right atrium as pressure in the left atrium is greater than in the right atrium and blood flows from an area of higher pressure to an area of lower pressure. This is an example of a left-to-right shunt and results in enlargement of the right atrium and ventricle, along with dilatation of the pulmonary trunk. The resulting increased blood flow through the pulmonary vasculature can result in pulmonary hypertension. A defect in the interventricular septum (in either its muscular or membranous part) is known as a ventricular septal defect (VSD). The majority of VSDs in the muscular part of the septum will close spontaneously; membranous VSDs are less likely to do so. Failure of a VSD to close leads to a left-to-right shunt, an increase in pulmonary blood flow and pulmonary hypertension. Defects in the membranous part are likely to be associated with defects in the formation of the valves.

Heart valves

The heart valves respond to pressure changes in the heart and ensure blood travels in one direction. There are two main groups.

Atrioventricular valves

The AV valves are positioned between the atria and ventricles. The right AV valve, commonly known as the tricuspid valve, allows flow from the right atrium to the right ventricle. The tricuspid valve has three cusps (anterior, posterior and septal).

On the left side of the heart, the left AV valve, known as the mitral valve, allows flow from the left atrium to the left ventricle. The mitral valve is bicuspid with an anterior and posterior cusp.

The bases of the AV valves are attached to the fibrous ring of the skeleton of the heart, with the free edges of the cusps being attached to the papillary muscles via the chordae tendineae.

Semilunar valves

There are two semilunar (SL) valves, the pulmonary valve and the aortic valve. They prevent blood flowing back into the ventricles from their respective outflow tract. On the right side of the heart, the pulmonary valve allows communication of the right ventricle with the pulmonary artery. The pulmonary valve has three cusps (anterior, left and right). Above each cusp, the pulmonary artery bulges to form the pulmonary sinuses.

On the left side of the heart, the left ventricle communicates with the aorta through the aortic valve, which also has three cusps (posterior, right and left). Similar to the pulmonary valve, above each cusp of the aortic valve is a bulge in the aortic wall giving rise to the aortic sinuses. The right and left aortic sinuses give rise to the right and left coronary arteries respectively.

CLINICAL NOTES

VALVULAR DISEASE

Remember: When listening to the heart sounds, the first sound (S1) is the *closure* of the AV valves, and the second (S2) is the *closure* of the SL valves. Obstruction of flow through a valve or insufficiency of a valve will lead to an audible 'murmur' as blood passes through the pathological valve. For example, with aortic stenosis, there is an additional crescendo-like sound between S1 and S2, which reflects the blood moving through the narrowed aortic valve. This specific pathological heart sound is known as an ejection systolic murmur.

Blood supply to the heart

Fig. 3.14 illustrates the blood supply of the heart. The right and left coronary arteries are the first branches of the aorta, arising from the right and left aortic sinuses. The coronary arteries give off a series of important branches, supplying the myocardium and epicardium (the blood supply to the endocardium comes directly from the chambers of the heart). The left coronary artery (LCA) is short and quickly divides into circumflex and anterior interventricular (commonly known as the left anterior descending artery (LAD)) branches. The circumflex branch passes posteriorly in the coronary groove, supplying the left atrium and left ventricle, before anastomosing with the right coronary artery in the coronary groove. The anterior interventricular branch runs in the anterior interventricular groove, supplying both ventricles and the interventricular septum, before anastomosing at the apex of the heart with the posterior interventricular artery.

The right coronary artery (RCA) gives off branches to the right atrium and right ventricle as it descends in the coronary groove. A right marginal branch runs along the inferior border of the heart to supply the right ventricle. On the inferior surface of the heart, the RCA anastomoses with the circumflex artery of the LCA. It also gives off a posterior interventricular (or right posterior descending) branch, which runs in the posterior interventricular groove and supplies both ventricles and the interventricular septum. The RCA supplies the sinoatrial node via a sinoatrial branch in 60% of individuals and the AV node in 90% of individuals. It also supplies the AV bundle (of His) and its

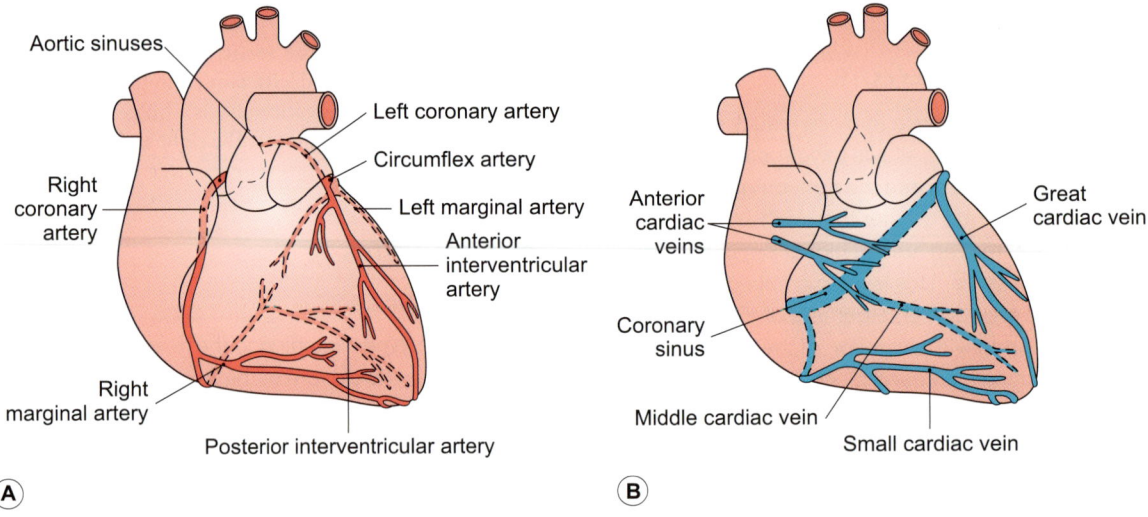

Fig. 3.14 Blood supply of the heart. (A) Coronary arteries; (B) cardiac veins.

right terminal branch. The left terminal branch is supplied by both the RCA and LCA.

Left and right dominance of the heart refers to the coronary artery from which the posterior interventricular branch arises. Right dominance is more common.

CLINICAL NOTES

ISCHAEMIC HEART DISEASE

Ischaemic heart disease results from lipid deposition (atheroma) within the tunica intima and tunica media of the coronary arteries. The result is stenosis (narrowing) of the coronary arteries, reducing the blood, and hence oxygen supply, to the myocardium. This leads to reduced exercise tolerance, angina pectoris, or if the vessel lumen is completely occluded, a myocardial infarction. The anterior interventricular artery (left anterior descending artery) is most commonly affected. Stenosis or occlusion can be overcome via percutaneous coronary intervention, which involves the insertion of a balloon catheter into the region of stenosis or occlusion, via either the femoral or radial artery. The balloon is inflated, compressing the area of atheroma. This is followed by the insertion of a stent, which ensures the affected region remains patent. Alternatively, a coronary artery bypass grafting operation may be performed. The internal thoracic, gastroepiploic and radial arteries and the long saphenous vein are commonly used as grafts to bypass the affected regions.

Venous drainage of the heart

Most of the venous blood from the heart drains into the coronary sinus, which lies in the posterior part of the coronary sulcus, and drains into the right atrium close to the IVC (Fig. 3.14). The great cardiac vein accompanies and drains the territory of the anterior interventricular artery and empties directly into the coronary sinus. The middle cardiac vein accompanies the posterior interventricular artery and empties directly into the coronary sinus. The small cardiac veins drain the myocardium of the right atrium and empty directly into the coronary sinus, just before it enters the right atrium. The remaining blood is returned to the heart via the anterior cardiac veins, which drain into the right atrium, and other small veins (venae cordis minimae), which open directly into the heart chambers.

Conducting system of the heart

The continual and rhythmic beating of the heart at approximately 72 beats per minute when at rest is due to autorhythmic fibres that repeatedly generate action potentials. Specialized myocytes have the ability to conduct these electrical impulses in a coordinated fashion to control the beating of the heart. One beat of the heart is conducted as follows (Fig. 3.15):

1. Spontaneous depolarization in the sinoatrial (SA) node results in the pacemaker potential. The SA node, also known as the pacemaker of the heart, lies in the upper part of the sulcus terminalis in the right atrium, near the entrance of the SVC.

2. When depolarization reaches the threshold, it generates an action potential (AP) in the myocytes.

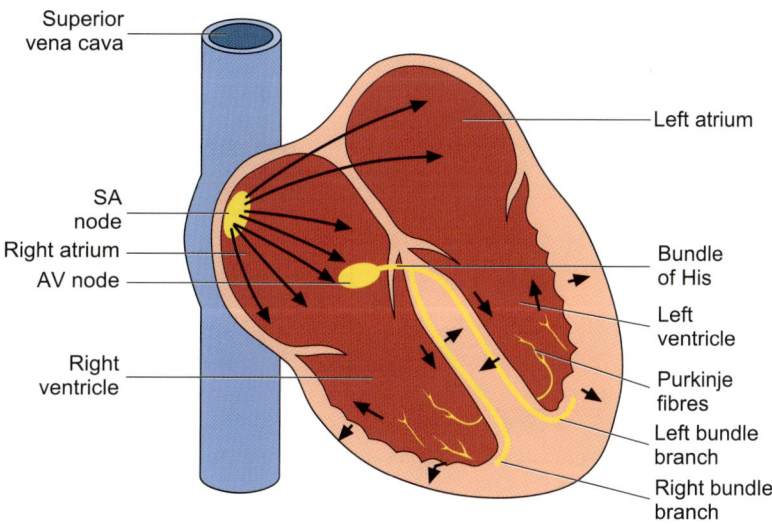

Fig. 3.15 Conducting system of the heart. AV, *Atrioventricular*; SA, *sinoatrial*.

3. The AP propagates to both atria via the gap junctions. This causes the atria to contract in synchrony and pump blood into the ventricles.
4. The AP travels along the cardiac muscle to the AV node, which is located in the AV septum (superior to the origin of the coronary sinus).
5. The AP then enters the bundle of His, located in the membranous part of the interventricular septum, carrying it from the atria to the ventricles.
6. The AP enters the left and right bundle branches, which extend through the interventricular septum towards the apex of the heart. The right bundle conducts impulses to the right ventricles. The left bundle divides into an anterior and posterior fascicle, conducting impulses to the left ventricle.
7. The AP eventually reaches the Purkinje fibres: A network of fine fibres through the ventricular walls. The AP causes synchronous contraction of the ventricles, pushing blood from the right ventricle into the pulmonary artery and from the left ventricle into the aorta.

Action potentials
Myocyte action potential
The three key stages to the formation of an AP in the contractile fibres (Fig. 3.16) are as follows:

1. *Rapid depolarization:* The resting membrane potential of a cardiac cell is $-90\,mV$ because the cells are more permeable to K^+ than to Na^+ (see Chapter 2). When threshold is reached and an AP occurs, voltage-gated Na^+ channels open for a few milliseconds, allowing the entry of Na^+. This produces a rapid depolarization and the fast upstroke. The channels then close.
2. *Plateau:* Voltage-gated slow Ca^{2+} channels then open in the membrane of the sarcoplasmic reticulum, allowing the influx of Ca^{2+} to the cell cytoplasm. This phase influences the strength of contraction. Concurrently, K^+ channels close, causing a decrease in K^+ permeability and a brief depolarization. The Ca^{2+} influx is also responsible for the refractory period of the cell, making it less likely to start another contraction. This is important, as contraction needs to be coordinated or the heart will not have enough time to refill with blood.
3. *Repolarization:* Voltage-gated K^+ channels open, which increases the efflux of K^+. This restores the resting membrane potential of $-90\,mV$ and causes the muscle to relax.

Sinoatrial node action potential
The SA node AP is different from the myocyte AP. It has an unstable resting membrane potential, so when it reaches the threshold value, it triggers an AP (Fig. 3.16). The upstroke is due to the entry of Ca^{2+}. The SA node is regulated by the autonomic nervous system and the hormones epinephrine (adrenaline) and thyroxine; these alter the rate at which the threshold potential is achieved and subsequently the heart rate (HR). There are a number of factors that alter the HR through modulating SA node activity; these can be seen in Table 3.4.

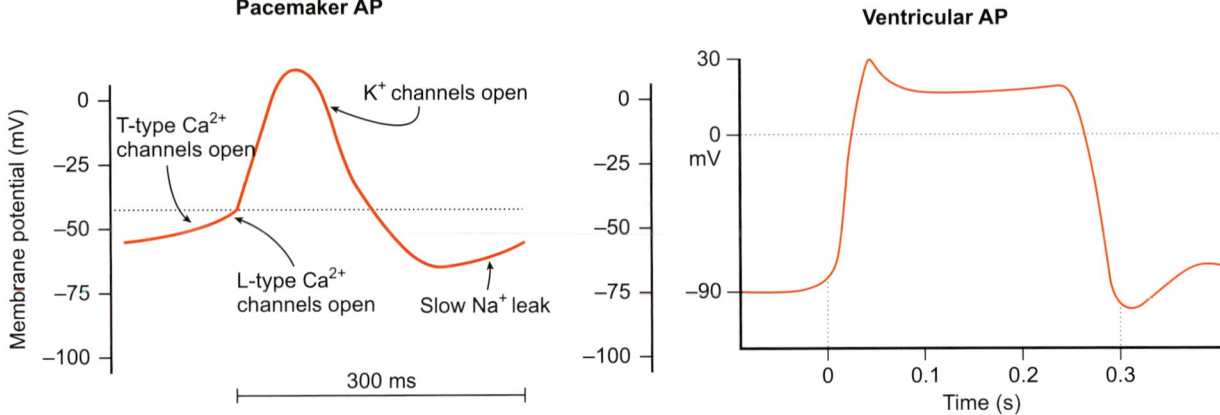

Fig. 3.16 Action potential in a sinoatrial node pacemaker cell and ventricular myocyte AP, *Action potential*.

Table 3.4 Factors increasing and decreasing heart rate via sinoatrial node

Increased rate	Decreased rate
High sympathetic tone	High vagal tone
Hyperthyroidism	Hypothyroidism
Hypokalaemia	Hyperkalaemia
	Hypoxia
Antimuscarinics, e.g. atropine	β-Blockers

CARDIAC CYCLE

The cardiac cycle is the sequence of pressure and volume changes that occur with one complete heartbeat.

Events of the cardiac cycle

The events of the cardiac cycle are as follows (Fig. 3.17):

1. Atrial and ventricular filling (diastole): all the chambers of the heart are relaxed, and there is passive filling of both the atria and ventricles.
2. Atrial contraction (atrial systole) lasts for 0.1 second, adding about 25 mL to the relaxed ventricles, producing a final volume of ~130 mL. The ventricles are still relaxed at this stage.
3. Ventricular systole (lasts for 0.3 second): both ventricles contract. The pressure inside the ventricles increases and closes the AV valves. For about 0.06 second, both the SL and AV valves are shut. This is when the cardiac muscle fibres are contracting but not yet shortening (isovolumetric contraction).
4. When the ventricular pressure exceeds aortic and pulmonary pressure, both SL valves open (ventricular

ejection) and blood is expelled into the aorta and pulmonary trunk. The amount of blood ejected per ventricle (around 70 mL) is called the stroke volume (SV). The volume remaining in the ventricles after ventricular systole is called the end-systolic volume (ESV).

Regulation of cardiac output

Definitions

- Cardiac output (CO) = the volume of blood ejected by one ventricle into its respective artery each minute. Hence, pulmonary blood flow = systemic blood flow in the aorta.
- Stroke volume (SV) = the volume of blood ejected in one ventricular contraction.
- Heart rate (HR) = number of ventricular contractions in 1 minute.
- End-diastolic volume (EDV) = volume of blood in the ventricle immediately prior to contraction.
- End-systolic volume (ESV) = volume of blood in the ventricle after contraction.
- Central venous pressure (CVP) = pressure of blood in the great veins as it enters the right atrium.
- Systemic vascular resistance (SVR) = resistance of blood flow in the circulatory system.
- Mean arterial blood pressure (MAP) = $CO \times SVR$.
- CO (mL/min) = SV (mL/beat) $\times HR$ (beats/min).

Three things directly affect CO:

1. EDV of the right heart.
2. Resistance to outflow.
3. Functional state of the heart–lung unit.

In a typical adult male, SV averages 70 mL/beat and HR 75 beats/min, so CO = 5.25 L/min. This value is close to the total blood volume. So, effectively, it takes 1 minute for the whole

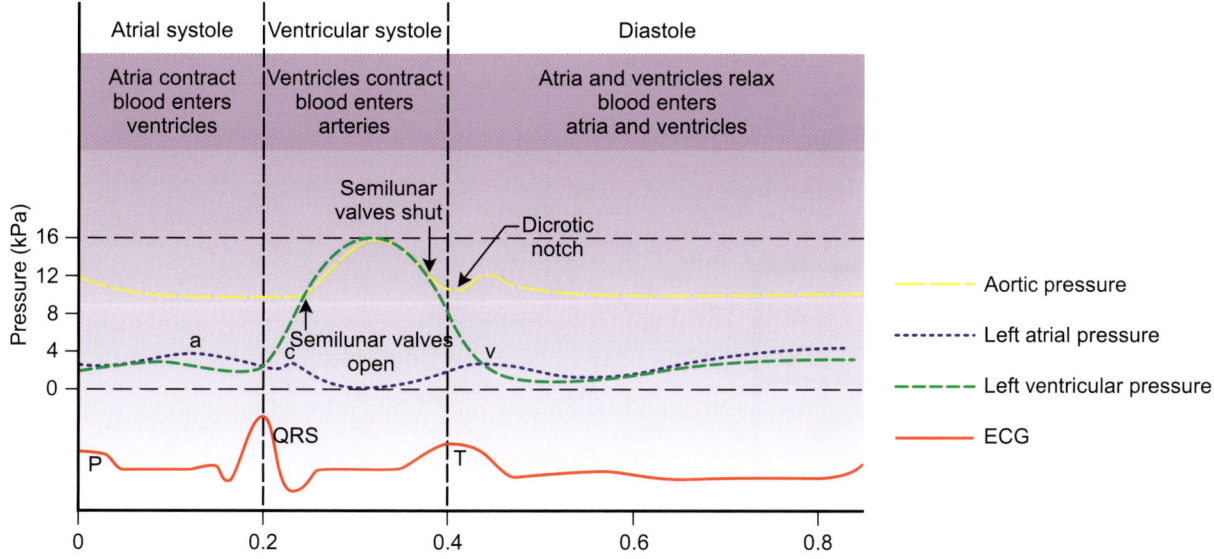

Fig. 3.17 Events in the cardiac cycle with the corresponding electrocardiogram *(ECG)* and atrial and ventricular pressures. a, *Atrial systole*; c, *closure of the mitral valve and its bulging into the left atrium*; v, *atrial filling against closed mitral valve.*

circulation to flow through the pulmonary and systemic systems (Fig. 3.18).

SV is regulated by:

- Preload
- Contractility
- Afterload

Preload

Preload is the degree to which the heart stretches prior to contraction. Within reason, the more the heart stretches, the stronger the force of contraction will be. This is known as Starling's law of the heart (Fig. 3.19). The more blood that enters the heart during diastole, the more the heart will stretch and hence the greater the contraction. Preload is determined by the duration of diastole and volume of venous return. The longer the diastole, the more the ventricles fill. Furthermore, the more blood that is returned to the heart by the venous system, the more it will fill and strengthen contraction. However, if preload becomes excessive in pathological states, that is when fluid gets overloaded during heart failure, the fibrils of the heart become extended beyond physiological limits and thus past their optimum configuration for contraction. This causes a reduction in SV beyond the threshold of optimum preload.

HINTS AND TIPS

Think of an elastic band. The greater the stretch, the faster and more forcefully it will contract. The same effect can be seen in the heart where, within reason, a greater stretch of the myocardium will lead to a more forceful contraction.

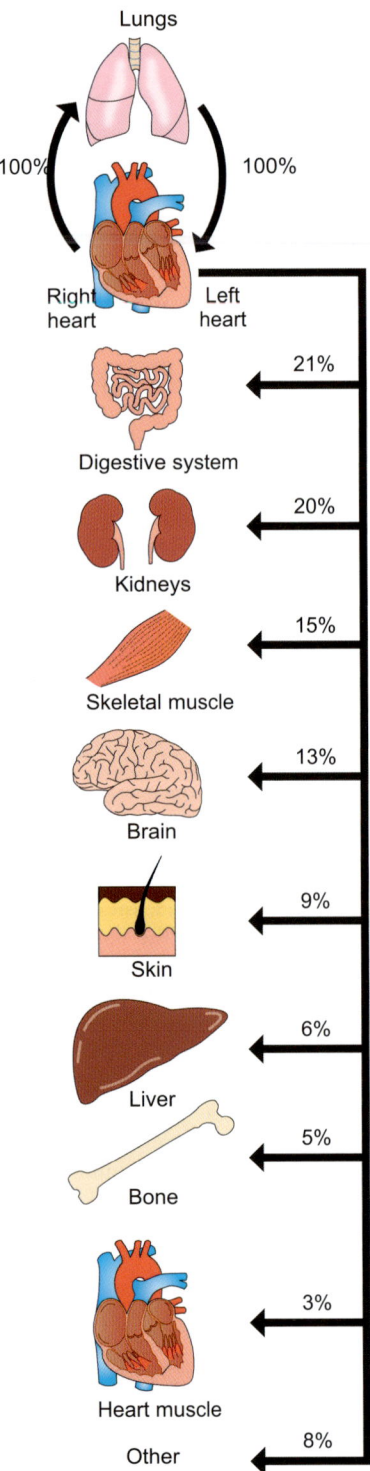

Fig. 3.18 Distribution of cardiac output when at rest.

Lungs

100%   100%

Right heart   Left heart

21% Digestive system

20% Kidneys

15% Skeletal muscle

13% Brain

9% Skin

6% Liver

5% Bone

3% Heart muscle

8% Other

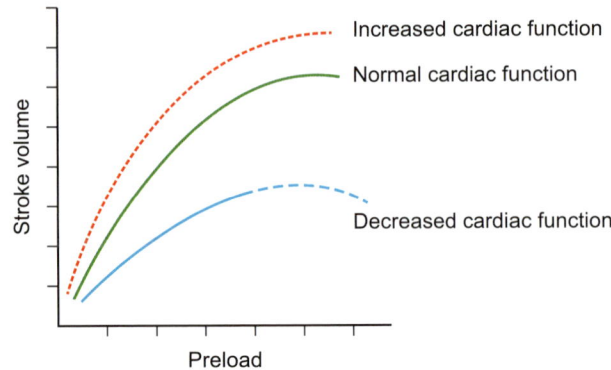

Fig. 3.19 Starling's curve.

Increased cardiac function

Normal cardiac function

Decreased cardiac function

Stroke volume

Preload

Contractility

Contractility can be affected by many factors, such as the length of the muscle fibre and inotropic (referring to the strength of contraction of the heart) agents. Positive inotropes (increase contractility) usually work by increasing Ca^{2+} inflow during the AP. These include:

- Noradrenaline (norepinephrine) binds to myocyte β_1-adrenergic receptors and increases Ca^{2+} via G protein activation.
- Cardiac glycosides, for example, digoxin.

  Negative inotropes decrease contractility. Examples include:

- Ca^{2+} channel blockers (e.g. verapamil), β-blockers (e.g. atenolol) and anaesthetic agents (e.g. propofol).

Afterload

This is the pressure across the left ventricular wall required to overcome any resistance to the ejection of blood. Anything that increases afterload will cause SV to decrease as less blood will be ejected and more will remain in the ventricle. Hypertension and atherosclerosis are common conditions that increase the afterload. Any increase in afterload causes the ventricles to work harder to overcome the increased resistance, and hence hypertrophy of ventricular muscle occurs. This can eventually lead to muscle weakness and failure. Right ventricular failure due to obstructed pulmonary circulation (cor pulmonale) is a common complication of emphysema and chronic bronchitis.

CLINICAL NOTES

TACHYCARDIA

Tachycardia is an early sign of maintaining blood pressure through increasing heart rate (HR). After that, stroke volume can be increased through increasing preload (fluid) and contractility through inotrope. Babies

---

have a physiologically higher resting HR than adults. This leads to a reduced ability to maintain an adequate cardiac output when blood volume loss occurs, that is bleeding, given that their reserves to mount a compensatory tachycardia are reduced compared with adults.

STRUCTURE AND FUNCTION OF THE BLOOD VESSELS

Given the varying functions of blood vessels throughout the body, their relative wall composition and resistance to flow differ, as highlighted in Table 3.5.

Great vessels of the thorax

Aorta

The ascending aorta originates as the outflow from the left ventricle and becomes the aortic arch at the level of the sternal angle. The arch extends posteriorly and to the left of the vertebral column. It becomes the descending aorta, again at the level of the sternal angle. The aortic arch has three branches to the head, neck and upper limbs: the brachiocephalic trunk, left common carotid artery and left subclavian artery. The brachiocephalic trunk bifurcates into the right common carotid and subclavian arteries. The subclavian arteries give rise to the vertebral, internal thoracic arteries, thyrocervical trunk, costocervical trunk and dorsal scapular artery.

Pulmonary trunk

The pulmonary trunk is the continuation of the right ventricle and branches into the right and left pulmonary arteries at the level of the sternal angle.

Superior vena cava

The SVC (Fig. 3.20) forms from the right and left brachiocephalic veins behind the right first costal cartilage. It runs behind the right sternal border and enters the right atrium of the heart behind the right third costal cartilage. The azygos vein drains into the SVC at the level of the second costal cartilage.

Inferior vena cava

The IVC enters the thorax through the diaphragm at the level of T8. It has a short thoracic segment before draining into the right atrium (Fig. 3.20).

Azygos system of veins

The azygos system comprises the azygos vein, the hemiazygos vein and the accessory hemiazygos vein. The azygos vein is formed from the lumbar veins and right intercostal veins. Its counterpart on the left-hand side is the hemiazygos vein, which drains into the azygos vein. Above T8, the left intercostal veins drain into the accessory hemiazygos vein, which drains into the azygos vein at T8.

Arteries

Structure of the arterial wall

There are two main types of arteries. Muscular arteries, which do not contribute to systemic vascular resistance, and elastic arteries, which do.

The arterial walls have three layers (Fig. 3.21):
1. *Tunica intima:* The endothelium lining of the vessel.
2. *Tunica media:* Contains elastic fibres and smooth muscle.
3. *Tunica externa* (also known as tunica adventitia): Elastic fibres and collagen.

Function of the arterial wall

The artery walls are distended during systole, and this force is transmitted as the wall recoils in diastole to keep blood under pressure.

Arterioles

Arterioles branch from arteries and contain variable amounts of smooth muscle and elastin. They can control blood flow through vasodilatation/constriction and so are known as resistance vessels.

Capillaries

Capillaries form network beds that lie between arterioles and venules. Their function is to exchange nutrients and waste from the tissues. More metabolically active tissues thus have a higher density of capillaries.

Table 3.5 Features of blood vessels

Feature	Structure	Function
Conductance	Large arteries with very low resistance	Deliver blood to more distal vessels
Resistance	Arterioles with smooth muscle walls	Regulate local blood flow by vasodilation (increases flow) or vasoconstriction (decrease flow)
Exchange	Capillaries with very thin walls	Transfer of materials between blood and tissue
Capacitance	Thin-walled, low-resistance veins and venules	Reservoir of blood and can increase blood to the heart when required, e.g. during exercise

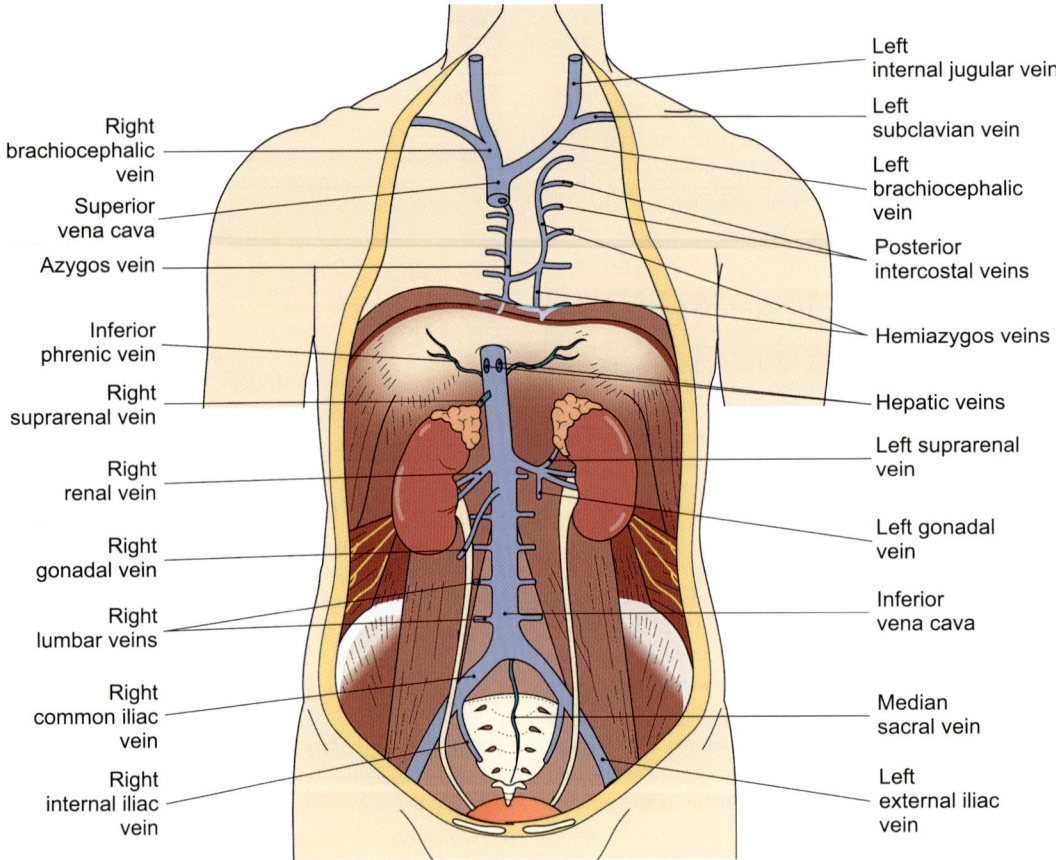

Right brachiocephalic vein
Superior vena cava
Azygos vein
Inferior phrenic vein
Right suprarenal vein
Right renal vein
Right gonadal vein
Right lumbar veins
Right common iliac vein
Right internal iliac vein

Left internal jugular vein
Left subclavian vein
Left brachiocephalic vein
Posterior intercostal veins
Hemiazygos veins
Hepatic veins
Left suprarenal vein
Left gonadal vein
Inferior vena cava
Median sacral vein
Left external iliac vein

Fig. 3.20 Superior and inferior vena cavae and their main tributaries.

Structure and functions of the capillary wall

To maximize nutrient and waste transport, the capillary wall is thin and consists of only a single layer of endothelium and a basement membrane.

The functions of the capillary wall include:

- Minimizing friction to promote laminar flow.
- Clotting.
- The inflammatory response.
- Controlling vessel tone (see later).

Venules

These vessels collect blood from the capillaries and are porous so that phagocytic leucocytes can pass into the tissues at sites of infection.

Veins

These share the same basic structure as arteries except they have a much thinner tunica media and no external elastic lamina. Their lumen is also much larger than arteries and contains valves to prevent backflow of blood.

The functions of veins are as follows:

- Transmit blood back to the heart.
- The storage of blood in distensible veins.

Vascular smooth muscle

Anatomy of vascular smooth muscle

Vascular smooth muscle (Fig. 3.22) has the following features:

- Length between 30 and 200 μm.
- It is thicker in the middle and thinner at the ends.

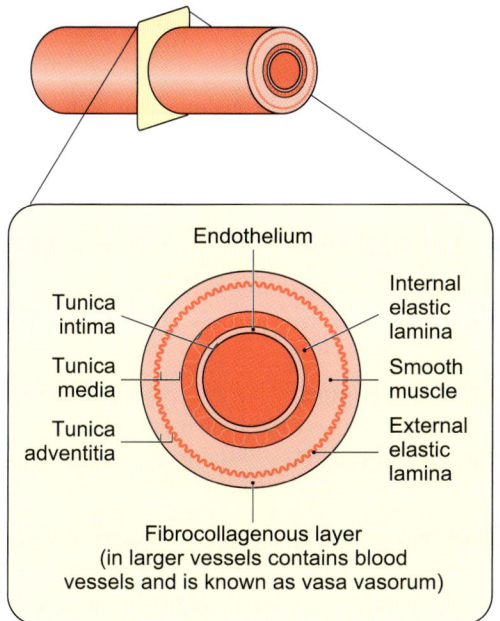

Fig. 3.21 Cross-section showing the layers (tunics) of an arterial wall.

- Each fibre has a single nucleus.
- It has no transverse tubules and only a rudimentary sarcoplasmic reticulum.
- It contains thick, intermediate and thin filaments.

Smooth muscle contraction

Smooth muscle contraction occurs by the following steps:

- There is an increase in Ca^{2+} from the interstitium and sarcoplasmic reticulum.
- Ca^{2+} binds to calmodulin.
- The Ca–calmodulin complex activates the light chain of myosin kinase, which phosphorylates the myosin head using adenosine triphosphate (ATP).
- The myosin head then binds to actin to cause contraction.

Smooth muscle relaxation

For relaxation to occur, the Ca^{2+} concentration must fall, which is achieved via two mechanisms:

- Hyperpolarization of the cell membrane, which prevents calcium channel opening.
- Cyclic adenosine monophosphate- and cyclic guanosine monophosphate (cGMP)-mediated vasodilatation.

Smooth muscle tone

Prolonged contraction of smooth muscle is achieved through slow entering and exiting of Ca^{2+} through the cell membrane.

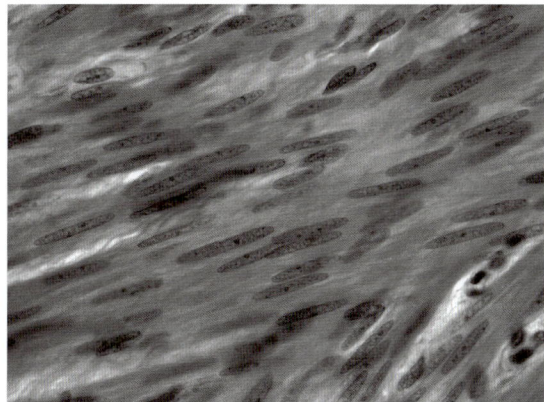

Fig. 3.22 Photomicrograph of smooth muscle.

Haemodynamics

Regulation of blood flow

The volume of blood travelling through a tissue per unit of time is known as blood flow. Ohm's law applied to physics states that:

Flow = pressure difference/resistance.

The principles for blood flow through a vessel to a tissue are also governed by the same factors. Thus this means blood flow is altered by changes in blood pressure (BP) and vascular resistance.

Pressure changes

Blood travels from areas of high pressure to low pressure. The highest pressure is in the aorta during systole and the pressure drops further into the vascular tree. The greatest drop in pressure is seen in the arterioles, so large arteries (e.g. the brachial artery) have a similar pressure to the aorta and so can be used for BP measurement.

Resistance of blood flow

The resistance to blood flow is governed by three factors, described in Poiseuille's law (pressure difference having been described previously):

$$\text{Flow rate} = \frac{(\pi \times \text{pressure difference} \times \text{lumen diameter}^4)}{(8 \times \text{viscosity} \times \text{vessel length})}$$

Lumen diameter flow is proportional to radius to the power of 4 so that only small changes in radius cause large changes in blood flow.

- *Blood viscosity:* Viscosity was described by Newton as a 'lack of slipperiness'. It is influenced by number of red blood cells, protein concentration (globulins and albumin) and fluid content in the blood plasma. For example, polycythaemia increases the number of red blood cells and dehydration reduces the fluid content, both of which will increase viscosity.

- *Vessel length:* Vessel length is directly proportional to resistance so that a longer vessel will have higher resistance.

Haemodynamics of the venous system

The veins and venules are thin walled and act as a reservoir for blood. The volume of blood in the venous system depends on venous pressure and wall tension.

Venous pressure

Venous pressure moves blood back to the heart. A pressure difference of 15 mm Hg exists between the venules and the right atrium to move blood back to the heart.

Active wall tension

Sympathetic tone causes constriction of the vessels to regulate venous volume. If the vessels dilate, for example during a hot bath, more blood pools in the venous system rather than returning to the heart, which causes dizziness (a 'head rush') when standing.

Posture and gravity

When a person changes from lying to standing, gravity pulls blood into the veins, which the body must overcome to ensure continued venous return to the heart. There are several mechanisms to achieve this:

- *Venous valves:* These restrict the backflow of blood.
- *Baroreceptor reflexes:* A drop in cardiac output caused by decreased venous return will activate the carotid and aortic baroreceptors and increase sympathetic nervous system activity to increase the BP.
- *Skeletal muscle pump:* Contraction of skeletal muscles in the legs compresses the veins and pushes blood towards the heart. Movement of blood towards the feet is prevented by the valves.
- *Respiratory pump:* Inspiration results in downward contraction and flattening of the diaphragm, which increases intraabdominal pressure and pushes blood towards the heart.

CLINICAL NOTES

POSTURAL HYPOTENSION

Postural hypotension occurs when the baroreceptors become less sensitive (as part of the ageing process). The body fails to raise its blood pressure when standing, dropping perfusion to the brain and causing lightheadedness. This can cause patients to fall and suffer serious injuries.

Capillary dynamics and transport of solutes

Capillaries have a single-layer endothelium with a basement membrane, which reduces the distance over which solutes must diffuse.

Starling's forces and capillary exchange

Blood plasma and tissue interstitial fluid exchange readily through the capillary walls. The two factors that govern this exchange are the hydrostatic pressure in the capillaries and the colloid osmotic pressure.

Hydrostatic pressure

The capillary wall acts as a filtration barrier that keeps most of the fluid (and electrolytes) within the vessel lumen, although some filters through, driven by the pressure difference between the capillary lumen and the interstitial fluid. Under normal circumstances, lipids and proteins stay within the capillary.

The hydrostatic pressure changes along the capillary bed, with the arteriolar end measuring 35 mm Hg, decreasing down to 15 mm Hg at the venule end. The balance between the hydrostatic pressure forcing fluid out and the oncotic pressure (see later) drawing water back into the capillary determines the net flow of movement.

Osmotic forces in the capillaries (colloid osmotic pressure)

As stated previously, the capillary wall is impermeable to proteins so they stay in the capillary and create an osmotic pressure, which draws fluid back into the capillary. Proteins are negatively charged molecules and further draw cations back into the blood via electrical attraction.

When the hydrostatic and osmotic forces become imbalanced, fluid accumulates in the tissues.

- Left-sided heart failure increases the pulmonary capillary pressure, preventing fluid from being absorbed from lung tissue. This results in pulmonary oedema.
- Liver disease or starvation reduces the amount of protein in the blood and so the oncotic pressure falls, causing widespread tissue oedema.
- Increased capillary permeability owing to histamine release allows proteins to leak out of the capillary and so the oncotic pressure gradient is lost.

Capillary transport

The movement of substances between the capillary and interstitial fluid is governed by three mechanisms.

Simple diffusion through the endothelial cell membrane

Simple diffusion occurs with substances such as O_2, CO_2, glucose and amino acids down a concentration gradient. Lipid-soluble molecules can diffuse directly through the cell membrane lipid bilayer.

Diffusion through pores and fenestrations

Pores and fenestrations are present in all cell membranes and allow diffusion of water-soluble molecules. The blood–brain barrier is unique in that it has a thickened basement membrane, tight junctions between endothelial cells and astrocyte foot processes. All of these restrict the diffusion of molecules through membrane pores.

Active transport by transcytosis

Some substances, for example insulin, move through the cell membrane wrapped in a vesicle that is actively transported by transcytosis.

LYMPH AND THE LYMPHATIC SYSTEM

The lymphatic system is part of the immune system and comprises lymphatic fluid, lymph nodes, lymph vessels and organs (e.g. the spleen). Lymphatics are found in all tissues of the body except for the central nervous system, the eyeballs, the internal ear, cartilage, bone and the epidermis. Approximately 8 L of fluid per day is filtered from the blood into the interstitial space. This is owing to hydrostatic pressure, and the fluid not immediately reabsorbed because of oncotic pressure is returned to the blood via the lymphatics.

Structure

The structure of the lymphatic system is outlined in Fig. 3.23. Lymph capillaries are blind-ending bulbous tubes lined with endothelium. Lymph capillaries merge to form a network of vessels that contain smooth muscle to help move the lymph fluid forward. During its movement through the network, the lymph flows through lymph nodes containing B and T cells where the lymph fluid is presented to the immune system. Efferent lymph vessels drain the nodes into lymph trunks (lumbar, intestinal, mediastinal, subclavian, jugular and bronchomediastinal). Lymph then passes into the right and left (thoracic) lymphatic ducts, which, in turn, drain the fluid back into the bilateral subclavian veins. The movement of lymph is enhanced by the skeletal muscle and respiratory pumps.

Functions of the lymphatic system

- Drainage of surplus tissue fluid back into the blood.
- Transporting dietary lipids (including fat-soluble vitamins) from the gut to the blood. Fats are absorbed from the gut lumen into lacteals where they mix with lymph fluid to form chyle.
- Immunity and presentation of antigen in the tissue fluid to the immune system.

CONTROL OF THE CARDIOVASCULAR SYSTEM

Control of blood vessel diameter

Controlling the flow of blood is required to ensure that adequate nutrients are delivered to meet the tissues metabolic requirements. The factors altering blood flow are intrinsic and hormonal.

Intrinsic control

This refers to intrinsic factors working locally, and they are independent of nerve supply and hormones.

Local temperature

Local temperature control is mostly seen in the skin, where increased temperature causes arteriole vasodilatation to aid heat loss. At temperatures below 15°C, α_1-adrenoceptors are stimulated to cause vasoconstriction.

Transmural pressure

This is the pressure across the wall of the vessel.

- External pressure can be applied during muscle contraction or compartment syndrome.
- Internal pressure forces, that is a rise in BP, cause the vessel to dilate. This stretches the smooth muscle, stimulating muscle contraction and vessel constriction, which reduces blood flow. This autoregulatory mechanism is called the *myogenic response*.

Local metabolites

Increased concentrations of cellular activity metabolites will induce vasodilatation. The increased blood flow will *wash out* the vasodilating metabolites until the vessel diameter (and thus blood flow) reaches a steady state. These include:

- Hypoxia (partial pressure of arterial oxygen (PaO_2)).
- Acidosis (from CO_2 or lactate).
- K^+ (especially in contracting muscles or active brain neurons).
- ATP breakdown products.
- Increasing osmolality.

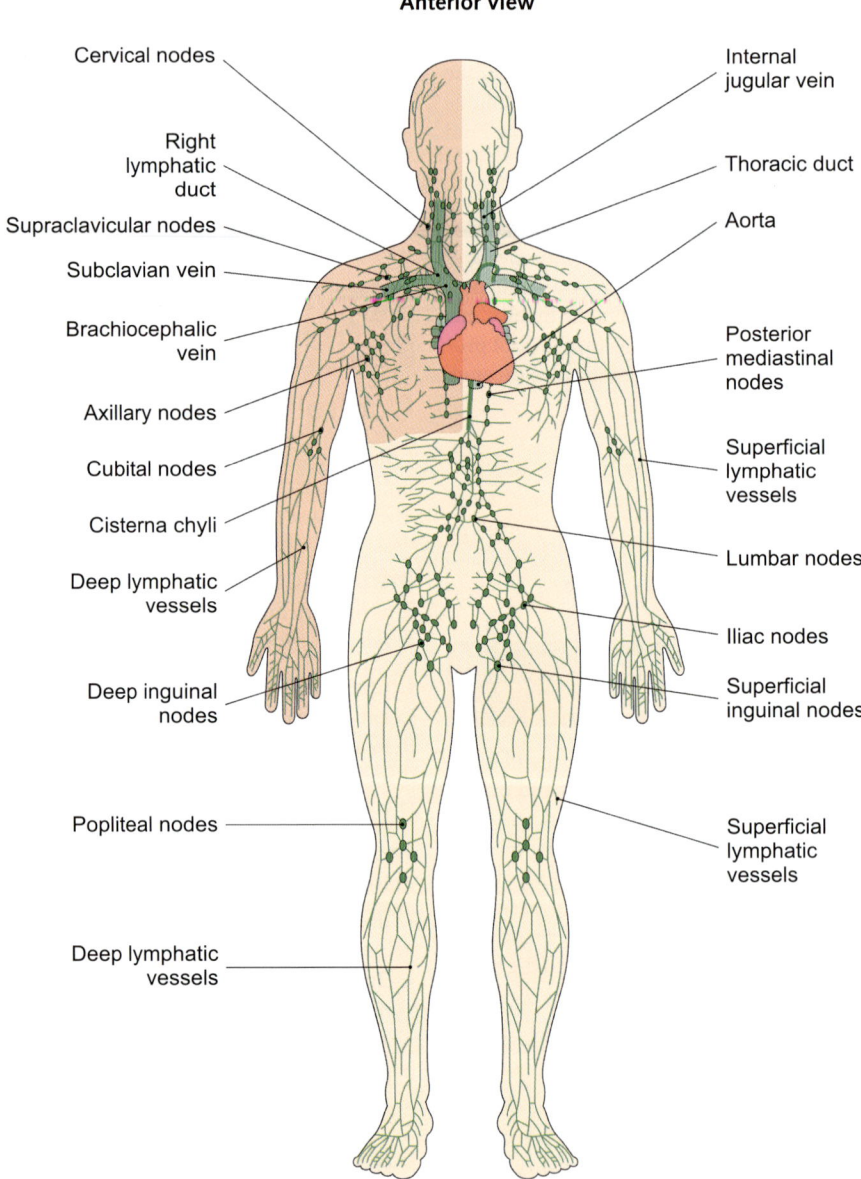

Anterior view

Cervical nodes

Internal jugular vein

Right lymphatic duct

Thoracic duct

Supraclavicular nodes

Aorta

Subclavian vein

Brachiocephalic vein

Posterior mediastinal nodes

Axillary nodes

Cubital nodes

Superficial lymphatic vessels

Cisterna chyli

Lumbar nodes

Deep lymphatic vessels

Iliac nodes

Deep inguinal nodes

Superficial inguinal nodes

Popliteal nodes

Superficial lymphatic vessels

Deep lymphatic vessels

Fig. 3.23 The lymphatic system. The majority of the body's lymphatics drain into the thoracic duct except the *shaded area,* which drains into the right lymphatic duct.

Different tissues have differing sensitivity to different metabolites, with coronary vessels more sensitive to hypoxia and adenosine, and cerebral vessels responsive to H^+, K^+ and partial pressure of carbon dioxide (PCO_2).

Cytokines

Cytokines are molecules whose production is increased in response to trauma to help control the local blood flow as part of the body's host defence.

- *Histamine:* Released from mast cells and causes arteriole vasodilatation (through H_1 receptors) and venous vasoconstriction (through H_2 receptors).
- *Bradykinin:* Causes vasodilatation via nitric oxide (NO) production.
- *Serotonin:* Released from activated platelets and causing vasoconstriction. This is a key component in haemostasis following trauma to blood vessels.

- *Prostaglandins (PG):* Released from leucocytes and the endothelium. They are synthesized from arachidonic acid via the cyclooxygenase enzymes. PGF causes vasoconstriction, whereas PGE and PGI_2 are vasodilators.
- *Thromboxane A_2:* Another vasoconstrictor released from activated platelets that is also important for haemostasis.
- *Leucotrienes:* Produced by leucocytes from arachidonic acid via lipoxygenase enzymes. They cause vasoconstriction and increase vascular permeability.
- *Platelet-activating factor:* Causes vasodilatation.

Endothelium-dependant relaxation and contraction

The endothelium produces several mediators to control vessel size.

- *Endothelium-derived relaxation factor (EDRF):* Later discovered to be NO, which is produced from arginine by NO synthase under the control of numerous cytokines. EDRF/NO diffuses locally into the smooth muscle to cause vasodilatation via cGMP second messengers.
- *Endothelium-constricting factor:* Released in response to smooth muscle stretch and/or hypoxia.
- *Endothelin:* A peptide causing a potent, long-lasting vasoconstriction. It is released in response to smooth muscle stretching as well as thrombin and adrenaline.

Hormonal control
Sympathetic nervous system

Adrenaline and noradrenaline are released from the adrenal medulla (in a 3:1 ratio) on activation of the sympathetic nervous systemic in response to fight or flight situations. Both are β-adrenoceptor agonists that increase HR and myocardial contractility (note that adrenaline has a higher affinity for β-adrenoceptors, whereas noradrenaline has a higher affinity for α-adrenoceptors).

They also cause vasoconstriction when postganglionic sympathetic nerves to the blood vessels release noradrenaline onto $α_1$-receptors causing smooth muscle contraction. This effect is most pronounced in the skin, gut and kidneys. The adrenaline from the adrenal medulla also stimulates $β_2$-receptors in the heart, lungs and skeletal muscles to cause vasodilatation. The net effect of sympathetic activation is to direct blood towards organs in which metabolic demand is higher during intense physical activity.

The parasympathetic nervous system

Parasympathetic nerves cause vasodilatation in the head, salivary glands, gastrointestinal mucosa, bladder and genitals. Their overall effect on BP is limited.

Nitrergic vasodilator nerves—A subset of parasympathetic fibres works on the male and female genitals to release NO, which promotes vasodilatation. This causes the penile and clitoral erection during sexual activity.

Antidiuretic hormone—Antidiuretic hormone is a peptide produced by the hypothalamus and released by the posterior pituitary gland in response to increased plasma osmolality or sympathetic nervous activity. In addition to its effects of free water retention in the kidney, it is also a potent vasoconstrictor in nearly all of the body's tissues (except for the heart and brain where it is a vasodilator).

Renin–angiotensin–aldosterone system

Renin is produced by the renal juxtaglomerular cells and converts angiotensinogen into angiotensin I in the liver (Fig. 3.24). The lungs then convert angiotensin I into angiotensin II using the angiotensin-converting enzyme (ACE).

Renin production is increased by:

- Decreased afferent arteriolar pressure in the renal glomerulus.
- Increased sympathetic activity.

The effects of angiotensin II are as follows:

- Stimulates the adrenal zona glomerulosa to release aldosterone, which causes salt and water retention in the kidneys thus increasing circulating blood volume.
- Vasoconstriction of the vascular smooth muscle.
- Increases noradrenaline release.
- Increases myocardial contractility.

Atrial natriuretic peptide

Stretching the cardiac atria due to increased blood volume will release atrial natriuretic peptide, which promotes water excretion in the kidneys thus lowering BP.

HINTS AND TIPS

A common exam question might ask you to consider why a patient with atrial fibrillation with a raised heart rate (140 beats/min) may be passing large quantities of urine overnight. This is because when the atria become overstressed, atrial natriuretic peptide is released, causing a diuresis effect.

CLINICAL NOTES

ANTIHYPERTENSIVE DRUGS

Many antihypertensive drugs work to reduce BP by opposing the RAAS. Ramipril is a common example of an ACE inhibitor that reduces BP by decreasing the conversion of angiotensin I to angiotensin II. Losartan is a common example of an angiotensin II receptor blocker that blocks the activation of angiotensin II receptors found on numerous different cell types.

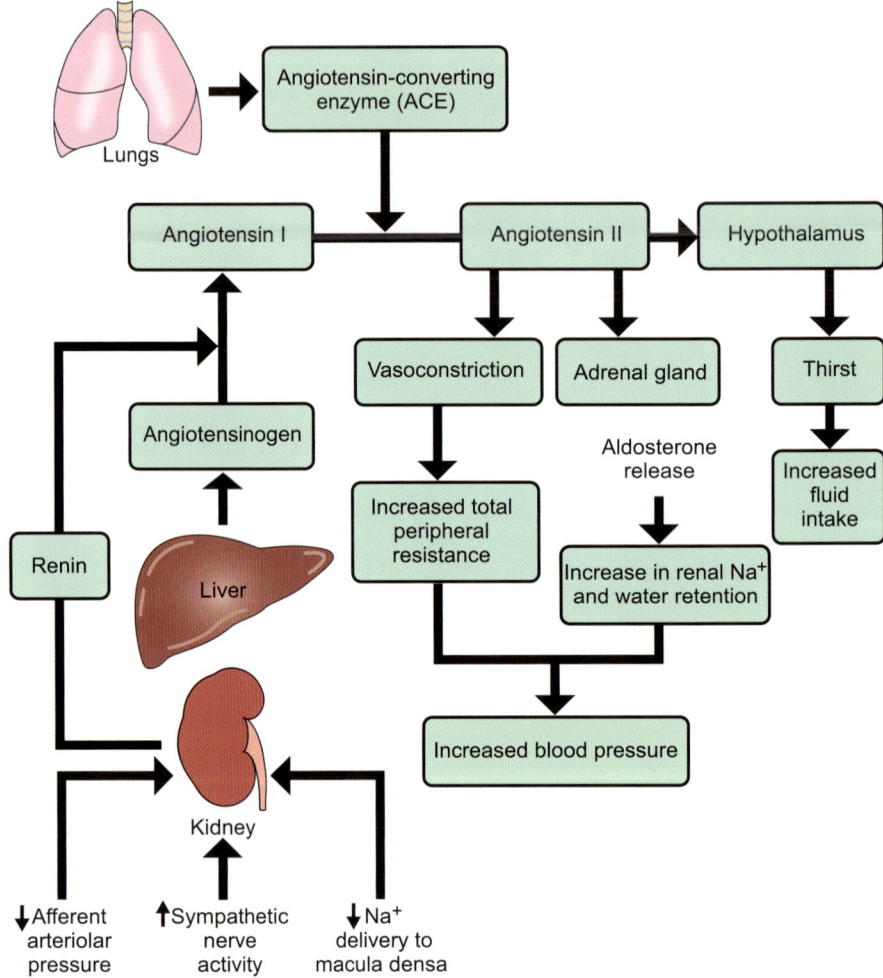

Fig. 3.24 Renin–angiotensin–aldosterone system.

Baroreceptors and the medulla oblongata

The main baroreceptors are found in the internal carotid arteries and the aortic arch. They are continuously firing, but this firing rate increases as they are stretched due to increasing BP. These firing signals are then transmitted to the medulla oblongata via the glossopharyngeal nerve (for carotid signals) and the vagus nerve (for aortic signals).

The cardiovascular centre in the medulla oblongata coordinates these afferent impulses and will reduce sympathetic and increase parasympathetic activity. Sympathetic activity is modulated through fibres in the brainstem, as well as fibres communicating with the hypothalamus. The nucleus accumbens is the main parasympathetic outflow nucleus in the medulla through which parasympathetic activity is controlled.

The sensitivity of the baroreceptors is altered by:

- *Age:* Compliance of arterial walls decreases with age so they are harder to stretch.
- *Chronic hypertension:* Arterial walls are also harder to stretch due to changes in the vessel wall structure.

The set point at which baroreceptors fire faster can be controlled by central and peripheral factors:

- *Central:* During exercise, the neurons that drive inspiration will block the vagal outflow so bradycardia will not occur as the BP rises.
- *Peripheral:* Chronic hypo-/hypertension will change the set point.

Hypothalamus

This has four areas of interest:

1. *Depressor area:* This can produce the baroreceptor reflex.
2. *Defence area:* This is responsible for the flight-or-fight response and governs central sympathetic outflow.
3. *Temperature-regulating area:* Regulates skin vascular tone and sweating.
4. *Vasopressin-secreting area:* Produces antidiuretic hormone (ADH) for release from the pituitary as described previously.

Cardiopulmonary receptors

Numerous cardiopulmonary receptors are connected to afferent fibres innervating the heart, great veins and pulmonary arteries. When these are stimulated, they cause bradycardia, vasodilatation and hypotension. There are four main types.

Venoatrial stretch receptors

Located where the great veins join the atria, venoatrial stretch receptors are connected to myelinated vagal fibres. Stimulation produces reflex tachycardia by increasing sympathetic drive to the pacemaker and increasing salt and water excretion.

Unmyelinated mechanoreceptor fibres

These are located in the atria and left ventricle and travel in the vagal and sympathetic nerves. Large distension stimulates these receptors, causing an inhibitory effect. Reflex bradycardia and peripheral vasodilatation occur.

Chemosensitive fibres

Some unmyelinated vagal and sympathetic afferents are chemosensitive. They can be stimulated in response to substances such as bradykinin. Respiration also increases, causing bradycardia and peripheral vasodilatation.

Chemoreceptors

Chemoreceptors are located in close proximity to baroreceptors in the carotid sinus and aortic arch. The chemoreceptors are nerve terminals sensitive to changes in oxygen, carbon dioxide and hydrogen ions. They send impulses to the medulla, which cause arterioles to vasoconstrict and increase BP. Impulses are also sent to the respiratory centre to modify the rate of breathing.

REGULATION OF CIRCULATION IN INDIVIDUAL TISSUES

Coronary circulation

The coronary circulation originates in the right and left coronary arteries, and together they meet the high metabolic demand of the heart (9 mL/100 g/min). The myocardial oxygen requirement can increase fivefold during exercise. The coronary circulation is adapted for this by:

- Having a high capillary density so there is a shorter distance for oxygen exchange.
- Having a high concentration of myoglobin, which has a higher affinity for oxygen than haemoglobin. This increases oxygen extraction from the blood.
- Having anastomoses between some arteries, which allows continued blood supply if an artery becomes blocked.

Skeletal muscle

Oxygen delivery and metabolite removal need to increase in skeletal muscle during exercise, just like heart activity. The skeletal muscle is adapted in the following ways:

- Modified capillary density: Higher in postural muscles than tonically active ones (e.g. biceps).
- Myoglobin concentrations are higher in postural muscles than in tonic ones.
- β-Adrenoceptors to increase blood flow.
- Muscle pump: This encourages venous return by pushing blood through one-way valves in the veins.

Cutaneous circulation

The skin is a reserve source of blood that can be diverted towards the heart or skeletal muscles during exercise or blood loss. The skin also contains arteriovenous anastomoses that can divert blood away from the surface to reduce heat loss from the skin. These anastomoses are under sympathetic control. Prolonged exposure to cold temperatures causes paradoxical vasodilatation as the neurotransmitter release is paralyzed and vasoconstriction halts. This reduces the damage to the skin by extreme cold.

Alongside noradrenaline, ADH and angiotensin II will cause cutaneous vasoconstriction, which explains why the skin looks pale and cold when a patient is hypovolaemic or shocked. A reactive hyperaemia will make the skin pink, or even sunset coloured, when reperfusion occurs after prolonged ischaemia.

Pulmonary circulation

The pulmonary circulation is adapted to increase gas exchange between the capillary and the alveoli:

- High capillary density.
- Shorter, thinner-walled arterioles, which reduces pulmonary vascular resistance and provides a shorter distance for gases to diffuse over.

Renal circulation

The kidneys also have a high oxygen demand (6 mL/100 g/min) and so the renal circulation is autoregulated to maintain constant perfusion. Renal blood flow is altered by:

- Noradrenaline, which constricts arterioles.
- Prostaglandins causing afferent arteriole vasodilatation. Strong nonsteroidal antiinflammatory drugs, which inhibit prostaglandin production, are thus contraindicated in patients with impaired renal function.

Mesenteric circulation

Mesenteric blood flow reduces with sympathetic activity. Blood flow through the mucosa is increased by the presence of food owing to:

- Digestive hormones such as gastrin and cholecystokinin.
- Local amino acids and glucose.
- Vagal activity.

COMPUTED TOMOGRAPHY SCANNING OF THE THORAX AND ANGIOGRAPHY OF THE GREAT VESSELS

1. Axial computed tomography (CT) chest at the level of T4 (Fig. 3.25).
2. Coronary angiogram with contrast demonstrating the major coronary arteries (Fig. 3.26).
3. Arteriogram of the aortic arch (Fig. 3.27).

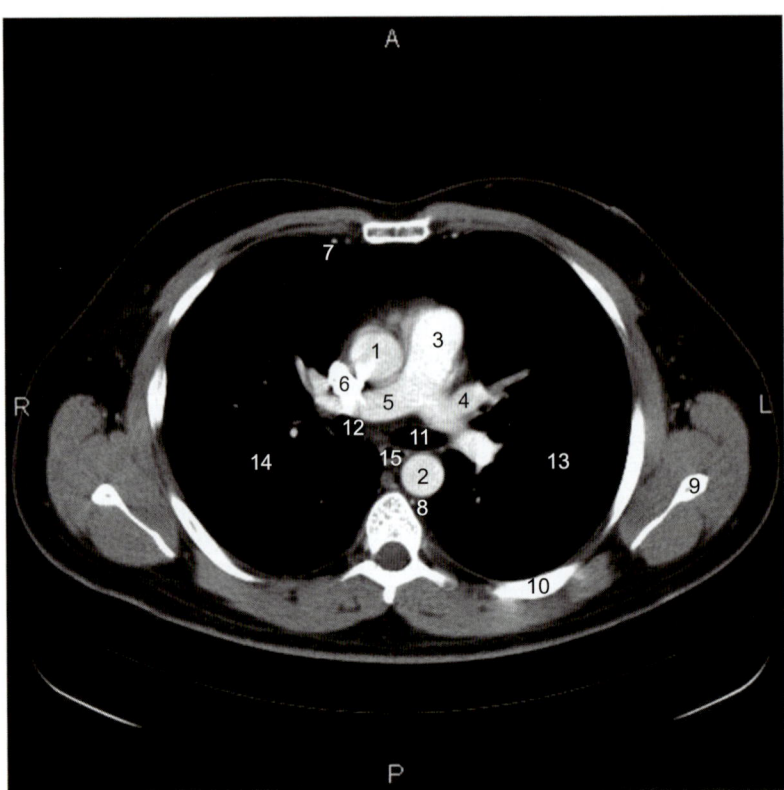

1. Ascending aorta
2. Descending aorta
3. Pulmonary trunk
4. Left pulmonary artery
5. Right pulmonary artery
6. Superior vena cava
7. Internal thoracic artery
8. Posterior intercostal arteries
9. Scapula
10. Rib
11. Left main bronchus
12. Right main bronchus
13. Left lung
14. Right lung
15. Oesophagus

Fig. 3.25 A computed tomography scan (transverse section) of the thorax at the level of the T4 vertebra. A, *Anterior*; L, *left*; P, *posterior*; R, *right*.

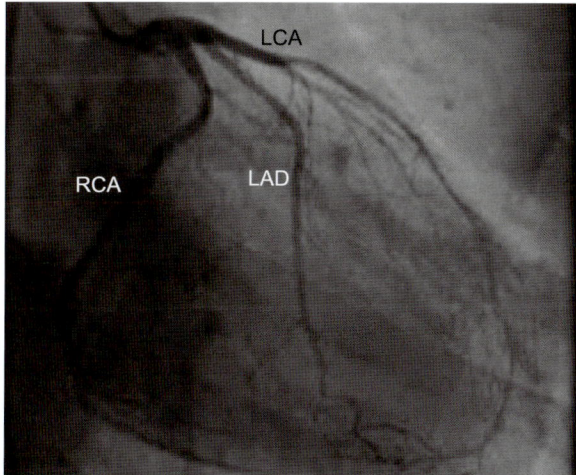

Fig. 3.26 Anterior view of the coronary angiogram. LAD, *Left anterior descending artery*; LCA, left circumflex artery; RCA, right coronary artery.

ELECTROCARDIOGRAPHY

Electrocardiography (ECG) is a simple noninvasive investigation that measures the electrical activity of the heart over time. It involves small electrodes being placed in specific positions over a patient's chest and limbs to detect the electrical signals generated by the heart from different angles. ECG is a useful investigation because correct interpretation gives an understanding of the electrophysiological function of the heart (Fig. 3.28).

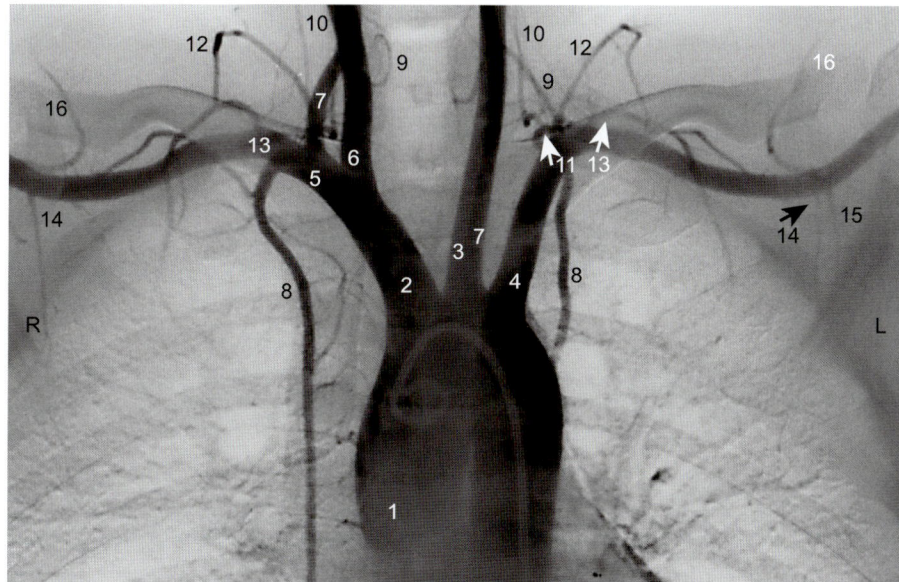

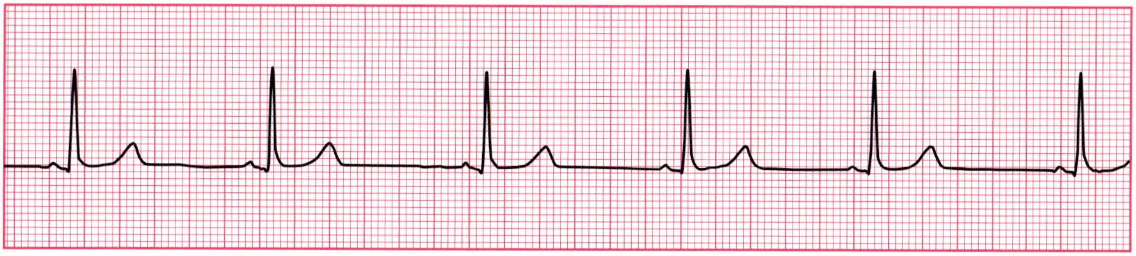

1. Ascending aorta
2. Brachiocephalic trunk
3. Left common carotid artery
4. Left subclavian artery
5. Right subclavian artery
6. Right common carotid artery
7. Vertebral artery
8. Internal thoracic artery
9. Inferior thyroid artery
10. Ascending cervical artery
11. Thyrocervical trunk
12. Suprascapular artery
13. Costocervical trunk
14. Superior thoracic artery
15. Lateral thoracic artery
16. Deltoid branch of the thoracoacromial artery

Fig. 3.27 Digital subtraction arteriogram of the aortic arch. L, *Left*; R, *right*.

Fig. 3.28 An electrocardiography tracing showing normal sinus rhythm.

VENTILATION AND GASEOUS EXCHANGE

Lung volumes

The average total lung capacity in adult males and females is 6.0 L and 4.2 L, respectively. Four volumes make up the total lung capacity (volumes are quoted for an average-size male/average-size females):

- *Tidal volume:* The volume of air moved in one breath at rest (500 mL/500 mL).
- *Inspiratory reserve volume:* The volume of air that can be forcibly inhaled at the end of a normal inspiration (3.1 L/1900 mL).
- *Expiratory reserve volume:* The volume of air that can be forcibly exhaled at the end of normal exhalation (1.2 L/700 mL).
- *Residual volume:* The volume of air left in the lungs at the end of maximal exhalation (1.2 L/1.1 L).

These volumes can be combined to describe other functional lung volumes (see Fig. 3.29).

Ventilation

Ventilation is the movement of air into and out of the lungs. It is caused by changes in intrapleural pressure, and thus the volume of the lungs, as the chest wall/diaphragm moves.

Anatomical dead space

The anatomical dead space is the volume of the airways through which ventilation occurs but that does not contribute to gaseous exchange with the pulmonary circulation. This comprises the conducting airways down to the terminal bronchioles. The volume is 150 mL in the textbook man or 2 mL/kg in nonobese people. This volume increases during inspiration as the airways stretch with increasing lung volume.

The dead space causes air to be reused because during expiration, dead space air is expelled first and some of the alveolar air goes to fill the dead space. During the next inspiration, this old air gets pulled back into the alveoli. The volume of the dead space can be measured using Fowler's method of inspiring pure oxygen and measuring the volume of exhaled nitrogen.

Physiological dead space

The physiological dead space is made of the anatomical dead space plus the volume of any alveoli that are ventilated but not perfused (alveolar dead space). The alveolar dead space is usually small (<5 mL) in healthy adults.

Minute ventilation

Minute ventilation is the total volume of air moved into and out of the lungs in 1 minute. It is calculated by multiplying the tidal volume (anatomical dead space + alveolar volume) by the respiratory rate. The normal tidal volume is 500 mL, and the respiratory rate is 12 to 20 breaths per minute.

Alveolar ventilation

This is the volume of air that reaches the alveoli in 1 minute. It is the alveolar volume multiplied by the respiratory rate.

Variation of ventilation in the lung

There are regional inequalities in how well parts of the lungs are ventilated, with the lower zones better ventilated than the upper ones when a person is upright. This can be demonstrated by inhaling radioactive xenon and imaging the lungs to view how much radiation is released.

Effects of disease on lung volume

Lung volumes are affected in particular patterns, depending on the disease process. The key measurements used are:

- *Forced expiratory volume in 1 second (FEV1):* The volume of air expelled in 1 second with maximum expiratory effort.
- *Forced vital capacity (FVC):* The total volume of air that the person can exhale (Table 3.6).

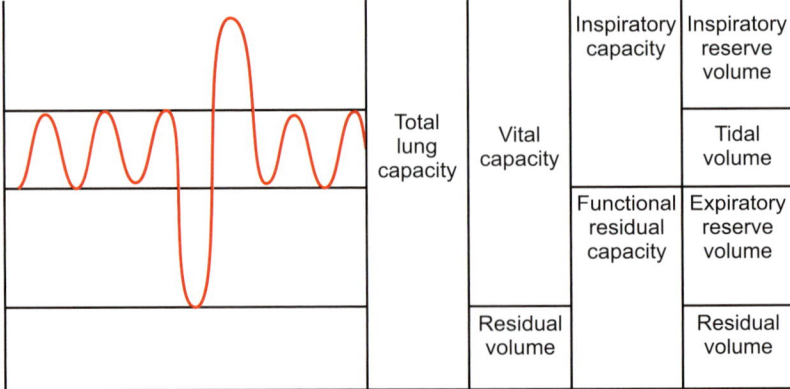

Fig. 3.29 Spirometry trace illustrating lung volumes and capacities.

Table 3.6 Comparison of obstructive versus restrictive diseases

	Obstructive	Restrictive
Aetiology	Airway obstruction occurs due to blockage of the lumen, constriction of the airways or external compression of the airways.	Restrictive diseases are caused by increased stiffness of the lung, which reduces the amount of expansion.
Spirometry findings	FEV1 decreases with a preserved FVC and increased residual volume. An FEV1:FVC ratio of <0.7 is diagnostic of obstructive lung disease.	The FEV1:FVC ratio will be preserved but the FVC will be decreased.
Examples	• Bronchiectasis: lumens blocked with mucous • Cystic fibrosis: viscous secretions block lumens • Asthma/COPD: airway constriction and inflammation narrows the lumen • Tumour: It can be intraluminal or external compression	• Pulmonary fibrosis • Silicosis • Asbestosis • Sarcoidosis • Scoliosis • Neuromuscular diseases

COPD, *Chronic obstructive pulmonary disease*; FEV, *forced expiratory volume*; FVC, *forced vital capacity*.

The mechanics of breathing

Flow of air into the lungs

The flow of air into the lungs is determined by the difference in air pressure between the atmosphere and the alveoli. As atmospheric pressure is fixed, the body changes alveolar air pressure to move air. During inspiration, alveolar pressure is less than atmospheric so that air flows into the lungs, and the reverse happens on expiration. The mechanism for reducing alveolar pressure is as follows.

Before inspiration, the intrapleural pressure trying to pull the lungs open is negative ($-4\,cm\,H_2O$) and is balanced with the force created by the elastic recoil of the lungs so no air is moved.

Contraction of the respiratory muscles increases thoracic volume, and intrapleural pressure decreases, further overcoming the elastic recoil of the lungs. This causes the lungs to be 'pulled' open to fill the larger thoracic volume, and thus the lung volume increases. The larger alveolar volume with the same amount of air reduces the alveolar air pressure (Boyle's law) and air is drawn into the alveoli.

Muscles of respiration

Inspiratory muscles

The muscles of inspiration create a larger thoracic volume and lower intrapleural pressure required for air movement.

- *Diaphragm (see previously for anatomy)*: Contraction of only 1 to 2 cm increases the thoracic length and is responsible for 70% of volume change during quiet respiration. The diaphragm can contract up to 10 cm during forced inspiration.
- *External intercostal muscles*: Span the intercostal space and slope downward and forward. Contraction pulls the ribs up and outward like a bucket handle, as the ribs are hinged on the vertebral attachment. The contraction also reinforces the intercostal spaces so that they do not get sucked inwards, which would reduce the thoracic volume. Paralysis of the intercostals has minimum effect on breathing if the diaphragm is still functioning.
- *Accessory muscles*: Scalenes and sternocleidomastoids. They only have a role in forced inspiration during times of respiratory distress.

When breathing becomes increasingly laboured, other changes to assist inspiration include:

- Flexion of erector spinae muscles to arch the back and increase thoracic volume.
- Scapulae become fixed by the levator scapulae, trapezius and rhomboid muscles.
- Ribs become raised by the pectoralis minor and serratus anterior muscles to increase thoracic volume.

Expiratory muscles

Expiration during normal breathing is passive, as the muscles relax and the elastic recoil of the lungs pulls the chest wall back to its original position. Expiratory muscles are only used for forced expiration, as seen during exercise, coughing or sneezing.

- *Internal intercostal muscles*: Pull the ribs down and inwards (the opposite of external intercostals).
- *Abdominal muscles*: Contraction increases intraabdominal pressure, which forces the diaphragm upwards.

Elastic properties of the lung

The elastic properties of the lung are generated by the collagen and elastin of the lung tissue, as well as surfactant in the alveoli. These elastic properties create the opposing force that must be overcome during inspiration.

Compliance

Compliance describes the ease with which an object can be stretched. It is defined as the change in volume per unit change in pressure. It is the inverse of elasticity. Compliance can be measured under static conditions (no breathing where values are independent of time) and dynamic conditions.

Lung compliance

This refers to the change in lung volume per change in pressure (either transmural or transpulmonary). When plotted on a graph, the line is not straight because compliance varies with lung volume. At low volumes (below residual volume), the compliance is low; compliance then increases with lung volume until all the alveoli are stretched and then compliance again reduces.

Lung compliance varies in different regions of the lung. At the apex, the alveoli are pulled open by the weight of the lung so the compliance is further along the curve. The reverse is true at the base of the lungs. The same pressure is applied to the whole lung during a breath, so the more compliant base of the lung will expand more.

An important note is that the compliance curve for lung expansion is not the same as when the lung is deflating. This is called hysteresis and is due to the extra energy required to recruit and inflate additional alveoli as the lung inflates.

Chest wall compliance

The elastic forces of the chest wall act in an outwards direction and thus oppose the elastic recoil of the lungs acting inwards. The 'resting position' of the lungs is when these forces are equal and is seen when the lungs are stretched to roughly two-thirds of the total lung capacity. At functional residual capacity (FRC), the chest wall compliance is $0.1 \, \text{L/cm} \, H_2O$.

Effect of disease on compliance

The lungs are more susceptible to changes in compliance than the chest wall. However, the chest wall can still be affected by structural changes such as scoliosis or obesity. Diseases such as emphysema, which destroy the alveoli including their elastic fibres, will increase compliance, whereas compliance will be reduced in diseases that stiffen the lungs such as congestion or pulmonary fibrosis.

SURFACE TENSION AND SURFACTANT

Surface tension

Surface tension is the property of a liquid that minimizes the area of the liquid at the liquid–gas interface. In the spherical alveoli, the surface tension would act as an inward force to reduce the surface area exposed to the air and thus collapse the alveoli. This relationship is described by the law of Laplace, which details that smaller alveoli have higher pressure so air will flow out of them into larger alveoli, causing the smaller one to collapse. It would

subsequently take a much larger force to open the collapsed alveoli during inspiration, owing to their lower compliance.

Law of Laplace

$P = 2 \, T/r$
P = pressure within the sphere
T = surface tension in the alveolar wall
r = radius

A phospholipid called surfactant is secreted by type 2 pneumocytes that lower the surface tension in the alveoli. Unlike water, the surface tension of surfactant changes with surface area. The presence of surface tension leads to alveolar stability and hysteresis and prevents pulmonary oedema.

Lowering surface tension

Surfactant molecules have both hydrophilic and hydrophobic entities so that the hydrophobic ends align facing the air. This interferes with the attractive forces between water molecules, which are repelled from the hydrophobic parts of the surfactant. As the surface area decreases, the distance between surfactant molecules decreases so that the repulsive forces are higher.

Alveolar stability

Surfactant lowers the surface tension in smaller alveoli and thus lowers the pressure inside them. This creates more equal pressures between different-sized alveoli and thus stops them from collapsing. The second component in alveolar stability is mechanical tethering to the adjacent alveoli so that if one collapses it is pulled open by its neighbour.

Prevention of pulmonary oedema

Pulmonary oedema is the pressure of excess fluid in the lung tissue and alveoli. Surfactant decreases surface tension, which would otherwise be accompanied by 20 mm Hg of unopposed pressure that would promote transudation of fluid from the capillary into the lung tissue/alveoli.

Hysteresis

The density of surfactant molecules is higher during expiration when the alveoli are smaller, compared with inspiration. Surface tension, and thus compliance, is different during the different phases of respiration.

CLINICAL NOTES

INFANT RESPIRATORY DISTRESS SYNDROME

Surfactant is produced at 34 weeks' gestation, and babies born before this have higher surface tension and reduced compliance in their alveoli. This requires higher pressures and higher work of breathing to ventilate and, thus, the secretion of a proteinaceous exudate that forms hyaline membranes within the alveoli.

Dynamic resistance of breathing

When air moves through the respiratory system during ventilation, there is dynamic resistance to inflation of the lungs.

- 80% of resistance is the resistance of the airways to air flow.
- 20% of resistance is friction between lung tissues during expansion.

The sum of the pressure required to overcome the dynamic resistance and the lung compliance is the total force of ventilation.

Airway resistance

The pattern of airflow through the tube will influence the resistance. Airflow (like all fluids through a tube) can be either laminar or turbulent (Fig. 3.30).

Pattern of flow

Laminar flow occurs at low flow rates and describes streamlined airflow moving in parallel to the vessel walls. Air will flow more slowly closer to the walls owing to resistance against the wall. Poiseuille's law can be applied to laminar flow:

$$\text{Poiseuille's law} - V = P\pi r^4/8\eta l$$

V = flow
P = pressure
r = vessel radius
η = fluid viscosity
l = vessel length

The radius of the vessel is critical to both flow rate and resistance. Doubling the radius will increase flow rate 16-fold.

Turbulent flow describes the breakdown of laminar flow so that air moves at right angles to the vessel walls with eddy currents moving in random directions. Turbulent flow occurs because of high flow rates, high gas density or wide diameter vessels.

Transitional flow is a mix of laminar and turbulent flow and is seen at branch points of vessels.

Site of airway resistance

- 40% is from the upper airways (less in mouth breathing).
- 60% is from the lower airways (of which 80% is the trachea and main bronchi).

It would be assumed that the smaller airways would have laminar flow and thus higher resistance. However, the parallel arrangement of so many airways means that the total resistance

is kept low. During normal breathing, it is the medium-sized airways that provide the greatest resistance.

Factors determining airway resistance

These factors are lung volume and bronchial smooth muscle contraction.

- *Lung volume:* The airways are tethered to the alveoli so that when the lungs are expanded the airways are pulled open and resistance decreases.
- *Smooth muscle contraction:* Smooth muscle contraction is under the control of the autonomic nervous system.

Bronchoconstriction is caused by:

- *Stimulation of parasympathetic fibres:* These also increase mucous secretion.
- Inflammatory mediators such as leukotrienes and prostaglandins.
- Local irritants such as smoke or dust.
- Decreased CO_2 in the conducting airways.

Bronchodilation is caused by:

- Stimulation of adrenergic sympathetic fibres working on β_2-receptors.
- Nitric oxide.
- Increased CO_2 in the conducting airways.

CLINICAL NOTES

ACUTE ASTHMA ATTACK

During an acute exacerbation of asthma, airway resistance is increased due to bronchoconstriction, airway inflammation and mucous production, among other factors. The inhaled drug salbutamol works as a short-acting β_2-adrenergic receptor agonist acting on airway smooth muscle. Salbutamol induces bronchodilation and therefore reduces airway resistance and relieves shortness of breath.

Effect of transmural pressure on airway resistance

Transmural pressure is important in holding open the small airways, which lack cartilaginous support.

Transmural pressure = alveolar pressure − pleural pressure

Alveolar pressure is positive and pleural pressure is either positive (expiration) or negative (inspiration). During inspiration, the transmural pressure is positive and thus the airways stay open. During expiration (particularly forced expiration) when the intrathoracic pressure is positive, the airways are at risk of collapsing if the transmural pressure becomes negative. Tethering of the airways to the surrounding lung tissue keeps the airways open in this circumstance.

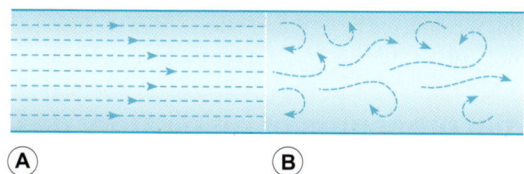

Fig. 3.30 Laminar (A) and turbulent (B) flow.

Dynamic compression occurs during forced expiration when transmural pressure becomes negative and the airways begin to collapse, so that the increasing force of expiration is balanced against the increasing airway collapse and a maximum flow rate is reached. This effect is more pronounced at low lung volumes when the mechanical tethering of the airways will be less.

CLINICAL NOTES

DYNAMIC COMPRESSION IN DISEASE

Exaggeration of dynamic compression occurs in certain diseases where the maximal airflow is reached at lower levels of flow. Reduced lung volume or destruction of the lung as seen in chronic obstructive pulmonary disease will reduce the mechanical tethering and allow airway collapse at lower pressures.

Measuring airway resistance

- *Peak expiratory flow rate (PEFR):* A single breath into a peak flow meter using maximal effort from the total lung capacity.
- *Spirometry:* Creates a maximal inspiratory and expiratory flow loop from which the FEV1 and the forced expiratory volume can be calculated. This technique is of clinical importance in separating obstructive from restrictive patterns of respiratory disease.
- *Plethysmography:* A patient breathes into a mouthpiece to measure lung volumes and capacities. It is a more accurate, but less practical method than the two above.

CLINICAL NOTES

PEAK EXPIRATORY FLOW RATE

Peak expiratory flow rate (PEFR) is used to monitor the severity of asthma, particularly during exacerbations, and the response to treatment. PEFR involves the patient blowing as hard and fast as they can into a peak flow meter, which measures the maximum speed of expiration in litres per minute.

The work of breathing

The work of breathing is the energy required to move the lungs and chest wall. It is proportional to the pressure change (needed to overcome dynamic resistance and lung compliance) and the volume change.

Work of breathing is increased if:

- Volume is increased (e.g. chronic obstructive pulmonary disease (COPD)).
- Pressure is increased because of reduced compliance or increased dynamic resistance.

During quiet respiration, the body uses 5% of its energy for respiration, which increases to 30% during vigorous exercise. The work of breathing can be reduced by bronchodilators (such as salbutamol), which reduces dynamic resistance.

GASEOUS EXCHANGE IN THE LUNGS

After the alveoli have been ventilated, the next stage is the exchange of gases between the alveoli and the bloodstream. This process occurs by diffusion and is dependent on the partial pressures of gases.

Diffusion

Diffusion is the net movement of molecules from an area of high concentration to low concentration until a dynamic equilibrium is reached. In the lungs, the net movement of gases is dependent on the partial pressure of gases in the alveoli and capillary blood and is described by Fick's law of diffusion. Diffusion across a membrane (i.e. the alveolar wall) is described by Graham's law.

Fick's and Graham's laws

Fick's law

$$J = \frac{A \times D \times (P_1 - P_2)}{T}$$

Graham's law

$$D = solubility / \sqrt{molecular\ weight}$$

- J = rate of diffusion
- A = surface area of membrane
- D = gas diffusion coefficient
- $(P_1 - P_2)$ = difference in partial pressure across the membrane
- T = membrane thickness

The rate of diffusion is increased by:

- Increased surface area.
- Increased partial pressure difference.
- Increased gas solubility.
- Decreased thickness of membrane.
- Decreased molecular weight.

The alveolar membrane is adapted to maximize diffusion, owing to its large surface area (50–100 m²) and a thickness of only 0.3 µm. The higher solubility of CO_2, despite its larger molecular weight, means that it diffuses 20 times faster than oxygen. However, this is countered by its slower release from the blood and the shallower partial pressure gradient across the alveolar membrane.

Partial pressures of respiratory gases

In a mixture of gases, each gas behaves as if it were alone in that space. This is shown by Dalton's law, which states that the pressure of a gas is equal to the sum of the partial pressures of its constituent gases. It follows that the partial pressure is equal to the total pressure of the gas multiplied by the percentage composition of that gas.

Using oxygen as an example:

101 kPa (pressure of air at sea level)

$\times$ 0.21 (fraction of oxygen in the air)

= 21 kPa (partial pressure of oxygen)

At high altitude when the total air pressure decreases, the partial pressure of oxygen drops but there is still 21% oxygen in the air.

Water vapour pressure

As it passes through the upper airways, the inspired air is heated and humidified, as water vapour is added to the mixture of gases in the air. The addition of the water vapour decreases the percentage of oxygen in the air.

Diffusion limitation and perfusion

The exchange of gas across the alveolar membrane into the capillary blood is dependent on the diffusion time across the membrane as well as the capillary perfusion.

Diffusion limitation

Diffusion of gas across the membrane is the rate-limiting step in gas exchange, as the gases are soluble and readily bind with haemoglobin (Hb). Fick's law of diffusion explains the limitations of gas transfer:

- Diffusion coefficient depends on solubility and molecular weight.
- Partial pressure gradient depends on the partial pressure of gas in the venous blood (as partial pressure is fixed in the air).

Normally, the transit time for an erythrocyte through the alveolar capillary is 0.7 to 1.2 s. If this transit time is very short (<0.2 s), equilibrium between capillary and alveolar partial pressures might not have time to be reached. As there is an excess erythrocyte transit time, any gas transfer becomes limited by diffusion.

Perfusion limitation

This refers to the transfer of gases that readily diffuse across the alveolar–capillary membrane, but transfer is limited by plasma solubility and weak/no binding to Hb. An insoluble gas will diffuse in the blood, causing the plasma concentration to rise, and equilibration with the alveolar concentration will occur quickly. This will remove the concentration gradient and thus the driving force for further diffusion. This equilibrium will occur early in the capillary, and no further gases are transferred for the rest of the capillary length; thus the rate of alveolar perfusion limits the amount of gas transport.

Nitrous oxide (N_2O) is a good example of a perfusion-limited gas. It traverses the alveolar–capillary barrier with ease, it has low plasma solubility and it does not combine chemically with Hb or any other blood component.

The time course for O_2 transfer is normally perfusion limited. At rest, equilibrium between alveolar and capillary partial pressure of oxygen (PO_2) occurs when the erythrocyte is one-third of the way along the capillary, so no partial pressure gradient after this point = no driving force. In some diseases where the diffusion properties of the lung are impaired—typically by thickening of the diffusion membrane or reduced surface area (e.g. emphysema)—equilibrium is not reached by the time blood has reached the end of the capillary (partial pressure of oxygen in the artery (PaO_2) < partial pressure of oxygen in the alveoli (P_AO_2)), so there is some diffusion limitation.

Oxygen uptake in the capillary network

As mentioned above, pulmonary PaO_2 (40 mm Hg) equilibrates with P_AO_2 (100 mm Hg) in 0.25 s, that is one-third of the transit time of capillary blood (0.75 s) at normal resting cardiac output. Therefore the transit time is surplus to the requirements for adequate O_2 transfer. During strenuous exercise, the transit time is decreased to 0.25 s because cardiac output results in faster flow rates through the pulmonary capillaries. In the absence of disease, there is very little change in end capillary PaO_2 (see Fig. 3.31).

During exercise, there is increased total O_2 transfer from:

- Improved ventilation–perfusion matching as more of the lung is ventilated with deeper inspiration.
- Greater gaseous exchange surface area due to an increased pulmonary capillary network: there is capillary distension and use of previously unperfused capillaries at rest.

If there is a diffusion limitation of O_2 transfer owing to greater diffusion distance (fibrotic thickening or interstitial oedema), PaO_2 values may be maintained at rest but cannot be maintained with exercise because of the loss of surplus perfusion time required to compensate for the increased diffusion distance.

Carbon dioxide transfer

As already mentioned, the diffusion coefficient (D) component of Fick's law of diffusion (see diffusion, gaseous exchange in the lungs, Chapter 3) implicates solubility and molecular weight (solubility/molecular weight) in the rate of diffusion. Graham's law is the basis for this coefficient with respect to molecular weight.

Pulmonary $PaCO_2$ (45 mm Hg) equilibrates with alveolar P_ACO_2 (40 mm Hg) in 0.25 s—the same time as for O_2 (see Fig. 3.31). CO_2 has a much higher diffusion coefficient than O_2; however, this is countered by the lower partial pressure gradient for CO_2 and its slow release from the blood.

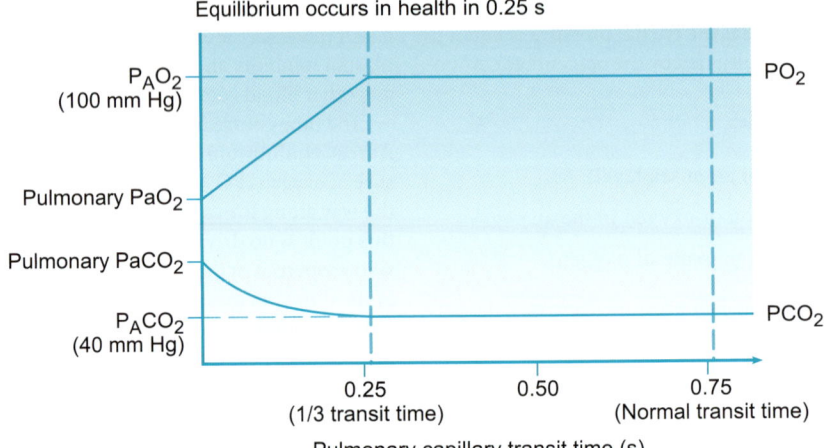

Fig. 3.31 Pulmonary PaCO₂ and PaO₂ variation with pulmonary capillary transit time.

CO$_2$ transfer is normally perfusion limited, although an abnormal gaseous exchange membrane, as seen with some diseases, may cause it to be diffusion limited.

LUNG PERFUSION

Presentation of blood for effective gaseous exchange is a complicated process. Most of the cardiac output is directed through the pulmonary circulation, where it flows in very close proximity with air in the alveoli. As well as a thin membrane between blood and air, a low-pressure circulation is needed to avoid fluid being driven as a transudate into the alveolar space. There must also be a ventilation–perfusion match, as gaseous exchange will be ineffective if non- or underventilated alveoli are perfused or, similarly, if there is very little perfusion of well-ventilated alveoli (i.e. if either of the two media—blood or air supply—is inadequate).

Pulmonary blood flow

Mechanics of the circulation

At rest, the pulmonary circulation constitutes 3 to 5 L blood/min/m² of body surface area. A large compliance enables the pulmonary arteries to accommodate two-thirds of the right ventricular stroke volume. In addition, the very small amount of smooth muscle in the pulmonary arterial walls means that the pulmonary circulation offers little resistance to the low-pressure blood leaving the thin-walled right ventricle (25 mm Hg systolic). The pulmonary arteries are therefore very compliant and distensible.

Pulmonary arterioles and capillaries are the main resistors. However, they permit further drops in pressure because their large number amount to a considerable total cross-sectional area for flow. At rest, pulmonary vascular resistance (PVR) is split evenly among pulmonary arteries, capillaries and veins.

Pulmonary blood flow and PVR are subject to:

- Vascular effects: including hydrostatic pressure within the vessel and vascular smooth muscle.
- Extravascular effects: including lung volume and intrapleural pressure, the influences of which are based on the concept of a transmural pressure gradient.

Hydrostatic pressure

The hydrostatic pressure dictates pulmonary arterial or venous pressure and provides the driving force for flow. When this pressure rises, PVR decreases further by two mechanisms:

- *Recruitment:* Blood flows through previously unused capillaries, which were either closed or open but without blood flow. When they open, the cross-sectional area to flow is increased, thereby lowering resistance. Recruitment occurs when pulmonary artery pressure increases from low levels.
- *Distension:* Individual capillary segments dilate, thereby increasing the radius and lowering the resistance fourfold (Poiseuille's law). Distension occurs at higher hydrostatic pressures than recruitment.

Recruitment and distension usually occur in unison. These effects are best illustrated at the higher hydrostatic pressures in the gravity-dependent (lower) regions of the lung.

Vascular smooth muscle

Vascular smooth muscle determines the calibre of extraalveolar vessels: contraction will decrease vessel radius and increase PVR.

Smooth muscle is subject to both neural and humoral influences. Constriction, and hence increased PVR, is caused by:

- Catecholamines: epinephrine (adrenaline) and norepinephrine (noradrenaline)
- Serotonin
- Histamine

Dilatation, and therefore reduced PVR, is caused by:

- Acetylcholine
- Isoprenaline (β-adrenergic agonist)
- Nitric oxide

Effects of transmural pressure gradients

The transmural pressure gradient (pressure inside the vessel – pressure outside the vessel) will dictate vessel diameter. As transmural pressure increases, the vessel diameter will increase and so the PVR decreases.

For the alveolar capillaries residing within alveolar walls, the transmural pressure gradient (and thus their diameter) is determined by the pressure within the capillaries and alveolar pressure outside. During normal inspiration, increased alveolar volume and stretching causes elongation of the capillaries and therefore a reduction in radius. Furthermore, the higher alveolar pressure compresses pulmonary capillaries, and the combined effect is greater vascular resistance of the alveolar vessels at higher lung volumes.

Lung volume

This affects PVR (Fig. 3.32) through the following:

- The effect of lung volume on transmural pressure.
- The individual effects on alveolar and extraalveolar vessels.

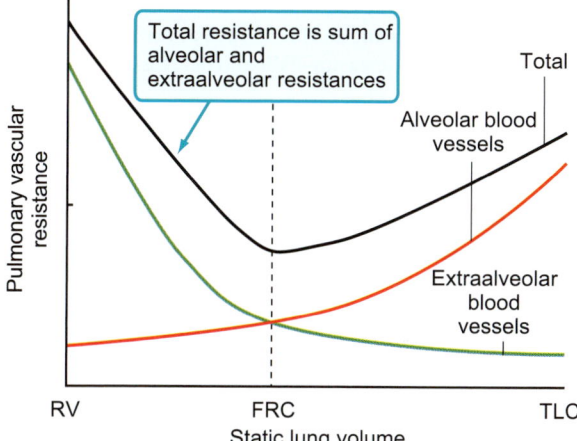

Fig. 3.32 Pulmonary vascular resistance variation with lung volume of alveolar and extraalveolar vessels. FRC, *Functional residual capacity*; RV, *residual volume*; TLC, *total lung capacity*.

At low lung volumes, the PVR of extraalveolar vessels is large as a result of effective smooth muscles in their walls, which resist distension. However, alveolar pressure and distension are minimal, so alveolar vessels have low levels of resistance. During deep inspiration, alveolar pressure rises and there is stretching of alveolar walls, both of which increase alveolar PVR. In addition, capillary hydrostatic pressure falls owing to more negative intrapleural pressure surrounding the heart. Hence, the transmural pressure gradient is greatly decreased, possibly negative, with squashing of the alveolar vessels. Without the effects of transmural pressure, PVR would still be elevated by stretching and thinning of the alveolar walls. Meanwhile, extraalveolar vessels are distended by increased radial traction.

As the resistance of the vessels adds up, total PVR will be highest at extremes of lung volume corresponding to maximal PVR of either group.

Distribution of blood within the lung

A gradient of regional perfusion exists, from the apex with the least blood flow to the base where blood flow is highest owing to the effects of gravity. The pulmonary system can be considered as a continuous column of blood, the hydrostatic pressure of which can be calculated by the following equation:

$$P = ghr$$

P = hydrostatic pressure
g = gravitational acceleration
h = height of column (distance from the top)
r = density of substance

This hydrostatic pressure is greater at lower regions with higher blood flow and responsible for lowering PVR in these areas by distension and recruitment of capillaries, as described previously. In addition, the capillary transit time is less in lower regions (i.e. increased blood flow rate).

From the above equation, it would be expected that ventilation would be better at the base where alveolar compliance is higher. However, comparatively, air has a very low density, so the hydrostatic pressure differences in different parts of the lungs are much less than for blood.

Zones of the lung (West's zones)

The lungs can be divided into four different zones depending on variations in three different pressures:

- P_A: alveolar pressure
- Pa: arterial pressure
- Pv: venous pressure

The lung is split vertically into four zones, across which differences in the three pressures listed above will lead to varying degrees of gas exchange (Fig. 3.33). These zones are frequently called 'West's zones'.

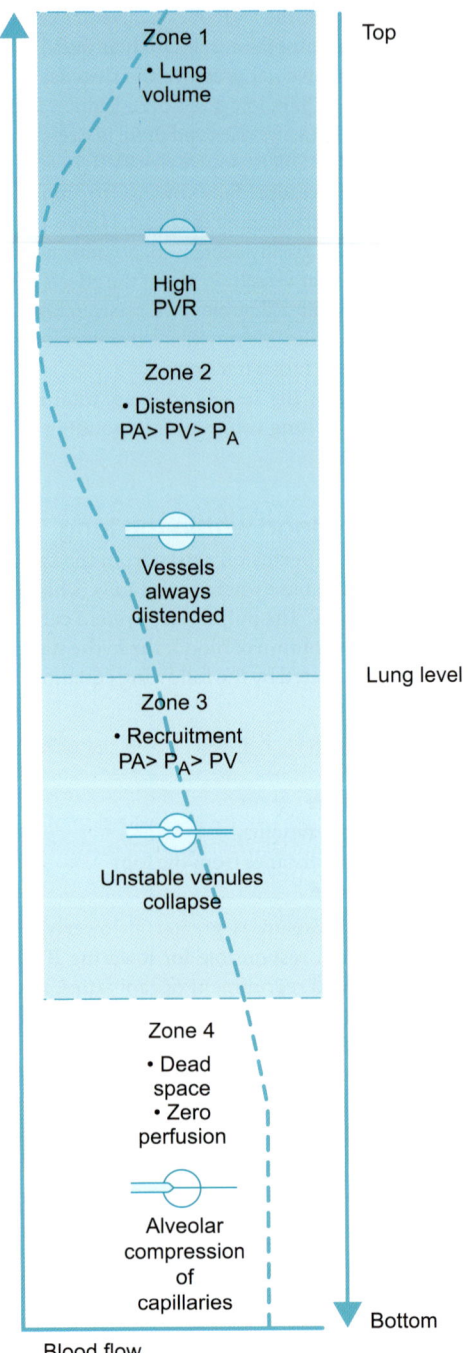

Fig. 3.33 Blood flow within the vessel zones and levels of the lung. PA, *Alveolar pressure*; Pa, *arterial pressure*; Pv, *venous pressure*; PVR, *pulmonary vascular resistance*.

Zone 1 (apex)—P_A > Pa. Capillary compression (dead space)

Dead space refers to lung tissue that is ventilated but not perfused. This happens if alveolar pressure is greater than arterial pressure. Under normal physiological conditions, this does not happen. Although the lung apex is approximately 15 cm above the right ventricle, pulmonary arterial pressure here is just enough to allow blood flow. However, areas of the lung may become dead space under conditions such as:

- Hydrostatic pressure (BP) drops, as seen in haemorrhage or shock.
- Alveolar pressure increases (positive-pressure ventilation).

Zone 2—Pa > P_A > Pv. There is blood flow in this region, which is lower down in the lung than zone 1. Pa is increased due to higher hydrostatic pressure, which causes the recruitment of capillaries. Pa and P_A still determine blood flow. Opening and closing of postcapillary venules occur with systole and diastole, respectively.

Zone 3—Pa > Pv > P_A. The arteriovenous pressure difference accounts for continuous blood flow. Distension owing to the higher hydrostatic pressure lower in the lung is particularly important in this zone and will decrease PVR with a resultant increase in mean vessel width.

Zone 4 (base)—A small section at the base of the lung is referred to as zone 4. The volume here is smaller than elsewhere because the lungs are compressed, which causes extraalveolar vessel compression and therefore high PVR, so that blood flow is less than in zone 3.

Control of pulmonary blood flow

As already mentioned, blood flow within the lung can be altered by passive or active means:

- *Passive effects:* Owing to change in hydrostatic pressure and include recruitment and distension of capillaries to alter PVR.
- *Active effects:* Include modification of vascular smooth muscle tone and humoral effects, such as contraction by catecholamines, increasing PVR and decreasing pulmonary blood flow.

Apart from these mechanisms, reduced alveolar PO_2 is also important in controlling pulmonary circulation. A decrease in P_AO_2 to <70% of normal values results in adjacent precapillary smooth muscle contraction. The function of this phenomenon is that blood is not wasted in perfusing poorly ventilated areas where there is air trapping and where no effective gaseous exchange would occur.

The ventilation–perfusion relationship

The ventilation–perfusion ratio is an important clinical measure of gaseous exchange.

Alveolar partial pressures are dictated by:

- Alveolar perfusion (Q)
- Ventilation rate (V)

However, neither of these two factors are uniformly distributed in the lungs; therefore the V/Q ratio will vary throughout the lung.

In general, alveolar minute ventilation and pulmonary blood flow can be substituted as values for V and Q, respectively, to give a normal V/Q value of 0.84. V/Q values are bordered at either end of the range by extreme numbers:

- V/Q = 0: there is no ventilation (V = 0). This corresponds to alveolar dead space.
- V/Q = ∞: there is no perfusion (Q = 0). This can be caused by shunts (see below).

Ventilation/perfusion shunts

Shunts refer to deoxygenated blood bypassing ventilated regions of the lung. They can be either physiological or pathological.

Physiological shunts

Blood from the bronchial circulation and thebesian vessels (small coronary vein) drains directly into the pulmonary veins and left ventricle, respectively, thereby avoiding the pulmonary capillaries and not undergoing gas exchange in the lungs. The consequence of adding this blood to the blood in the pulmonary veins—known as venous admixture—is a small depression of PaO_2 and only a slight elevation of $PaCO_2$, as the shunt accounts for 2% to 5% of cardiac output only.

Pathological shunts

This can occur with one of the following:

- *Intrapulmonary shunt:* Whereby totally unventilated or collapsed alveoli are perfused.
- *Anatomical shunt:* This is usually described as a right–left shunt owing to structural abnormalities of the heart and great vessels (e.g. septal defects). Venous blood from the right side of the heart mixes directly with arterial-quality blood from the left side rather than travelling through the lungs, and thus the arterial blood in the left-sided heart becomes 'diluted' before being pumped around the rest of the body.

As with all shunts, the result of a larger than normal venous admixture is to reduce the concentration of O_2, which disproportionately reduces the PO_2 of the arterial blood.

Unexpectedly, $PaCO_2$ is not usually raised despite the relatively high partial pressure of carbon dioxide (PCO_2) of the venous admixture because chemoreceptors sense the elevated $PaCO_2$ and stimulate ventilation. This decreases the PCO_2 of unshunted blood below its normal value, and thus, $PaCO_2$ is not grossly elevated in the venous admixture. However, PaO_2 is not corrected even if the patient is given 100% O_2 because the shunted blood does not undergo gaseous exchange with higher P_AO_2 and the unshunted blood is already almost maximally saturated with O_2. Although it has a higher than normal level of dissolved O_2, which serves to increase PaO_2, below-normal values are still expected for the concentration of oxygen inspired.

Effects of ventilation/perfusion mismatch on alveolar partial pressure and gaseous exchange

V/Q = 0: no ventilation

No ventilation can occur when the airway leading to the alveolus is occluded, such as with a tumour or sputum (Fig. 3.34). Gas trapped in the alveolus will undergo exchange with blood until the Pa and P_A equilibrate for respective PO_2 and PCO_2 values. Over time, the alveolus will collapse, and this unit (alveolus with its blood) will function as an intrapulmonary shunt.

V/Q = ∞: no perfusion

Nonperfusion of a ventilated alveolus can occur when the blood vessel is occluded, as with pulmonary embolus. No blood means no gaseous exchange; no O_2 is swept away and no CO_2 is released into the alveolus. Physiologically, this occurs with dead space/ zone 1 (see previously). Therefore there is no difference between alveolar and inspired gas.

Gaseous exchange

CO_2 removal:O_2 uptake ratio at the blood–gas interface, known as the exchange ratio (R), varies with V/Q values (Fig. 3.35). This is explained by the dissociation curves of Hb for these gases. For this reason:

- *R is high when V/Q is high:* Well-ventilated alveoli will remove more CO_2 from the blood in comparison to O_2 uptake by the blood, as Hb is already almost fully saturated.
- *R is low when V/Q is low:* Blood exchanging with less well-ventilated alveoli will take up more O_2 in comparison to CO_2 released into the alveoli because the gradient of the O_2 dissociation curve corresponding to lower PO_2 is steeper than that for the CO_2 dissociation curve.

Regional variation of ventilation/perfusion

Although the lower regions of the lung receive more ventilation than the higher regions, greater hydrostatic effects of blood mean that (Fig. 3.36 and Table 3.7):

- Lower regions are relatively overperfused (V < Q).
- Upper regions are relatively underperfused (V > Q).

Lung apex: high ventilation/perfusion

V/Q can be as high as three in the upper regions of the lung. This means R is also high, so more CO_2 is released (blood CO_2 load is less owing to underperfusion, so proportionally more is extracted from the blood) than O_2 is taken up (less O_2 can be removed from the alveoli owing to underperfusion) (Table 3.4).

Lung base: low ventilation/perfusion

V/Q here can be as low as 0.6. R is also low, meaning less CO_2 is removed compared with O_2 uptake.

Carbon dioxide: Unmatched ventilation does not clear the relatively large load of CO_2 presented by the rich perfusing blood

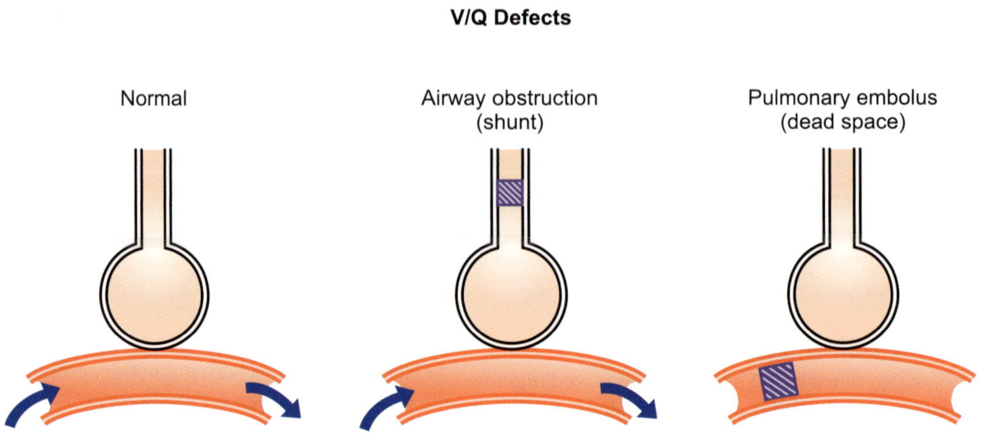

V/Q Defects
Normal
Airway obstruction
(shunt)
Pulmonary embolus
(dead space)

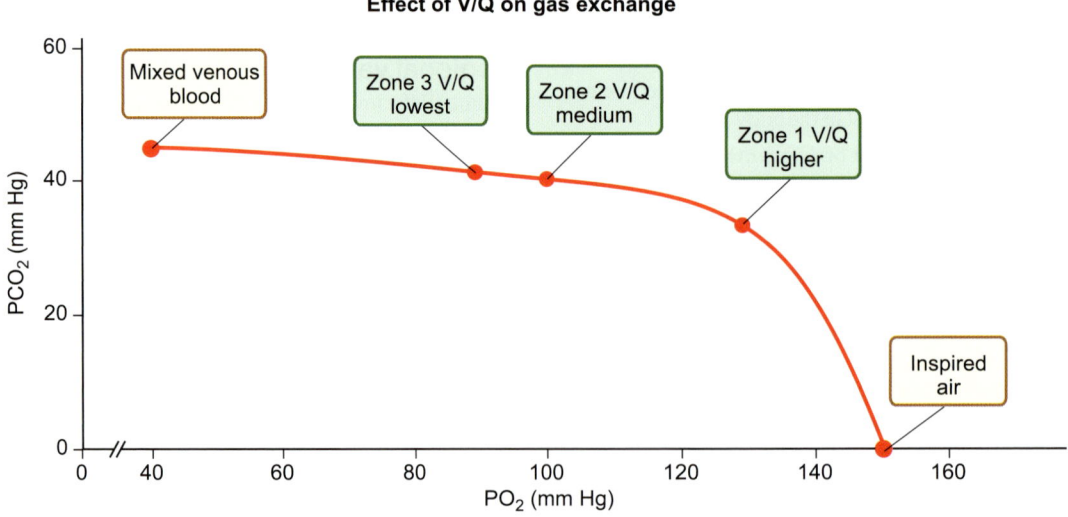

	Normal	Airway obstruction (shunt)	Pulmonary embolus (dead space)
V/Q	0.8	0	∞
P_AO_2	100	40	150
P_ACO_2	40	46	0
PaO_2	100	40	–
$PaCO_2$	40	46	–

Fig. 3.34 Effect of ventilation/perfusion defects on gaseous exchange in the lungs.

Effect of V/Q on gas exchange
Mixed venous blood
Zone 3 V/Q lowest
Zone 2 V/Q medium
Zone 1 V/Q higher
Inspired air
PCO2 (mm Hg)
60
40
20
0
0
40
60
80
100
120
140
160
PO2 (mm Hg)

Fig. 3.35 Effect of ventilation/perfusion *(V/Q)* on gaseous exchange.

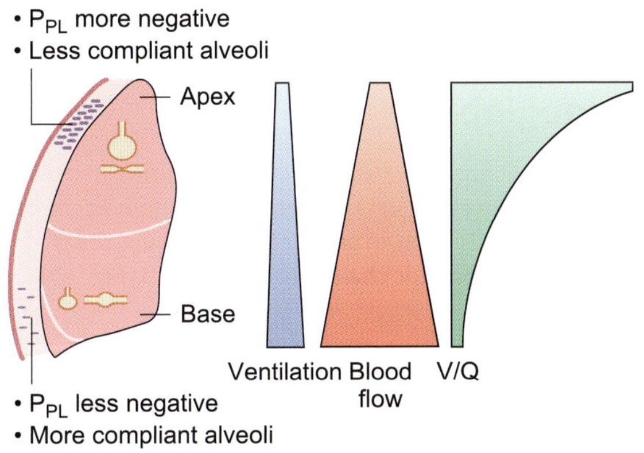

- P$_{PL}$ more negative
- Less compliant alveoli

Apex

Base

Ventilation Blood V/Q
flow

- P$_{PL}$ less negative
- More compliant alveoli

Fig. 3.36 Variation of ventilation, blood flow and ventilation/perfusion *(V/Q)* values according to lung level. P$_{PL}$, *Pleural pressure*.

Table 3.7 Differences between apical and basal gaseous exchange

Gaseous exchange at apex	Gaseous exchange at base
V > Q	Q > V
Less blood flow	More blood flow
↑ PAO$_2$	↓ PAO$_2$
↓ PACO$_2$	↑ PACO$_2$
↑ PaO$_2$	↓ PaO$_2$
↓ PaCO	↑ PaCO

Remember, a greater amount of gaseous exchange takes place in more basal regions.

Q, *Alveolar perfusion;* V, *ventilation rate.*

supply. Hence, P$_A$CO$_2$ tends to rise and is relatively high compared with the apical regions. Consequently, PaCO$_2$ will also be higher, owing to diffusion. P$_A$CO$_2$ is still less than PaCO$_2$ because V/Q is greater than zero (in which case the two values would be the same after equilibrating).

Oxygen: Greater perfusion transports away relatively more O$_2$ from the alveolus than at the apex. As ventilation is less in lower regions, P$_A$O$_2$ is lower at the base than at the apex. Consequently, PaO$_2$ will be lower.

Effect of regional variation in ventilation/perfusion on overall gaseous exchange

The fact that there is more blood flow through the basal regions, which comprise a greater volume of the lung, is of no

consequence for systemic CO$_2$, as the combined blood from different levels of the lungs has a 'normal' CO$_2$ content.

However, it is critical for O$_2$ that V/Q values do not differ too greatly as a result of unequal perfusion. The blood from the apex has a high PaO$_2$ and low PaCO$_2$; however, this is a relatively small volume and the Hb is saturated, so the O$_2$ content of this blood is not significantly higher than normal values. This then mixes with a large volume of blood with a lower O$_2$ content from the bases.

The narrow range of V/Q ratios must be maintained and ventilation best matched to perfusion to avoid depression of PaO$_2$ in the left atrium (the majority of which drains from the lung bases). Distribution of ventilation and blood flow follows a bell-shaped curve, with the greater proportion of all ventilation and perfusion directed to regions where V/Q is nearer 1. This can change in disease when areas with low V/Q ratios are perfused well.

Measurement of ventilation and perfusion
V/Q scan

This consists of two separate scans of ventilation and perfusion, respectively, which are then compared for any mismatch or 'filling defects' (Fig. 3.37). Typically, such mismatches occur in pulmonary embolus, where this investigation is particularly useful.

CLINICAL NOTES

PULMONARY EMBOLUS INVESTIGATION

The investigation of choice for pulmonary embolism is a computed tomography pulmonary angiogram (CTPA) because of its higher accuracy and ability to better visualize the lungs. However, V/Q scans are often still used to investigate for pulmonary emboli in pregnant females to avoid the radiation dose of a CTPA.

Ventilation scan: This involves whole-lung scintillation images after inhalation of a radioactive gas mixture such as ^{133}Xe or technetium-labelled diethylene triamine penta-acetic acid (^{99m}Tc DTPA). Ventilated areas will take up the radioactive gas and will therefore show up on the scan.

Perfusion scan: As with the measurement of pulmonary blood flow, ^{99m}Tc-labelled macroaggregates of albumin (MAA) are used to demonstrate any perfusion defects. A gamma camera is used to scan the positions of the MAA. As these have a larger diameter than the pulmonary capillaries, they are wedged within the capillaries for several hours.

Disordered perfusion or ventilation can be seen in respiratory diseases such as asthma or COPD. However, in such cases, any defects in ventilation are geographically matched to defects on the perfusion scan.

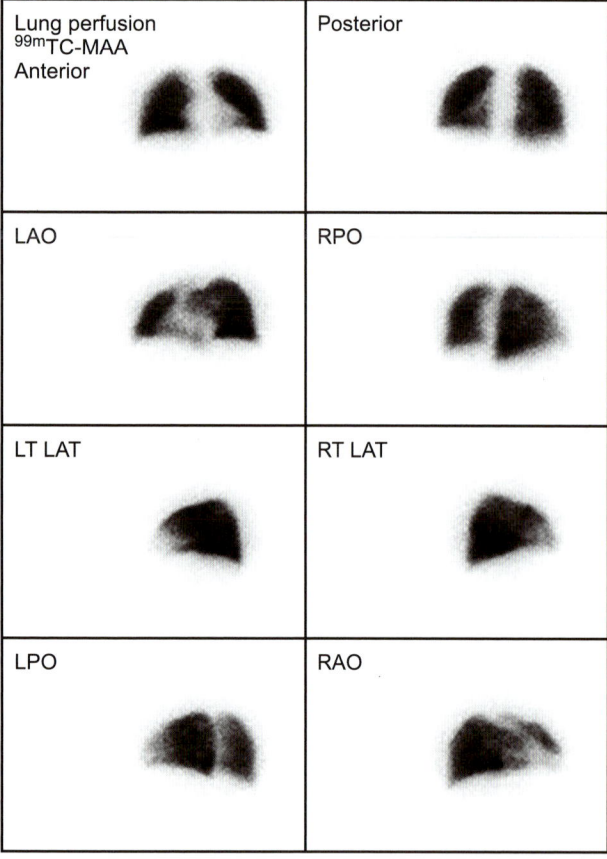

Lung perfusion 99mTC-MAA Anterior	Posterior
LAO	RPO
LT LAT	RT LAT
LPO	RAO

Fig. 3.37 Normal ventilation/perfusion lung scan. LAO, *Left anterior oblique*; MAA, *macroaggregates of albumin*; RAO, *right anterior oblique*; LT LAT, *left lateral*; RT LAT, *right lateral*; LPO, *left posterior oblique*; RPO, *right posterior oblique*.

GAS TRANSPORT IN THE BLOOD

Oxygen transport

The factors that determine oxygen delivery to the tissue are as follows:

- The volume of blood flow as determined by vasoconstriction or vasodilatation.
- The amount of oxygen carried by the blood (dissolved and bound to Hb).

Ninety-eight per cent of oxygen in the blood is bound to Hb, and the remainder is dissolved in the plasma. The amount of dissolved oxygen is governed by the partial pressure (as per Henry's law) and, owing to its poor solubility, is usually 3 mL of oxygen per litre. This would not be enough to meet the body's oxygen demand of 250 mL/min, hence the need for Hb to carry oxygen.

Haemoglobin

Hb is a protein with four subunits (i.e. a quaternary protein), each of which can carry an O_2 molecule. Each subunit comprises a polypeptide chain with an attached haem group (the O_2-binding site). The polypeptide chains are either α or β (Fig. 3.38).

> **CLINICAL NOTES**
>
> **IRON DEFICIENCY ANAEMIA**
>
> Iron deficiency is the most common cause of anaemia. If the body loses or uses iron faster than it can be absorbed, then the production of haemoglobin and myoglobin is impaired. This results in anaemia, which can present with lethargy, pallor and shortness of breath on exertion.

Haemoglobin binding

Oxygen binding is cooperative, so that binding of the first molecule makes it easier for the second to bind and so on, creating the sigmoid-shaped curve for oxygen dissociation. The plateau of the curve is reached at $PO_2 > 70$ mm Hg, which creates a redundancy that allows for complete saturation of the Hb when alveolar concentration of oxygen falls.

The binding of oxygen converts deoxyhaemoglobin to oxyhaemoglobin. The O_2 carrying capacity of Hb is 1.34 mL/g, which includes the small amount of Hb in the Fe^{3+} state and that which is bound to carbon dioxide—neither of which can bind oxygen.

Considering the average amount of Hb in the body (150 g/L for males and 130 g/L for females), the total O_2 carrying capacity will be:

$$\text{Males } 150 \times 1.34 = 201 \text{ mL } O_2/L$$
$$\text{Females } 130 \times 1.34 = 174 \text{ mL } O_2/L$$

> **CLINICAL NOTES**
>
> **CYANOSIS**
>
> Cyanosis is caused by increased levels of deoxyhaemoglobin in the blood from impaired oxygenation of the blood. On examination, a bluish tinge of the finger nails, lips and oral mucosa can be seen.

The oxygen dissociation curve

In addition to the partial pressure of oxygen, the dissociation curve (Fig. 3.39) is affected by:

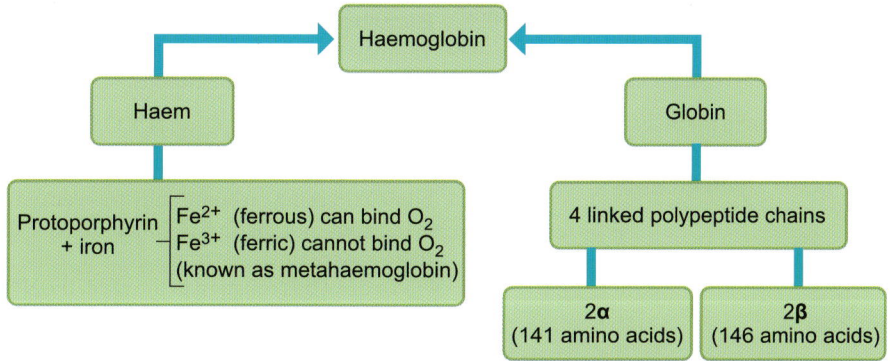

Fig. 3.38 Components of haemoglobin.

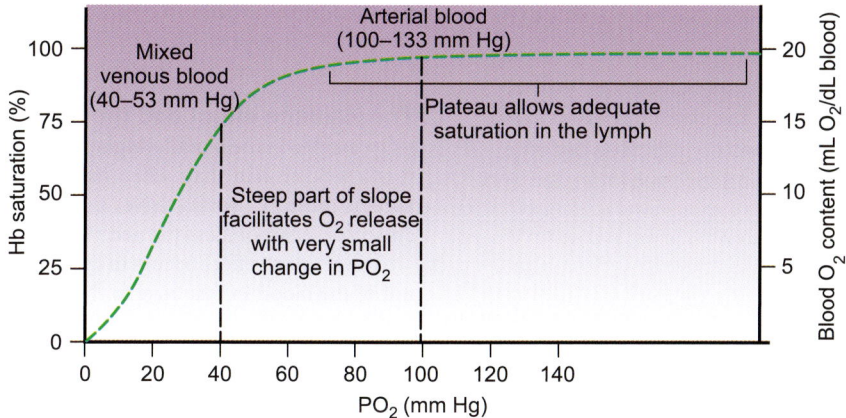

Fig. 3.39 Oxygen dissociation curve. Hb, *Haemoglobin*.

- pH
- Temperature
- 2,3-Diphosphoglycerate (DPG)

Right shift

When there is a reduced affinity of oxygen to Hb, the dissociation curve shifts to the right. This means that it is easier for oxygen to be unloaded from the Hb into the tissues. A right shift is created by the following conditions:

- Lower pH
- Increased temperature
- Increased PCO_2 (the Bohr effect)
- Higher 2,3-DPG

Left shift

A left shift of the dissociation curve allows for easier binding of oxygen and thus better uptake of oxygen in the lungs. It is influenced by the same factors as the right shift but in reverse.

Effects of 2,3-diphosphoglycerate

2,3-DPG is a by-product of metabolism and functions to allow greater offloading of O_2 into metabolically active tissues. It works by binding to the Hb β-chain and reducing its affinity for oxygen. 2,3-DPG is lost in stored blood, which reduces the ability of transfused blood to offload oxygen.

Other forms of haemoglobin
Myoglobin

This is formed of a haem unit with a polypeptide chain and is found in muscles. It differs from Hb in the following ways:

- Higher affinity for oxygen. Aids O_2 offloading from the blood. It cannot be used for blood transport of O_2 because its affinity is so high that the O_2 would never be offloaded.
- Can transport and temporally (for a few seconds) store O_2 in the skeletal muscle.

Foetal haemoglobin

The foetal circulation has a lower PO_2 than the maternal circulation, so an Hb with a higher affinity for oxygen is required to maintain Hb saturation. The foetal Hb differs in that the β-chains are replaced by γ-chains.

Sickle haemoglobin

Sickle haemoglobin has a mutation in the β-chain that reduces its affinity for oxygen. In its deoxygenated state, it has poor solubility, causing it to polymerize and distort the shape of the erythrocyte into a sickle or crescent shape.

Thalassaemias

Mutations in either α- or β-chains create defective synthesis in the production of either globin chain.

Carbon monoxide poisoning and carboxyhaemoglobin

When CO binds to Hb, it forms carboxyhaemoglobin. CarboxyHb competes with O_2 for the haem-binding site, but its affinity is 250 times that of O_2. This means that even small amounts of CO can significantly impair O_2 carriage. This shifts the dissociation curve to the left so that both O_2 loading in the lungs and offloading in the tissue are impaired. Inspiring only 0.1% CO reduces O_2 binding by 50%.

Carbon dioxide transport

CO_2 is transported in the blood in the following forms:

- Dissolved in plasma
- Bicarbonate ions
- Carbamino compounds

Dissolved CO_2

Between 5% and 10% of CO_2 is dissolved in the plasma, which is governed by its pCO_2. The solubility of CO_2 is 20 times more than that of O_2 so that the amount of dissolved CO_2 is 27 mL CO_2 per litre of plasma.

Bicarbonate ions

The majority of CO_2 (90% in arterial and 60% in venous) blood is transported as bicarbonate ions.

$$CO_2 + H_2O \rightleftharpoons H_2CO_3 \rightleftharpoons H^+ + HCO_3^-$$

The initial phase in this reaction converts the CO_2 into carbonic acid using carbonic anhydrase enzyme found in erythrocytes (but not plasma), which makes this reaction occur thousands of times faster.

To drive this equation to the right, the H^+ ions become bound to Hb and the HCO_3^- ions are transported out of the red blood cells (RBC) in exchange for Cl^- (the Hamburger phenomenon).

Carbamino compounds

In the tissues, CO_2 reacts with the terminal amino group on proteins to form a carbamino compound. This accounts for 30% of venous CO_2 transport. This reaction does not use an enzyme and CO_2 is readily released in the lungs.

The Haldane effect and the Bohr effect

CO_2 carriage in the blood is higher when deoxygenated because it is a weaker acid than when oxygenated. This means that it accepts more H^+, which drives the above reaction to the right, and more bicarbonate is formed.

The Haldane effect occurs in the lungs when CO_2 is dumped out of the blood in response to the sudden oxygenation of Hb, and conversely, in the tissues, when the extraction of oxygen for metabolism creates an uptake of CO_2.

The Bohr effect is a shift of the oxygen dissociation curve to the right in response to CO_2 and acidity in metabolically active tissues, meaning more oxygen is released.

CONTROL OF RESPIRATORY FUNCTION

Control of ventilation

Control of ventilation is vital for maintaining arterial blood gases while meeting the variable requirements of the body. Generally, control of ventilation is involuntary or automatic, resulting from impulses originating in the brainstem, which generates the normal quiet breathing cycle of rhythmic inspiration and expiration.

The control system adjusts its output in response to alterations in ventilation or chemical markers such as H^+ or $PaCO_2$.

The respiratory control system consists of three basic components (Fig. 3.40):

1. *Sensors:* Detect changes and feedback information to the central control.

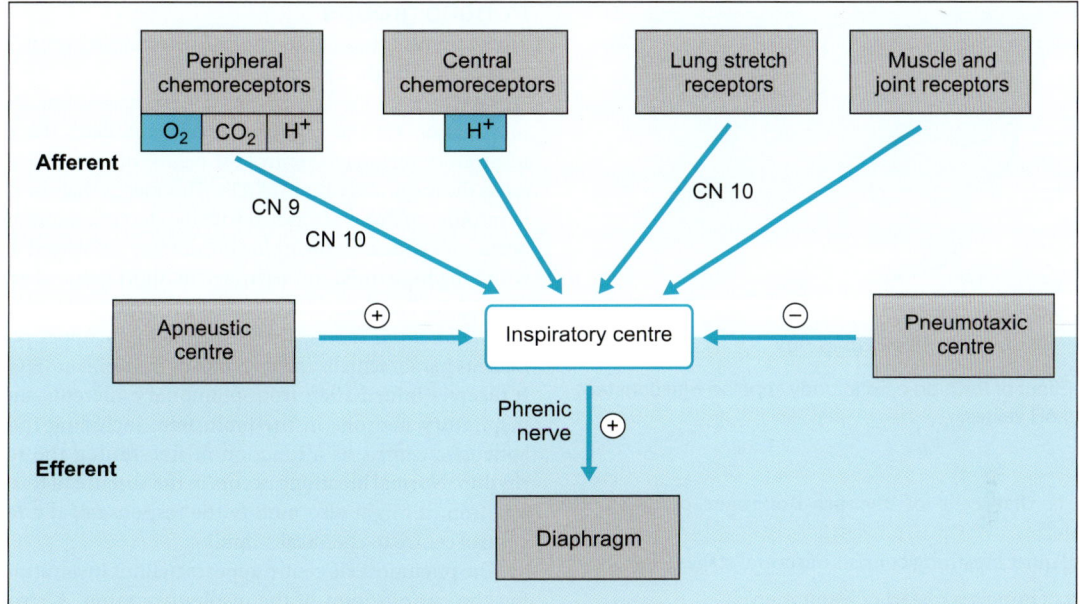

Fig. 3.40 Simplified ventilatory system. CN, *Cranial nerve.*

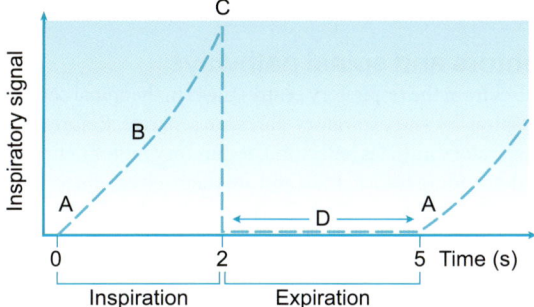

Fig. 3.41 Schematic representation of dorsal and ventral respiratory group circuits.

2. *Central control:* Produces a modifiable breathing pattern and sends command discharges to the effectors.
3. *Effectors:* Perform ventilation and modifications to breathing and tidal volume as dictated by the central control.

Central control of breathing

Brainstem collections of neurons, also known as respiratory centres, generate the breathing cycle. Several functional groups concerned with breathing control are recognized in the medulla and pons (Fig. 3.41):

- Medullary groups: Located in the reticular formation beneath the floor of the fourth ventricle bilaterally:

- *Dorsal respiratory group (DRG):* Mainly involved with inspiration.
- *Ventral respiratory group (VRG):* Mainly involved with expiration.
- Pontine groups:
  - *Apneustic centre:* modifies inspiration.
  - *Pneumotaxic centre (also known as pontine respiratory group):* modifies inspiration.

Medullary respiratory centre
This is believed to be essential to generate breathing. DRG and VRG are not completely anatomically discrete, with intermingling of their neurons.

Dorsal respiratory group
The DRG is located mostly in the nucleus of tractus solitarius, which is where the sensory parts of the glossopharyngeal nerve (cranial nerve (CN) 9) and vagus nerve (CN 10) terminate. The information the DRG receives from receptors/sensors is thought to be integrated, and breathing control is influenced by this area as well as by the VRG, which receives collaterals from the DRG.

The DRG is believed to be primarily responsible for establishing rhythmic breathing by the periodic, repeated production of APs that excite (contralateral) lower motor neurons of inspiratory muscles such as the intercostals and diaphragm. Early evidence suggested that these APs were generated in the absence of any known afferent signal. However, more recent

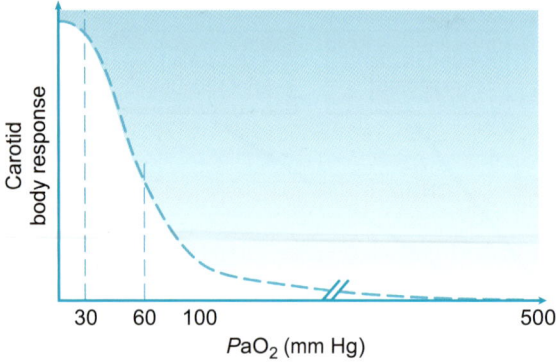

Fig. 3.42 Effect of PaO_2 on carotid body impulse with constant $PaCO_2$ and pH values.

evidence is that cells of the pre-Botzinger complex are responsible.

Normal quiet breathing consists of several stages (Fig. 3.41):

- A: Start of impulses = start of inspiration.
- B: Increase in impulses in crescendo style = increasing muscle activity and lung volume.
- C: Abrupt cessation of impulses = diaphragm contraction ceases with limit reached in lung volume.
- D: No impulses = expiration with diaphragm relaxation permitting elastic recoil of chest wall.

Thus lung volume steadily increases with increasing signal intensity (Fig. 3.42).

Ventral respiratory group

The VRG is located anterolateral to the DRG and involve the:

- Nucleus retroambiguus
- Nucleus ambiguus
- Retrofacial nucleus

There are both inspiratory and expiratory neurons in each of the above.

Nucleus retroambiguus: Contains two types of inspiratory neurons, which:

- Project within the medulla to other inspiratory cells.
- Stimulate contralateral external intercostals and the phrenic nerve supplying the diaphragm.

Nucleus ambiguus: Contains expiratory and inspiratory vagal motor neurons. Parasympathetic innervation of upper respiratory structures concerned with airway patency (laryngeal, pharyngeal and tongue muscles).

Retrofacial nucleus: Consists mainly of expiratory neuron clusters—known as the Botzinger complex—the functions of which include:

- Inhibition of DRG inspiratory cells.
- Inhibition of some phrenic motor neurons.

Pontine groups

The main function of the pontine respiratory groups is to fine-tune or modify the breathing rhythm.

Apneustic centre: This is located in the lower pons and receives information via the vagus nerves. It stimulates the medullary inspiratory regions to control the degree of inspiration and prolongs the inspiratory ramp of APs. This means that the abrupt halt in inspiration that is associated with the start of expiration does not occur and apneustic breathing occurs (i.e. prolonged inspiration with lung hyperinflation separated by short gasps of expiration). This type of breathing also occurs when vagal nerves are not intact.

Pneumotaxic centre: This is located in the upper pons, in the nucleus parabrachialis medialis and in the Kolliker–Fuse nucleus. It receives information from pulmonary afferents and inhibits inspiratory neurons in the brainstem, including those in the apneustic centre, as a function of fine-tuning the respiratory rhythm. Normal breathing occurs in the absence of this centre. In addition, it might also modify the response of the respiratory control centre to chemical stimuli.

The pneumotaxic centre appears to limit inspiration by altering the cut-off point of the inspiratory ramp. A strong signal from the pneumotaxic centre results in a dramatic shortening of inspiration, with a secondary effect of increasing the respiratory rate. A weak signal from this region will cause lung hyperinflation and a very slow respiratory rate.

Effectors and spinal pathways

Impulses from the respiratory centres travel in the spinal cord, where the inspiratory and expiratory fibres are separate. Before reaching the respiratory muscles (effectors), respiratory motor neurons integrate descending information and are themselves subject to spinal reflexes. Hence, once this information reaches the effectors, coordination between the muscle groups is assured so that expiratory muscles are not active during inspiration and vice versa.

Sensors

- *Chemoreceptors:*
  - Both central and peripheral.
  - Report chemical changes associated with matching ventilation to the body's needs.
- *Lung receptors:*
  - Three main types of receptor: pulmonary stretch, irritant and juxtacapillary (J) receptors.
  - Travel via the vagus nerve.
- *Others:*
  - Chest wall receptors, which use muscle spindle reflex.
  - Include baroreceptors and pain.

Chemoreceptors

These report variations in blood chemistry, stimulating the respiratory control system to ensure homoeostasis of PaO_2, $PaCO_2$

and plasma H^+ as markers of ventilation. Chemoreceptors are either:

- *Central:* Lie within the central nervous system (CNS); their effects bypass respiratory centres.
- *Peripheral:* Lie outside the CNS; they send afferents to the respiratory centres.

In general, the effects of the chemoreceptors are to increase ventilation in response to the following:

- *Hypercapnia ($PaCO_2$):* Detected mainly by central chemoreceptors.
- *Hypoxia (PaO_2):* Mostly mediated by peripheral chemoreceptors.
- *Acidosis (plasma H^+):* Central and peripheral chemoreceptors.

Central chemoreceptors: Chemosensitive areas on the ventral medullary surface, separate from the VRG and DRG, provide 80% of the ventilatory drive and mediate hyperventilation in response to surrounding extracellular fluid (ECF) increase in H^+. Low H^+ inhibits ventilation. Factors affecting the ECF content are cerebrospinal fluid (most important), local blood flow and local tissue metabolism. These are not in direct contact with arterial blood and do not respond to hypoxia.

Response to $PaCO_2$: CO_2 has an indirect effect on the central chemoreceptor by changing H^+ in the cerebrospinal fluid (CSF). CO_2 diffuses freely across the blood–brain barrier into the CSF and reacts with H_2O to liberate H^+ via the following reaction:

$$CO_2 + H_2O \rightleftarrows H_2CO_3 \rightleftarrows HCO_3^- + H^+$$

Importantly, CSF contains very little protein so it does not buffer pH changes as well as blood (plasma proteins and RBC Hb are buffers). Hence, for a fixed change in PCO_2, the effect on pH is greater in CSF than in blood.

Response to plasma H^+: The effect of increased plasma H^+ on central chemoreceptor stimulus is less than that of PCO_2 because of the relative impermeability of the blood–brain barrier to H^+ and HCO_3^-, which penetrate very slowly.

CSF has a normal pH of 7.32, which varies more easily than blood and returns more quickly to normal levels (compared to renal compensatory effects on blood pH). However, if the pH of the CSF is altered for a long time, as is the case in persistent hypercapnia, it returns to nearly normal values. This is because slow HCO_3^- diffusion through the blood–brain barrier buffers the protons; it explains why some patients with COPD have inappropriately low ventilation.

Peripheral chemoreceptors: These are also known as arterial chemoreceptors and are located in the carotid and aortic bodies. They are responsible for all increases in ventilation due to hypoxaemia. They are also sensitive—to a lesser extent—to the following:

- Hypercapnia
- pH change
- Blood flow

Information from the peripheral chemoreceptors is sent to the respiratory centres and ventilation is altered. The hypercapnic stimulus is less important than it is with the central chemoreceptor, contributing 10% to 20% of the steady-state response to elevated PCO_2. That said, the peripheral chemoreceptors respond faster than the central ones to changes in arterial gases.

The carotid bodies are the principal peripheral chemoreceptors and are located at the bifurcation of the common carotid arteries. They measure arterial values only. A high blood flow rate (estimated at $200\,mL/100\,g$ tissue per minute) means the arteriovenous difference is small despite its own very high metabolic rate. The response of the carotid bodies is sensitive and rapid: information relating to variation in arterial blood gases between each breathing signal is relayed via the glossopharyngeal to the respiratory centres.

Each carotid body contains a rich blood supply and islands consisting of two different types of cells:

- Type 1 (glomus) cells:
  - Monitor PaO_2.
  - Lie in close proximity to the carotid sinus nerve (afferent): a branch of the glossopharyngeal nerve.
  - Hypoxia promotes the release of catecholamine granules.
  - The principal signal transmitter appears to be dopamine, which excites dopamine receptors.
- Type 2 cells:
  - Supportive function that is believed to be comparable to that of CNS glia.
  - Surround type 1 cells.

Response to PaO_2: The carotid bodies are sensitive to PaO_2, which ranges from 0 to 500 mm Hg (Fig. 3.42).

- Response is increased below PaO_2 <100 mm Hg.
- Most sensitive when 30 mm Hg < PaO_2 < 60 mm Hg, with the greatest change in ventilation.

As carotid bodies derive their O_2 supply from dissolved O_2, they respond to vascular stasis (decreased rate of O_2 delivery) and cyanide (an inhibitor of cellular aerobic respiration). They do not respond to factors affecting O_2 carriage by Hb, such as anaemia.

Response to other stimuli: The carotid, but not aortic, bodies respond to a fall in arterial pH. Also, the peripheral chemoreceptor stimuli interact so that hypoxic ventilatory drive is increased when there is concurrent hypercapnia and acidosis.

The carotid bodies have both parasympathetic and sympathetic innervations, which can modulate the hypoxic response. In addition, sufficient nicotine will activate chemoreceptors and possibly increase K^+, as shown by experimental studies and supported by the positive effects of exercise, which increase plasma K^+.

Lung receptors

Three main types of receptors in the lung relay information, via the vagus nerve, to the respiratory control centre:

1. Pulmonary stretch receptors.
2. Irritant receptors.
3. Juxtacapillary receptors: including bronchial C-fibre receptors.

Pulmonary stretch receptors—These are located in the bronchi and bronchiolar smooth muscle and respond to changes in transmural pressure during lung inflation/deflation. Stretch receptors project to the DRG and pontine groups, providing them with information on lung volume; increasing lung volume increases the firing of APs in the inhibitory respiratory centres.

Because they respond only to lung inflation, displaying very little adaptability, these receptors are known as slowly adapting pulmonary stretch receptors. Their role has been described generally as to limit the tidal volume by terminating inspiration and to extend the expiratory phase. Two reflexes are associated, providing negative feedback on respiratory activity:

1. Hering–Breuer inflation reflex—Lung inflation inhibits the activity of the inspiratory muscles. This appears to be more important in minimizing the work of breathing in infants and babies, as the reflex occurs within their normal tidal volume. In adults, this reflex is triggered by tidal volume >1.0 L—more than occurs with normal quiet breaths, but probable in exercise.
2. Hering–Breuer deflation reflex—Deflation stimulates inspiration. Hyperpnoea results from decreased receptor activity, with the possible involvement of other lung receptors. This reflex is thought to be important in maintaining the FRC in infants, who have a greater tendency to collapse the lungs owing to (inward) lung recoil > (outward) chest wall recoil.

Rapidly adapting pulmonary stretch receptors—Those stretch receptors located at branch points in the tracheobronchial tree have mechanoreceptor functions. These are known as rapidly adapting pulmonary stretch receptors, and they respond to the rate of change in lung volume. Hence, there is a transient firing of impulses with lung volume change and also rapid adaptability, as the impulse frequency quickly drops to background levels if the volume is maintained.

Normal breathing is interrupted approximately every 10 minutes by a deep slow breath, which serves to prevent the slow lung collapse that would otherwise occur.

Mechanical or chemical stimuli can also elicit the following reflexes:

- *Sneeze:* Occurs in response to stimulation of nasal receptors, which send afferents via the trigeminal and olfactory nerves. Such stimulation brings about sneeze, bronchoconstriction and a BP increase.
- *Cough:* Occurs as a result of stimulation of receptors in the upper and lower airways, which send afferents via the vagus nerve. Responses include bronchoconstriction and cough.

Irritant receptors—Irritant receptors are thought to be located between epithelial cells throughout the respiratory tract (possibly including the alveoli). They respond to inhalation of noxious gases and vapours, such as cigarette smoke, dust and ammonia, sending impulses via the vagus nerve (except the nasal receptors, which send afferents via the trigeminal and olfactory nerves).

Juxtacapillary receptors and bronchial C-fibres—Both of these receptor types comprise nonmyelinated C-fibre endings that project to the respiratory centres via the vagus nerve.

Juxtacapillary receptors
- Located in the pulmonary capillary walls or interstitium, these are stimulated by:
  - Pulmonary vascular congestion.
  - Interstitial fluid (ISF) (oedema).
  - Factors released by lung damage: histamine, prostaglandins and bradykinin.
  - Reflex action: rapid, shallow breathing (tachypnoea) and cardiovascular effects (hypotension and bradycardia).
- Intense stimulation results in apnoea.
- Probably responsible for dyspnoea (sensation of difficulty in breathing) in pulmonary oedema and pulmonary vascular congestion secondary to heart failure.

Bronchial C-fibres
- Supplied by the bronchial circulation.
- Stimulated by injection of chemicals into the bronchial circulation, such as capsaicin.
- Reflex action: tachypnoea, bronchoconstriction and mucus secretion.

Other receptors

Chest wall: The receptors of the chest wall are muscle spindles, which function via a feedback mechanism to adjust the strength of muscular contraction. This can be important in altering ventilatory muscle output to meet increased workloads, such as decreased compliance.

Joint and muscle receptors: Limb proprioceptive and tendon organ receptors can send information to the respiratory centres. In addition, proprioceptive receptors stimulated by moving limbs are believed to increase ventilation, especially during the early stages of exercise.

Arterial baroreceptors: These function as stretch receptors in the carotid sinuses and aortic arches and are stimulated by increased arterial BP:

- An increase in BP results in hypoventilation or a brief period of apnoea, bronchodilation and bradycardia.
- A decrease in BP results in hyperventilation.

Pain: The effects of pain on respiration depend on the type of pain:

- Visceral pain (e.g. internal organ distension) causes decreased ventilation or apnoea.

- Somatic pain (e.g. skin laceration) causes rapid shallow breathing.

Voluntary control of breathing

Automatic control of breathing can be overridden by voluntary control from higher centres. Information from the cortex bypasses the brainstem structures and is relayed directly to the spinal nerves, driving respiratory muscles via the corticospinal tract. Higher brain centres mediate control in the case of emotion, speech or singing.

Coordinated responses of the respiratory system

Response to CO_2

CO_2 is the most important factor in ventilatory control through its action on chemoreceptors as described previously. A rise in $PaCO_2$ stimulates ventilation, increasing the rate of CO_2 excretion and reducing $PaCO_2$ to normal values (40 mm Hg). $PaCO_2$ is precisely controlled within very fine limits so that even small changes will trigger a ventilatory response.

- Increasing inspired CO_2 increases minute ventilation in a linear fashion, by elevating both depth and rate of inspiration.
- Minute ventilation is most sensitive to inspired CO_2 of 5% to 10%.
- Elimination of CO_2 becomes difficult when inspired air is similar to alveolar values with respect to PCO_2.
- Inspired CO_2 >10% to 15% has little effect on ventilation.

The physical response to this gas is dictated by inspired concentration:

- Low concentrations (>0.3%) cause increased ventilation.
- Higher concentrations (5–10%) cause:
  - dyspnoea (feeling of difficulty breathing)
  - greatly increased ventilation
  - cerebral vasodilation, causing headache
  - restlessness
- Very high concentrations (15–20%) cause:
  - respiratory depression
  - coma (CO_2) narcosis
  - rigidity and tremor
- Grossly high concentrations (>20%) cause generalized convulsions.

The CO_2 ventilatory response is reduced in certain circumstances:

- Non-rapid eye movement (REM) sleep
- Trained athletes
- Narcotics and anaesthetics
- Increased work of breathing
- Old age

CO_2 ventilatory response is increased in:

- Metabolic acidosis
- Hypoxia

Response to O_2

The ventilatory response to reduced PaO_2 increases significantly below 50 to 60 mm Hg (with normal $PaCO_2$ values). These are much lower than occur normally; thus the hypoxic stimulus is usually not a significant contributor to ventilatory drive. Experiments have demonstrated that PaO_2, which relates to dissolved O_2 and not to blood O_2 content (e.g. low Hb), determines this response. The increase in ventilation is brought about via peripheral chemoreceptor afferents (in particular, those from the carotid bodies).

The hypoxic response is subject to $PaCO_2$; a greater ventilatory response occurs at any PaO_2 when $PaCO_2$ is greater than normal, and with significant hypercapnia, $PaO_2 < 100$ mm Hg will actually result in some ventilatory stimulus. As the ventilation response to the two conditions in combination is greater than the sum of their separate effects, hypercapnia is said to interact with hypoxia (Fig. 3.43).

The hypoxic drive becomes the chief ventilatory stimulus in some severe lung diseases such as COPD, where chronic CO_2 retention and resetting of ECF pH have rendered the central chemoreceptors relatively insensitive to hypercapnia. Therefore patients with COPD might have concurrent hypoxaemia, on which they rely to breathe.

CLINICAL NOTES

OXYGEN IN COPD

Treating patients with COPD with too much supplementary oxygen is potentially harmful. If a patient has chronic hypercapnia and a subsequent hypoxic drive, then the supplementation of oxygen will increase their blood oxygen levels, causing a consequential reduction in their respiratory effort. To counter this risk, oxygen supplementation in patients with COPD should be titrated according to the patient's oxygen saturation, aiming for 88% to 92%.

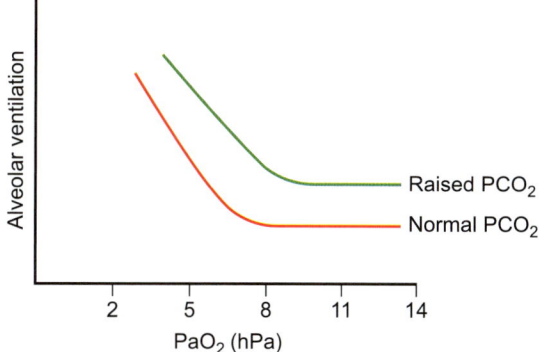

Fig. 3.43 The hypoxic response at differing carbon dioxide concentrations.

Response to H+

Ventilation is stimulated by decreased pH/raised H^+, with the resultant lowering of PCO_2 as alveolar ventilation increases.

H^+ concentration is sensed by the peripheral chemoreceptors because the blood–brain barrier is relatively impermeable to ions, which limits its effect on the central chemoreceptors. However, if there is a significant change in blood pH, the permeability of the blood–brain barrier increases somewhat, so H^+ does exert some influence on central chemoreceptor activity.

Lowered pH usually occurs in association with elevated $PaCO_2$, so that it is difficult to separate responses to the two stimuli. However, animal experiments demonstrate increasing ventilation by increasing H^+ while maintaining PCO_2.

CLINICAL NOTES

KUSSMAUL BREATHING
Metabolic acidosis (e.g. diabetic ketoacidosis) will stimulate the respiratory drive, so-called Kussmaul breathing.

Response to exercise

The increased demands of exercise require a prompt ventilatory response that closely matches elevation in O_2 consumption and CO_2 production. Increases in both tidal volume and respiratory rate can create a minute ventilation of up to 120 L/min, 15 times that at rest. The ventilatory responses to exercise can be considered under the following headings:

- Immediate: at the start of exercise.
- During aerobic-only exercise (<60% maximum work capacity).
- During strenuous exercise with anaerobic metabolism (>60% maximum work capacity).

Immediate response

Neural influences are likely, as they would permit the instantaneous response seen. There is involvement of the following:

- *Higher centre:*
  - Motor cortex neurons send information to skeletal muscles and collaterals to the respiratory centre.
  - Conditioned learned response to exercise exists.
- *Limb proprioceptors:* Send afferents to the respiratory centre.
- *Hypothalamic 'exercise' centre:* May contribute to the initial response to exercise.

During aerobic exercise

There is a linear increase in minute ventilation in association with increased O_2 consumption and CO_2 production. Blood gases change very little during this phase:

- PaO_2 may rise.
- $PaCO_2$ is maintained.
- pH is maintained.

Role of CO_2 oscillations: It has been suggested that peripheral chemoreceptors respond to the greater amplitude of oscillations in $PaCO_2$ and PaO_2 during exercise, even though the mean values remain constant. The periodic nature of ventilation is responsible for fluctuations, which become wider about their mean with increasing tidal volume (as is the case with exercise). The slow ventilatory increase during this phase of exercise in those who have undergone surgical removal of their carotid bodies lends support to this hypothesis.

Role of potassium: Exercising muscle cells release K^+ into the bloodstream, elevating its concentration, which makes the peripheral chemoreceptors more sensitive to hypoxia and so increases respiratory drive.

During strenuous exercise with anaerobic activity

Sixty per cent of an individual's maximum work capacity is typically the threshold above which anaerobic metabolism will begin. After this point, the rise in ventilation is greater than the rise in O_2 consumption but remains proportional to CO_2 production. In this phase, the blood gases change:

- PaO_2 may drop.
- $PaCO_2$ increases.
- pH falls due to lactic acid.

The CO_2 production rises beyond O_2 consumption because the lactic acid drives the equation to the left:

$$CO_2 + H_2O \rightleftarrows H_2CO_3 \rightleftarrows HCO_3^- + H^+$$

Abnormal periodic breathing

Periodic breathing is an abnormal type of ventilation characterized by a cycle of short periods of deep breathing followed by apnoea or hypoventilation. Cheyne–Stokes breathing is the most common example of periodic breathing, consisting of alternating equal length (20–30 seconds each) periods of hyperventilation then apnoea.

The tidal volume waxes and wanes with significant variations in PaO_2 and $PaCO_2$. It is commonly seen in disease states and in various conditions:

- High altitude, especially when asleep.
- Congestive cardiac failure.
- Brain disease.

Several factors might have a role:

- Prolonged circulation from lungs to brain: the negative feedback mechanism from lung to brain is delayed.
- Increased sensitivity to $PaCO_2$: apparently due to disruption of the inhibitory pathways and is seen mainly in patients with brain damage where it is a preterminal sign.

OVERVIEW OF THE GASTROINTESTINAL SYSTEM

Structure

The abdominal cavity contains the majority of the organs of the gastrointestinal (GI) tract together with its accessory organs (liver, gallbladder and pancreas) (Fig. 4.1). The abdominal cavity is separated from the thoracic cavity by the diaphragm. The domes of the diaphragm arch above the costal margin, meaning some of the abdominal organs (liver, spleen, upper poles of the kidneys and suprarenal glands) are protected by the bony thoracic cage. The pelvis surrounds the lower part of the abdominal cavity. The abdominal cavity is lined by parietal peritoneum with visceral peritoneum covering many of the organs. Some organs lie posterior to the parietal peritoneum, in what is called the retroperitoneal space.

Function

The GI system (also known as the alimentary canal) is a mucosal-lined muscular tube extending from the mouth to the anus. It has three major functions:

1. Digestion of food material, starting with chewing (mastication) and continuing in the stomach and duodenum.
2. Absorption of the products of digestion in the small intestine.
3. Absorption of fluid and formation of solid faeces in the large intestine, which are subsequently eliminated.

In addition, the GI system has endocrine and immunological roles.

The process of digestion begins in the mouth, with mastication and secretion of salivary enzymes (amylase and lipase). In the stomach, acid and enzyme secretion continue the process. In the second part of the duodenum, pancreatic enzymes, along with bile from the liver, complete digestion. The majority of absorption occurs in the jejunum, which has a large surface area owing to the presence of plicae circulares (folds), villi (finger-like projections) and microvilli (microscopic projections on individual cells). Carbohydrates and proteins enter the hepatic portal system (see later) via capillaries within the intestinal villi, and fats enter the lymphatic system via lacteals in the intestinal villi.

The liver has multiple functions including the production of bile (which is then stored in the gallbladder) and metabolizing a variety of nutrients, drugs and hormones which can then be excreted. The kidneys' primary function is to filter the blood. They play an integral role in balancing plasma electrolytes and water and thus regulate blood pressure as well as secreting water, ions, some metabolites and toxins via urine. Superior to the kidneys lie the adrenal glands which produce and release hormones.

Surface anatomy and nine abdominal regions

To aid description, the abdomen is divided into regions. A simple yet accurate method is to divide the abdomen into nine regions demonstrated in Fig. 4.2.

The linea alba is a midline depression running from the xiphisternum to the pubis. The linea semilunaris is a slightly curved line and represents the lateral margin of the rectus abdominis muscle on each side.

The inguinal ligament lies between the anterior superior iliac spine and the pubic tubercle. The deep inguinal ring lies at the midinguinal point (halfway between the anterior superior iliac spine and the pubic symphysis). The umbilicus lies at approximately the level of the L3 vertebra.

CLINICAL NOTES

ABDOMINAL INCISIONS (FIG. 4.3)

- A midline incision passes through the linea alba: This allows rapid access with minimal blood loss.
- A paramedian incision passes through the anterior wall of the rectus sheath, the rectus muscle is displaced laterally and the posterior sheath is then divided. Postoperatively, the rectus muscle covers and strengthens the scar on the posterior layer of the sheath.
- A subcostal incision is made 2.5 cm below and parallel to the costal margin (on the right for biliary surgery and on the left to expose the spleen).
- McBurney point is one-third of the distance from the umbilicus to the right anterior superior iliac spine. Each muscle layer is incised individually in line with its fibres, so the strength of the wall is virtually unaffected, although there is a risk of damaging the iliohypogastric and ilioinguinal nerves.
- Transverse incisions are made across the rectus abdominis muscle which is supplied segmentally, so there is no danger of denervation.

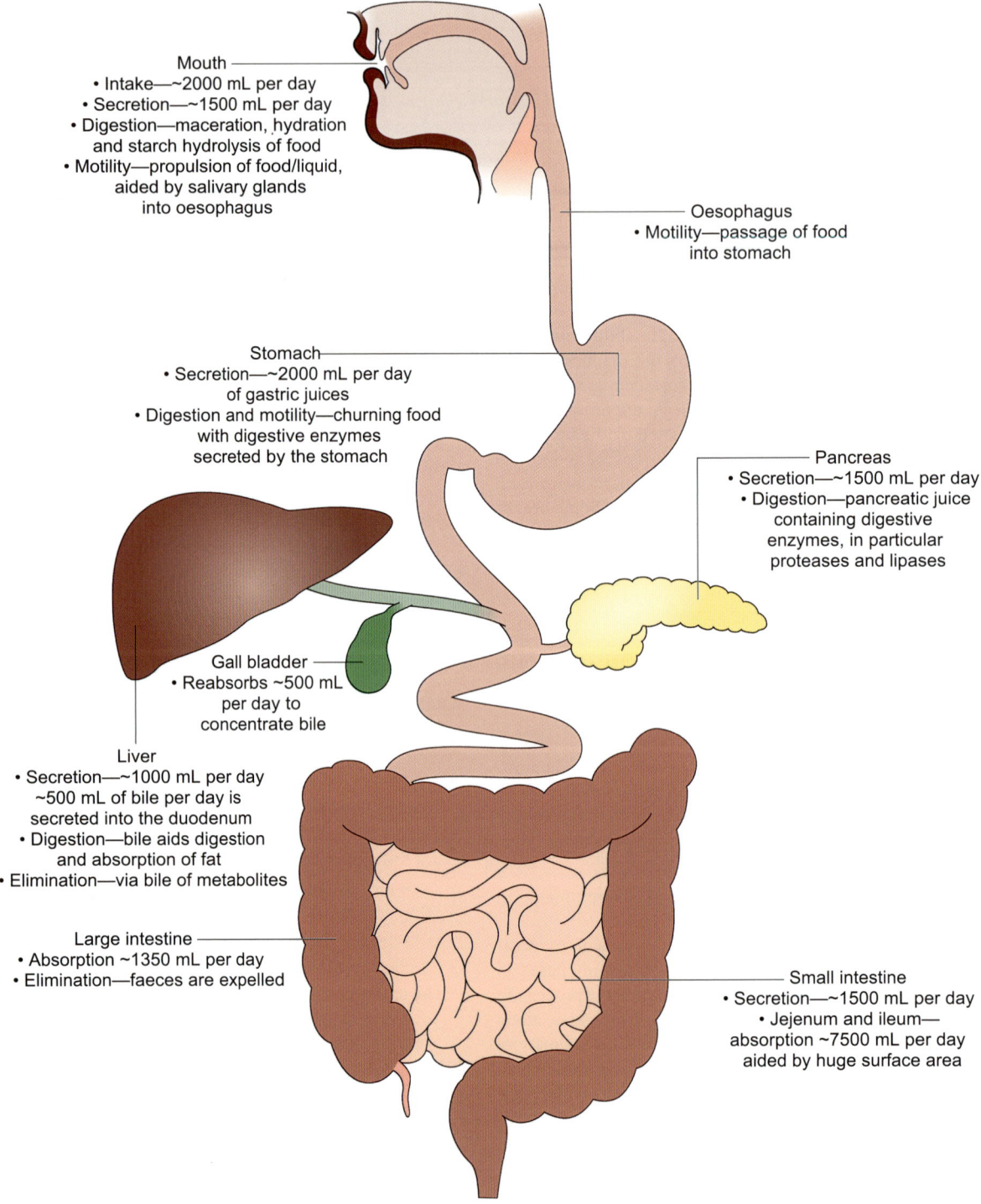

Mouth
• Intake—~2000 mL per day
• Secretion—~1500 mL per day
• Digestion—maceration, hydration
and starch hydrolysis of food
• Motility—propulsion of food/liquid,
aided by salivary glands
into oesophagus

Oesophagus
• Motility—passage of food
into stomach

Stomach
• Secretion—~2000 mL per day
of gastric juices
• Digestion and motility—churning food
with digestive enzymes
secreted by the stomach

Pancreas
• Secretion—~1500 mL per day
• Digestion—pancreatic juice
containing digestive
enzymes, in particular
proteases and lipases

Gall bladder
• Reabsorbs ~500 mL
per day to
concentrate bile

Liver
• Secretion—~1000 mL per day
~500 mL of bile per day is
secreted into the duodenum
• Digestion—bile aids digestion
and absorption of fat
• Elimination—via bile of metabolites

Large intestine
• Absorption ~1350 mL per day
• Elimination—faeces are expelled

Small intestine
• Secretion—~1500 mL per day
• Jejenum and ileum—
absorption ~7500 mL per day
aided by huge surface area

Fig. 4.1 Overview of structure and function of the gastrointestinal system.

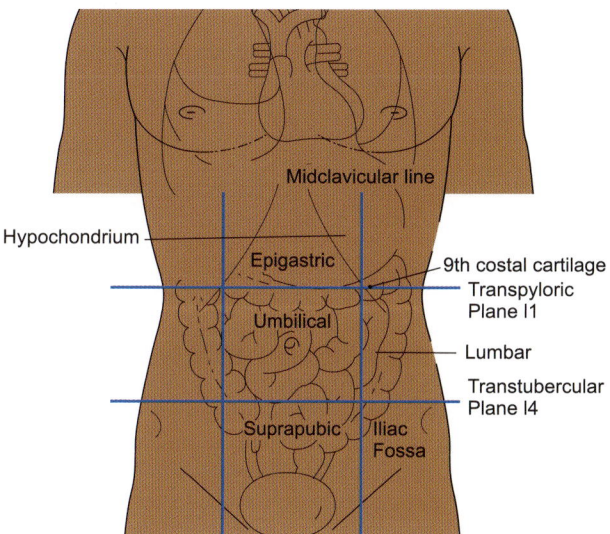

Fig. 4.2 Surface anatomy of the abdomen.

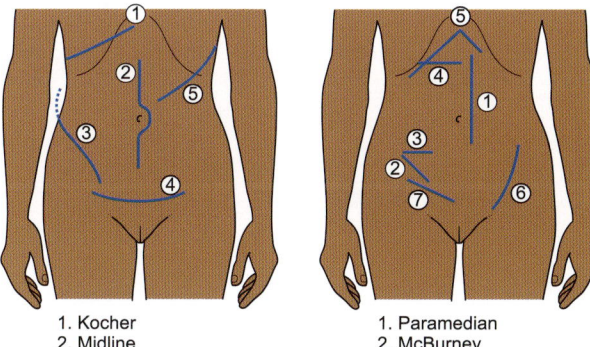

1. Kocher
2. Midline
3. Muscle splitting (ureter)
4. Pfannenstiel
5. Thoracoabdominal

1. Paramedian
2. McBurney
3. Lanz
4. Muscle-cutting transverse
5. Roof-top
6. McEvedy (femoral hernia)
7. Inguinal hernia incision

Fig. 4.3 Surgical incisions.

Liver

The inferior border of the liver extends from the 10th costal cartilage on the right, in the midclavicular line, to the fifth rib on the left, in the midclavicular line. The upper border runs between the left and right fifth ribs, both in the midclavicular line.

Fundus of the gallbladder

The fundus of the gallbladder lies posterior to the ninth right costal cartilage, at the intersection of the transpyloric plane with the costal margin.

Spleen

The spleen lies deep to the left 9th, 10th and 11th ribs, posterior to the midaxillary line. It is not palpable unless enlarged, in which case the spleen extends inferiorly and anteriorly below the costal margin.

Pancreas

The head of the pancreas lies in the 'C'-shaped concavity of the duodenum at the level of the L2 vertebra. The neck lies in the transpyloric plane (at the level of the L1 vertebra). The body of the pancreas extends left, curving upwards towards the hilum of the spleen.

Kidneys

The hilum of each kidney lies in the transpyloric plane. The upper pole of the kidneys lie deep to the 12th rib posteriorly. They lie opposite the L1 to L4 vertebrae (the right lies slightly lower than the left due to the presence of the liver).

Ureters

Each ureter begins at the hilum of the kidney, in the transpyloric plane. The ureter runs inferiorly over the psoas major muscle, anterior to the tips of the transverse processes of the lumbar vertebrae, as far as the sacroiliac joint, where it enters the pelvis.

Development of the gut

The majority of the anatomic formation of the GI tract is achieved in the fourth week of foetal life. The GI tract can be divided into three distinct regions (the foregut, midgut and hindgut) with each region having its own separate blood supply. Importantly, pain caused by pathology in an organ within each region may be felt in different locations of the body. With abdominal pain being very common, a good knowledge of embryology and anatomy will help in diagnosis.

Foregut

The foregut contains all organs of the GI tract proximal to and including the second part of the duodenum. This includes the oesophagus, stomach, liver, gallbladder, spleen, pancreas and parts one and two of the duodenum. It derives its blood supply from the coeliac trunk, with pain from the foregut referred to the epigastric region.

Midgut

The midgut follows on from the foregut at the third part of the duodenum and continues to roughly two-thirds along the transverse colon. It therefore includes parts three and four of the duodenum, jejunum, ileum, caecum, appendix and ascending colon, and the proximal two-thirds of the transverse colon. The midgut is supplied by the superior mesenteric artery (SMA), with pain felt in the umbilical region.

Hindgut

The hindgut begins roughly at the distal third of the transverse colon and includes the remainder of the GI tract, namely the descending colon, sigmoid colon, rectum and part of the anal canal. The inferior mesenteric artery (IMA) supplies the hindgut, with pain referred to the suprapubic region.

Histological overview of the gastrointestinal tract

The wall of the GI tract is composed of four basic layers, with areas of specialization reflecting function as illustrated in Fig. 4.4:

- Mucosa: It is the innermost layer of the GI tract. Modifications to this structure reflect the primary function of each area of the intestine, for example there are more folds and villi in the jejunum than in the ileum or colon, since the jejunum has a more important role in absorption.
- Submucosa: It is a connective tissue layer containing blood vessels, autonomic nerves and lymphatics. Within the submucosa lies the enteric nerve plexus and submucosal (Meissner) plexus.

- Muscularis externa: It is composed of an inner circular layer and a longitudinal outer layer of muscle. The myenteric (Auerbach plexus) lies between these two layers.
- Adventitia: It is the outer layer of the GI tract.

ARTERIAL SUPPLY OF THE GUT

The foregut, midgut and hindgut are supplied by the branches of the coeliac trunk, the SMA and the IMA, respectively. The coeliac trunk arises from the abdominal aorta at the level of T12. It gives off the left gastric, common hepatic and splenic arteries (Figs 4.5 and 4.6).

The SMA arises from the abdominal aorta at the level of L1 (transpyloric plane). It gives off the inferior pancreaticoduodenal, jejunal, ileal, ileocolic and right and middle colic arteries. The IMA arises from the abdominal aorta, opposite L3. It gives off the left colic, sigmoid and superior rectal arteries (Fig. 4.7).

VENOUS DRAINAGE OF THE GUT

Venous drainage of the intestine occurs via the hepatic portal system (Fig. 4.8). The hepatic portal vein is formed by the union of the superior mesenteric vein (SMV) and the splenic vein,

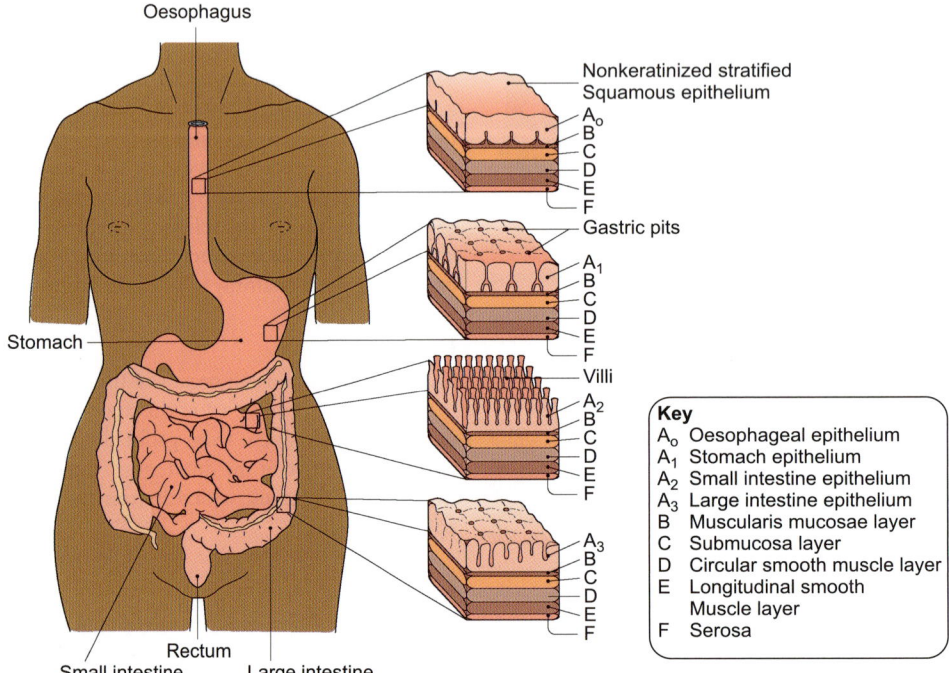

Fig. 4.4 Histology of the gastrointestinal system. The layers comprising the wall of the gastrointestinal tract are illustrated. Epithelial adaptions that dictate function are also shown.

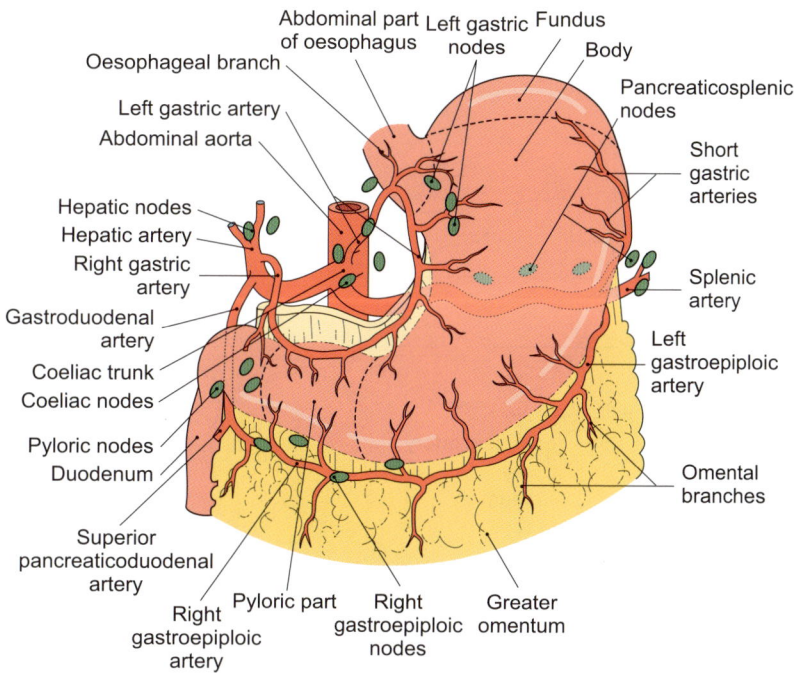

Fig. 4.5 Arterial supply and lymph nodes of the stomach.

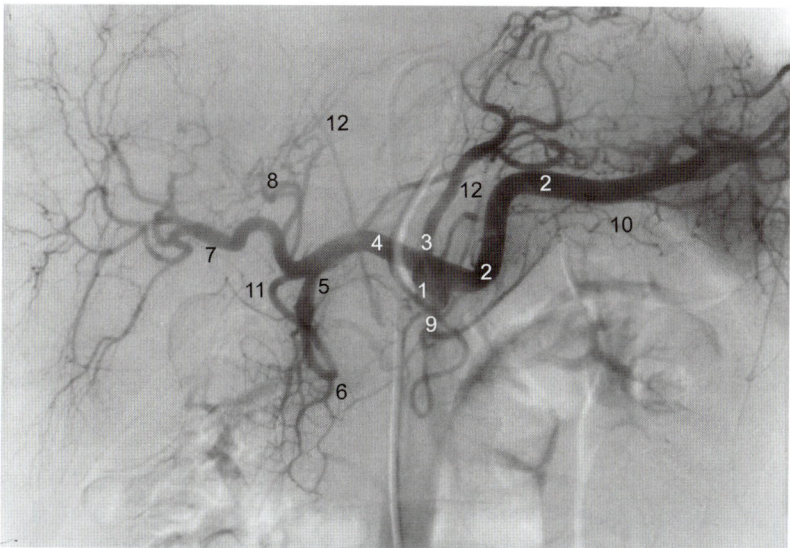

1. Tip of catheter in coeliac trunk
2. Splenic artery
3. Left gastric artery
4. Hepatic artery
5. Gastroduodenal artery
6. Superior pancreaticoduodenal artery
7. Right hepatic artery
8. Left hepatic artery
9. Dorsal pancreatic artery
10. Left gastroepiploic artery
11. Right gastroepiploic artery
12. Phrenic artery

Fig. 4.6 Digital subtraction angiogram of the coeliac trunk and its branches.

posterior to the neck of the pancreas. The inferior mesenteric vein (IMV) drains into the splenic vein.

The hepatic portal vein passes posterior to the first part of the duodenum, in the free edge of the lesser omentum. At the porta hepatis, the vein divides into left and right branches, supplying the left and right lobes of the liver. Within the sinusoids of the liver, hepatic portal blood and oxygenated blood from the hepatic artery mix together and come into contact with hepatocytes, where metabolites, such as the products of digestion, are exchanged. Blood from the sinusoids empties into hepatic veins draining the liver, which in turn drain into the inferior vena cava (IVC) and blood is returned to the heart.

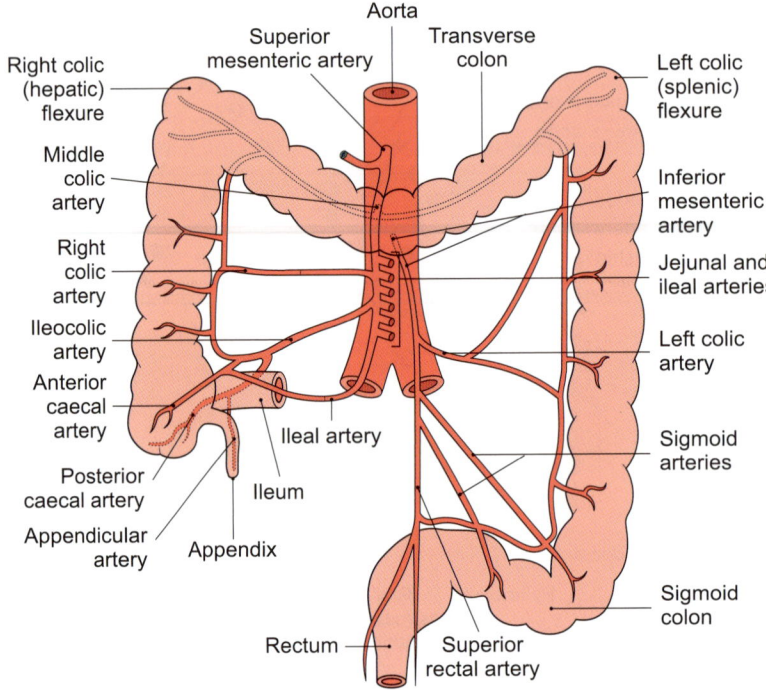

Fig. 4.7 The colon and its blood supply.

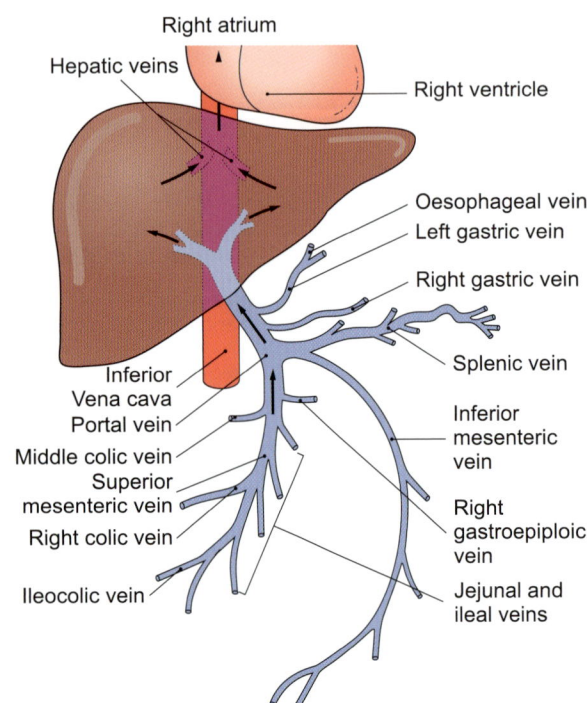

Fig. 4.8 Hepatic portal venous system.

CLINICAL NOTES

PORTAL HYPERTENSION AND AREAS OF PORTOSYSTEMIC ANASTOMOSIS

In portal hypertension, the pressure within the portal vein is elevated. This is usually owing to either increased blood flow or increased resistance to blood flow through the liver (e.g. in cirrhosis, where the liver becomes fibrosed and stiff, causing damage to the blood vessels). The consequence is that a large amount of the blood which would normally pass through the portal vein into the liver is shunted via collateral vessels, which provide an alternative route for the blood to return to the inferior vena cava. Dilatation of these vessels increases the risk of rupture and bleeding. There are several sites at which the portal circulation meets the systemic circulation (i.e. where shunting occurs). These are known as portosystemic anastomoses:

- The lower end of the oesophagus: Present between the oesophageal tributary of the left gastric vein and the oesophageal tributaries of the azygos vein—enlargement results in oesophageal varices, which may rupture, causing massive haematemesis.

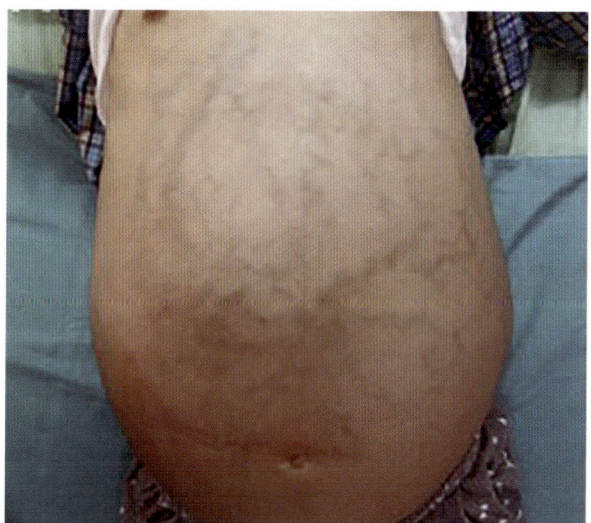

Fig. 4.9 Patients with cirrhosis-related portal hypertension may present with cutaneous manifestations such as visible varicose veins on the abdominal wall called caput medusae. (From Liu, C. H., & Hsu, C. H. (2011). Caput medusa. *Clinical Gastroenterology and Hepatology*, 9(9), A26–A26.)

CLINICAL NOTES — *Contd.*

- Anal canal: Present between the superior and middle/inferior rectal veins—enlargement results in rectal varices.
- Periumbilical region of the abdominal wall: Present between the paraumbilical veins and the superficial and inferior epigastric veins—enlargement causes caput medusae: visible, enlarged, systemic veins radiating outwards from the umbilicus (Fig. 4.9).
- Retroperitoneal anastomoses and anastomoses of the bare area of the liver: These are not clinically significant.

NERVE SUPPLY OF THE GUT

The gut tube receives sympathetic and parasympathetic nerves that travel with the gut arteries. The section 'Nerves of the posterior abdominal wall' has more detail.

LYMPHATIC DRAINAGE OF THE GUT

The majority of lymph from the GI tract drains to nodes close to the viscera in question (usually of the same name), then into either the paraaortic nodes (coeliac nodes, superior or inferior

mesenteric nodes) if the viscera is intraperitoneal, or to the lumbar nodes if the viscera is retroperitoneal. In the case of organs that are secondarily retroperitoneal (the pancreas, the ascending and descending colon), drainage is to the preaortic nodes. Lymph from the preaortic nodes drains to intestinal trunks, and lymph from lumbar nodes drains to lumbar trunks. Lymph from the intestinal and lumbar trunks then drains into the cisterna chyli and into the thoracic duct.

ANTERIOR ABDOMINAL WALL

Over the anterior abdominal wall, the superficial fascia is composed of two layers. The outer layer (Camper's fascia) is continuous with the superficial fascia of the thigh. Deep to Camper's fascia lies a thin membranous layer (Scarpa's fascia). The arrangement of these two layers allows the abdomen to expand. Scarpa's fascia fades over the thoracic wall superiorly, and inferiorly it fuses with the fascia lata of the thigh. In males, it continues into the scrotum and penis as the superficial perineal fascia (of Colles) and the superficial fascia of the penis, respectively. In the female, the superficial perineal fascia lines the labia majora and is perforated by the vagina.

The anterolateral abdominal wall is composed of three layers of muscle. These form an aponeurosis anteriorly to surround the rectus abdominis muscle.

Osteology

Fig. 4.10 shows the skeleton of the abdominal and pelvic cavities. For further details on the pelvis, please see Chapter 5 - Pelvis. The costal margin and floating ribs are described in Chapter 3 - Thorax..

Thoracolumbar fascia

The lumbar part of this fascia arises from the vertebrae in three layers:

1. The anterior layer: From the anterior aspect of the lumbar transverse processes.
2. The middle layer: From the tips of the lumbar transverse processes.
3. The posterior layer: From the tips of the lumbar spinous processes.

The anterior and middle layers enclose quadratus lumborum, and the middle and posterior layers enclose the erector spinae muscles. The three sheets fuse laterally and provide attachment for the internal oblique and transversus abdominis muscles. The thoracic part of the fascia consists of the posterior layer only. This attaches to the thoracic spinous processes and angles of the ribs.

Muscles of the anterolateral abdominal wall

Table 4.1 outlines these muscles. The conjoint tendon is formed by the lowest fibres of the internal oblique and transversus abdominis muscles, inserting into the pubic crest and the most medial part of the pectineal line.

Rectus sheath

Each rectus abdominis muscle is enclosed in a fibrous sheath, formed by the aponeuroses of the three muscles of the abdominal wall (Fig. 4.11). The composition of the rectus sheath changes at three points:

1. Above the costal margin, the sheath is composed of an anterior layer only—formed by the aponeurosis of the external oblique. The posterior aspect of the rectus muscle lies on the costal cartilage.
2. Between the costal margin and a point midway between the umbilicus and pubic symphysis, the internal oblique splits into an anterior and posterior layer. The anterior part of the

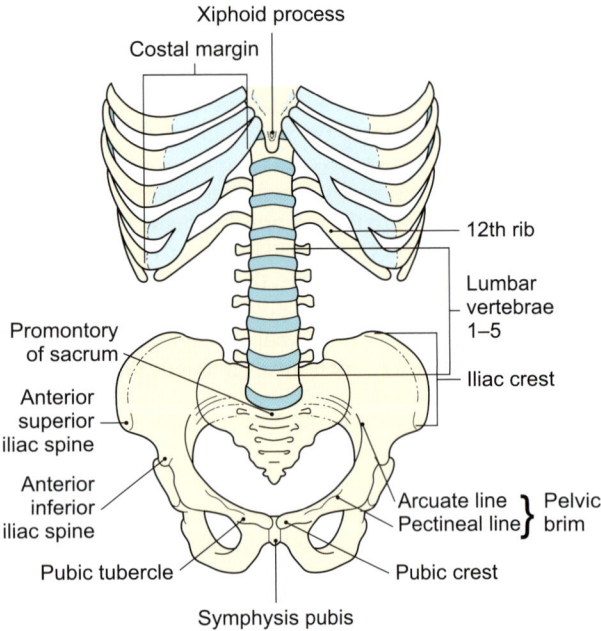

Fig. 4.10 Skeleton of the abdomen and pelvis.

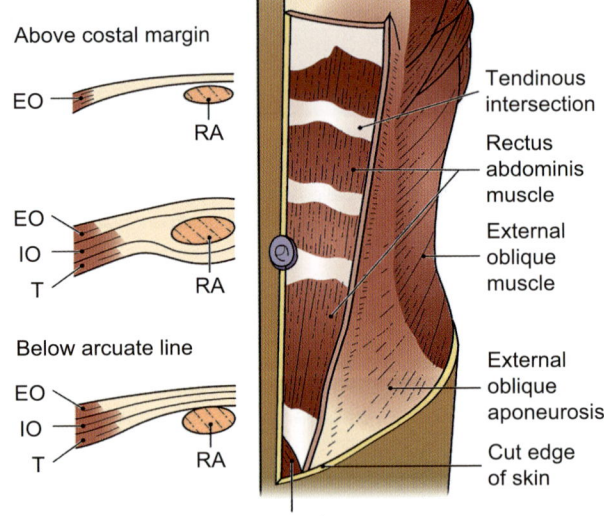

Fig. 4.11 Rectus sheath and rectus abdominis muscle. EO, *External oblique*; IO, *internal oblique*; RA, *rectus abdominis*; T, *transverse abdominis*.

Table 4.1 Muscles of the anterolateral abdominal wall			
Name of muscle (nerve supply)	**Origin**	**Insertion**	**Action**
External oblique (outermost layer) (T6–T12 spinal nerves)	Lower eight ribs	Becomes aponeurotic and attaches to the xiphoid process, linea alba, pubic crest, pubic tubercle, and iliac crest	Flexes and rotates trunk; pulls down ribs in forced expiration
Internal oblique (spinal nerves T6–T12, iliohypogastric and ilioinguinal nerves)	Thoracolumbar fascia, iliac crest, lateral two-thirds of inguinal ligament	Ribs 10–12 and costal cartilages, linea alba, pubic symphysis; forms conjoint tendon with transversus abdominis	Assists in flexing and rotating trunk; pulls down ribs in forced expiration
Transversus abdominis (innermost layer) (spinal nerves T6–T12, iliohypogastric and ilioinguinal nerves)	Lower six costal cartilages, thoracolumbar fascia, iliac crest, lateral third of inguinal ligament	Xiphoid process, linea alba, pubic symphysis: forms conjoint tendon with internal oblique	Compresses abdominal contents with external and internal oblique
Rectus abdominis (spinal nerves T6–T12)	Symphysis pubis and pubic crest	Costal cartilages 5–7 and xiphoid process	Compresses abdominal contents and flexes vertebral column

sheath is formed by the aponeurosis of the external oblique along with the anterior layer of the internal oblique. The posterior part of the sheath is formed by the aponeurosis of the transversus abdominis, along with the posterior layer of the internal oblique. The lower limit of the posterior part of the sheath is known as the arcuate line.

3. Inferior to the arcuate line, all three aponeuroses pass anterior to the rectus muscle, and the posterior wall of the sheath is composed only of transversalis fascia and peritoneum.

Nerve and blood supply of the anterolateral abdominal wall

The principal nerves and arteries of the anterolateral abdominal wall are shown in Fig. 4.12. The inferior epigastric artery and vein enter the sheath at the level of the arcuate line and pass superiorly, deep to rectus abdominis, to anastomose with the superior epigastric vessels. Nerves run in a 'neurovascular plane' between the transversus abdominis and internal oblique muscles. All the nerves give off anterior and lateral cutaneous branches, except for the ilioinguinal nerve, which gives off an anterior branch only.

Venous drainage of the anterolateral abdominal wall

The superficial veins of the abdominal wall include the superficial epigastric and thoracoepigastric veins, which ultimately drain into the femoral vein and axillary veins, respectively.

The superior and inferior epigastric veins and the deep circumflex iliac veins follow the course of the arteries and drain into the internal thoracic and external iliac veins.

Of the four lumbar veins, the lower two drain into the IVC. The upper two join to form the ascending lumbar vein and, with the subcostal vein, drain into the azygos vein on the right and hemiazygos vein on the left.

Inguinal region

Inguinal ligament

The inguinal ligament is formed from the lower edge of the aponeurosis of the external oblique. It extends from the anterior superior iliac spine (ASIS) to the pubic tubercle. It gives origin to the internal oblique and transverse abdominis muscles, and the fascia lata of the thigh.

Inguinal canal

The inguinal canal is a narrow passage, approximately 4 cm long, which lies superior and parallel to the medial half of the inguinal ligament. It runs inferomedially and extends from the deep inguinal ring (DIR) to the superficial inguinal ring (SIR) (Fig. 4.13). The DIR is an opening in the transversalis fascia approximately 1 cm superior to the midinguinal point and lateral to the inferior epigastric artery. The spermatic cord in males, the round ligament in females and the genitofemoral nerve in all sexes pass through the DIR to enter the inguinal canal. The ilioinguinal nerve also passes through the inguinal canal but enters it by piercing the transversalis fascia, that is it does not pass through the DIR. The SIR is a triangular opening in the external oblique aponeurosis, superolateral to the pubic tubercle. The contents of the inguinal canal exit through this ring. It has an anterior wall, a posterior wall, a roof and a floor (Table 4.2).

CLINICAL NOTES

INGUINAL HERNIAS

An inguinal hernia occurs when bowel, omentum or another organ protrudes through part of the inguinal canal.
- An indirect hernia occurs when the protrusion is through the DIR. It is typically a congenital condition.
- A direct hernia protrudes through the transversalis fascia and normally occurs in older males. The hernia passes through Hesselbach triangle (its boundaries are the rectus sheath, inferior epigastric vessels and the inguinal ligament), located in the posterior wall of the inguinal canal, medial to the inferior epigastric artery.

Either hernia may extend along the inguinal canal to exit the SIR and can enter the scrotum. A hernia can be

(Continued)

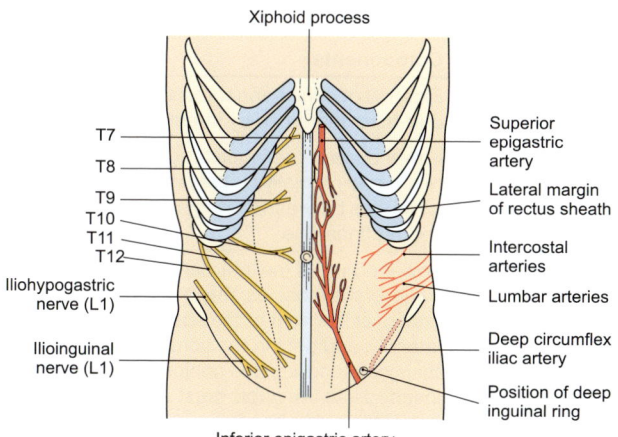

Xiphoid process

T7
T8
T9
T10
T11
T12
Iliohypogastric nerve (L1)
Ilioinguinal nerve (L1)
Inferior epigastric artery

Superior epigastric artery
Lateral margin of rectus sheath
Intercostal arteries
Lumbar arteries
Deep circumflex iliac artery
Position of deep inguinal ring

Fig. 4.12 Innervation (*left*) and arterial supply (*right*) of the anterolateral abdominal wall.

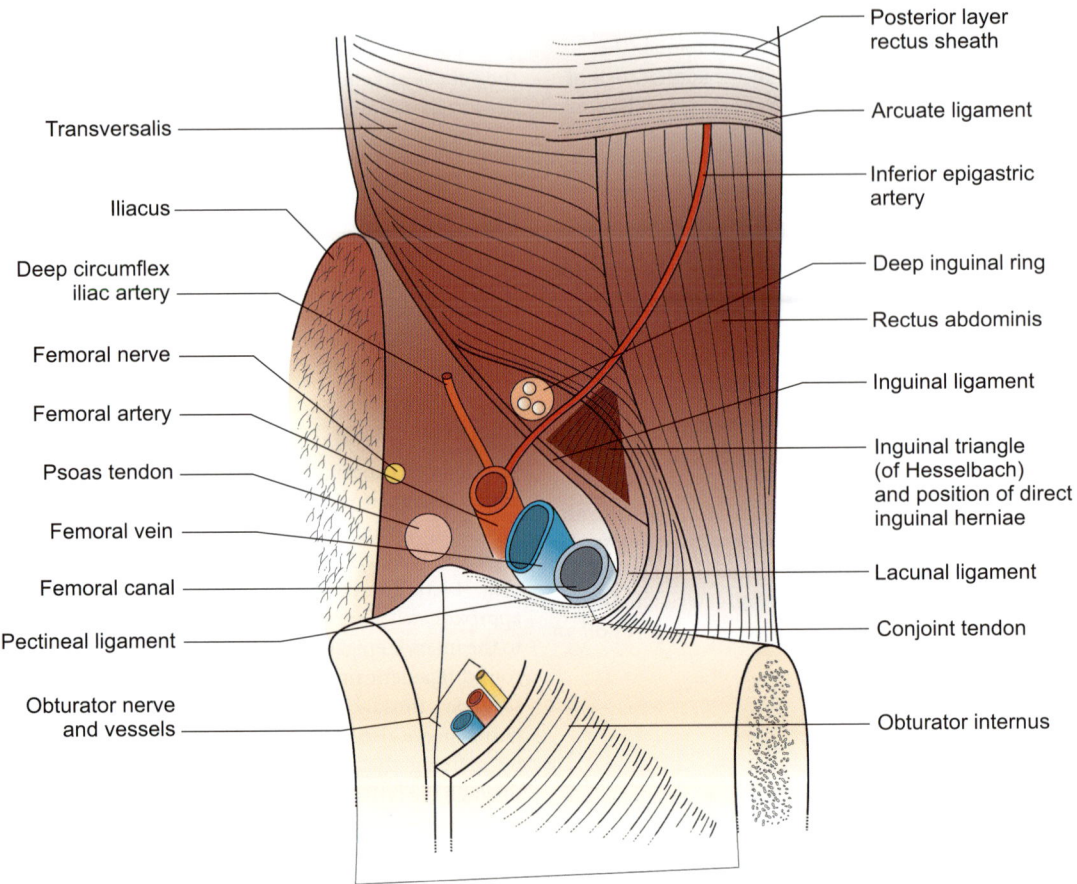

Fig. 4.13 The posterior aspect of the left anterior abdominal wall showing the relationship of the structures described in the text and illustrating the course of the inferior epigastric artery and the relative positions of the deep inguinal ring and the femoral sheath and canal.

CLINICAL NOTES — Contd.

elicited by coughing or straining and can normally be reduced back into the abdominal cavity with gentle pressure or manipulation. If a hernia cannot be reduced, it is referred to as an incarcerated hernia which may lead to partial or complete bowel obstruction accompanied by its associated symptoms (e.g. pain, nausea and vomiting). With an incarcerated hernia, the blood supply to the herniated tissue may become compromised, which is then referred to as a strangulated hernia. Clinically, the patient may present with symptoms similar to that of an incarcerated hernia. However, they are generally more unwell (tachycardic and pyrexial). Strangulated hernias require emergency surgery to prevent necrosis of the bowel.

Table 4.2 Boundaries of the inguinal canal

Region	Components
Anterior wall	External oblique aponeurosis; lateral one-third reinforced by internal oblique
Floor	Lower edge of the inguinal ligament; reinforced medially by the lacunar ligament, which lies between the inguinal ligament and the pectineal line
Roof	Lower edges of the internal oblique and transversus muscles: the muscles fibres arch over the front of the spermatic cord laterally, and behind the cord medially, where their joint tendon—the conjoint tendon—is inserted into the pubic crest and pectineal line of the pubic bone
Posterior wall	Conjoint tendon medially and the transversalis fascia laterally

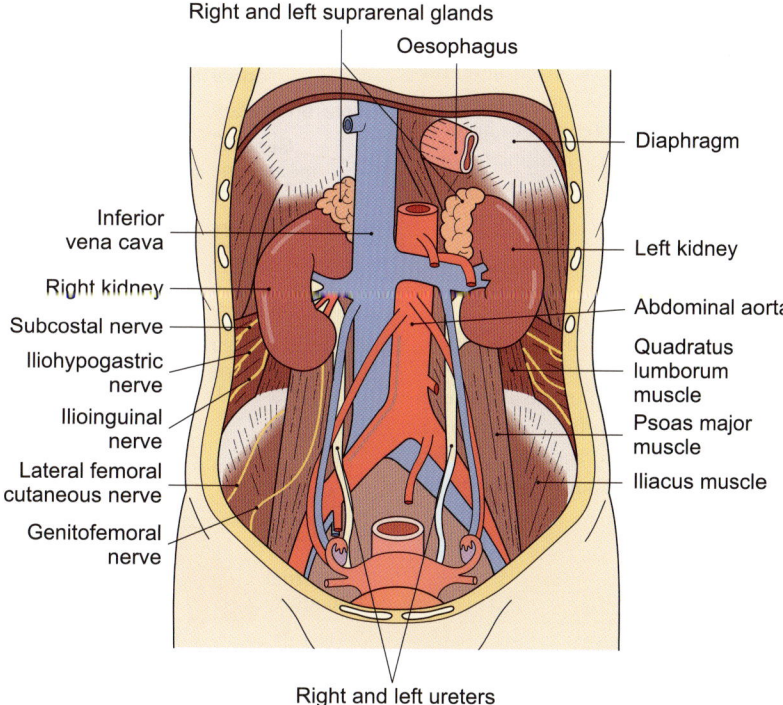

Fig. 4.14 Structures of the posterior abdominal wall.

Labels:
- Right and left suprarenal glands
- Oesophagus
- Diaphragm
- Inferior vena cava
- Left kidney
- Right kidney
- Abdominal aorta
- Subcostal nerve
- Quadratus lumborum muscle
- Iliohypogastric nerve
- Psoas major muscle
- Ilioinguinal nerve
- Iliacus muscle
- Lateral femoral cutaneous nerve
- Genitofemoral nerve
- Right and left ureters

POSTERIOR ABDOMINAL WALL

Posteriorly, the abdominal wall offers protection to the abdominal contents. Largely due to the presence of the vertebral column, the posterior abdominal wall provides a greater deal of protection compared with the anterolateral wall, which is muscular and, therefore, more vulnerable to injury (Fig. 4.14). The posterior abdominal wall is composed of:

- Bony structures: the 11th and 12th ribs, the bodies of the five lumbar vertebrae (and their intervertebral discs), which project forwards into the abdominal cavity and the medial region of the ilia.
- Muscular structures: the psoas major, iliacus and quadratus lumborum muscles. The iliolumbar ligament is a ligament passing from the transverse process of the L5 vertebra to the posterior part of the iliac crest. Table 4.3 details the muscles of the posterior abdominal wall.

Fascia of the posterior abdominal wall

Fascia covers the muscles of the posterior abdominal wall with psoas fascia covering psoas major and the three-layered thoracolumbar fascia already discussed on page 141.

Table 4.3 Muscles of the posterior abdominal wall

Name of muscle (nerve supply)	Origin	Insertion	Action
Psoas major (L1–L3)	Bodies, transverse processes and intervertebral discs of T12 and L1–L5 vertebrae	Lesser trochanter of femur	Flexes thigh on trunk
Quadratus lumborum (T12–L3)	Iliolumbar ligament, iliac crest, transverse processes of lower lumbar vertebrae	12th rib	Depresses 12th rib during respiration; laterally flexes vertebral column
Iliacus (femoral nerve)	Iliac fossa	Lesser trochanter of femur	Flexes thigh on trunk

Adapted from Snell, R. S. (1996). Clinical anatomy. An illustrated review with questions and explanations (2nd ed.) Little Brown & Co.

The superior edge of the thoracolumbar fascia forms the lateral arcuate ligament slung between the middle of the 12th rib and the transverse process of the L1 vertebra. From here, the medial arcuate ligament (the superior edge of the psoas fascia) extends to the side of the L1 or L2 vertebra. Tendinous fibres of the diaphragm pass in front of the aorta in the midline to form the median arcuate ligament.

Vessels of the posterior abdominal wall

Abdominal aorta

The abdominal aorta passes through the diaphragm at the level of T12. It passes inferiorly on the bodies of the lumbar vertebrae. Anterior to the L4 vertebrae, it divides into the right and left common iliac arteries. The branches of the abdominal aorta are illustrated in Fig. 4.15.

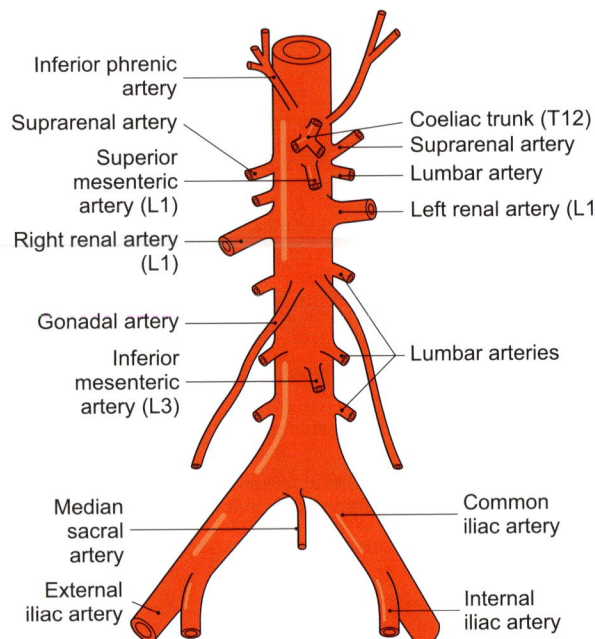

Fig. 4.15 Branches of the abdominal aorta.

> **CLINICAL NOTES**
>
> **ABDOMINAL AORTIC ANEURYSM (AAA)**
>
> An aneurysm is the pathological, localized balloon-like swelling of a blood vessel wall. When an AAA occurs, it is most commonly found infrarenally, that is distal to the branching of the renal arteries. AAAs may be detected as an incidental finding, felt as an expansile mass on the left of the midline or identified using imaging.
>
> Patients suspected of having an aneurysm undergo assessment to confirm the diagnosis and assess risk. Risk factors include being male; age above 65 years; having a family history of AAA; having coronary, cerebrovascular or peripheral artery disease, hyperlipidaemia or hypertension; and smoking. Symptoms may include abdominal or back pain, and if it ruptures, patients will likely be hypotensive and shocked.
>
> The larger the aneurysm, the higher the risk of rupture. Aneurysms less than 5 cm in diameter are generally monitored by means of regular ultrasound scans. Aneurysms over 5.5 cm or those growing at a rate greater than 1 cm per year may require surgery. Surgical management can be an endovascular repair or open surgery to stent the weakened area. Aneurysm rupture is associated with a high degree of blood loss and haemodynamic compromise and can often be fatal.

Inferior vena cava

The IVC is formed by the joining of the left and right common iliac veins (see Fig. 5.13) at the level of the L5 vertebrae. The IVC ascends to the right of the aorta, passes posterior to the liver and pierces the diaphragm with the right phrenic nerve at the level of T8. It then almost immediately enters the heart.

Nerves of the posterior abdominal wall

Somatic nerves

The L1 to L4 spinal nerves emerge from their intervertebral foramina and enter the psoas major muscle, which they supply. The ventral (anterior) rami of the nerves form the lumbar plexus (Fig. 4.16), which is mostly concerned with sensory and motor innervation to the lower limb. However, some branches are motor and sensory to the anterior abdominal wall, for example iliohypogastric nerve, and sensory to the parietal peritoneum, for example obturator nerve. The lumbosacral trunk joins the first three sacral nerves to contribute to the sacral plexus.

Autonomic nerves

The autonomic nerve supply of the abdomen is composed of the following:

- Parasympathetic supply from the vagal trunks and pelvic splanchnic nerves (S2–S4).

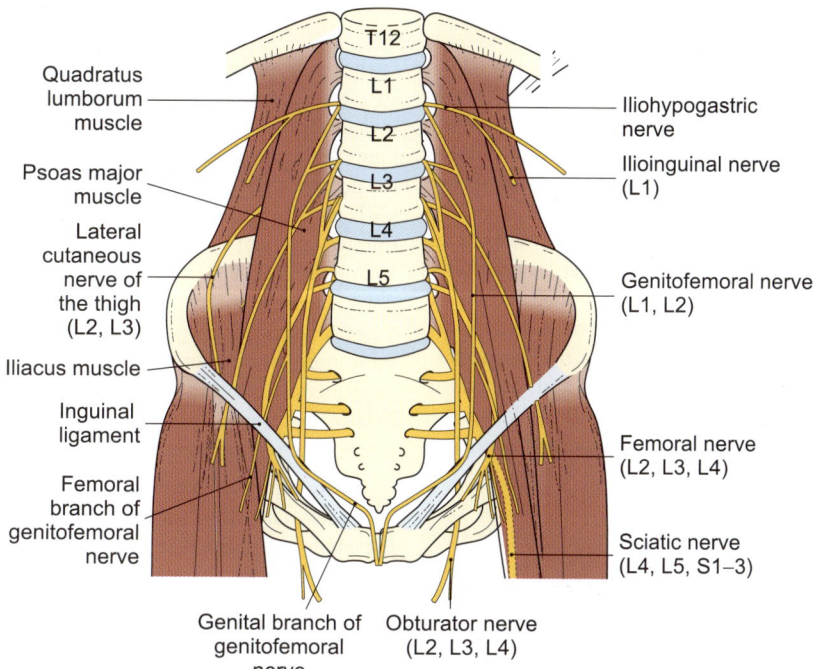

Fig. 4.16 Lumbar plexus and the relationship to the psoas muscle. Note that the sciatic nerve is not part of the lumbar plexus and is shown only for completeness.

- Sympathetic supply from the lumbar sympathetic trunks and the thoracic and lumbar splanchnic nerves.
- Prevertebral autonomic plexuses surrounding the aorta (coeliac, aortic and superior hypogastric), all of which distribute the nerve fibres.

Sympathetic nerves

The lumbar sympathetic trunk comprises preganglionic fibres from the lower thoracic trunk and from L1 and L2 nerves (via white rami). This trunk enters the abdomen posterior to the medial arcuate ligament of the diaphragm. It lies on the bodies of the lumbar vertebral bodies, along the medial border of psoas major.

There are usually four lumbar ganglia. These give somatic branches (grey rami communicantes) to all five lumbar nerves, supplying the body wall and lower limb, and visceral branches (lumbar splanchnic nerves) that join the prevertebral plexuses. Fibres from the third and fourth lumbar ganglia join with fibres from the aortic plexus in front of the L5 vertebra to form the superior hypogastric plexus. The superior hypogastric plexus divides into the right and left hypogastric nerves, which run into the pelvis to join the inferior hypogastric plexus. The sympathetic trunks in the abdomen do not give branches to the abdominal viscera, which are supplied by the greater, lesser and least splanchnic nerves.

The greater and lesser splanchnic nerves are preganglionic—they pierce the crura of the diaphragm to synapse in the coeliac ganglion. The least splanchnic nerves relay in a small renal ganglion close to the renal artery.

From the coeliac ganglion, postganglionic fibres form the coeliac plexus around the origin of the coeliac trunk. Fibres either pass directly or via superior and inferior mesenteric plexuses along branches of the aorta to supply all abdominal viscera.

The suprarenal gland also receives preganglionic fibres directly from the lesser splanchnic nerve—stimulation of which causes the release of adrenaline.

Functions of the sympathetic nerves include vasomotor, motor to the sphincters with inhibition of peristalsis, and carrying sensory fibres from all the abdominal viscera.

Parasympathetic nerves

The vagal trunks supply the foregut, midgut and hindgut: they enter the abdomen on the surface of the oesophagus, directly supplying the stomach. Branches to the coeliac plexus then supply the remainder of the gut as far as the distal two-thirds of the transverse colon. Branches to the renal plexus pass to the kidneys.

The pelvic splanchnic nerves (from S2 to S4) join the inferior hypogastric plexus. Some fibres pass up into prevertebral plexuses to be distributed to the distal part of the transverse colon, descending colon and sigmoid colon (hindgut). Parasympathetic activation of the gut causes stimulation of peristalsis and secretomotor activity of glands (remember 'rest and digest').

PERITONEUM

The peritoneum lines the abdominal and pelvic cavities. It consists of a parietal and visceral layer. The parietal peritoneum lines the anterior, posterior and lateral walls of the abdomen, the inferior surface of the diaphragm and the walls of the pelvic cavity. It reflects off the body wall to surround some of the abdominal viscera. The peritoneum extending from the body wall to the organs forms mesenteries and ligaments. Between the parietal and visceral peritoneum lies a potential space, the peritoneal cavity, filled with a small amount of serous fluid, to allow free movement of viscera. In males the peritoneal cavity is completely closed, whereas in females, the uterine (fallopian) tubes open into the peritoneal cavity and provide a connection to the exterior through the uterus and vagina. Within the abdomen, posterior to the peritoneum lie the retroperitoneal organs.

HINTS AND TIPS

Posterior to the peritoneum lie the retroperitoneal organs. The latter can be remembered with the mnemonic 'PEAR DUCKS' which stands for Pancreas, (o)Esophagus, Aorta and IVC, Rectum, Duodenum, Ureters, Colon (ascending and descending), Kidneys and Suprarenal glands (Fig. 4.17.)

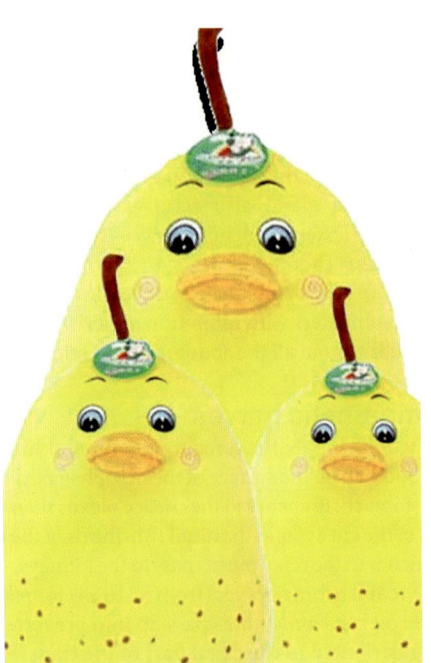

Fig. 4.17 Depiction of the pneumonic PEAR DUCKS. This terrifying image will hopefully mean the pneumonic never leaves your head! (Courtesy Dominic O'Brien.)

Embryology of the gut

In the embryo, the gut begins development as a simple tube-like structure. It develops into the foregut, midgut and hindgut, and invaginates into the peritoneal cavity (in a similar way to the lungs in the pleural cavity). The gut tube is then suspended from the posterior abdominal wall by the dorsal mesentery—the double layer of peritoneum connecting it to the body wall. Between the two layers of the peritoneum are blood vessels, lymphatics and nerves (Fig. 4.18). The dorsal mesentery eventually forms the dorsal mesentery of the small intestine and other named mesenteries, for example the greater omentum. Organs suspended from these mesenteries (and so almost entirely covered by visceral peritoneum) become intraperitoneal organs, while those that develop or come to lie on the posterior abdominal wall, posterior to the visceral peritoneum, are the retroperitoneal organs.

The foregut is also connected to the body wall via the ventral mesentery. Growth of the liver divides the ventral mesentery into the falciform ligament anteriorly and the lesser omentum posteriorly (Fig. 4.19).

CLINICAL NOTES

EMBRYOLOGY OF THE DIAPHRAGM

The diaphragm develops opposite the cervical spine, and its nerve supply is derived from spinal nerves C3 to C5 (C3, C4, C5—keep the diaphragm alive!). Although it moves inferiorly during foetal development, it retains this innervation. Irritation of the diaphragm by thoracic or abdominal pathology (e.g. infection in the subphrenic recess) may cause pain in the C4 dermatome which lies above the shoulder, owing to shared C4 root value—this is an example of 'referred pain'.

Nerve supply of the peritoneum

The parietal peritoneum is supplied segmentally by the nerves supplying the overlying muscles and skin. The peritoneum covering the inferior surface of the diaphragm is supplied by the intercostal nerves peripherally and by the phrenic nerve (C3–C5) centrally. The parietal peritoneum in the pelvis is supplied by the obturator nerve. The visceral peritoneum does not have a somatic innervation and thus is insensitive to pain. However, it receives sympathetic innervation, so it is sensitive to stretch, tension and ischaemia.

Peritoneal folds of the anterolateral abdominal wall

Peritoneal folds are reflections of peritoneum, forming ridges on the body wall. They are produced by an underlying vessel or duct,

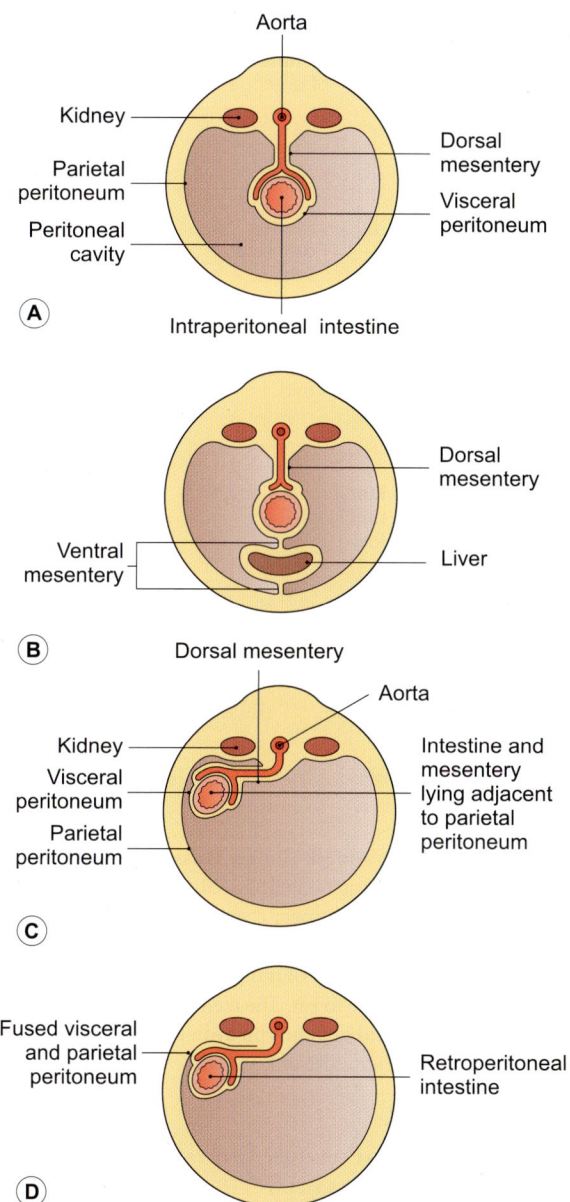

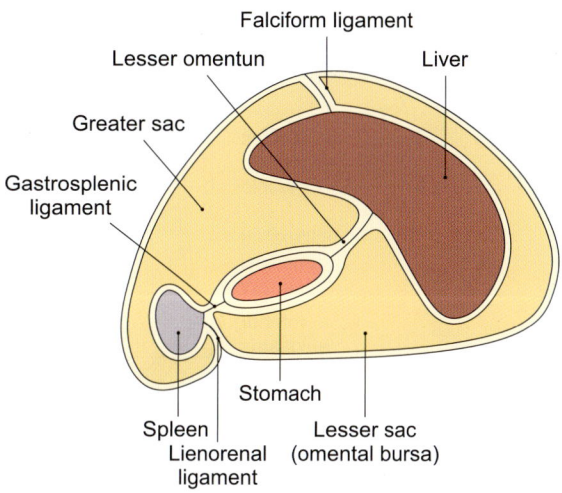

Fig. 4.19 Division of the ventral mesentery, forming the falciform ligament and the lesser omentum.

Fig. 4.18 The embryonic (A), dorsal (B) and ventral mesenteries (C and D) and the formation of the retroperitoneal part of the intestines.

or the remnant of a foetal vessel. There are five peritoneal folds on the abdominal wall (Fig. 4.20):

- Median umbilical fold: Contains the remnant of the urachus (median umbilical ligament).
- Two medial umbilical folds: Contain remnants of the umbilical arteries (medial umbilical ligaments).

- Two lateral umbilical folds: Contain the inferior epigastric vessels.

The falciform ligament is an anterior peritoneal fold (originally the ventral mesentery), lying between the diaphragm and the umbilicus, which contains the ligamentum teres (the remnant of the umbilical vein) in its free margin.

Greater and lesser sacs

During development, the peritoneal cavity is divided into greater and lesser sacs by growth of the liver (which rotates the stomach and duodenum to the right) and elongation of the dorsal mesentery. The lesser sac (omental bursa) is a sac of peritoneum lying posterior to the stomach. The remainder of the abdominal cavity forms the greater sac. The lesser sac communicates with the greater sac through the epiploic foramen. The boundaries of the epiploic (omental) foramen are:

- Superiorly: The caudate process of the liver.
- Anteriorly: The portal vein, hepatic artery and bile duct, in the free edge of the lesser omentum.
- Inferiorly: The first part of the duodenum.
- Posteriorly: The IVC.

For descriptive purposes, the greater sac is divided into compartments. The supracolic compartment lies superior to the transverse mesocolon (containing the stomach, liver and spleen). It is divided into left and right regions by the falciform ligament. The infracolic compartment lies inferior to the transverse mesocolon (containing the small bowel, the ascending and descending colon) (Fig. 4.21A). The infracolic compartment is further subdivided by the mesentery of the small intestine into right and left divisions. The supracolic and infracolic compartments

147

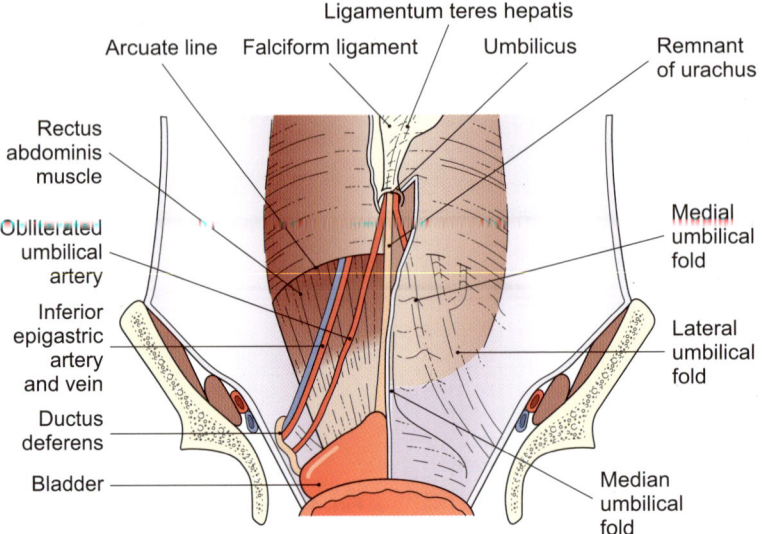

Fig. 4.20 Peritoneal folds of the anterior abdominal wall, viewed from the posterior.

Labels (clockwise from top): Ligamentum teres hepatis · Umbilicus · Remnant of urachus · Arcuate line · Falciform ligament · Rectus abdominis muscle · Medial umbilical fold · Obliterated umbilical artery · Lateral umbilical fold · Inferior epigastric artery and vein · Ductus deferens · Bladder · Median umbilical fold

communicate via the paracolic gutters, lying lateral to ascending and descending colon.

Between the upper surface of the liver and the diaphragm lies the subphrenic recess, divided into left and right halves by the falciform ligament. Inferior to the liver and superior to the right kidney lies the right subhepatic recess (the hepatorenal recess or Morrison pouch), which communicates with the right paracolic gutter (see Fig. 4.21B). The left subhepatic recess forms part of the lesser sac.

In the pelvic compartment, the peritoneum lies over and between the pelvic viscera. The peritoneal pouches formed differ between sexes. Males have a rectovesical pouch. Females have vesicouterine and rectouterine pouches (see Chapter 5).

Greater and lesser omenta

The greater omentum is the largest peritoneal fold, arising from the greater curvature of the stomach. It hangs like an apron over the intestines and is filled with fat. It is fused with the transverse mesocolon and with the anterior aspect of the transverse colon.

The lesser omentum extends from the inferior border of the liver to the lesser curvature of the stomach (known as the hepatogastric ligament) and from the proximal part of the duodenum to the liver (known as the hepatoduodenal ligament).

Peritoneal folds, sacs, recesses and omenta are important as they determine the distribution of intraperitoneal fluid and act as boundaries and conduits for disease (e.g. infection, tumours and trauma).

Food intake and its control

Definitions

- Hunger—craving for food. Hunger is associated with increased food-seeking behaviour, salivation and rhythmical stomach contractions (hunger cramps).
- Appetite—desire for certain foods that directs the choice of food. Can be independent of hunger.
- Satiety—lack of desire to eat. The feeling usually follows the ingestion of food and depends on individual energy stores.
- Anorexia—loss of appetite or hunger.

Central control

Feeding mechanisms are controlled by brainstem centres. Regulation of food intake occurs via:

- Higher centres: Involving the prefrontal cortex and amygdala. Implied importance of habit and conditioning to appetite.
- Hypothalamus: Appetite is regulated by interaction between two areas within the hypothalamus: the feeding centre (ventrolateral nucleus) and the satiety centre (ventromedial nucleus).

Feedback control

There are two main types of feedback control of appetite:

1. Short-term feedback involves mechanical feedback from the alimentary tract during feeding and limits the quantity of food eaten per meal.

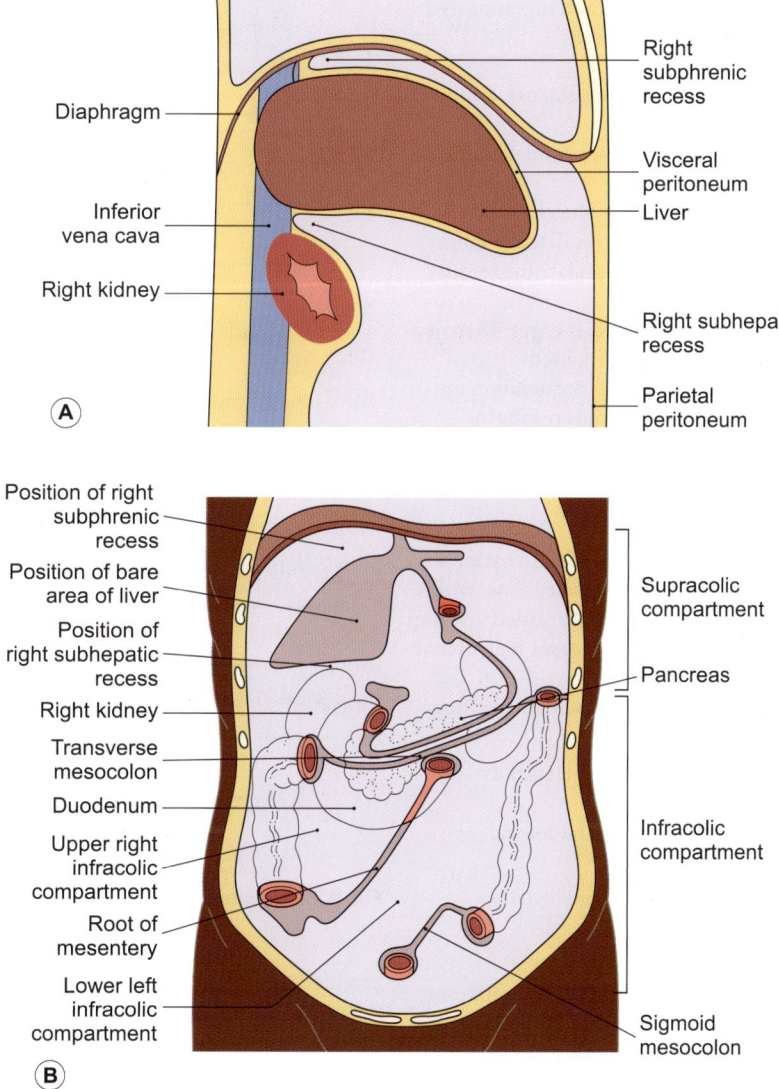

Fig. 4.21 (A) Sagittal section of the upper abdomen to show recesses of the right supracolic compartment. (B) Posterior abdominal wall showing lines of peritoneal reflection and the compartments of the greater sac (liver, stomach, small intestine, caecum, transverse and sigmoid colons have been removed). (Adapted from Williams, P. (Ed.). (1995). *Gray's anatomy* (38th ed.). Churchill Livingstone.)

2. Long-term feedback involves chemical feedback related to the body's nutritional status. Its function is to maintain the body's energy stores.

Short-term or alimentary feedback

- Oral activity: Including salivation, chewing, taste and swallowing. This inhibits the feeding centre for approximately 30 minutes.
- Stomach or duodenal distension (as detected by stretch receptors): Vagal afferents inhibit the feeding centre.

- Chemical content of food: GI hormones and humoral factors stimulate the release of:
  - Cholecystokinin: From fat ingestion.
  - Insulin and glucagon: From the pancreas.

All the above suppress feeding.

Long-term or nutritional feedback

- Temperature: interaction between the hypothalamus and temperature-regulating systems:

- Cold: Stimulates the feeding centre → food ingestion → ↑ metabolic rate (heat) and ↑ fat deposition
- Heat: inhibits the feeding centre.
- Blood concentration of nutrients, including glucose, amino acids and lipids:
  - A low concentration of any of the above stimulates an increase in feeding.
  - Hypothalamic glucoreceptors monitor glucose concentrations; high concentrations stimulate the satiety centre, whereas low concentrations stimulate the feeding centre.
- The amount of white adipose tissue (stored energy): There is negative feedback via the secretion of leptin, high concentrations of which indicate adiposity. Stimulation of leptin-specific receptors in the hypothalamus results in inhibition of food intake.

Mastication

Mastication involves the cutting and tearing of food by incisor teeth and grinding by molars, stimulating salivary flow, which then lubricates the food. Digestion is further aided by the removal of the indigestible fibrous coat that encases many plant materials.

Mastication involves two muscle groups, which are innervated by the trigeminal nerve motor branches:

1. Jaw-opening muscles: Digastric and lateral pterygoid muscles.
2. Jaw-closing muscles: Masseters, temporal and medial pterygoid muscles.

The tongue, gums and hard palate are also involved.

Chewing reflex

Brainstem reticular areas elicit and maintain chewing, with probable input from other structures, including the hypothalamus, amygdala and cortical sensory areas. The chewing reflex (Fig. 4.22) lasts about 1 second and consists of coordinated rhythmical jaw movements, the sequence of which is shown below.

Salivation and oral defence

Saliva is important for oral hygiene as well as for digestion. There are two secretions:

1. Serous: Contains ptyalin (α-amylase) and enzymes that can digest starch.
2. Mucoid: Contains mucin, which has lubrication and oral protective properties.

Composition and production of saliva

Saliva is composed of water, proteins (including enzymes) and electrolytes, and the exact concentrations of which depend on the

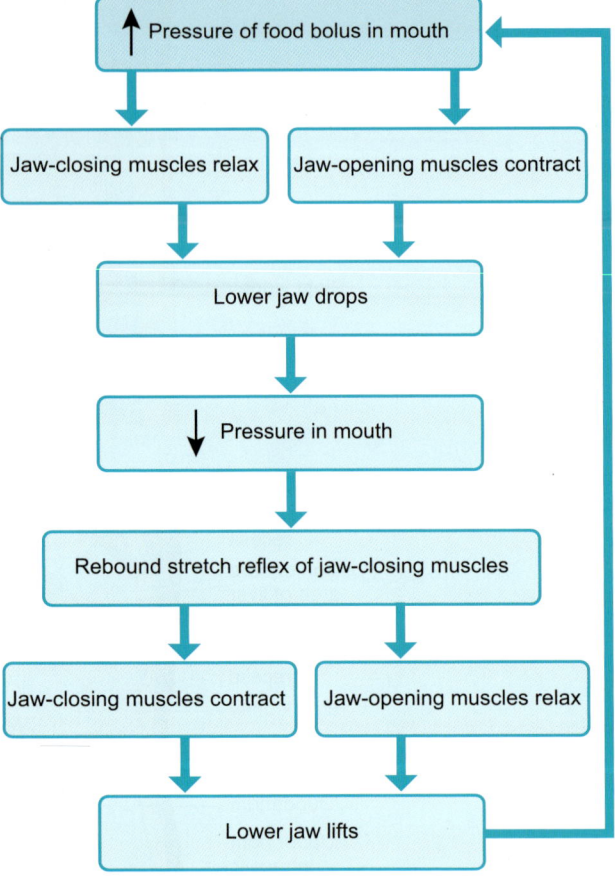

Fig. 4.22 Sequence of chewing reflex muscle movements.

production site and rate; it is always hypotonic. The two stages in the production of saliva occur in the salivary compound glands: the primary secretion in the acinus followed by secondary ionic modifications within the duct.

Nervous supply

Salivary glands receive both sympathetic and parasympathetic innervation; the parasympathetic nerves extending from the salivary nuclei in the upper medulla have more important effects. These nerves:

- Dilate blood vessels supplying the glands, increase the synthesis of ptyalin and mucins and enhance epithelial transport processes in the duct, causing hypersalivation.
- Receive cortical input: A greater response occurs with favourite foods.
- Are involved in stomach and small intestine reflexes: Nausea/irritant foods cause hypersalivation.
- Respond to tactile stimuli in the mouth and taste: Especially to acids (i.e. sour taste).

Sympathetic nerve supply from the superior cervical ganglia causes vasoconstriction and a transient increase in secretion.

Functions of saliva
Oral defence
- Rinses away some bacteria and their energy source, that is food particles.
- Saliva contains immunoglobulins and bactericidal substances, for example lysozyme and thiocyanate ions.
- Calcium and phosphate promote the mineralization of the teeth.
- Proteins provide a protective tooth covering known as an 'acquired pedicle'.
- High HCO_3^- neutralizes acid that can contribute to the formation of caries.
- Cools hot food and/or liquid that would otherwise damage the upper GI tract.

Digestion
Lubrication:
- Decreases friction of the food bolus, aiding swallowing.
- Moistens the mouth for speech, comfort and breastfeeding.
- Hydrolyzes polysaccharides.

CLINICAL NOTES

ROUTE OF ADMINISTRATION OF MEDICATIONS

Compared with oral medications, sublingual administration of drugs may allow a smaller dose of drug to be given because it permits rapid absorption directly into the systemic circulation through the rich capillary network of the mouth. Furthermore, this pathway bypasses initial metabolism by the liver (known as 'first-pass metabolism') which oral medications are subjected to. A common example of a sublingual drug is glyceryl trinitrate, which can rapidly relieve the symptoms of angina.

Oesophagus

Structure
The oesophagus is the continuation of the laryngopharynx (at the level of the C6 vertebra). In the thorax, the oesophagus lies between the trachea and the vertebral column. Accompanied by the vagus trunk, the oesophagus passes through the diaphragm at the level of the T10 vertebrae (known as the oesophageal hiatus), turns anteriorly and leftwards, and after 1 to 2 cm, enters the stomach. Fibres from the right crus of the diaphragm form a

sling around the oesophagus. The upper oesophageal sphincter, which is primarily composed of the cricopharyngeus muscle, lies at the C5 to C6 vertebral level. This is the narrowest part of the oesophagus.

Further constrictions of the oesophagus occur where it is crossed by the aortic arch, where it is crossed by the left main bronchus and where it pierces the diaphragm. The left atrium of the heart is an anterior relation of the oesophagus and may cause constriction if mitral valve incompetence is present (regurgitation of blood leads to dilatation of the left atrium).

The oesophagus is lined with nonkeratinized stratified squamous epithelium that can withstand regular trauma as liquids and solids descend (and sometimes ascend when vomiting!).

Muscular composition, blood supply, lymphatic drainage and nerve supply
The arterial supply and venous drainage of the oesophagus is complex as the oesophagus spans from the head and neck, through the thorax and into the abdomen (Table 4.4).

Swallowing

The movement of food from the mouth to the stomach is a complex event, which is initiated voluntarily but then proceeds through reflexes. As adults swallow about 600 times a day, this process must be closely coordinated with respiration. It consists of three phases:

1. Voluntary phase (closed mouth).
2. Pharyngeal phase.
3. Oesophageal phase.

Voluntary phase
Food is separated into a bolus by the tongue, which then propels it posteriorly and upwards against the hard palate towards the pharynx.

Pharyngeal phase
The food bolus exerts pressure near the opening of the pharynx, stimulating mechanoreceptors. These send afferents to the medullary swallowing centres via the trigeminal (cranial nerve (CN) 5), glossopharyngeal (CN 9) and vagus (CN 10) nerves to elicit the swallowing reflex. The stages in this phase are as follows:

- Soft palate rises → nasopharynx closed off, preventing reflux through this area.
- Palatopharyngeal folds move inwards (medially) → a channel for the food bolus is opened into the posterior pharynx.
- Vocal cords are pulled together, causing the epiglottis to tilt over the larynx → the trachea is closed off to prevent respiration.

Table 4.4 Muscle composition, blood supply, nerve supply and lymphatic drainage of the oesophagus

	Superior third	Middle third	Inferior third
Muscle composition of wall	Skeletal	Mixed (skeletal and smooth)	Smooth
Arterial supply	Inferior thyroid artery	Oesophageal branches of the aorta	Left gastric artery
Venous drainage	Brachiocephalic vein	Azygos vein	Oesophageal tributaries of the left gastric veins that drain into the portal vein
Nerve supply	Recurrent laryngeal nerves and sympathetic fibres from cell bodies in the middle cervical ganglion running on the inferior thyroid artery	Fibres from the anterior and posterior oesophageal plexus from the vagus nerves (cranial nerve 10); sympathetic fibres from the sympathetic trunks and greater splanchnic nerves	
Lymphatic drainage	Deep cervical nodes near the origin of the inferior thyroid artery	Tracheobronchial and posterior mediastinal nodes	Preaortic nodes of the coeliac group

Adapted from Hall-Craggs, E. C. B. (1995). Anatomy as a basis for clinical medicine. Williams & Wilkins.

- Larynx pulled anteriorly and upwards → entrance to the oesophagus is stretched and enlarged.
- Upper oesophageal sphincter relaxes for 0.5 to 1 seconds → food enters the upper oesophagus.

Oesophageal phase

The oesophageal phase of swallowing lasts 6 to 10 seconds. Immediately after upper oesophageal sphincter relaxation with each swallow, pressure increases, thereby promoting the one-way passage of the bolus of food. Conduction through the oesophagus occurs by both primary and secondary peristalsis.

Primary peristalsis

Primary peristalsis is a continuation of oropharyngeal swallowing. It consists of a sequence of nerve activation causing a ring of contraction and high pressure. It has a speed of 3 to 5 cm/s and the lower oesophageal sphincter (LOS) is reached 6 seconds later. Furthermore:

- Movement is aided by gravity.
- Passage is faster with warm liquids than with cold ones.
- The glossopharyngeal (CN 9) and vagus nerves (CN 10) control peristalsis in the pharynx and the upper third of the oesophagus, which are made up of striated muscle.
- The vagus nerve (CN 10) controls the smooth muscle of the lower two-thirds of the oesophagus.

Secondary peristalsis

Secondary peristalsis occurs in response to oesophageal distension caused by incomplete stomach emptying and reflux of stomach contents back into the oesophagus. It involves intrinsic myenteric circuits and pharyngeal reflexes that continue until the stomach is completely empty. Secondary peristalsis has no appreciable perception.

Lower oesophageal sphincter

The LOS consists of a circular ring 3 cm above the gastro-oesophageal junction. It is normally constricted, thereby protecting the oesophagus from acidic and proteolytic gastric secretions. The LOS relaxes for 5 to 10 seconds when it meets the peristaltic wave, permitting passage of the food bolus. During drinking, there is rapid swallowing with a relaxed LOS and no peristalsis until the last swallow.

Vomiting

Vomiting is the forceful expulsion of gastric (and sometimes duodenal) contents through the mouth. It occurs when the vomiting centres, which are located bilaterally in the lateral medulla, are stimulated by a variety of stimuli including distension, irritation or excitation of any part of the upper GI tract (Fig. 4.23). Impulses are sent to the vomiting centres from:

- Higher centres (including cerebral and limbic regions): In response to psychic stimulation (e.g. smells, emotions, disturbing sights) and raised intracranial pressure.
- Chemoreceptor trigger zones (CTZs): These respond to upper GI tract lesions, drugs (e.g. opioids) and metabolic conditions (e.g. uraemia). CTZs are located bilaterally on the fourth ventricle floor near the area postrema. In addition, they respond to prolonged vestibular nuclei stimulation resulting from rapid changing of rhythm or direction of motion (i.e. motion sickness).

When there is a gastric lesion, retrograde peristalsis from the small bowel occurs many minutes before vomiting. Consequently, food is unloaded into the stomach and duodenum, which distends and stimulates the vomiting centre.

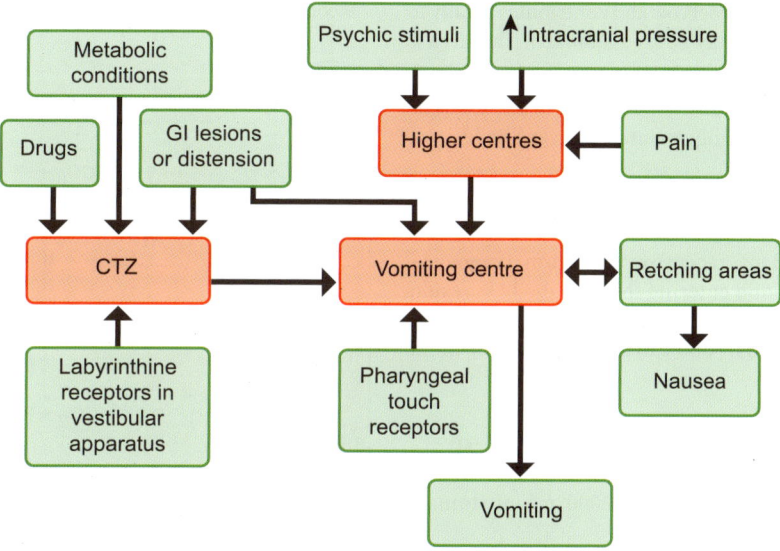

Fig. 4.23 Control of vomiting. CTZ, *Chemoreceptor trigger zone*; GI, *gastrointestinal*.

Staging of vomiting

Vomiting usually includes a prodrome of nausea—An accompaniment of autonomic symptoms that include sweating, hypersalivation and pallor. A sequence of events then follows:

- Deep inspiration.
- Closure of the glottis: This protects the airways and fixes the chest by holding the diaphragm down.
- Raising of the larynx and hyoid bone: This extends the opening of the oesophagus (oesophageal sphincter (UOS)).
- Elevation of soft palate: This seals off the nasopharynx.
- Strong contractions of abdominal skeletal muscles: → ↑ Intraabdominal pressure → diaphragm forced up into the thorax →↑ intrathoracic pressure.
- Relaxation of the LOS: This permits the stomach contents to enter the oesophagus.

The oesophagus can empty food back into the stomach, with recycling of the whole process if the UOS remains closed. However, when the UOS opens because of expulsive forces, vomit enters the mouth.

STOMACH

Anatomy of the stomach

The stomach lies intraperitoneally, in the left hypogastric and epigastric regions of the abdomen. It is a dilated muscular bag, which is relatively mobile, fixed only to the oesophagus and duodenum (see Fig. 4.5). It is composed of the cardia, fundus, body, antrum and pylorus. The gastro-oesophageal junction (between the oesophagus and the cardia) lies at the level of T10, and the pyloric sphincter (gastroduodenal sphincter) lies at the level of L1.

The mucosal lining of the stomach is thrown into folds or rugae, which allow considerable dilatation. The wall is muscular and comprises outer longitudinal, middle circular and inner oblique muscle layers.

The relations of the stomach are:

- Anteriorly: The anterolateral abdominal wall, left costal margin and diaphragm.
- Posteriorly: The left suprarenal gland, upper pole of the left kidney, pancreas, spleen, splenic artery and left colic flexure (forming the stomach bed).

The stomach and oesophagus are supplied by arterial branches of the coeliac trunk. Venous drainage of the stomach accompanies the arteries. Smaller veins drain into the SMV and the splenic vein, which combine to form the hepatic portal vein (some veins drain directly into the portal vein).

The hepatic portal vein carries blood to the liver. Lymph from the stomach drains to the coeliac nodes and eventually into the thoracic duct.

Innervation of the stomach is via the coeliac plexus (part of the autonomic nervous system): sympathetic supply arises from the greater and lesser splanchnic nerves. Parasympathetic innervation arises from the anterior and posterior vagal trunks.

Storage of food: the fundus

Storage of food is an important motor function that permits a controlled release of gastric contents into the duodenum. The fundus, in particular, acts as a reservoir and contributes greatly to the 1- to 1.5-L capacity of a fully relaxed stomach. This area is particularly suited to its distensible function as:

- The muscular wall is thinner than in other parts of the stomach.
- Intragastric pressure is roughly maintained over a wide range of gastric volumes.
- An additional oblique layer of stomach muscle facilitates expansion.

Storage is facilitated by receptive relaxation (vagovagal reflex) by the stomach. Food entering through the LOS results in decreased muscle tone of the fundus and upper stomach walls, which bulge outwards. Food can stay up to 1 hour in the fundus.

Gastric secretions and their control

There are two main components of the 2000 mL of stomach secretions produced every day:

1. Nonacid secretion: Alkaline material, which is released by mucous cells and coats the entire mucosal surface.
2. Acid secretion: Gastric juice released by parietal and chief cells in the oxyntic region.

Nonacid secretion

The alkaline secretion, which comprises mainly mucus and bicarbonate (HCO_3^-), adheres to the stomach lumen, forming a protective fluid barrier against the acidic gastric juice, which would otherwise cause autodigestion. The viscous secretion is isosmolar to plasma ultrafiltrate but, owing to its high HCO_3^- content, has an alkaline pH (7.7). Acid-resistant trefoil proteins in the GI tract mucosa offer further resistance to tissue damage.

Gastric juice

This is composed of mucus, hydrochloric acid (HCl), intrinsic factor (IF), pepsin and other enzymes. The pH of this fluid is low, with an increase in flow rate associated with an increase in acidity (reaching pH 1.0).

Mucus

Mucus is secreted principally in the antropyloric region and by surface mucous cells located throughout the stomach. The roles of mucus are:

- Lubrication of food.
- Protection against autodigestion.

Mucus is a gel, which permits HCO_3^- to be trapped within it. Therefore an alkaline barrier to H^+ diffusion back to the epithelium is created. Hence, a pH gradient is established between the lumen (pH 1.5) and the epithelial surface (pH 6.5).

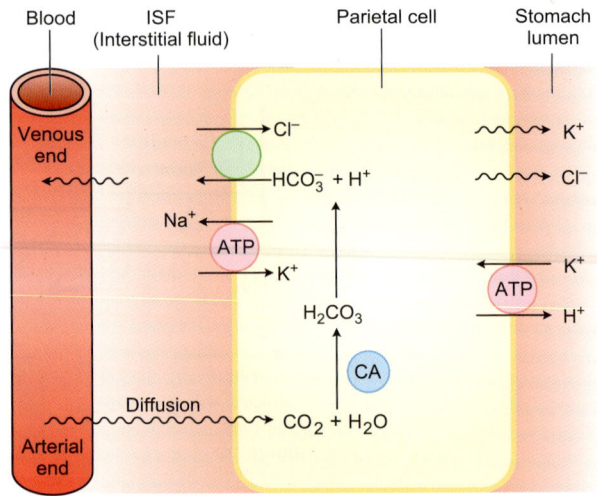

Fig. 4.24 Parietal cell secretion of hydrochloric acid. ATP, *Adenosine triphosphate*.

Prostaglandins and local irritation stimulate mucus production. Pepsin only modestly degrades mucus, as a low pH is required for optimal pepsin activity.

Hydrochloric acid

Parietal cells actively secrete HCl (Fig. 4.24), the functions of which include:

- Defence against ingested microorganisms.
- Activation of pepsinogen.
- Stimulation of bile and pancreatic juice flow.

Parietal cells are suited to this function as they contain:

- Abundant carbonic anhydrase: This catalyzes H^+ and HCO_3^- formation from diffused plasma CO_2. HCO_3^- is then exchanged with Cl^- from interstitial fluid and effluxed into the blood. Hence, parietal cell HCl secretion causes gastric venous blood to have a lower $[CO_2]$ than its arterial counterpart (alkaline tide).
- Large quantities of H^+/K^+ ATPase molecules: These permit H^+ extrusion against a huge concentration gradient: gastric juice $[H^+]$ can be 1.5×10^{-1} M, whereas plasma $[H^+]$ is 10^{-8} M. These pumps are associated with tubovesicular structures that move and fuse with the apical membrane when parietal cells are stimulated.

The rate of formation of HCl is directly related to histamine production by enterochromaffin cells, which in turn are stimulated by the following:

- Gastrin: An antral hormone, the production of which increases with protein consumption.
- Acetylcholine (ACh): From vagal nerve endings, which act via M_3 muscarinic receptors.
- ACh and gastrin also have direct effects on parietal cells acting via M_3 receptors and gastrin receptors on the surface membrane, respectively.
- Signal-transduction pathways for ACh and gastrin involve activation of protein kinase C and release of Ca^{2+} and for histamine (H_2 receptors) adenylyl cyclase, production of cyclic adenosine monophosphate and activation of protein kinase A.

Prostaglandins inhibit HCl secretion and also stimulate mucus production.

Intrinsic factor

Parietal cells produce IF, a glycoprotein that is essential for vitamin B_{12} (also known as cobalamin) absorption in the terminal ileum. Without IF, anaemia would develop once liver stores of B_{12} were depleted (after 2–3 years), given that vitamin B_{12} is required for the production of red blood cells. This is known as pernicious anaemia.

Pepsin

Chief cells secrete pepsinogen, the inactive precursor of pepsin. Under acidic conditions (pH <2), pepsinogen is rapidly converted to pepsin.

Pepsin is a proteolytic enzyme that degrades proteins into peptides. Stimulation by the vagus nerve (CN 10) containing ACh or gastric enteric plexus promotes the secretion of pepsinogen. The gastric enteric reflexes involved may in turn be influenced by the amount of HCl present.

Other enzymes

Small quantities of the following are secreted in gastric juice:

- Gastric lipase: Principally acts on butter fats.
- Gastric amylase: Plays a small role in starch digestion.
- Gelatinase: Aids in the hydrolysis of gelatin.

Control of gastric secretion

Gastric secretion occurs both continuously at rest (basal secretion) and as a response to food. Stimulation associated with feeding involves neural, hormonal and paracrine mechanisms and is divided into three phases:

1. Cephalic phase: Stimuli involve the brain.
2. Gastric phase: Stimulus is food or fluid within the stomach.
3. Intestinal phase: Stimulus is food in the small intestine.

Cephalic phase

- Responsible for 20% of the gastric secretion associated with feeding.
- Reflex gastric stimulation occurs with anticipation of eating (e.g. sight, smell and taste) and then continues up to 30 minutes after ingestion.
- Vagus nerve (CN 10) mediates gastric secretion in preparation for the meal involving central nervous system centres.
- Anger and hostility increase gastric secretion while fear and depression decrease gastric secretion.

Gastric phase

- Responsible for 70% of gastric secretion associated with feeding.
- Food entering the stomach accelerates gastric secretion in response to both chemical stimuli and distension.
- pH <3 inhibits gastrin release in response to distension or chemical stimuli via somatostatin release from antral mucosa D cells and secretin from the duodenal mucosa S cells, both of which inhibit HCl secretion through inhibition of gastrin release from the antral mucosa and, for somatostatin, by reducing histamine release.

Intestinal phase

- Responsible for <10% of total gastric acid secretion.
- Response to food (chyme) in the duodenum.

Fat, acid and hyperosmolar solutes within the duodenum are often inhibitory and mediated by the release of two inhibitory factors: gastric inhibitory peptide and cholecystokinin (CCK). Both suppress the secretion of HCl by parietal cells.

Gastric motility and emptying

The motor functions of the stomach are threefold:

1. Storage of food (see previously).
2. Mixing of gastric secretion with food to form a mixture known as chyme.
3. Controlled release of chyme into the small intestine.

Gastric motility

The proximal stomach stores food and presses it towards the distal region via low-amplitude, slow peristaltic waves, which occur at a rate of 3 to 4/min. These contractions are initiated and regulated by pacemaker cells in the middle of the stomach body. Initially, the waves travel at 1 cm/s but gather speed and amplitude towards the antropyloric region.

Generating very high pressure in the antrum is facilitated by a thicker muscle layer in the stomach, enabling small boluses of food to be ground. During antral peristalsis, pyloric contraction causes reflux of the antral contents to more proximal regions of the stomach. This is known as retropulsion, and has the following consequences:

- Breakdown of solid foods.
- Churning of food with secretions to form the semi-solid chyme.

Gastric emptying

- There is coordinated sequential contraction of the antrum, pylorus and then duodenum.
- The partially contracted pylorus regulates the amount of gastric emptying and prevents the reflux of potentially damaging bile into the stomach.
- Only small amounts of chyme pass through the pylorus into the duodenum, which has a limited capacity.

The rate of gastric emptying depends on factors (Table 4.5) relating to stomach contents and duodenal chyme (generally inhibits historic emptying):

- Stomach contents.
- Duodenal chyme which generally inhibits e mptying, and is known as the enterogastric reflex.

Protection of the gastric mucosa

In addition to stimulating the secretion of HCO_3^- and mucus, the inhibitory actions of prostaglandins and other factors on acid secretion serve to maintain the gastric mucosa. If the protective barrier is breached, H^+ penetrates the mucosa, causing local inflammation with epithelial cell necrosis and haemorrhage (ulcer). This can occur with the following:

Table 4.5 Factors involving stomach emptying

	Factor	
	Stomach content	Duodenal chyme
Energy content	Carbohydrates empty quickest Proteins empty slower Fats empty slowest	Fats
Bulk	Solid and coarse foods	Distension (duodenum)
Osmolality	Isosmolar ↑ in variation from isosmolar values further ↑ emptying	High osmolality
Temperature	Body temperature Cold or hot substances	
pH		<3.5

- Nonsteroidal antiinflammatory drugs (NSAIDs): Inhibit prostaglandin from arachidonic acid production, reducing HCO_3^- secretion and mucus.
- *Helicobacter pylori* infection: Disrupts the mucosal barrier, causing acute inflammation.
- Zollinger–Ellison syndrome: Characterized by multiple gastrinomas with acid hypersecretion.
- Lifestyle:
  - Alcohol: Increases barrier permeability by interfering with mucosal enzymatic processes.
  - Smoking: Chronic nicotine exposure.
  - Elevated stress.

LIVER, GALLBLADDER AND BILIARY TRACT

Anatomy of the liver, gallbladder and biliary tract

The liver is a wedge-shaped organ surrounded by a fibrous capsule and lies inferior to the right hemidiaphragm. It spans the right hypochondrium, the epigastrium and the left hypochondrium. It lies largely under the cover of the ribs, and it is covered by peritoneum except for the 'bare area' on the diaphragmatic surface of the liver.

The liver has four lobes, although this is a purely anatomical description and does not reflect functional subdivisions (Fig. 4.25). Anteriorly, the falciform ligament (visible on the anterior surface of the liver) attaches the liver to the anterior abdominal wall and also divides the liver into right and left lobes. Posteriorly, the caudate lobe lies superiorly, between the fissure for the IVC and the fissure for the ligamentum venosum. Inferior to this lies the quadrate lobe, between the gallbladder fossa and the ligamentum teres. The transverse fissure separates the caudate lobe from the quadrate lobe. Functionally, the quadrate and

Anterior view

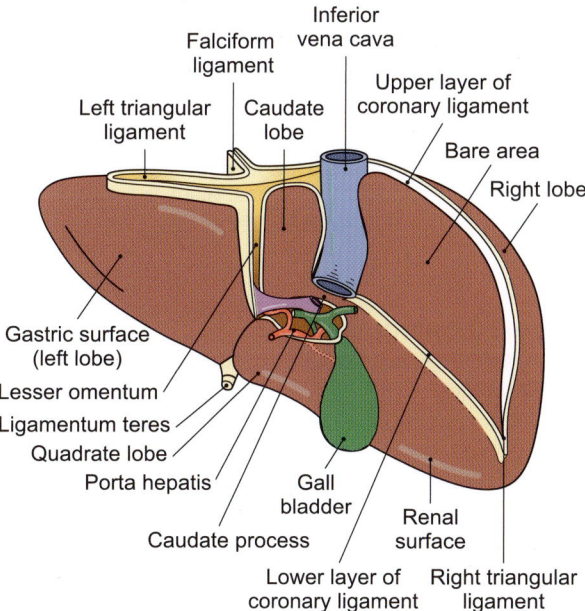

Inferior vena cava

Upper layer of coronary ligament

Anterior layer of lesser omentum

Posterior layer of lesser omentum

Oesophagus

Greater omentum

Left lobe

Left triangular ligament

Ligamentum teres in falciform ligament

Right lobe   Gall bladder

Posterior view

Falciform ligament

Inferior vena cava

Left triangular ligament

Caudate lobe

Upper layer of coronary ligament

Bare area

Right lobe

Gastric surface (left lobe)

Lesser omentum

Ligamentum teres

Quadrate lobe

Porta hepatis

Gall bladder

Renal surface

Caudate process

Lower layer of coronary ligament

Right triangular ligament

Fig. 4.25 Anterior and posterior views of the liver.

caudate lobes are part of the left lobe as they are supplied by the left hepatic artery and the left branch of the portal vein and deliver bile to the left bile duct.

The falciform ligament is the remnant of the embryonic ventral mesentery. On the superior surface of the liver, the falciform ligament forms the left and right triangular ligaments. The right layer forms the upper layer of the coronary ligament, the right

triangular ligament and the lower layer of the coronary ligament (see Fig. 4.25).

The area between the upper and lower parts of the coronary ligament is the bare area of the liver that lies in contact with the diaphragm. The right and left layers of peritoneum meet on the visceral surface of the liver to form the hepatogastric and hepatoduodenal ligaments, part of the lesser omentum. Between the caudate and quadrate lobes, the two layers surround the porta hepatis. The porta hepatis, the IVC, the gallbladder and the fissures of the ligamentum venosum and ligamentum teres form an H-shaped pattern. The ligamentum venosum is the remnant of the foetal ductus venosus, which transports blood from the portal and umbilical veins to the hepatic veins in foetal life.

The porta hepatis contains the following structures (see Fig. 4.25):

- The hepatic artery proper (a branch of the coeliac trunk) splits into the right and left hepatic arteries and supplies oxygenated blood to the liver. The right hepatic artery gives off the cystic artery, which supplies the gallbladder.
- The hepatic portal vein carries the products of digestion from the gut to the liver. This blood is also partially oxygenated.
- The right and left hepatic ducts drain bile into the common hepatic duct, which joins the cystic duct to form the common bile duct.

These three structures form the portal triad that lies in the right free margin of the lesser omentum. The porta hepatis also contains lymph nodes and nerves.

Venous drainage of the liver occurs via the hepatic veins, which pass directly from the posterior surface of the liver into the IVC, draining the liver.

Lymphatic drainage of the liver is to the hepatic nodes around the porta hepatis and on into the coeliac nodes. Lymphatics of the bare area drain into the posterior mediastinal nodes. Innervation is provided via sympathetic and parasympathetic nerve fibres (via the vagus nerves, CN 10) in the hepatic plexus, a branch of the coeliac plexus.

Anatomy of gallbladder and biliary tract

The gallbladder lies in a fossa on the visceral surface of the liver. It has a fundus, a body and a neck (Fig. 4.26). Bile secreted by the liver is concentrated and stored in the gallbladder (its capacity is approximately 50 mL). After the consumption of fat- or protein-rich food, cells of the duodenum release CCK, which stimulates the smooth muscle of the gallbladder wall and relaxes the hepatopancreatic sphincter (sphincter of Oddi—A layer of circular muscle surrounding the ampulla, controlling the flow of bile and pancreatic secretions), releasing bile into the duodenum.

The cystic duct drains the gallbladder and joins the common hepatic duct to form the common bile duct (CBD). The CBD passes through the free margin of the lesser omentum, posterior to the first part of the duodenum. It then enters the second part of the

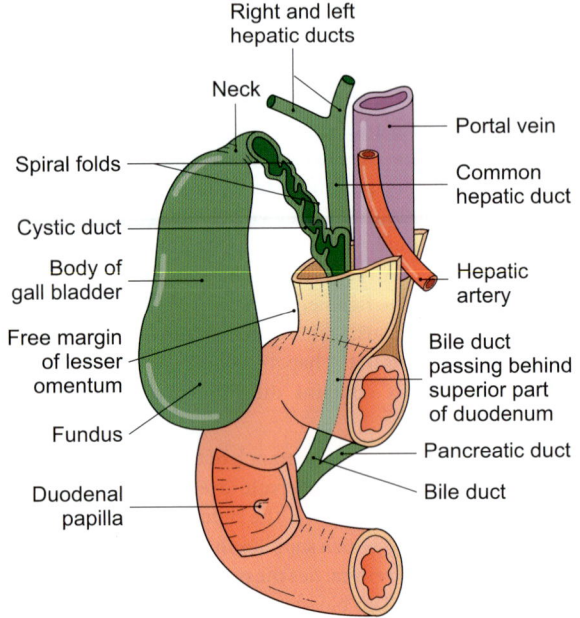

Fig. 4.26 Gallbladder and biliary tract.

Table 4.6 Overview of nutrient metabolism by the liver

Nutrient	Metabolic process
Carbohydrate	Utilization of major monosaccharides to synthesize other substances: fatty acids, amino acids, glycogen Glycogen breakdown and storage: <65 g/kg in liver tissue Gluconeogenesis (glucose production)
Lipid	Fatty acid synthesis and storage as triglycerides Ketogenesis from fatty acid oxidation and lipolysis (fat breakdown) Cholesterol synthesis from acetyl coenzyme A involving the enzyme hydroxymethylglutaryl-coenzyme A reductase Conversion of cholesterol to bile salts Secretion and metabolism of lipoproteins Metabolism and excretion of steroid hormones
Protein	Synthesis of plasma proteins: albumin and globulins, acute-phase proteins and complement Synthesis of clotting factors (V, VII, IX, X, prothrombin and fibrinogen) Generation of urea from ammonia Amino acid deamination
Vitamins	Storage of fat-soluble vitamins A, D, E and K (depending on production) Storage of a 2–3 year supply of vitamin B_{12} Storage of a few months' supply of folate Modification of most vitamins to active coenzyme forms

duodenum with the pancreatic duct at the hepatopancreatic ampulla (of Vater). The ampulla opens at the major duodenal papilla.

Blood supply to the gallbladder is via the cystic artery, a branch of the right hepatic artery. Venous drainage occurs via the cystic veins, which drain into the right hepatic vein. The majority of lymph drains to the hepatic nodes and ultimately into the coeliac nodes. The nerve supply arises from the coeliac plexus, the vagus nerve (CN 10) and the right phrenic nerve.

Overview of liver metabolism

The functions of the liver include:

- Production of bile, cholesterol, albumin and clotting factors.
- Detoxification of drugs and chemicals.
- Homoeostasis of blood glucose levels.
- Metabolism of carbohydrates, proteins, fats and vitamins.
- Storage of vitamins, cholesterol, fats, proteins, copper and iron.
- Destruction of erythrocytes.
- Production of heat.

The liver metabolizes a variety of substances including nutrients, drugs and hormones, which can then be excreted (Table 4.6).

Liver biotransformation and clearance occur in three stages.

Phase 1 (oxidation)

- Involves oxidation and reduction by enzymes (e.g. cytochrome P450).
- Increases polarity and water solubility which enables excretion via urine/bile.

Phase 2 (conjugation)

- Involves the conjugation with various groups (e.g. glucuronide).
- Decreases toxicity of substance.

Phase 3 (elimination)

- Active transport via ATPase pumps into the circulation.

Bile production and function

The liver produces and secretes up to ~1000 mL of bile daily, which flows equally into either the:

- Small intestine through the ampulla of Vater.
- Gallbladder which stores and concentrates bile until it is stimulated to empty into the intestine by a fatty meal.

Around 90% of the bile in the small intestine is recycled back to the liver via the mesenteric venous drainage through the portal vein—the enterohepatic circulation. The pathway of bile is shown in Fig. 4.27.

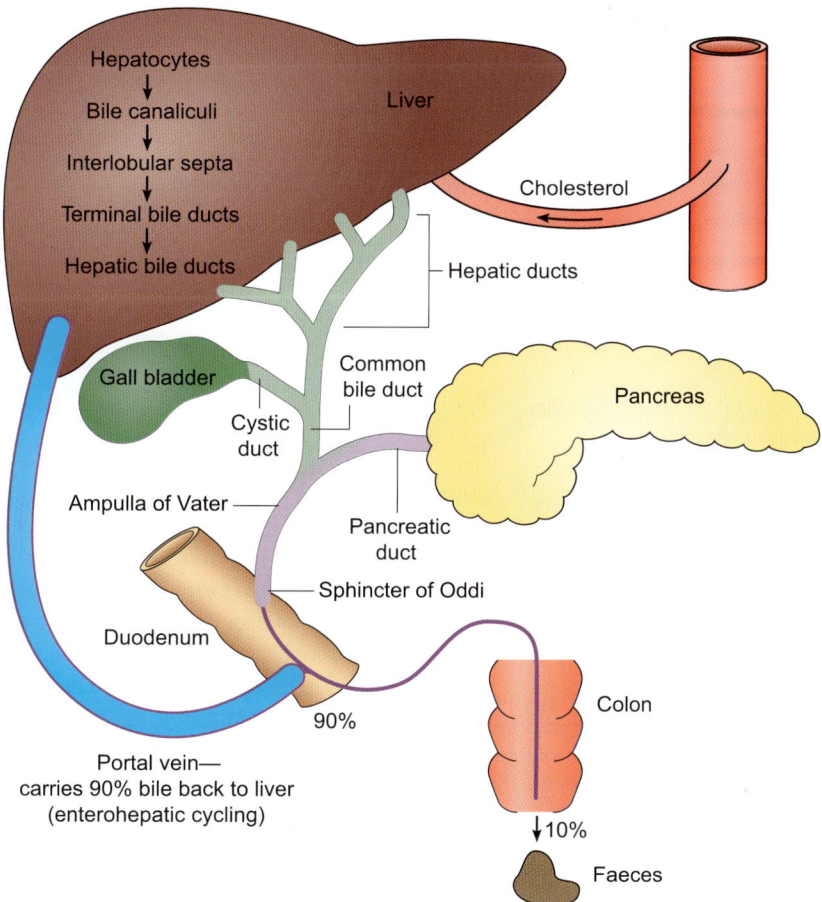

Fig. 4.27 Pathway of bile in and outside the liver.

Bile is an aqueous solution composed of bile salts, inorganic salts (electrolytes), bile pigments, phospholipids and cholesterol. It forms a medium for biotransformed substances and waste products, such as cholesterol and bile pigments (bilirubin and biliverdin), enabling their elimination. In addition, bile facilitates fat handling by:

- Emulsifying fat: Helping with digestion.
- Promoting absorption from the small intestine.

Bile salts

These refer to potassium and sodium salts of bile acids, notably cholic and chenodeoxycholic acid, which are synthesized from cholesterol and then conjugated before their secretion into bile. Cholesterol 7-α-hydroxylase is the rate-limiting factor in the production of bile salts (Fig. 4.28).

Over 24 hours, 0.2 to 0.4 g of bile salts are synthesized and recycled six to eight times via the enterohepatic circulation. Hepatic uptake is by a secondary active process involving Na+/bile salt cotransporter powered by basolateral Na+/K+-ATPase. Interruption of bile salt circulation—either by inadequate production or exclusion from the small intestine—results in severe fat malabsorption inclusive of fat-soluble vitamins.

Properties of bile salts

Amphipathic properties (hydrophobic and a hydrophilic end) enable bile salts to perform two special actions:

- Detergent function: Surface tension is reduced, permitting lipid emulsification with the aid of lecithin (a phospholipid).
- Micelle formation: Micelles are spherical aggregates with a hydrophilic shell and a hydrophobic core. Bile salts can form mixed micelles by incorporating phospholipids, to transport lipids, which are normally very water insoluble. Cholesterol, fatty acids and monoglycerides can thus be maintained in solution, and their absorption greatly assisted.

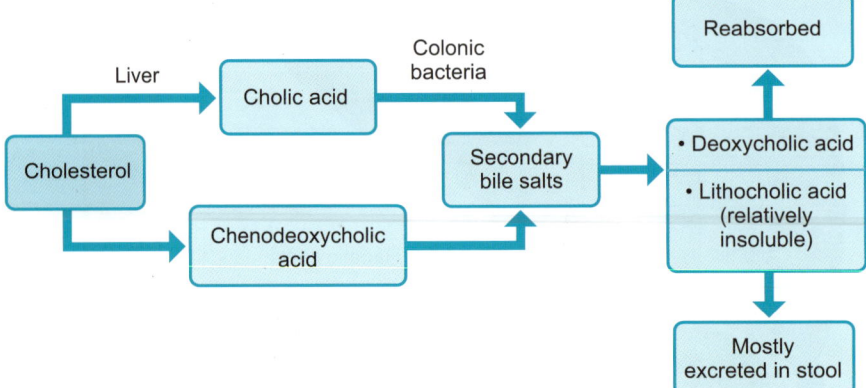

Fig. 4.28 Synthetic pathway of bile salts.

In addition, bile salts stimulate the secretion of water and electrolytes via the:

- Stimulation of bile: When secreted by the liver.
- Production of diarrhoea: If present in the colon.

Bile pigments

The primary bile pigment is bilirubin. It is derived from the breakdown of haem, which is formed principally from haemoglobin (85%), as well as others (e.g. myoglobin). Bilirubin is bound to albumin unconjugated and is therefore relatively insoluble.

Most bilirubin dissociates into its free form in the liver. It is then taken up by the liver cells (hepatocytes) in exchange for Cl⁻ via an anion transporter. In the hepatocytes, cytoplasmic proteins (ligandins) bind to bilirubin, which is then conjugated with glucuronate via glucuronyl transferase (UDP glucuronosyltransferase) → bilirubin diglucuronide (conjugated bilirubin).

Conjugated bilirubin has a higher water solubility than free bilirubin and is actively transported into the bile canaliculi. A small amount escapes into the blood, where it is lightly bound to albumin and excreted in the urine. Most of the conjugated bilirubin is excreted, in the bile, into the small intestine, the wall of which is permeable to free bilirubin and urobilinogen but impermeable to conjugated bilirubin. Here intestinal bacteria convert conjugated bilirubin into urobilinogen and a little free bilirubin, some of which passes through the bowel wall before circulating back to the liver (via the enterohepatic circulation). However, most conjugated bilirubin remains in the bowel.

Urobilinogen in the gut is partially reoxidized to stercobilinogen, which is then lost via faeces.

CLINICAL NOTES

JAUNDICE

Jaundice results from an increased level of bilirubin in the blood. It accumulates in the skin and mucous membranes, including the conjunctiva of the eye. The causes of jaundice may be classified as prehepatic, usually related to increased breakdown of bilirubin; hepatic, disease within the liver; and posthepatic, disruption to the flow of bile. Obstruction of the biliary tree is most commonly caused by gallstones but may occur secondary to carcinoma of the head of the pancreas. If the biliary tree is obstructed, causing posthepatic jaundice, bilirubin cannot enter the intestine (bile pigments give stools their brown colour); therefore it is reabsorbed into the blood, filtered by the kidney and excreted in the urine. This produces the characteristic features of obstructive jaundice—dark urine and pale stools.

Control of bile synthesis and secretion

Both bile acid concentration and hormones affect the secretion and flow of bile.

The concentration of bile acids in the portal vein

- Low concentrations: Stimulate bile acid secretion and inhibit bile acid synthesis.
- High concentrations: Inhibit bile acid secretion and stimulate bile acid synthesis.

Hormones

- Secretin: Sstimulates bile duct-dependent secretion of bile.
- CCK:
  - ↑ Bile acid secretion during digestion (intestinal phase).
  - ↑ Flow of bile into the duodenum.

Role of the gallbladder

Between digestive periods, there is increased resistance to bile flow due to constriction of the sphincter of Oddi. Meanwhile, bile is preferentially diverted towards the cystic duct and the relaxed gallbladder. Storage within the gallbladder serves to concentrate bile to up to 20-fold that of hepatic bile. The epithelium actively transports Na^+ out of bile which is followed by a secondary absorption of Cl^-, water and other solutes, including HCO_3^-. This reabsorption of HCO_3^- reduces the bile pH. As there is a large volume reduction of bile, the gallbladder can store 12 hours' worth of bile secretions despite its capacity of only 50 to 60 mL.

Gallbladder emptying

Contraction of the gallbladder occurs intermittently to release bile into the duodenum. It does this between digestion as well as in response to a meal. This response is mediated via the following processes:

- During the cephalic phase of digestion: Resistance by the sphincter of Oddi decreases, and the gallbladder begins to empty with the early digestion of food.
- In the stomach: Antral distension and gastrin secretion stimulate gallbladder contraction via nerve reflexes.
- Fatty acids (and amino acids) in the duodenum: Stimulate the release of CCK, which acts to greatly increase gallbladder emptying.

Gallbladder relaxation results from the following:

- The presence of bile acids.
- Vasoactive intestinal peptide (VIP).
- Pancreatic polypeptide.
- Sympathetic stimulation of the gallbladder.

PANCREAS

The pancreas has both exocrine and endocrine functions.

Anatomy of the pancreas

The pancreas is a retroperitoneal organ, lying posterior to the stomach (Fig. 4.29). It spans the epigastrium and left hypochondrium. It has a head, neck, body and tail:

- The head lies in the concavity of the duodenum, anterior to the IVC and left renal vein. The bile duct travels through it.
- The uncinate process is an extension of the head, and the SMA and SMV pass anterior to the uncinate process.
- The neck lies anterior to the point at which the SMV and splenic vein join to form the portal vein.
- The body is related to the stomach anteriorly, and to the aorta, splenic vein, left kidney and renal vessels, and left suprarenal gland posteriorly.
- The tail passes into the splenorenal ligament, reaching the hilum of the spleen, accompanied by the splenic vessels and lymphatics.

The main pancreatic duct begins in the tail of the pancreas. In the head of the pancreas, the pancreatic duct joins with the CBD to form the ampulla of Vater. This then opens into the duodenum at the major duodenal papilla. Approximately 2 cm proximal to this, the accessory pancreatic duct opens into the duodenum at the minor duodenal papilla. It drains the head of the pancreas.

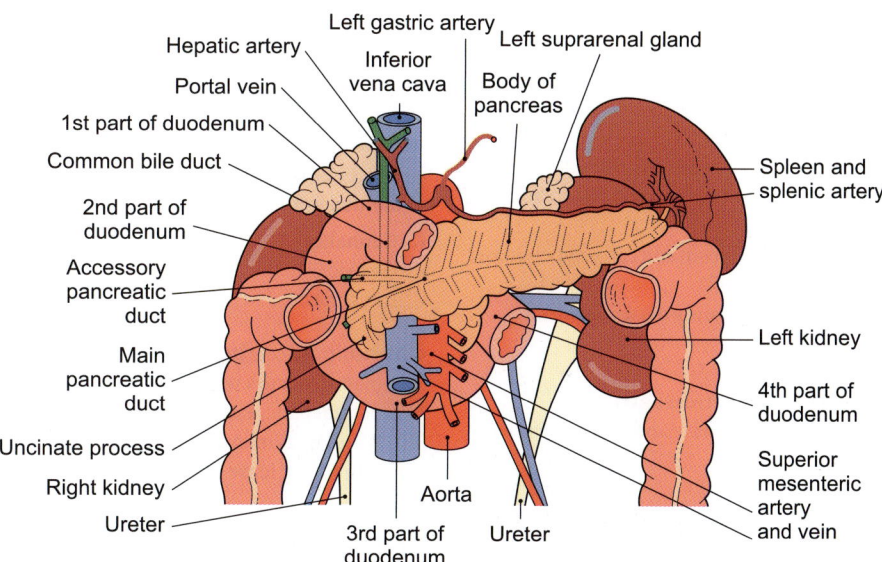

Fig. 4.29 Relations of the duodenum. Note the splenic vein runs posterior to the pancreas and is, therefore, not visible. The inferior mesenteric vein has been omitted for clarity.

The splenic artery (a branch of the coeliac trunk) supplies the neck, body and tail of the pancreas. The superior and inferior pancreaticoduodenal arteries supply the head. The splenic vein and SMV drain the pancreas. Lymphatics drain into superior and inferior pancreatic nodes and then to coeliac and superior mesenteric nodes. Nerve supply to the pancreas arises from the vagus nerves (parasympathetic, CN 10) and the splanchnic nerves (sympathetic) arising from the coeliac and superior mesenteric plexuses.

Pancreatic secretions

Exocrine pancreatic secretion has two components:

1. Aqueous alkaline fluid: Secreted by duct cells.
2. Organic, for example inactive digestive enzymes: Secreted by acinar cells.

When it enters the duodenum, the pancreatic fluid regulates the pH and helps with the digestion of fats, proteins and nucleic acids.

Alkaline secretions

Alkaline fluid is iso-osmolar at all rates of secretion. Its main component is aqueous bicarbonate (HCO_3^-), and smaller quantities of other solutes are also present. HCO_3^- secretion by epithelial cells is an active process requiring adenosine triphosphate (ATP). Concentrations of bicarbonate can rise to five times plasma value with high rates of pancreatic fluid secretion.

Enzyme secretion

Acinar cells secrete the following groups of enzymes:

- Peptidases:
  - Digest proteins to form peptides.
  - Form the most abundant of enzymes secreted.
  - Are secreted in precursor form to prevent pancreatic autodigestion.
  - Examples are trypsin, chymotrypsin and carboxypeptidase.
- Amylases:
  - Hydrolyze carbohydrates to mainly disaccharides.
  - Main example: α-amylase.
- Lipases:
  - Digest fat to release monoglycerides and fatty acids.
  - Examples are lipase, phospholipase and cholesterol esterase.
- Nucleases:
  - Examples: Ribonuclease and deoxyribonuclease, which act on RNA and DNA, respectively.

When it enters the duodenum, trypsinogen is converted to trypsin by brush-border enterokinase, thus activating the other peptidases (Fig. 4.30).

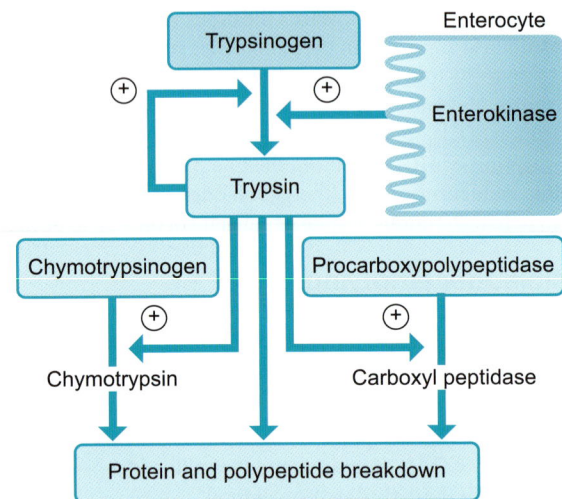

Fig. 4.30 Peptidase activation within the duodenum.

Control of pancreatic secretion

Pancreatic secretion is subject to both neural and hormonal effects.

Hormonal control

The most powerful stimulant of ductal cell HCO_3^- secretion is secretin. Acetylcholine (ACh) and cholecystokinin (CCK) also stimulate its release. Somatostatin potently inhibits all pancreatic secretions via direct and indirect mechanisms involving the above hormones.

Neural control

Sympathetic stimulation: Globally inhibits secretions from the pancreas, mainly through gland arteriolar vasoconstriction. Parasympathetic stimulation: via vagal ACh, increases both enzyme and alkaline fluid secretion.

The phases of secretion occurring in response to a meal can be divided into:

- Cephalic.
- Gastric.
- Intestinal.

Cephalic secretion

Stimulation occurs with anticipation of feeding and accounts for 15% of total pancreatic secretion. At this stage, both alkaline fluid (10%) and enzymes (25%) are secreted. It is mediated by parasympathetic release of ACh and inhibited by sympathetic activity.

Gastric secretion

In response to food entering the stomach and antral distension, predominantly enzymes are secreted (5%–10%) during this phase. It is mediated by a vasovagal stomach reflex and gastrin release.

Intestinal secretion

The greatest volume of pancreatic secretion occurs during this stage in response to gastric chyme entering the duodenum. It is mediated by:

- Secretin
  - Responsible for large amounts of alkaline fluid secretion.
  - Present in duodenal and jejunal mucosal cells.
  - Released in response to acidic chyme.
- CCK
  - Present in duodenal and jejunal mucosal cells. CCK is responsible for copious enzyme secretion.
  - CCK is released in response to fatty acids and amino acids (protein breakdown products) in chyme.

SMALL INTESTINE

The small intestine comprises the duodenum, jejunum and ileum.

Anatomy of the small intestine

Duodenum

The duodenum is approximately 40 cm long and C-shaped, curving around the head of the pancreas. It is divided into four parts (the first part is intraperitoneal, the remainder is retroperitoneal):

- The first part passes anterolateral to the L1 vertebra and travels superiorly and posteriorly.
- The second part passes inferiorly. The major duodenal papilla (the opening of the bile duct and main pancreatic duct) opens into this part at the level of the L2 vertebra.
- The third part lies horizontally and crosses the vertebral column at the level of L3. It is crossed by the SMA and SMV.
- The fourth part travels superiorly to the level of the L2 vertebra and joins with the jejunum.

Fig. 4.29 shows the relations of the duodenum. Blood supply to each of the four parts arises from the superior and inferior pancreaticoduodenal arteries, branches of the gastroduodenal artery (a branch of the hepatic artery) and SMA, respectively. Venous drainage occurs via the SMV and the splenic vein. Lymphatic drainage of the duodenum is via the coeliac and superior mesenteric nodes. Its nerve supply arises from the vagus (CN 10) and sympathetic nerves via the coeliac and superior mesenteric plexuses.

CLINICAL NOTES

PEPTIC ULCER DISEASE

Peptic ulcers include ulceration of the stomach (gastric) or duodenum (duodenal). A gastric ulcer in the posterior stomach wall may erode into the splenic artery, causing massive haemorrhage into the lesser sac. It may also erode into the pancreas, causing referred pain in the back.

Ninety-five per cent of duodenal ulcers occur in the posterior wall of the first part of the duodenum. Perforation causes the duodenal contents to enter the abdominal cavity, causing peritonitis. An ulcer may also erode the gastroduodenal artery, causing major haemorrhage. An anterior ulcer may be sealed off by the greater omentum.

Jejunum and ileum

The jejunum and ileum are intraperitoneal. They are attached to the posterior abdominal wall by the mesentery of the small intestine. The root of the mesentery extends along the posterior abdominal wall from the left of the L2 vertebra to the right sacroiliac joint and contains blood vessels, fat, lymph nodes and nerves.

Table 4.7 outlines the differences between the jejunum and ileum. Of note are lymphoid nodules known as Peyer patches, found mostly, but not exclusively, in the ileum. They play a role in generating the immune response, containing many of the cells of the immune system.

The jejunum and ileum are supplied by jejunal and ileal arteries (branches of the SMA) which form anastomotic loops known as arterial arcades. Vasa recta (straight arteries) arise from the arcades to supply the walls of the intestine. The vasa recta are end arteries—occlusion may result in infarction. Venous drainage

Table 4.7 Differences between the jejunum and ileum

Characteristic	Jejunum	Ileum
Colour	Deep red	Paler pink
Wall	Thick and heavy	Thin and light
Vascularity	Greater	Less
Vasa recta	Long	Short
Arcades	A few large loops	Many short loops
Peyer patches (aggregated lymphoid follicles)	No	Yes
Plicae circulares (mucosal folds increasing surface area)	More and larger	Less and smaller/absent
Fat	Less—stops at the mesenteric border with the jejunum	More—encroaches onto the ileum

occurs via the SMV. Lymphatic drainage of the jejunum and ileum is to the superior mesenteric nodes.

Innervation arises from the posterior vagal trunks (parasympathetic) and the greater and lesser splanchnic nerves (sympathetic).

Overview of digestion

Food enters the GI tract as complex chemicals: fats, proteins and carbohydrates. Digestion represents the breakdown of these substances into simpler subunits, involving hydrolysis.

Digestion begins in the mouth through physical (mastication) and enzymatic actions (secreted salivary amylase) as previously discussed. Food is then processed in an orderly fashion as it travels along the alimentary tract. The small intestine is the principal site for digestion, which occurs by enzymatic activity, mainly in the duodenum:

- Intraluminally: By secreted enzymes.
- At the cell (enterocyte) surface: By brush-border enzymes.
- Within the cytoplasm of intestinal mucosal cells (enterocytes).

The products of digestion are then transported across the wall of the small intestine by various processes. The jejunum and ileum have mainly absorptive functions, facilitated by their huge surface areas.

Intestinal circulation

The intestines receive 10% of cardiac output via the splanchnic circulation, most of which supplies the mucosa (Fig. 4.31):

- The coeliac trunk supplies the proximal duodenal half.
- The SMA (extensive branching network) supplies the remainder of the small intestines.

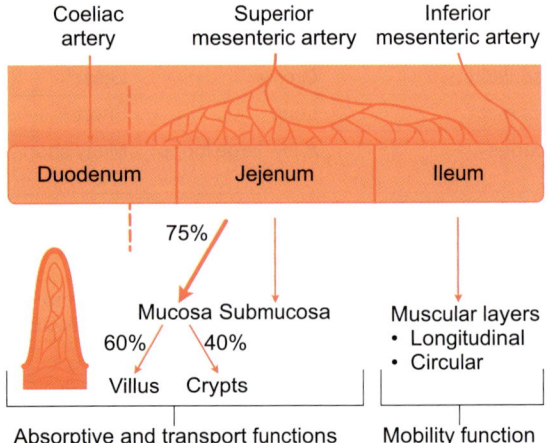

Fig. 4.31 Blood supply and distribution of the small intestines.

- The IMA contributes a small amount of blood to the terminal ileum.

Variation in intestinal circulation

The autonomic nervous system is one of the factors affecting the blood supply:

- Decreases in splanchnic circulation can result from sympathetic nervous stimulation → shunting of blood away from the intestines, for example during exercise or shock. Mediators include catecholamines, angiotensin II and antidiuretic hormone.
- Increases in splanchnic circulation can result from a response to a meal or functional hyperaemia, involving:
  - Peptide hormones: CCK, VIP, gastrin and secretin.
  - Kinins: Released by GI glands into the gut wall.
  - Digestive products within chyme: Glucose and long-chain fatty acids cause localized intestinal hyperaemia. Bile salts cause direct vasodilation in the terminal ileum.
  - Decreased intestinal wall O_2 tension: Secondary to increased gut metabolic activity, with subsequent rise in adenosine concentrations.

Local activity dictates the distribution of blood flow. The mucosal blood supply is greater with increased absorption or secretion. The blood supply to the muscular layers is greater during increased motility. There are two main functions of the intestinal circulation:

1. It provides a readily available blood reservoir that can be mobilized on demand.
2. It provides a countercurrent system within the villus.

Circulation within the villus

The villus represents the absorptive unit within which arterial and venous blood lie in close proximity but flow in opposite directions (Fig. 4.32). This anatomical arrangement facilitates diffusion between arterioles and venules. O_2 diffuses directly between the two, with a significant amount bypassing the capillaries supplying the villus. The partial pressure of arterial oxygen (PaO_2) is higher where the arteriole enters the base of the villus than the tip of the ascending limb, with no harmful effects under normal conditions. Ischaemia, leading to necrosis of the villus tip (extending to the whole villus in some cases), can interfere with the absorptive capacity of the intestine.

As with the countercurrent system in the kidneys, the tip of the hairpin loop (villus tip) is hyperosmolar. There is net diffusion of substances between arteriole and venule such that nutrient-rich venous blood leaves the gut via the portal vein to the liver.

Factors that control absorption

Absorptive mechanisms involve:

- Diffusion: ~80% of the 9.0 L of water entering the small intestine per day is absorbed by diffusion.

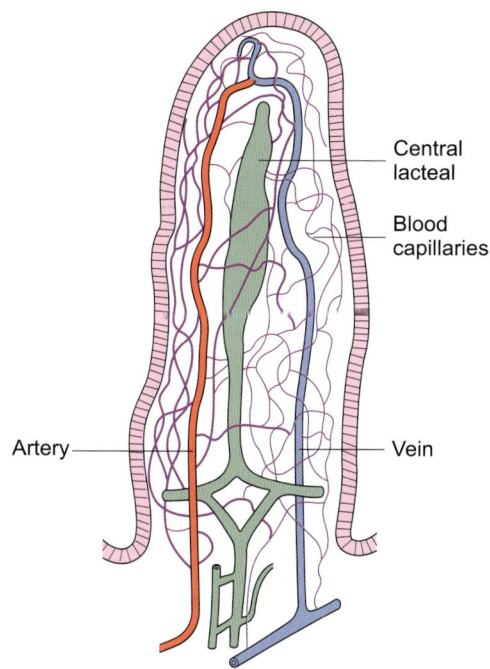

Fig. 4.32 The countercurrent mechanism in the villi of the small intestine. This enables absorption of electrolytes and water.

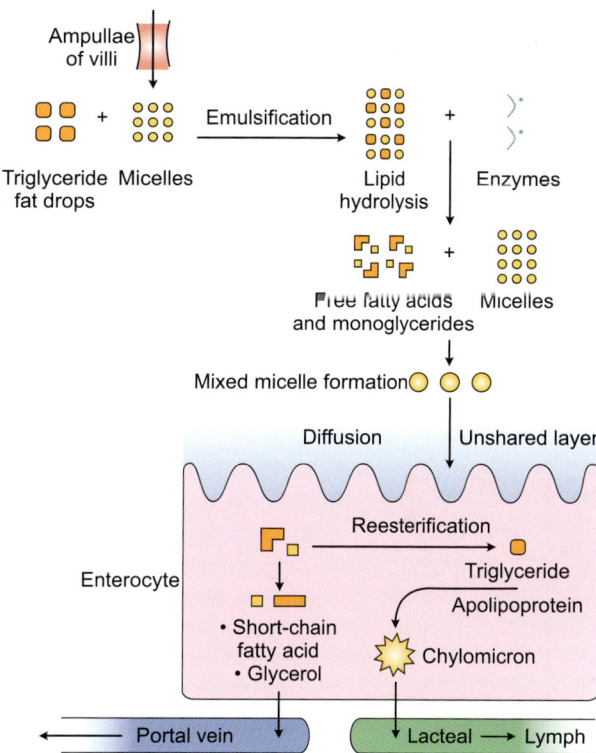

Fig. 4.33 Overview of intestinal fat digestion and absorption.

- Solvent drag: The flow of water (solvent) results in secondary 'dragging' of solute with it.
- Active transport: Large amounts of nutrients are absorbed via membrane carrier proteins.

Absorption and rate of transport are facilitated by:

- Increased surface area: Villi greatly multiply the surface area of the gut available for transport.
- Vascular supply: The countercurrent system permits the rapid uptake of fluid, electrolytes and nutrients. Rates of blood flow are adequate to not limit absorption.
- High cell turnover: Increased food intake itself stimulates mucosal growth, which in turn improves substance absorption.
- Carrier protein density: Nutrient absorption relies on carrier molecules and plentiful brush-border enzymes.
- Permeability gradient: Mucosal permeability decreases along the small bowel, and absorption is high in the duodenum and low in the ileum.

Handling of water and electrolytes is affected in particular by:

- Osmotic gradient: This depends on the intracellular osmolality.
- Tight junction selectivity: Monovalent cations (Na^+) pass more readily than anions (Cl^-) or divalent cations (Mg^{2+}).

- Mineralocorticoids: Aldosterone increases intestinal Na^+ absorption and K^+ secretion.
- Autonomic control: Absorption is increased and decreased by sympathetic and parasympathetic stimulation, respectively.

Intestinal digestion and absorption of different components of the diet

Fats

The arrival of lipids (triglycerides) in the duodenum serves as a stimulus for the secretion of bile. Bile contains phospholipids and bile salts, which form micelles. A minimum bile acid concentration is required for micelle formation (critical micelle formation occurs at 5 mmol/L).

Micelles function as detergents by breaking the fat globules into tiny emulsified droplets, thus presenting a greater surface for hydrolysis by pancreatic lipase, cholesterol esterase and phospholipase (Fig. 4.33). The breakdown products—fatty acids and 2-monoglycerides—are incorporated into mixed micelles, which have longer fatty acids at their centre.

Micelles transport lipids through an unstirred layer of fluid at the enterocyte surface. Lipid then passively diffuses across the intestinal cell wall whereupon it is taken up by smooth endoplasmic reticulum. Here, rapid reesterification mostly occurs, reforming triglycerides. Triglycerides, phospholipids and cholesterol are then combined with lipoprotein (in particular apolipoprotein B) to form chylomicrons, which consist of:

- Outer coat: Composed of phospholipids and apolipoprotein.
- Inner core: Composed of fatty acids, cholesterol and cholesterol ester.

Chylomicrons exocytose from the epithelial basolateral surface and enter the villus lacteal to be transported to venous blood via the lymph system. A minority of lipid digestion products, including short-chain fatty acids and glycerol, pass into the portal system to the liver. The digestion of the fat-soluble vitamins A (retinol), D, E (via the lymph system) and K follow the same principles.

Carbohydrates

Digestion of carbohydrates begins in the mouth, where starch is broken down by the action of salivary amylase (also known as ptyalin), which is subsequently destroyed by the low pH in the stomach. The α-1,4 linkages in up to 50% of the ingested starch are hydrolyzed in the stomach to produce maltose. Thus carbohydrate enters the duodenum in a variety of forms:

- Complex carbohydrates (starch).
- Disaccharides (sucrose, lactose and maltose).
- Monosaccharides (glucose, galactose and fructose).

Digestion continues with the release of pancreatic α-amylase, which, like its salivary form, requires a neutral or mild alkaline pH and chloride for optimum activity.

The appropriate oligo- and disaccharidases (e.g. lactase) in the intestinal epithelial brush border act to release monosaccharides. Free concentrations of these subunits at the mucosal surface are likely to be adequate for the passive process of facilitated absorption. As concentrations fall, however, other transport processes are necessary. Apical membrane-associated transporters powered by basolateral Na^+/K^+-ATPase are employed—Na^+/glucose cotransporters (SGLT1) that also bind galactose. Entry of fructose, independent of Na^+ movement, and much slower than glucose and galactose, is by facilitated diffusion utilizing GLUT 5, a member of another group of protein transporters (GLUT 1–5).

Monosaccharides move out of the epithelial cells by facilitated diffusion utilizing the GLUT 2 transporters in the basolateral membrane and enter the capillaries of the villi.

Proteins

In the stomach, proteins are denatured by acidic gastric juice before hydrolysis by pepsin to produce polypeptide fragments. These then pass into the duodenum, where pancreatic bond-specific proteolytic enzymes, including chymotrypsin, elastin and carboxypeptidases, continue the hydrolysis of peptide bonds. The resultant mixture of free amino acids and small peptides is then transported into the intestinal cells by a series of carrier systems. Di- and tripeptides are either:

- Absorbed intact by secondary active transport mechanisms with Na^+ (compared with SGLT), although not all protein transporters are Na^+ dependent.
- Broken down into free amino acids by the action of peptidases on the microvillus membrane (brush-border enzymes) before absorption by active transport.

Peptides are hydrolyzed within the epithelial cells into amino acids, which, along with other amino acids, pass into the capillaries of the villus.

Acidic amino acids serve as energy substrates for enterocytes; they do not appear to exit via carrier proteins.

Water and water-soluble vitamins

The small intestine absorbs about 80% of the 9 L of water that enters it per day. This is achieved by solvent drag through paracellular and transcellular routes consequent on sodium uptake (in association with carbohydrate and amino acid absorption). Passive diffusion accounts for a significant amount of water-soluble vitamin uptake, although there are other mechanisms.

Vitamin C (ascorbic acid)

Secondary active transport mechanisms employing Na^+ cotransport in the proximal ileum.

Folate

Carrier-mediated facilitated diffusion.

Vitamin B 'complex'

- Biotin, riboflavin and choline are absorbed by facilitated diffusion.
- Thiamin, inositol and nicotinic acid rely on Na^+-dependent active transport.

Vitamin B_{12} (cobalamin)

On entering the duodenum, B_{12}-R protein complexes are degraded. B_{12} then binds to IF, which is secreted by the gastric parietal cells in the stomach, enabling the absorption of vitamin B_{12} in the terminal ileum. The ileal epithelial brush border contains receptors that bind the IF–B_{12} complexes, enabling cobalamin uptake.

Vitamin B_{12} crosses the basolateral border and enters the portal blood by an unknown mechanism. It is then bound to a globulin—transcobalamin II—as a complex before being taken up by the liver and other tissues. Passive diffusion throughout the small intestine accounts for 1% to 2% of vitamin B_{12} absorption.

Ions and minerals
Sodium

The distal small bowel and colon are largely responsible for absorbing 95% of the sodium load entering the gut. The four mechanisms implicated are powered by basolateral Na^+/K^+-ATPase, enabling Na^+ diffusion into the cells from the lumen via passive and coupled means.

Chloride

Rapid diffusion in the proximal small bowel and distal colon occurs through Cl^- channels via both transcellular and paracellular routes powered by the electrochemical gradient secondary to Na^+ absorption. Cl^- absorption also occurs via apical Cl^-/HCO_3^- exchange.

Bicarbonate

The absorption of HCO_3^- is important because large quantities are secreted by the pancreas and in bile: significant loss in faeces will lead to metabolic acidosis. The mechanism of absorption is the same as that in some renal tubules: luminal HCO_3^- combines with H^+ exchanged for Na^+ to form H_2CO_3. This then dissociates into H_2O and CO_2; the latter is absorbed into the blood and contributes to plasma HCO_3^- homoeostasis.

Calcium

Absorption occurs:

- Passively: High chyme $[Ca^{2+}]$ via the paracellular pathway.
- Actively: Low chyme $[Ca^{2+}]$ and is rate limited.

Active absorption occurs throughout the small intestine in balance with the body's needs. It is subject to:

- Parathyroid hormone, which activates vitamin D, which in turn enhances Ca^{2+} absorption.
- Vitamin D, which stimulates the synthesis of basolateral Ca^{2+}-ATPase pumps and binds to enterocyte nuclear receptors to stimulate the synthesis of brush-border and cytosolic calcium-binding proteins.

Diffusion of luminal Ca^{2+} into the enterocyte through Ca^{2+} channels is facilitated by a reduction in the intracellular $[Ca^{2+}]$ that is brought about by basolateral transport proteins and calbindin, which binds to two calcium ions before entering the cell.

Iron

Haem represents the majority of iron consumed by nonvegetarians. Iron exists in two forms:

1. Fe^{2+} (ferrous): Present in haem and more easily absorbed as it has a lower tendency to form insoluble complexes.
2. Fe^{3+} (ferric): Reduced by ascorbic acid or HCl, both secreted by the stomach, to Fe^{2+}. It is less well absorbed, more readily forming insoluble complexes with tannins and phytins.

Only the proximal 10 cm of the small intestine absorbs haem and Fe^{2+}:

- Haem: Uptake is via facilitated diffusion. Intracellular xanthine oxidase releases Fe^{2+} ions.
- Fe^{2+}: Duodenal and jejunal epithelial cells secrete transferrin, each of which binds with two Fe^{2+} ions. Brush-border

transferrin receptors bind to the complex and are then endocytosed. Fe^{2+} ions are released inside the cell, and transferrin and the receptor are returned to the lumen.

Within the enterocyte, iron is either:

- Stored: In combination with apoferritin, known as ferritin (majority).
- Transported: To the basolateral membrane where it binds to a receptor 'mobilin'. The iron is then bound to transferrin and released in the blood.

Cells with a large ferrous store take up this ion less readily, discouraging iron overload.

The intestinal flora

Bacteria colonize most of the GI tract, exceptions being the stomach, gallbladder and salivary glands. The majority of these microflora are commensal (do not have adverse effects) and differ according to site. Although there are skin flora and bacteria in the mouth, the harsh acidic conditions result in a low bacterial count in the duodenum.

The bacterial count increases distally from the duodenum, and there are progressively fewer aerobic bacteria, which favour the more aerated, better-oxygenated conditions that predominate in the proximal small bowel.

Duodenum

- Contains few microflora.
- Species include gram-positive cocci and rods.

Jejunum

- Contains more bacteria.
- Examples include *Enterococcus faecalis*, lactobacilli and diphtheroids.

Ileum

- Contains a large number of flora.
- Species include *Bacteroides*, *Clostridia* and *Bifidobacterium*.

Colon

- Contains more bacteria than the small intestines by a factor of $\sim 10^3$.
- Over 400 species, including *Bacteroides* and coliforms (e.g. *Escherichia coli*, *Enterococcus faecalis*).
- Large microflora is maintained by relatively low peristalsis activity.
- Bacterial residues contribute a third of the dried weight of faeces.

Functions of colonic bacteria

- Immunity: Commensal bacteria compete with pathological types for food and space, thus keeping them under control.

- Bilirubin metabolism: The bacteria in the small bowel assist in the enterohepatic cycling of bilirubin by converting conjugated bilirubin back into its free form. They also form urobilinogen, which can be reabsorbed, excreted in urine, or further acted on to produce stercobilinogen (which is excreted in the faeces).
- Production of vitamins: Bacterial activity forms B vitamins (riboflavin and thiamin). Anaerobes are particularly important for the production of vitamin K, which would be insufficient for coagulation if relying on ingested amounts alone.

LARGE INTESTINE

The large intestine consists of the caecum and appendix, colon, rectum and upper part of the anal canal.

Anatomy of the caecum and appendix

The caecum and the vermiform appendix lie in the right iliac fossa. The caecum is a blind pouch invested by peritoneum. It is the first part of the large intestine, continuous with the ascending colon. The ileum enters the caecum at the ileocaecal valve (not a true valve).

The appendix is a blind-ending tube, 6 to 9 cm long, and rich in lymphoid tissue. It opens into the posteromedial wall of the caecum, 2 cm inferior to the ileocaecal junction. It is suspended by a mesentery (the mesoappendix). The taeniae coli (bands of smooth muscle that correspond to the outer, longitudinal layer of muscle elsewhere in the GI tract) of the caecum merge at the base of the appendix—this is a useful landmark during surgery. The position of the body of the appendix varies—the majority are retrocaecal (65%) or pelvic (30%), with the remainder (5%) occupying a variety of positions. Swelling of the appendix may obstruct the artery, resulting in necrosis and perforation. The arterial supply, venous and lymphatic drainage, and nerve supply of the caecum and appendix are detailed in Fig. 4.7 and Table 4.8.

CLINICAL NOTES

APPENDICITIS

Appendicitis occurs when the appendix is obstructed by faecoliths or by swelling of lymphoid tissue (often after a viral infection). As the appendix becomes inflamed, it produces periumbilical pain (the appendix is part of the midgut and visceral pain from this region is felt around the umbilicus). Pain subsequently becomes sharper and localized to the right iliac fossa, owing to irritation of the parietal peritoneum. The treatment of appendicitis is with antibiotics, with or without an appendicectomy, the surgical removal of the appendix.

Untreated appendicitis can result in rupture, peritonitis (with increased pain, nausea/vomiting and abdominal rigidity), the formation of an appendix abscess and sepsis.

Anatomy of the colon

The colon has several characteristic features:

- Three bands of smooth muscle run longitudinally along the wall of the colon—the taeniae coli. They correspond to the outer longitudinal layer of the muscularis externa in other regions of the GI tract.
- Haustra: Pouches along the length of the colon, formed by the taeniae coli, which 'bunch together' in the colonic wall.
- Appendices epiploicae: Pouches of peritoneum filled with fat project from the external surface of the colon.

CLINICAL NOTES

MECKEL DIVERTICULUM

This is a remnant of the vitelline duct (a connection between the gut tube and the embryonic yolk sac). It projects from the ileum, approximately 60 to 70 cm from the ileocaecal junction in roughly 2% of people. It is twice as common in males than females. It may contain ectopic mucosa (gastric, pancreatic or colonic). It may cause ulceration with pain, bleeding or diverticulitis, producing symptoms similar to those of appendicitis.

CLINICAL NOTES

DIVERTICULAE

Outpouchings of mucous membrane may herniate through the perforations in the muscle layer of the colon made by the blood vessels between the taeniae coli. The outpouchings are known as diverticulae and are most common in the sigmoid colon. The presence of diverticulae is known as diverticulosis. Inflammation of the diverticulae, resulting in pain in the left iliac fossa and pyrexia, is known as diverticulitis.

The colon is composed of the following regions:

- Ascending colon: This occupies a retroperitoneal position, and extends from the ileocolic junction to the right colic (hepatic) flexure. The right paracolic gutter lies on its lateral side.

- Transverse colon: This extends from the right colic (hepatic) flexure to the left colic (splenic) flexure, the former being lower due to the right lobe of the liver. It is intraperitoneal suspended by the transverse mesocolon.
- Descending colon: This extends from the left colic (splenic) flexure to the sigmoid colon. It lies retroperitoneally. The left paracolic gutter lies on its lateral side.
- Sigmoid colon: This extends from the descending colon and becomes continuous with the rectum inferiorly. It hangs free from the sigmoid mesocolon. The mesocolon is an inverted V-shape (see Fig. 4.21B), the base of which lies over the sacroiliac joint. From here, one part runs to the midinguinal point along the external iliac vessels and the other runs to the level of the S3 where the rectum begins.

The arterial supply, venous and lymphatic drainage, and nerve supply of the colon are illustrated and detailed in Fig. 4.7 and Table 4.8.

CLINICAL NOTES

ISCHAEMIC BOWEL AND HIRSCHPRUNG DISEASE

The terminal branches of the superior mesenteric artery (SMA) and inferior mesenteric artery (IMA) form an anastomotic network (important in the event of arterial occlusion), known as the marginal artery. Vasa recta arise from the marginal artery to supply the colon.

The splenic flexure is the watershed area between the arterial supply of the SMA and IMA. Anastomoses here are often weak or absent, and so this region is an area particularly prone to ischaemia and infarction.

Hirschsprung disease generally presents in infancy or childhood. It arises owing to an absence of nerve plexuses within the wall of the gut, most commonly in the rectosigmoid region. This results in constipation, bowel obstruction and vomiting. It is normally confirmed by biopsy. Treatment consists of surgical removal (resection) of the affected area of the colon.

Transport and secretion in the large intestine

The colon represents a 1.5-m reservoir that has important functions in the absorption, secretion, motility and elimination of faeces.

Water and electrolyte transport

Approximately 90% of water is absorbed from the 1.5 L of fluid chyme that enters the colon. Most of this occurs in the proximal colon, leaving ~150 mL per day to be excreted in faeces.

Water absorption is by solvent drag, following the passage of electrolytes which themselves employ active transport. As in the

---

Table 4.8 The arterial supply, venous and lymphatic drainage, and nerve supply of the caecum and appendix

	Arterial supply	Venous drainage	Nerve supply	Lymphatic drainage
Caecum	SMA → ileocolic artery → anterior and posterior caecal arteries	Ileocolic veins → SMV → portal vein	Parasympathetic fibres from the vagus nerves (cranial nerve 10) and sympathetic fibres from the superior mesenteric plexus	Superior mesenteric nodes
Appendix	SMA → ileocolic artery → appendicular artery	Appendicular vein → SMV → portal vein		
Ascending colon	SMA → ileocolic and right colic arteries	Ileocolic and right colic veins → SMV → portal vein		
Transverse colon	Proximal two-thirds: SMA → middle colic artery. Distal one-third: SMA → left colic artery	Proximal two-thirds: middle colic vein → SMV → portal vein. Distal one-third: left colic vein → IMV → portal vein	Proximal two-thirds: sympathetic and vagus nerves (CN 10) in the superior mesenteric plexus. Distal one-third: sympathetic via inferior mesenteric ganglion, parasympathetic via pelvic splanchnic nerves	
Descending colon	IMA → left colic and sigmoid arteries	Superior rectal veins → IMV → portal vein	Sympathetic via inferior mesenteric ganglion, and parasympathetic pelvic splanchnic nerves	Inferior mesenteric nodes
Sigmoid colon	IMA → sigmoid arteries and superior rectal arteries	Superior rectal veins → IMV → portal vein		

IMA, Inferior mesenteric artery; IMV; inferior mesenteric vein; SMA, superior mesenteric artery; SMV, superior mesenteric vein.

small bowel, basolateral Na^+/K^+-ATPase is key to permitting Na^+ influx by secondary active transport.

Although the mechanisms for water absorption are similar to those operating to concentrate bile in the gallbladder, there are some important differences. The colonic mucosa has relatively small pores compared with the small bowel and offers high resistance to the passage of water. Hence, passive water movement into the intercellular spaces is much slower than electrolyte transport. Water absorption is promoted by the following:

- Aldosterone: Stimulates electrogenic Na channels and increases basolateral Na^+/K^+ ATPase pumps.
- Angiotensin II: Increases Na^+ and water absorption.
- Glucocorticoid: Stimulates electroneutral NaCl absorption.

Mucus secretion

Thick mucus, rich in HCO_3^- and K^+, is secreted by the abundant goblet cells of colonic mucosa. Mucus lubricates the colon and serves to minimize mechanical trauma from the passage of faeces. Secretion is promoted by:

- Distension or mechanical irritation: probably involving VIP and ACh.
- Parasympathetic stimulation.

Secretion of mucus is inhibited by:

- Sympathetic stimulation: Mediated by adrenaline and somatostatin.

The motility of the large intestine

Colonic movements resemble a reduced and slow version of the small intestine. These are adequate for its main functions of absorption in the proximal half and storage in the distal half. The large intestine has both mixing and propulsive contractions:

- Mixing: haustration: no net movement of chyme.
- Propulsive:
  - Segmental propulsion: Movement of chyme from one segment to another.
  - Peristalsis: Propagated wave of contraction behind a relaxed area.
  - Mass movement: Contraction of a large length of bowel at once.

Haustration

Contraction of the circular muscles in one portion of the colon causes distension of the distal segment. Hence, mixing of the contents with mucosal contact is enabled, facilitating absorption.

Segmental propulsion

Contraction of the three longitudinal muscle bands in the wall of the colon (known as the taeniae coli) results in sequential

haustration. This slowly moves the intestinal contents (8–15 hours from the ileocaecal valve to the transverse colon) towards the anus. Distension of the longitudinal bands of the muscularis externa itself stimulates contraction. Movement is initiated by ACh and the release of substance P.

Peristalsis

Contractions are less frequent than in the small bowel and hence are slower, although they do propel chyme further.

Mass movement

This refers to the intense contraction that occurs between the transverse colon and the sigmoid colon between one and three times a day, shortly after ingestion of a meal. The colonic contents are pushed towards the anus and the urge to defecate is experienced when there are faeces in the rectum, usually during a period following a large meal. This is known as the gastrocolic reflex, and involves the coordination of physical, hormonal and neuromyoelectric mechanisms of bowel movement:

- Parasympathetic stimulation (vagal and pelvic nerves): Increases proximal colonic contraction.
- Sympathetic stimulation (inferior mesenteric and hypogastric plexi): Decreases colonic movement and is responsible for reflex relaxation of bowel adjacent to a contracting portion: colocolonic reflex.

Defaecation

Continence is maintained though the action of both internal and external sphincters (Fig. 4.34).

- Internal sphincter: Thickened continuation of circular muscle inside the anus, which is under involuntary control.
- External sphincter: Striated voluntary muscle extending more distally than the internal sphincter and surrounding it.

Defaecation occurs as an intrinsic reflex in response to faeces distending the rectum. However, it is subject to input from

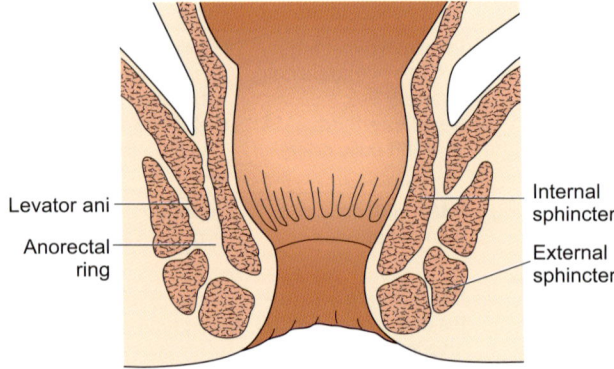

Fig. 4.34 Rectum and anal canal.

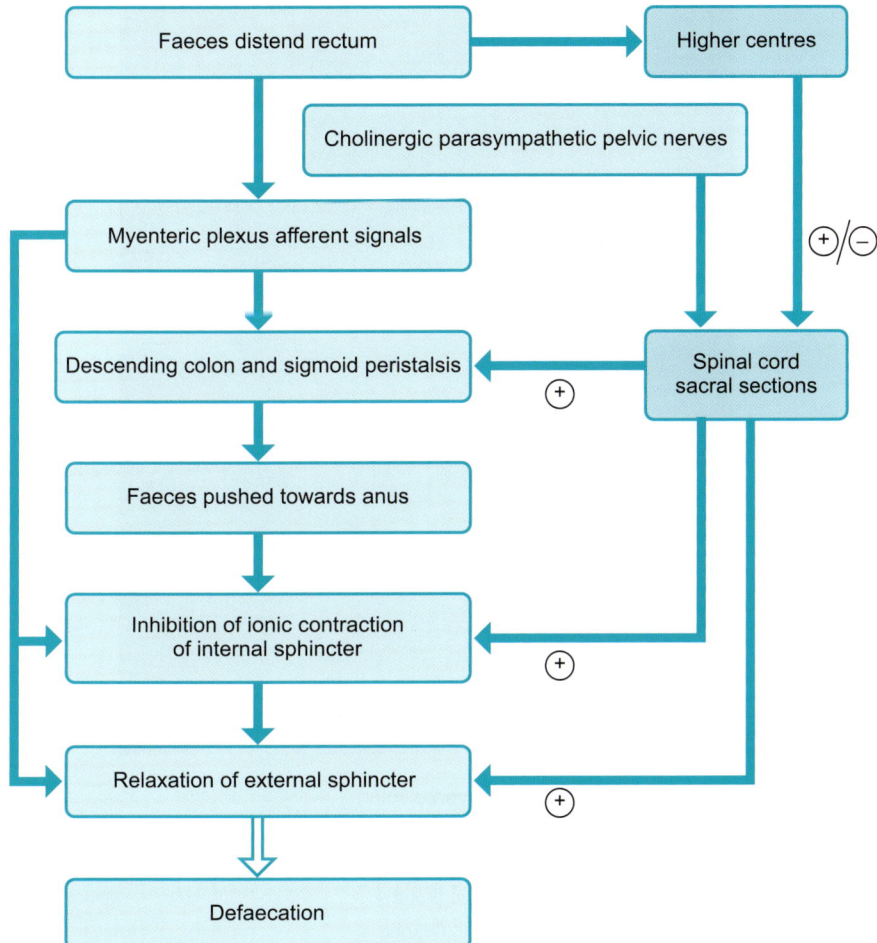

Fig. 4.35 Sequence of events in defaecation.

higher centres, so defaecation occurs when socially acceptable (Fig. 4.35).

Autonomic reflexes involving the parasympathetic system augment this intrinsic pathway to further increase distal colon motility.

SPLEEN

Anatomy of the spleen

The spleen is a large lymphoid organ, located in the left hypochondrium, inferior to the diaphragm. It is only palpable when enlarged. It has a convex diaphragmatic surface and on its concave visceral surface lies the hilum—the site of entry and exit of the splenic vessels. The visceral surface is also related to the

stomach, kidney, colon and tail of the pancreas. Its anterior and superior borders are notched and sharp, but its posterior and inferior borders are rounded.

It is connected to the greater curvature of the stomach by the gastrosplenic ligament, and to the posterior abdominal wall at the left kidney, by the splenorenal (lienorenal) ligament. It is completely enclosed by peritoneum except at the hilum.

Its arterial supply arises from the splenic artery (a branch of the coeliac trunk), a tortuous vessel which passes along the superior border of the pancreas and anterior to the left kidney. As it does so, the splenic artery gives off short gastric and left gastroepiploic arteries to the stomach and branches to the pancreas. Between the layers of the splenorenal ligament, the splenic artery divides into terminal branches which enter the hilum of the spleen.

Venous drainage occurs via the splenic vein, which runs along the posterosuperior aspect of the pancreas, and is joined by

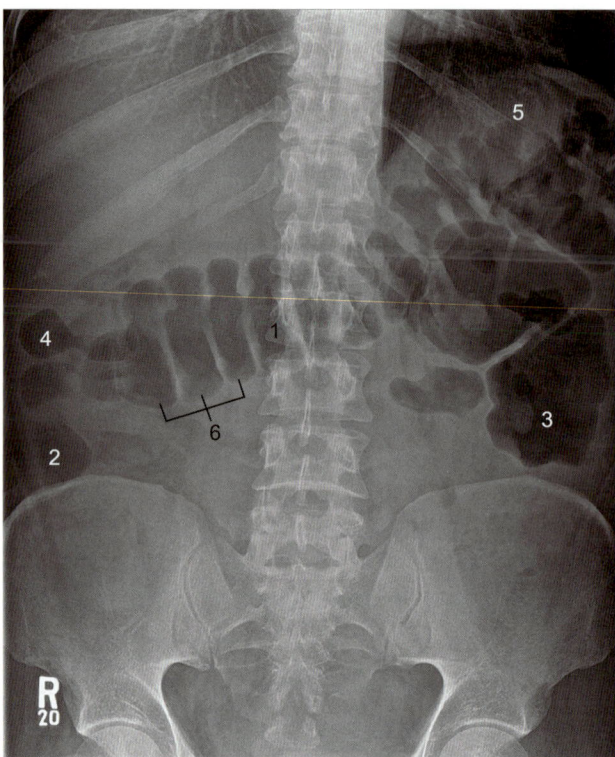

1. Transverse colon
2. Ascending colon
3. Descending colon
4. Hepatic flexure
5. Splenic flexure
6. Haustra

Fig. 4.36 Abdominal radiograph—supine projection. (Courtesy Dr Malcolm Johnston.)

the IMV posterior to the body of the pancreas. Posterior to the neck of the pancreas, the vein unites with the SMV to form the hepatic portal vein.

Lymphatic drainage is to the splenic nodes and, subsequently, the coeliac trunk. Its nerve supply arises from the coeliac plexus.

CLINICAL NOTES

RUPTURED SPLEEN AND SPLENECTOMY

The spleen can be damaged by blunt trauma or rib fractures (particularly of the 9th–11th ribs). Splenic rupture can lead to massive blood loss and hypovolaemic

shock. Emergency splenectomy is required. Patients who have undergone a splenectomy are vulnerable to infection (due to the role of the spleen in immunity) and so they must ensure that they are vaccinated against appropriate diseases. They may also be advised to take lifelong antibiotics.

Function of the spleen

The spleen removes damaged or antibody-coated cells from the blood and assists in mounting immunological responses against blood-borne pathogens. It is a site of haematopoiesis in the foetus and a potential site of haematopoiesis in the adult.

CLINICAL NOTES

RADIOLOGY OF THE GASTROINTESTINAL SYSTEM

Imaging the gastrointestinal system can be done in a variety of ways:
- Plain abdominal x-ray (Fig. 4.36).

   Abdominal x-rays (AXRs) are most commonly requested for patients who present with an 'acute abdomen'. They are typically readily available and can be obtained quickly for acutely unwell patients. AXRs are normally anteroposterior (AP) films, taken with the patient in a supine position. AXRs can be difficult to interpret, with a degree of ambiguity even for experienced practitioners, yet they remain an important first-line investigation and should not be underestimated.

   They are not generally used to diagnose a perforated viscus; this is normally diagnosed by an erect chest x-ray, where air will be visible under the diaphragm (usually more easily seen on the right side).
- Abdominal contrast studies: Barium.

   The use of contrast medium (barium sulphate) enhances images produced by plain abdominal x-ray. Depending on the area of the gut to be assessed, one of the following may be performed:
   - Barium swallow: Barium is swallowed to detect problems in the oesophagus.
   - Barium meal: Barium is swallowed to detect problems in the stomach and duodenum.
   - Barium follow-through: Barium is swallowed to detect problems in the small intestine (Fig. 4.37).
   - Barium enema: Barium is introduced via the rectum to detect problems in the colon (Fig. 4.38).

Both a barium meal and a barium enema can be further enhanced by the introduction of air into the gastrointestinal tract (a double-contrast barium meal/enema).

- Abdominal contrast studies—gastrografin.
- Ultrasound.

   Ultrasound examination is quick and simple to perform; therefore it is often a first-line investigation in the diagnosis of many abdominal diseases, for example testicular swellings, inflammation of the gallbladder, gallstones and abdominal aortic aneurysm.

- Computed tomography (CT)/magnetic resonance imaging (MRI) scanning of the abdomen.

   CT and MRI scans of the abdomen are performed to diagnose or provide more detail of diseases within the abdomen such as tumours, inflammatory bowel disease, vessel disease (e.g. abdominal aortic aneurysm) and trauma. CT scans are quick and typically readily available, making them useful for a detailed assessment of acute/emergency gastrointestinal and intraabdominal pathology. CT scans can also be invaluable for operative planning and decision-making. CT is also used to guide biopsies (e.g. a liver biopsy) or drainage of abscesses. A transverse CT scan of the abdomen at the level of L1 is shown in Fig. 4.39.

   MRI of the gastrointestinal tract is highly detailed and typically ordered only by specialists, given the time, cost and often lesser availability of MRIs. It is frequently used for the diagnosis of abnormalities such as fistulae, certain neoplasia and inflammation.

   Angiography involves the injection of radioopaque contrast into blood vessels while taking multiple x-ray images. Abdominal angiography can provide information on blood flow through arteries and organs, where flow may be limited by stenosis or thrombus, or active bleeding from vessels or an organ. Interventions can then be made during the procedure including stenting stenoses, repairing aneurysms and embolization. Fig. 4.36 shows the branches of the coeliac trunk and its branches during angiography.

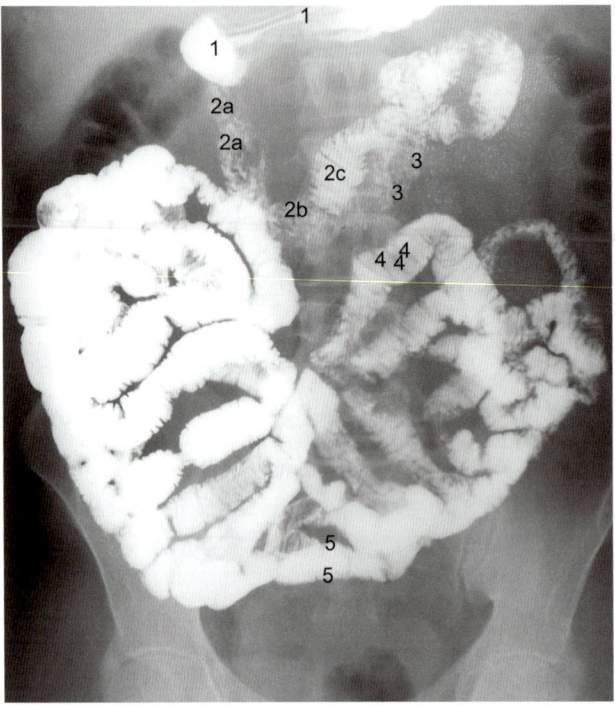

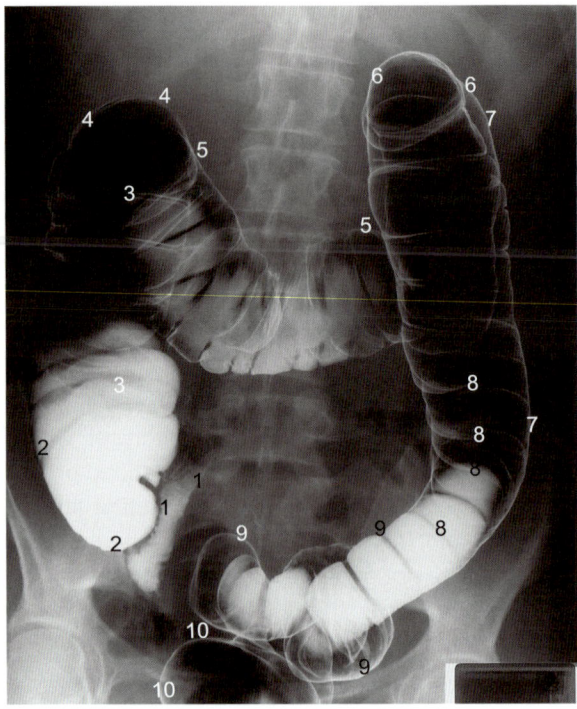

1. Stomach
2a. Descending (second) part duodenum
2b. Horizontal (third) part of duodenum
2c. Ascending (fourth) part of duodenum
3. Proximal jejunum
4. Valvulae conniventes (plicae circulares) of jejunum
5. Proximal ileum

Fig. 4.37 Abdomen barium follow-through showing duodenum and small intestine.

1. Terminal ileum
2. Caecum
3. Ascending portion
4. Right colic (hepatic) flexure
5. Transverse portion
6. Left colic (splenic) portion
7. Descending portion
8. Sacculations (haustrations)
9. Sigmoid colon
10. Rectum

Fig. 4.38 Abdomen double-contrast barium enema of colon.

KIDNEYS AND URETERS

Anatomy of the renal tract

Kidney

The kidneys are paired organs with dimensions of $12 \times 7 \times 3$ cm and weighing 140 g each. They are situated in the retroperitoneal space covered by the costal margins. They extend from T12 to L3 with the right kidney lower than the left owing to the presence of the liver. The hilum of the left kidney is at the level of L1. The internal structure of the kidneys is shown in Fig. 4.40. Grossly, the kidney is separated into the cortex which has the tubules and filtering capsules, and the medulla which has the vasa recta, loops of Henle and collecting ducts.

Each kidney is surrounded by three layers, which from superficial to deep are renal fascia, perinephric fat and renal capsule (Fig. 4.41).

The arterial supply to the kidneys comes from the renal arteries, which are paired arteries branching from the lateral aspect of the abdominal aorta between the L1 and L2 vertebral levels. Each renal artery gives suprarenal and ureteric branches. In the kidney, the renal artery divides into the anterior and posterior branches and further into segmental, arcuate and interlobular branches (end arteries). Venous drainage is the reverse process of the arterial supply, with the renal veins draining into the inferior vena cava. The left renal vein also receives a branch from the left gonadal vein. The orientation of the renal arteries is shown in Fig. 4.42.

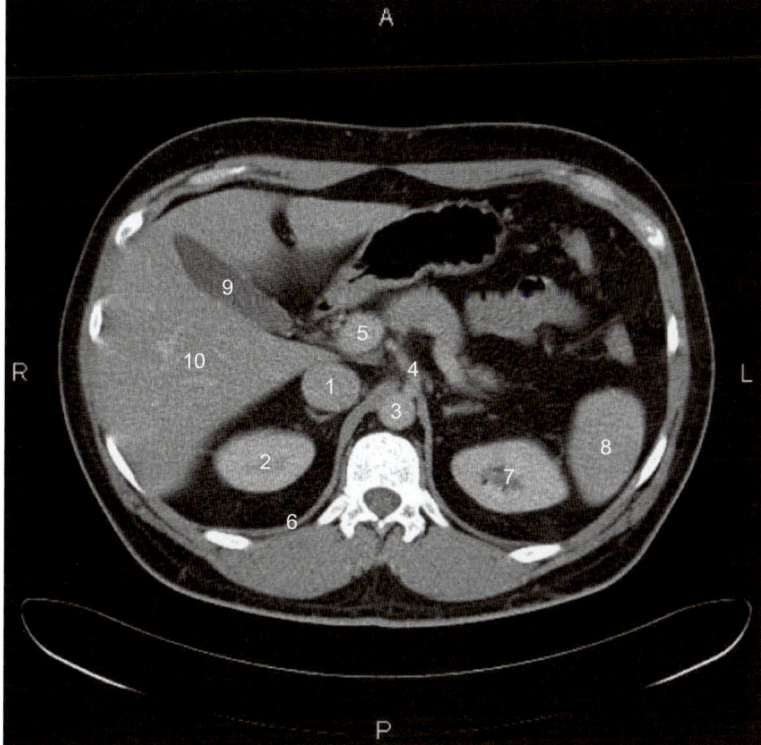

1. Inferior vena cava
2. Right kidney
3. Descending aorta
4. Coeliac trunk
5. Portal vein
6. Right crura of diaphragm
7. Left kidney
8. Spleen
9. Gallbladder
10. Liver

Fig. 4.39 Computed tomography scan (transverse section) of the abdomen at the level of L1.

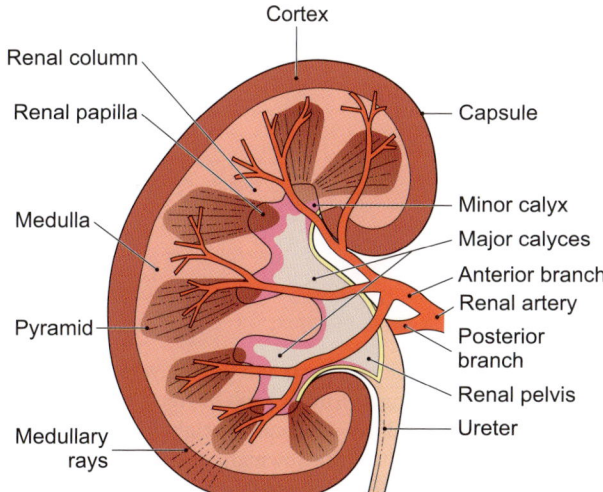

Fig. 4.40 Macroscopic structure of kidney.

CLINICAL NOTES

VARICOCELE

Left-sided varicocele (distended venous plexus in the testicle) can be a sign of left renal carcinoma, owing to obstruction of drainage of the gonadal vein into the left renal vein.

The nephron

The nephron is the single functional unit of the kidney (Fig. 4.43), and there are one million in each kidney. The nephron can be divided into the following key components:

- Renal corpuscle: glomerulus and Bowman capsule.
- Renal tubule: proximal convoluting tubule, loop of Henle (LoH), distal convoluting tubule, collecting duct (DC).

Eighty per cent of nephrons are cortical and only just penetrate into the medulla. The remaining nephrons are juxtamedullary and

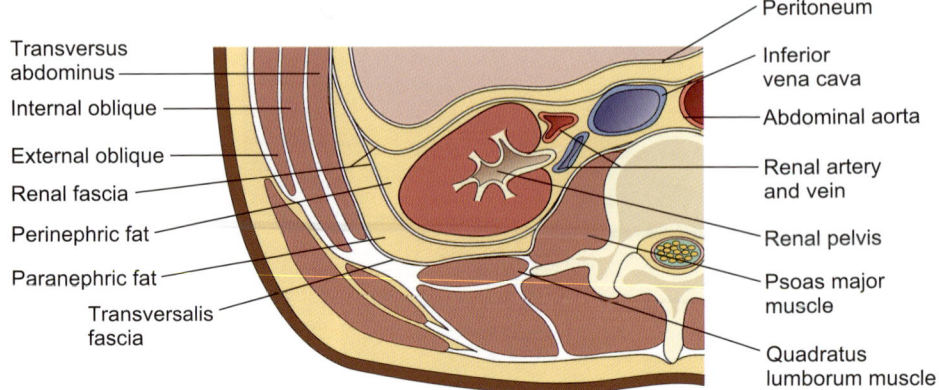

Fig. 4.41 Cross section of kidney and surrounding structure.

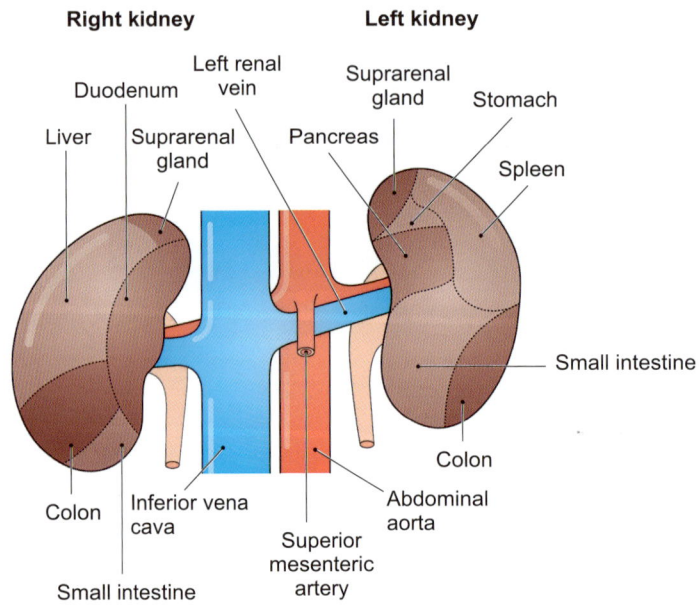

Dark shading = structures directly related
Light shading = structures indirectly related

Fig. 4.42 Arterial supply and venous drainage of the kidneys.

have loops deep into the medulla which can create very dilute or concentrated urine.

Glomerulus and Bowman capsule

The glomerulus is a ball of capillaries fed by the afferent arteriole which drains into the efferent arteriole. The glomerulus is pushed into a cup-like structure called the Bowman capsule, which is 200 μm in diameter. As blood travels through the glomerulus, fluid and substrates are filtered out of the capillaries and into the capsule. The volume of filtrate formed per unit time is known as the glomerular filtration rate (GFR).

Structure of the glomerular filter

The glomerular capillary wall acts as a three-layered sieve (Figs 4.44 and 4.45), allowing a virtually protein-free filtrate containing inorganic ions and low-molecular-weight (LMW) organic solutes to pass through into the Bowman capsule. The properties of this filtration barrier are accounted for by its three layers:

Glomerular capillary endothelium

A high plasma filtration rate is facilitated by thousands of small holes or fenestrae perforating the thin, flat endothelial cells and

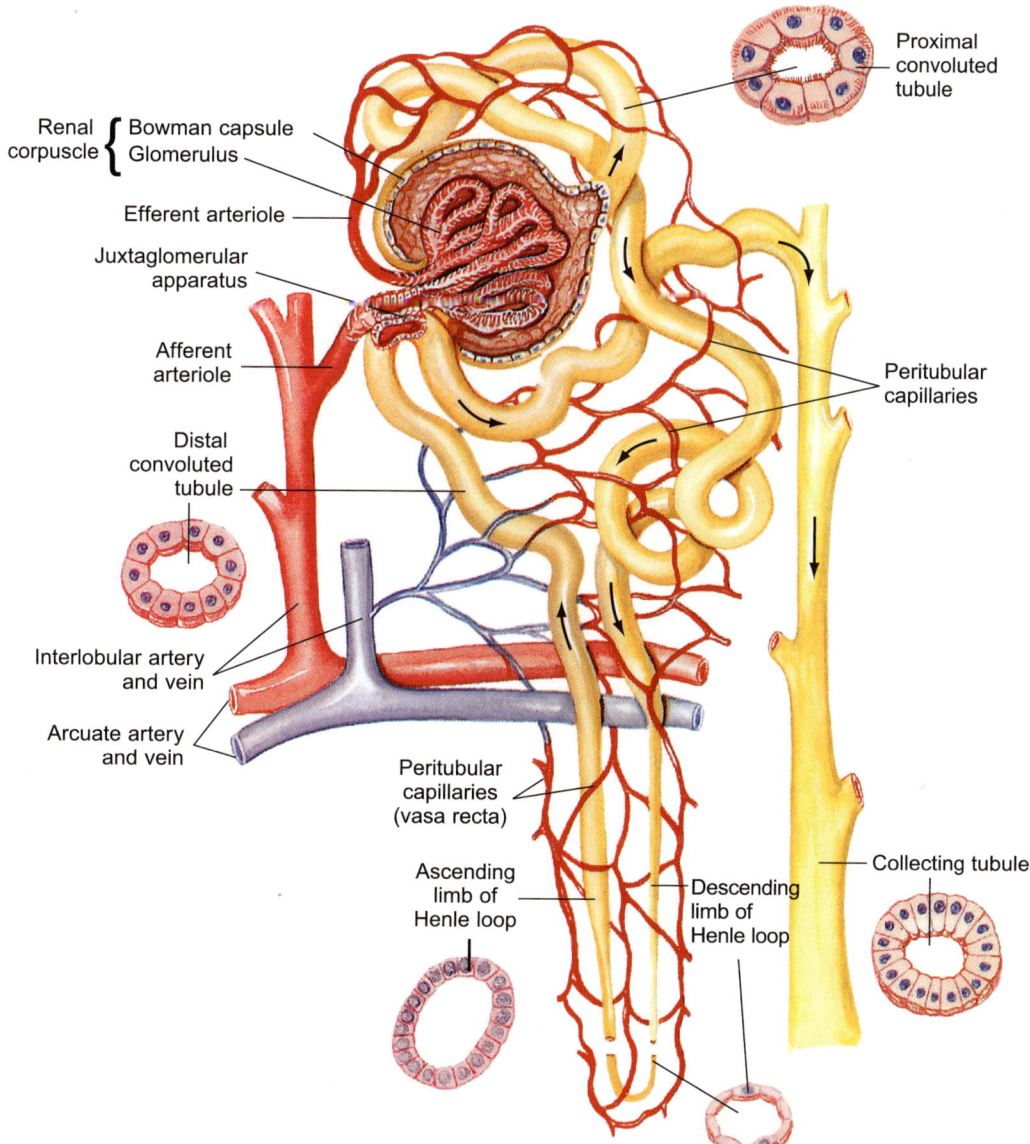

Fig. 4.43 Structure of the nephron. (From Thibodeau, G. A., Patton, K. T. (1996). *Anatomy & physiology* (3rd ed.). Mosby.)

occupying approximately 10% of the endothelium surface. Their diameter is 60 nm, which allows only small molecules to pass through and keeps blood cells and platelets in the vascular compartment. In addition, the endothelial cells are lined with fixed negatively charged ions that further discourage the passage of anionic plasma proteins.

Basement membrane (connective tissue)

The collagen and proteoglycan meshwork of the basement membrane has a strong negative charge which limits any further passage

of plasma proteins through electrical repulsion. At the same time, it permits water and small solutes through its large spaces.

Bowman capsule epithelial cells (podocytes)

This final layer comprises negatively charged cells called podocytes, providing a further barrier to plasma proteins. These podocytes are named so because of their long, foot-like processes embedded in the basement membrane, encircling the capillary. At the end of these extensions are small 'toe-like' processes, called pedicels, which

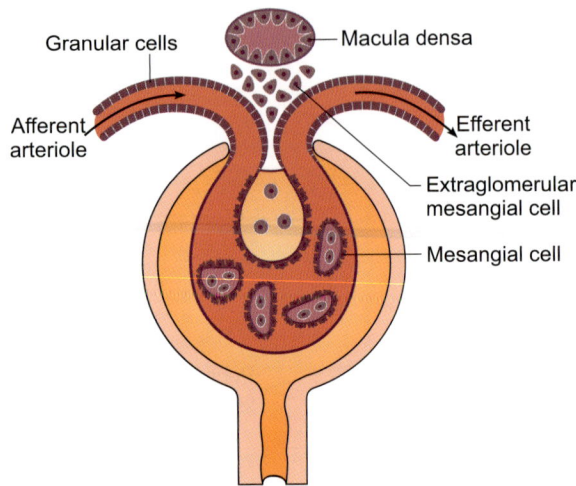

Fig. 4.44 The Bowman capsule and juxtaglomerular apparatus.

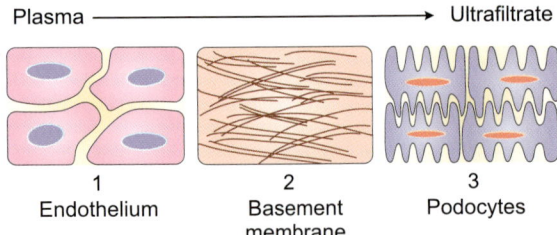

Fig. 4.45 The three layers of glomerular filter.

interdigitate with the pedicels of neighbouring podocytes. The gaps formed are called *slit pores*, and the glomerular filtrate passes through these into the Bowman capsule. These cells are also involved in macromolecular phagocytosis.

The mesangium

The mesangial matrix and mesangial cells—which lie between the glomerular capillaries—are also part of the renal corpuscle. Mesangial cells have several properties and they:

- Act as phagocytes, preventing buildup in the basement membrane of escaped macromolecules from the capillaries.
- Have a supportive function in maintaining the delicate structure of the glomerulus.
- Can alter the surface area of the glomerular capillaries available for filtration using their large amounts of myofilaments to contract in response to various stimuli.
- Can secrete extracellular matrix and prostaglandins (PGs).

Process of glomerular filtration

Glomerular filtration is the first step in the formation of urine. It involves the passive flow of solvent through a molecular sieve, as

described previously. The filtrate formed is known as glomerular *ultrafiltrate* (because the filter operates at the molecular level) and is composed of only LMW substances from plasma, at the same concentrations as in plasma.

Glomerular filtration rate

All the blood flow of the kidney passes through the glomeruli. The volume of filtrate formed (fluid from the blood which passes into the glomeruli) per unit time is known as the glomerular filtration rate (GFR).

Normal GFR = 90 to 125 mL/min. GFR is used to indicate renal function: very low values are a cardinal sign of renal failure.

This value correlates with body surface area, so 125 mL/min is an appropriate value for an average male, while in females, the GFR is always 10% less than in males, even after correcting for surface area.

The total volume filtered is 180 L/day and the normal urine volume is 1 to 2 L/day, that is most ultrafiltrate is reabsorbed. The advantage of such a high GFR is to permit rapid excretion of waste from the body and also to repeatedly filter and process all the body fluids each day. Hence, the kidney can tightly and swiftly control both the volume and composition of body fluids.

Molecular size

The glomerular filter acts selectively, filtering by electrical charge and molecular size. Although all three layers of the filter have a negative charge, they exert an inhibitory effect on macromolecules, not negative small ions. Smaller positive molecules may also remain in the capillaries if they are protein bound. In terms of molecular weight, molecules less than 70 kDa are generally filtered freely. Shape can also be a factor, with filtration affected by radius:

- Radius <20 Å (Angstroms): Freely filtered.
- 20 Å < radius < 40 Å: Filtered to various degrees depending on molecular weight and charge.
- Radius >36 Å: Generally not filtered.

Albumin—the smallest of the plasma proteins (radius = 35.5 Å)—is partially filtered but only ~0.01% of the plasma albumin ends up in the ultrafiltrate. However, almost none appears in the urine as it is avidly reabsorbed by the proximal tubule (PT). Significant amounts of protein in the urine (proteinuria) indicates kidney disease. Many diseases can cause proteinuria by affecting the negative charges of the layers of the glomerular filter, in particular that of the basement membrane. In general, a total of ~30 g/day protein enters the lymphatic channels within the kidney and is returned to the vascular space.

Forces governing tissue fluid formation and glomerular filtration rate

Filtration across the glomerular capillaries is determined by the same factors that determine filtration across all capillaries—Starling forces:

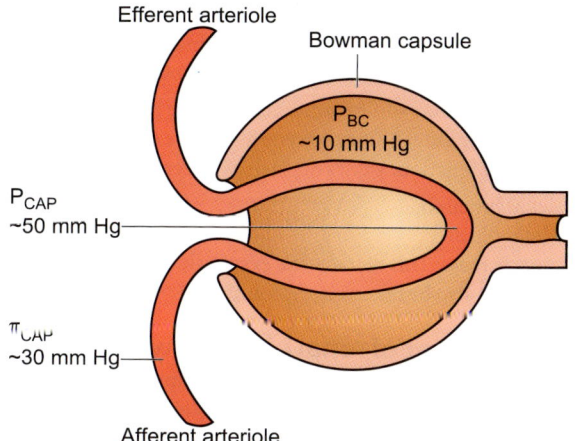

Fig. 4.46 Starling forces acting in glomerular capillaries.

GFR is increased by
- ↑ k$_F$ mesangial cell relaxation causes ↑glomerular surface area
- ↑ Renal plasma flow
- ↑ P$_{CAP}$↑↑↑Renal arterial pressure
  - ↓Afferent arterial resistance
  - ↑Efferent resistance

GFR

GFR is decresased by
- ↑ P$_{BC}$ obstruction of tubule or extrarenal urinary system
- ↑ π$_{CAP}$
  - ↓ Renal plasma flow

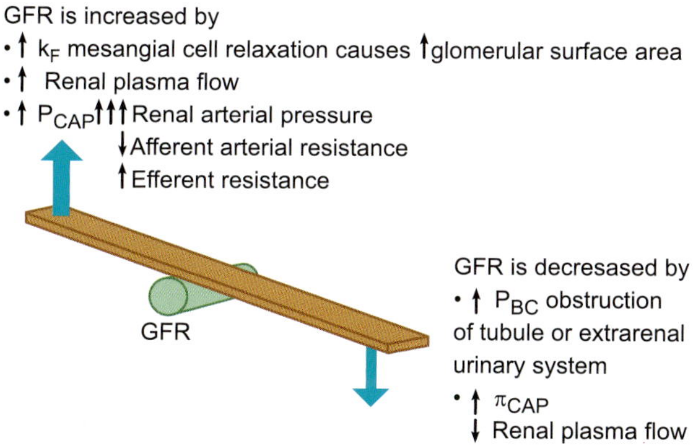

Fig. 4.47 The effects of Starling forces on glomerular filtration rate (*GFR*). k$_f$, *Coefficient of filtration*; P$_{BC}$, *Bowman capsule hydrostatic pressure*; P$_{CAP}$, *glomerular capillary hydrostatic pressure*; π$_{CAP}$, *glomerular capillary oncotic pressure*.

P: Hydrostatic pressure (from water): Favours filtration out of that space.

π: Oncotic (osmotic) pressure (exerted by proteins): Opposes filtration out of that space.

The narrow capillary of the glomerulus creates a resistance to flow, thus increasing hydrostatic pressure above oncotic pressure so that fluid is forced out (filtration) through the highly permeable cells. Fluid continues to move out of the capillaries until hydrostatic pressure has decreased to a value lower than oncotic pressure. The opposite is also true when oncotic pressure is greater than hydrostatic pressure, the fluid moves back from the Bowman capsule into the vascular space. This usually happens at the venule end of the capillary.

In the nephron, the formation of filtrate depends on the balance of hydrostatic and oncotic pressures of both the glomerular capillary and Bowman capsule (Fig. 4.46). Changes in these forces will change the GFR.

As the filtrate in Bowman capsule is virtually protein free (due to the filtering mechanism described above), there is a negligible oncotic pressure in the capsule (π$_{BC}$), which can therefore be disregarded when calculating net glomerular filtration force. Therefore the GFR is calculated as:

$$GFR = k_f(P_{CAP} - P_{BC} - \pi_{CAP})$$

where GFR = glomerular filtration rate, k$_i$ = coefficient of filtration, P$_{CAP}$ = glomerular capillary hydrostatic pressure, P$_{BC}$ = Bowman capsule hydrostatic pressure and π$_{CAP}$ = glomerular capillary oncotic pressure.

The elements of this equation can be altered, as shown in Fig. 4.47.

The surface area of the glomerular capillaries is relatively large when compared with normal systemic capillary beds such as the peritubular capillaries. However, the hydrostatic pressure within the glomerular capillary does not decline along the capillary as in systemic capillaries, and it is maintained essentially constant because the efferent arteriole acts as a secondary resistance vessel.

From the above equation, it follows that net filtration will occur until the sum of the hydrostatic pressure within Bowman capsule (P$_{BC}$) and the oncotic pressure within the capillary (π$_{CAP}$) is in equilibrium with the hydrostatic pressure of the capillary.

Feedback control of glomerular filtration

Although GFR can be altered by various mechanisms, renal blood flow (RBF) is the major determinant. RBF, and thus GFR, can be maintained over a large range of arterial systolic pressures, approximately 90 to 180 mm Hg, through autoregulation. This autoregulation occurs by adjusting vascular resistance—namely that of the afferent arteriole—through two mechanisms:

1. Myogenic mechanism: Affected by arterial pressure changes.
2. Tubuloglomerular feedback: Affected by changes in the flow rate of tubular fluid.

Myogenic mechanism

Myogenic regulation relies on the property of smooth muscle to contract in response to stretching so that as arterial pressure increases and the smooth muscle in the arteriole vessel wall is stretched, it responds by contracting to reduce vessel diameter.

Flow = change in pressure/resistance

RBF and hence GFR are kept constant if changes in arterial pressure and flow are the same. If the pressure difference at the beginning and end of the capillary changes (i.e. owing to rising or falling systemic arterial pressure), there must be a compensatory change in the resistance (i.e. vessel diameter change) to maintain a contact blood flow.

Tubuloglomerular feedback

Tubuloglomerular feedback from the tubules to the glomerulus relies on the relationship between the filtration rate and the amount of Na^+ escaping reabsorption in the PT and LoH. The more Na^+ entering the capsule and PT, the more Na^+ that remains in the tubular fluid and enters the distal tubule (DT), where its levels are detected by the macula densa of the juxtaglomerular apparatus (JGA). The macula densa acts as both a detector (of osmolality, Na^+ and/or Cl^- load, or tubular flow) and effector:

- Higher GFR causes higher Na^+ and Cl^- loads in the distal tubular fluid.
- This change in load increases cellular NaCl transport which is sensed by macula densa cells.
- Macula densa cells release signals (adenosine, adenosine diphosphate (ADP), adenosine triphosphate (ATP) or thromboxane) into the interstitial space.
- These transmitters decrease filtration by causing vasoconstriction of the afferent arteriole thus hydrostatic pressure in the glomerular capillaries decreases.
- Signals also result in mesangial cell contraction which further reduces filtration.

Overall, these mechanisms lead to GFR being reduced.

Renal blood flow and the glomerular filtration rate

Clearance

The GFR can be calculated by measuring the clearance of a substance (C):

$$C = (U \times V)/P$$

where C = volume of plasma cleared of a particular substance in a unit time, U = urine concentration of substance (mg/mL), V = urine flow rate (mL/min) and P = plasma concentration of substance (mg/mL).

For clearance of a compound to be used as an accurate estimate of GFR, the compound must be completely eliminated by the kidney meaning the compound must:

- Be freely filtered.
- Be unaffected by tubular processing, that is it is not reabsorbed or secreted.
- Not be synthesized or metabolized by the kidney.

Inulin is a polysaccharide of fructose found in Jerusalem artichokes and dahlia tubers and has a molecular weight of 5500. It meets all of the above criteria for measuring GFR. However, although inulin clearance is equal to GFR, the method involved is invasive and seldom used clinically. Instead, the clearance of creatinine, a product of muscle metabolism, is used to estimate GFR in clinical practice.

A small amount of creatinine is secreted by the tubules; therefore GFR is slightly overestimated (overestimation of plasma creatinine concentration by the methods used is thought to negate this).

Since plasma creatinine concentrations are reciprocally related to GFR, plasma creatinine concentrations are commonly used to reflect renal function. Values of plasma concentration depend on:

- Renal function.
- Metabolism.
- Muscle mass: This dictates the exact value, so size, age and sex must also be taken into account.

Measurement of renal blood flow

Approximately 20% of an adult's cardiac output is directed to the kidneys, giving an RBF of roughly 1100 mL/min. The calculation of RBF clinically is based on Fick's principle: blood flow to an organ can be calculated as the amount of a substance removed by the organ (e.g. filtered by the kidney) divided by the difference in the arterial and venous concentrations of the substance. Concerning the kidney, the amount of substance filtered by the kidney per unit time is equal to that appearing in the urine. Specifically, the kidney filters plasma so renal plasma flow (RPF) is calculated by this method:

$$\text{Renal plasma flow} = (V \times U)/(\text{Arterial} - \text{Venous})$$

where V = urinary flow rate, U = urinary concentration of substance, Arterial = arterial concentration of substance and Venous = venous concentration of substance.

Infusion of para-aminohippuric acid (PAH) can be used to calculate RPF. As 90% of PAH in arterial plasma is removed after a single passage through the kidneys (either filtered or secreted into the tubules), the extraction ratio (or arteriovenous concentration difference) is said to be sufficiently high for the venous concentration value to be ignored. Therefore RPF can be calculated by dividing the amount of PAH in urine (volume × concentration) by the amount of plasma PAH, noting this calculates the 'effective renal plasma flow' as renal venous plasma is ignored.

$$C = (V \times U)/P$$

Normal RPF is 600 mL/min which can be converted to RBF by using the haematocrit value (total percentage of total blood volume composed of erythrocytes). If the haematocrit is 45%, 55% must be plasma. So:

$$\text{Normal RBF} = \text{RPF} \times \frac{1}{(1 - \text{Haematocrit})}$$
$$= 600 \times \frac{1}{0.55}$$
$$= 1100 \text{ mL/min}$$

This value only relates to blood going through the renal cortex and does not account for blood in the renal arteries that supplies the capsule, perirenal fat, medulla, tubules and glomeruli.

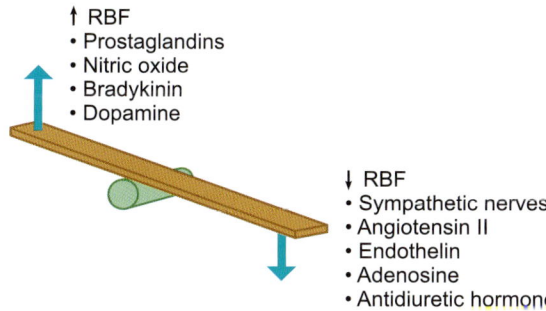

Fig. 4.48 The effects of vasoactive substances on renal blood flow (*RBF*).

Filtration fraction

The filtration fraction describes how much of the plasma passing through the glomerulus is filtered, which is normally about 20%.

$$\text{Filtration fraction} = \text{GFR}/\text{RBF}$$

Fractional excretion

Fractional excretion (FE) is used to determine whether a freely filtered substance undergoes net reabsorption or secretion, by comparing the amount excreted in the urine with the amount filtered.

Regulation of RBF

Autoregulation of RBF and thus GFR involves changes in the tone of the afferent and efferent arterioles as described previously. Normal values are:

- RBF: 1100 mL/min.
- RPF: 600 mL/min.
- GFR: 120 mL/min.

As the perfusion pressure increases over the autoregulatory range of 90 to 180 mm Hg, so too does resistance to flow, owing to myogenic mechanisms. Additionally, a high-protein diet leads to increases in RBF, glomerular capillary pressure and GFR.

Vasoactive substances (Fig. 4.48) are particularly important in maintaining renal perfusion, as in cases of acute haemorrhage, where increased sympathetic activity leads to vasoconstriction and decreased blood flow. In this situation, intrarenal prostaglandin production prevents excessive vasoconstriction, preserving blood flow.

It is the afferent arteriole diameter with respect to the efferent that separates the control of RBF and GFR (Fig. 4.49).

- RBF: Changes reflect changes in total arteriolar resistance.
- GFR: Increases by relative constriction of the efferent arteriole compared with the afferent.

Age-related changes in renal blood flow and glomerular filtration rate
Renal blood flow

RBF is 5% of the cardiac output in the newborn, rising to 20% in the adult. RPF cannot be measured reliably using PAH clearance

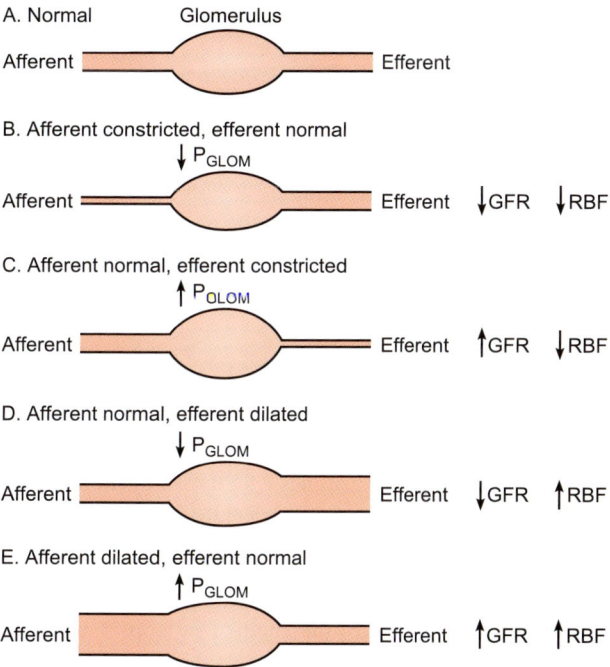

Fig. 4.49 The effect of afferent and efferent vessel constriction on glomerular filtration. GFR, *Glomerular filtration rate*; RBF, *renal blood flow*.

in infants, as its extraction is lower than that in adults owing to immature tubular secretory mechanisms.

Changes in glomerular filtration rate with age
- Filtration of fluid and urine production: contributing to amniotic fluid, starts in week 10 of gestation.
- 25 mL/min in the newborn.
- Progressive increase in GFR from 1 month.
- Adult values reached by 1 year of age.
- Progressive decline with old age.

RENAL TUBULES, LOOP OF HENLE AND COLLECTING DUCTS

The proximal tubule

The proximal tubule (PT) is continuous with the Bowman capsule (see Fig. 4.43). This tubule is 15 mm long but only 55 μm in diameter. The PT is the site where most reabsorption takes place, especially the reabsorption of water and solutes from the filtrate. It is divided into two parts: the pars convoluta and pars recta.

The cells making up the first portion of the PT, the pars convoluta, lie immediately distal to the glomerulus and have the following features:

- Tight junctions at their luminal surfaces.
- Extensive interdigitations.
- Magnified absorptive surface area due to the microvillus-dense brush border.
- Extracellular space between bases of cells (the lateral intercellular spaces).
- Large numbers of mitochondria.

The second straight part of the PT is the pars recta, which has less structural complexity, and fewer microvilli and mitochondria than the pars convoluta. It is continuous with the first part of the LoH.

LOOP OF HENLE

The LoH is a hairpin structure (see Fig. 4.43) with the following parts:

- A thin descending limb that ends at the tip of the hairpin loop.
- A thin ascending limb of variable length (20 μm diameter). It differs from the preceding part with respect to permeability.
- A thick ascending limb: This is about 12 mm long, with an abrupt transition from the thin ascending limb. Its start position is determined by the length of the loop.

The loop (up to about 14 mm long) can superficially enter the medulla or extend as far down as the renal pelvis in the case of some juxtamedullary nephrons. The LoH works with the high solute/ionic concentration of the medulla to drastically concentrate urine at the bottom of the hairpin, and then dilute it as it ascends.

Role of the loop of Henle

The LoH functions primarily as a site for reabsorption by using a countercurrent multiplier system, which serves to increase the osmolality of the medullary interstitial fluid (ISF) and promote reabsorption.

Proportionally more Na^+ and Cl^- are reabsorbed than water: 25% versus 15% of the filtered loads. There is a differential permeability to substances of the ascending and descending limbs:

- Descending limb: Reabsorbs H_2O but not NaCl (very H_2O permeable).
- Ascending limb: Reabsorbs NaCl but not H_2O (H_2O impermeable).

Countercurrent multiplier

The actions of the countercurrent multiplier set up an osmotic pressure gradient between the ascending and descending limbs:

- Descending limb: Increasing tubular fluid concentration as water flows out into the hyperosmolar interstitium.
- Ascending limb: Progressively removes solutes into the interstitium as the fluid moves away from the tip of the hairpin.

Tubular fluid enters the loop isosmolar to the plasma but water is drawn out of the tubules and into the hyperosmolar interstitium. The fluid thus becomes more concentrated. As the fluid enters the ascending limb, it is hyperosmolar and so has the solute concentration necessary to pump solutes into the interstitium. This creates the hyperosmolar interstitium necessary for water reabsorption and the cycle continues.

It is the nature of the two parallel tubules in continuity separated by the interstitium that creates this countercurrent system.

Microstructure of the loop

The LoH consists of three functionally distinct parts:

1. Thin descending limb.
2. Thin ascending limb: Only present in very long loops.
3. Thick ascending limb.

Osmolarities at various sections of the LoH can be seen in Fig. 4.50.

Thin descending limb

- Thin, flat epithelia without brush borders, minimal metabolic activity and hence few mitochondria.
- Highly permeable to H_2O.
- Relatively low permeability to Na^+, Cl^- and urea.
- The main function is simple diffusion through its epithelia:
  - H_2O diffuses by osmosis down its concentration gradient owing to the hypertonic medullary interstitium. This accounts for ≈15% of filtered H_2O reabsorption and is the primary reason for osmotic equilibration between luminal fluid and medullary ISF.
- Some Na^+, Cl^- and urea (UT2 transporter) can enter the lumen but in limited amounts.

This continues until an osmotic equilibrium between tubular fluid and medullary interstitium is reached (at the tip of the hairpin).

Thin ascending limb

- Epithelial cells are similar to those of the thin descending limb.
- They are quite impermeable to H_2O owing to a lack of aquaporins but they exhibit some permeability to Na^+, Cl^- and urea.
- Previous H_2O reabsorption in the descending limb concentrates luminal Na^+ so that small amounts of passive Na^+ and Cl^- reabsorption occur via the paracellular route plus urea (UT2 transporter) entry.

Thick ascending limb

- Large cells with plenty of mitochondria, which suit the high metabolic activity required for active transport.
- Reabsorption of ≈25% filtered Na^+, Cl^- and K^+. This occurs via the apical $Na^+/K^+/2\,Cl^-$ transporter, which:
  - Depend on the Na^+ gradient established by the basolateral Na^+/K^+-ATPase (primary active transporter).

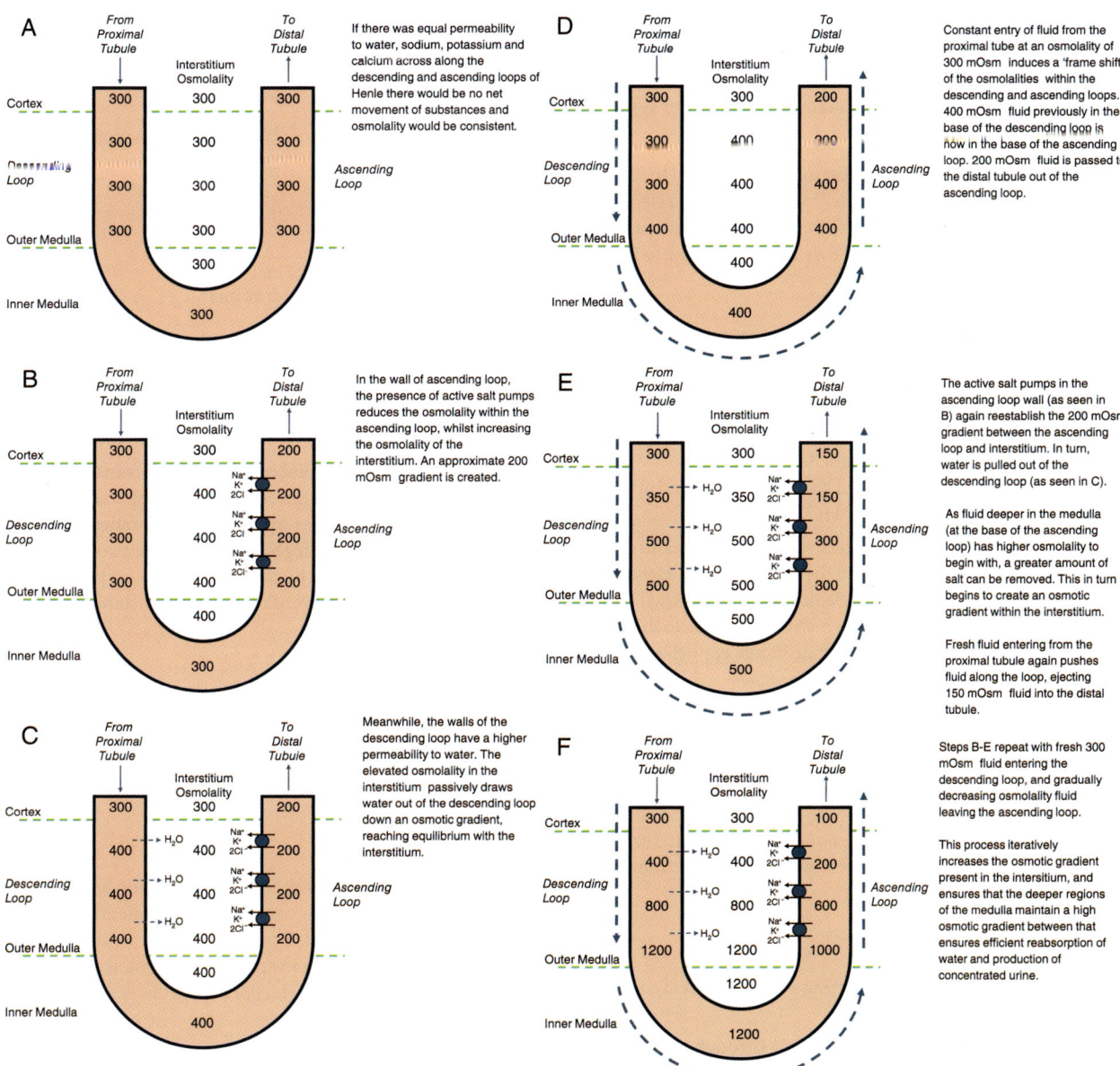

Fig. 4.50 The establishment of the countercurrent multiplier. DT, *Distal tubule*. (Courtesy Dr Oli Steele.)

- K^+ leaking back through apical K^+ channels and Cl^- efflux across the basolateral membrane through Cl^- channels.

The H_2O impermeability of the thick ascending limb means that H_2O cannot move down the osmotic gradient generated by the accumulation of mainly NaCl in the medullary ISF. This prevents dilution of the interstitium and keeps it hyperosmolar, for fluid to be absorbed through the descending limb.

The thick ascending limb can be thought of as the initiator and driving force behind the countercurrent multiplier system.

Distal tubule

The distal tubule (DT) is a continuation of the LoH in the cortex of the kidney, and it is approximately 5 mm long. The cells forming this segment are concerned with hormone-sensitive water balance. The terminal portions of 8 to 10 DTs coalesce to form a collecting duct (CD).

Collecting ducts

In the cortex, the CD is ~20 mm long and predominantly composed of principal (P) and intercalated (I) cells:

- P cells: They have few organelles and are involved in Na^+ and antidiuretic hormone (ADH)-mediated water reabsorption.
- I cells: They contain more organelles, including mitochondria, than P cells, and they secrete H+ and are involved with the transport of HCO_3^-.

The cortical CD becomes progressively larger as it passes downwards through the medulla to form the medullary CD. Here, pairs of CDs join, forming the ducts of Bellini. These ducts then empty into the renal papillae and calyces which deliver urine to the pelvis of the kidney, a structure lined with transitional epithelium.

Transport processes in the renal tubules

On leaving the Bowman capsule, ultrafiltrate journeys from the PT to the collecting ducts to become urine. Along the way, it is modified significantly by various reabsorption and secretion mechanisms. The key cell surfaces and fluid compartments are shown in Fig. 4.51.

Transport mechanisms

Solute can cross the epithelial lining of the tubule by passing either between or through the cells:

- Paracellular movement (around cells): Through the matrix of tight junctions between cells, driven by molecule concentration, electrical and osmotic gradients.
- Transcellular movement (through cells) is osmotic and relies on two factors:
  - Solute crosses the apical membrane (in contact with filtrate), then the basolateral wall (facing the capillary at an angle). Water follows down the osmotic gradient.

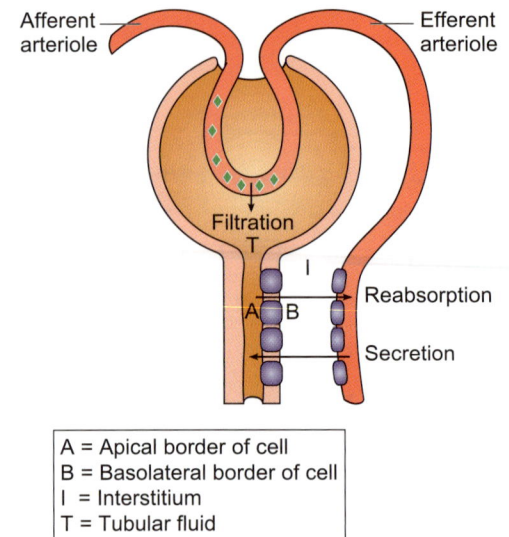

A = Apical border of cell
B = Basolateral border of cell
I = Interstitium
T = Tubular fluid

Fig. 4.51 Cell surfaces involved in secretions and reabsorption.

- Polarization of epithelial cells (crucial to transcellular movement): Proteins differ between the apical and basolateral membranes so that the membranes have different electrical charges. Hence net influx of Na^+ from tubular fluid to the cell is permitted—a process crucial to the transport of most other substances (see later).

Diffusion

This is the passive simple movement of a substance down its electrochemical gradient. Substances that are lipid soluble, such as blood gases and steroids, diffuse through the membrane driven by their gradient.

Facilitated diffusion

Facilitated diffusion is faster than simple diffusion and the passage of substances down their concentration gradients requires a transporter (a specific carrier protein located within the cell membrane). Examples within the proximal convoluted tubule are GLUT 1 and GLUT 2 transporters of the basolateral membrane (cell to ISF) which move glucose.

Primary active transport

Primary active transport refers to the direct coupling of ATP hydrolysis with a transport process concerned with the movement of a substance against its electrochemical and concentration gradients. It uses energy derived from hydrolysis of the terminal phosphate bond of the ATP molecule, which itself forms part of the protein structure of the transporter.

In the nephron, the key example is the 3 Na$^+$/2 K$^+$-adenosine triphosphatase (ATPase) pump located on the basal membranes of the tubular epithelium: for every molecule of ATP hydrolyzed, 3 Na$^+$ are moved out of the cell into the ISF while 2 K$^+$ are simultaneously pumped inwards, both against their electrochemical gradients. This keeps the intracellular sodium concentration low.

Other important primary active transport systems are:

- H$^+$-ATPase: Moves protons out of cells into tubular fluid.
- Ca^{2+}-ATPase: Moves calcium out of cells.
- H$^+$/K$^+$-ATPase: Moves H$^+$ into the lumen and K$^+$ into cells.

Secondary active transport

Transporters that require energy but do not hydrolyze ATP are called secondary active transporters. Instead, they rely on the ionic gradient established by the ATPases. This is best illustrated by the basolateral Na$^+$/K$^+$-ATPase, which causes the cell to have a low Na$^+$ relative to the lumen (Fig. 4.52). Na$^+$ will now diffuse along its electrochemical gradient into the cell from the tubular fluid. The processes involved are:

Symport (cotransport)

Movement of solute by protein carriers down the Na$^+$ gradient or in the same direction as Na$^+$. Examples include:

- PT:
  - Na$^+$/glucose: (SGLT2; lumen to cell): SGLT1 to 4: a family of protein transporters.

Na$^+$/3 HCO$_3^-$ (cell to ISF).

- Thick ascending limb of LoH: Na$^+$/K$^+$/2 Cl$^-$ (triple transporter; lumen to cell).

Antiport (exchange/countertransport)

Protein carriers move solute in the opposite direction to Na$^+$. Examples include:

- Na$^+$ (into cell)/H$^+$ (into lumen).
- Na$^+$/Ca^{2+} exchange.

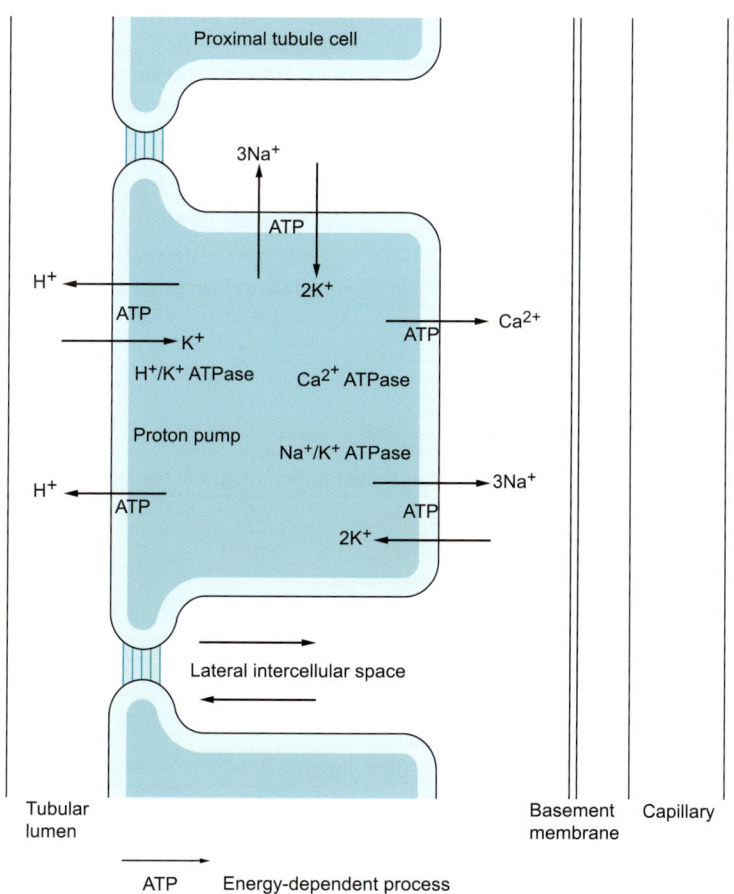

Fig. 4.52 Active transporters in the proximal tubule. ATP, *Adenosine triphosphate*.

Ion channels

Within the epithelial membrane are proteins which form ion channels. They permit much faster transport (10^6–10^8 ions/s) than both the relatively abundant ATPases and transporter molecules (100 ions/s). However, ion channels are greatly outnumbered by the active transporters (100 vs. 10^7 per cell). In addition to the Na^+/K^+-ATPase pump in the basolateral membranes, specific Na^+, Cl^- and K^+ ion channels are located in the apical membranes of all parts of the nephrons.

Handling of sodium by the kidney

Free filtration in the Bowman capsule means that filtrate Na^+ = plasma Na^+. Modification of filtrate as it passes through the successive segments of the nephron means that 99% of filtered Na^+ is reabsorbed into the circulation (Table 4.9). The mechanisms of Na^+ transport occur via both paracellular and transcellular routes using the movement via Na^+ ion channels and symports, which rely on the ATPase pump keeping the intracellular environment relatively negative.

In addition to the conservation of Na^+ in the body, the concentration of other solutes whose transport processes are dependent on Na^+ reabsorption are also maintained:

- Glucose.
- Amino acids.
- Lactate.
- Cl^-.
- HCO_3^-.
- PO_4^{3-}.

Transport of sodium and chloride

Movement of sodium into the interstitial space

The key to PT reabsorption is the Na^+/K^+-ATPase pump on the basolateral membrane, which actively transports Na^+ into the interstitial space. Most (70%) of the reabsorption of Na^+ from the filtrate occurs in the early portion of the PT. However, cell junctions are leaky and unable to maintain a secure concentration gradient, as the PT is highly permeable to Na^+ in both directions. However, the more distal parts of the PT can establish a better concentration gradient because the cell junctions are tighter, even though less reabsorption takes place here.

Sodium entry into the cell

The ATPase pump has already established:

- Low Na^+ (<30 mmol/L) within the PT tubular cells.
- A relatively negative transmembrane potential (−70 mV) compared to the lumen.

Table 4.9 Sodium reabsorption by different sections of the kidney

Nephron segment	% Na⁺ reabsorbed	Route and mechanism of apical Na⁺ entry	Hormone involved
Proximal tubule	67	Paracellular	Angiotensin II
		Transcellular Na^+/H^+ exchange	
		Cotransport with glucose, amino acids, PO_4^{3-} HCO_3^-/Cl^- anion exchange	
Thick ascending limb of the loop of Henle	25	Paracellular	Aldosterone
		Transcellular $Na^+/K^+/2Cl^-$ symport	
Early distal tubule	4	Na^+/Cl^- symport	
Late distal tubule and collecting ducts	3	Na^+ channels	Aldosterone Atrial natriuretic peptide

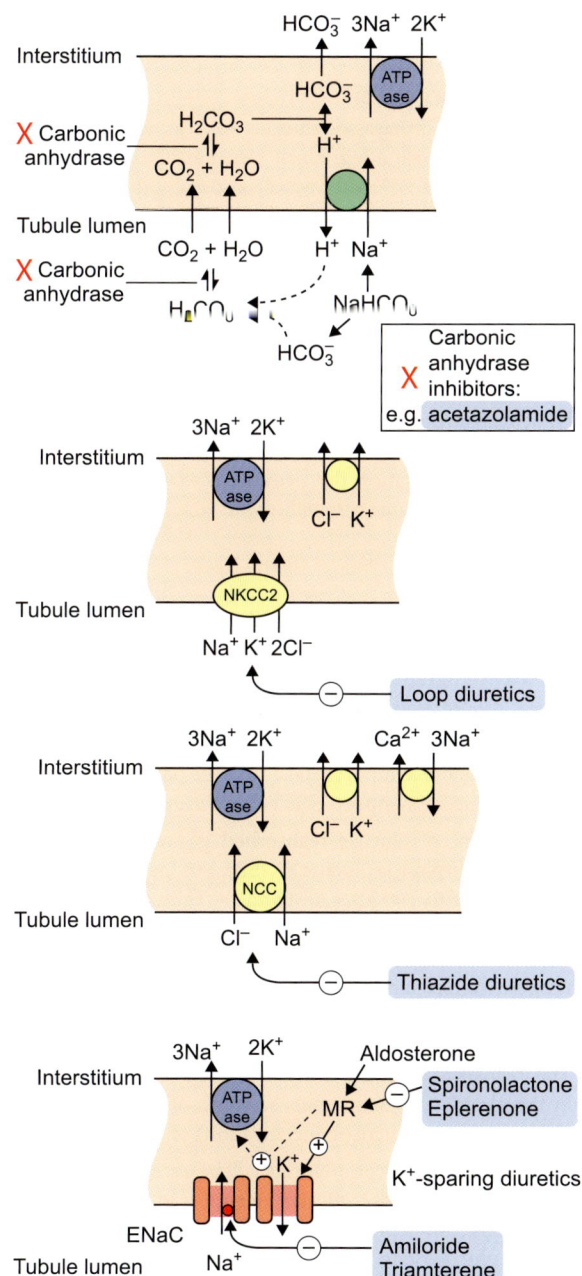

Fig. 4.53 Sites of action of diuretics. Osmotic diuretics increase osmotic pressure through the tubule, reducing electrolyte reabsorption across the luminal membrane. Other drugs gain access to their sites of action after secretion into the tubule by the organic anion transporters (*OATs*) in the proximal tubule. Acetazolamide inhibits carbonic anhydrase and is a weak, self-limiting diuretic, now largely used for other conditions such as glaucoma. Loop diuretics such as furosemide block the luminal $Na^+/K^+/2Cl^-$ cotransporter (*NKCC2*) and inhibit up to 20% to 25% of filtered Na^+ reabsorption. The thiazide diuretics inhibit the luminal Na^+/Cl^- cotransporter (*NCC*) and reduce reabsorption of 3% to 5% of filtered Na^+. The aldosterone antagonists spironolactone and eplerenone compete with aldosterone for the mineralocorticoid receptor (*MR*), blocking the induction by aldosterone of the expression and activity of the epithelial Na^+ channel (*ENaC*) and the basolateral Na^+/K^+-ATPase pump. Amiloride and triamterene act directly on ENaC to block Na^+ reabsorption. Potassium-sparing diuretics inhibit the reuptake of less than 2% of filtered Na^+. (Adapted from Hitchings, A., Sampson, A., & Waller, D. G. (2022). *Medical pharmacology and therapeutics* (6th ed.). Elsevier.)

Both serve to drive Na^+ intracellularly along its electrochemical gradient from the tubular fluid (Fig. 4.54). In the first half of the PT, this is coupled with the movement of other solutes:

- Symport with glucose, amino acids, phosphate, lactate and so on.
- Antiport with H^+ (which is linked to HCO_3^- reabsorption).

Little of the glucose or other solutes symported with Na^+ remain in the later portion of the PT. Chloride ions are the main method for Na^+ reabsorption in late PT because there is a relatively high Cl^- concentration owing to the preferential HCO_3^- reabsorption in the early PT.

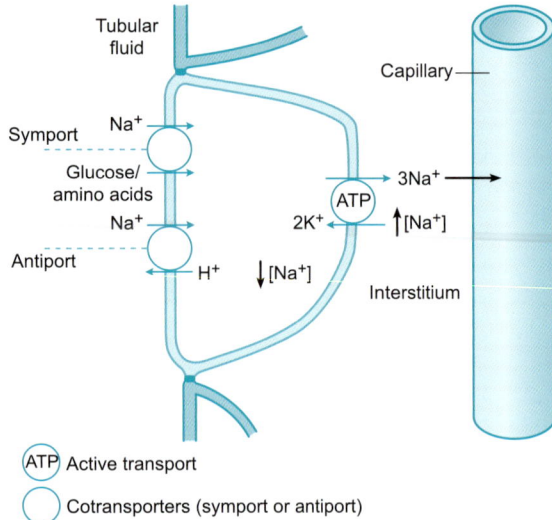

Fig. 4.54 Sodium transporters in the proximal tubule. ATP, *Adenosine triphosphate*.

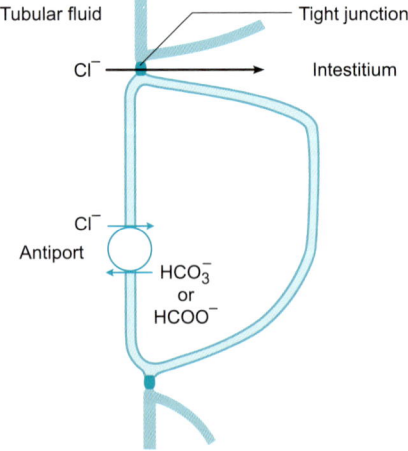

Fig. 4.55 Chloride transport in the proximal tubule.

Chloride reabsorption

In the early PT, the relatively negative transmembrane potential opposes intracellular Cl^- entry from the tubular lumen. Coupling of HCO_3^- with Na^+ reabsorption maintains osmolality in this section, although Cl^- rises. A concentration gradient that favours Cl^- diffusion into the cell is thus established in the middle to late portions of the PT.

- 60% of Cl^- reabsorption occurs in the middle to late PT.
- Most Cl^- diffusion is paracellular.

Smaller amounts of Cl^- enter by Cl^-/HCO_3^- and $Cl^-/HCOO^-$ antiporters (Fig. 4.55). Both HCO_3^- and $HCOO^-$ are continuously

generated in the cell by dissociation of H_2CO_3 and HCOOH, respectively, which then drives the antiport to bring Cl^- into the cell.

Water reabsorption

In the PT, there is a strong association between Na^+ reabsorption with water following the osmotic gradient. Hence as 70% of the sodium is reabsorbed in the PT, 70% of the water is also reabsorbed. In addition, there is a high H_2O permeability within this section of the nephron owing to the presence of aquaporins (water pores), which permit small changes in osmolality to affect H_2O reabsorption.

Note that glomerular filtration causes a high plasma protein concentration within the peritubular capillaries as the water is filtered from the blood but the proteins remain. This equates to a high oncotic pressure and this Starling force causes H_2O from the ISF to be reabsorbed into these capillaries.

Although the main function of the PT is reabsorption, it does not alter the concentration: fluid leaves this section of the nephron having virtually the same osmolality with which it entered.

Transport of other solutes

Glucose

Overall, almost all of the filtered glucose is reabsorbed in the PT. Only a few milligrams at most may be excreted in the urine per 24 hours. The transport systems within the PT for glucose reabsorption are by secondary active transport (SGLT1 and SGLT2):

- 1 Na^+/1 glucose symport (SGLT2) in the pars convoluta.
- 1 Na^+/1 glucose symport (SGLT1) in the pars recta.

The amount of glucose reabsorbed is proportional to the amount filtered (plasma glucose $\times$ GFR). Plasma glucose concentrations transiently rise after meals and so the amount of glucose filtered will rise. However, glucose reabsorption mechanisms can become saturated. This means that if plasma glucose is above a certain concentration, such that the amount filtered exceeds the reabsorptive capacity of the SGLT of the PT cells, glucose will be excreted in the urine (glycosuria).

The reabsorptive limit differs between nephrons, ranging from thresholds at plasma glucose levels of 10 to 20 mmol/L; therefore at plasma glucose concentrations of:

- 10 mmol/L: Reabsorption limits will be exceeded for a few nephrons and glucose will start to appear in urine.
- 20 mmol/L: No nephrons will be able to reabsorb their entire filtered glucose load.

Glycosuria (Table 4.10) occurs if:

- The renal threshold is exceeded by the filtered glucose load: This is seen with the elevated plasma glucose concentration of uncontrolled diabetes mellitus.
- Glucose absorption capacity is lower than normal: This occurs in certain inherited tubular diseases and pregnancy. Hence, glycosuria will appear with plasma glucose concentration <10 mmol/L.

Table 4.10 Summary of organic solute transport in the proximal tubule

Substance	Normal plasma values (mmol/L)	% Reabsorbed (normal)	% Excreted (normal)	Factors affecting excretion
Glucose	5	100	0	Low T_m Diabetes mellitus
Amino acids	2.5	>99	Negligible	High plasma concentration Fanconi syndrome
PO_4^{3-}	1	80	21	Plasma >1.2 mmol/L
				Hypoparathyroidism Acidosis Glucuronidases Vitamin D
Urea	2.5–7.5	40–50	50–60	Antidiuretic hormone

Amino acids

Plasma amino acids are continuously being absorbed from the gut, while at the same time, their steady removal for restructuring/building maintains a concentration of 2.5 mmol/L. Their small size means that they undergo free filtration by the glomerulus. Most amino acids are reabsorbed, primarily in the PT by symport with Na^+ (i.e. a secondary active process). The PT has the capacity for the reabsorption of a significant amino acid load, meaning a negligible amount is excreted in the urine. However, aminoaciduria can occur if this mechanism is saturated, or in Fanconi syndrome (see Table 4.10) where the mechanism is faulty.

In the PT, there are at least five different systems, depending on the character of the amino acids:

1. Glycine.
2. Imino acids.
3. Glutamate and aspartate.
4. Neutral amino acids.
5. Cystine and basic amino acids.

Phosphate

Phosphate is essential for mineralized tissue structure (bones and teeth) and 80% of the body PO_4^{3-} content is found in the skeleton. The remaining 20% is distributed mainly in the intracellular fluid (ICF) and least of all in the plasma, the concentration of which is approximately 1 mmol/L.

PO_4^{3-} is freely filtered, the amount filtered being proportional to plasma values. Eighty per cent of filtered PO_4^{3-} is reabsorbed in the PT with Na^+ by the 2 Na^+/1 PO_4^{3-} symporter of the apical membrane. The rate of PO_4^{3-} uptake is hormonally regulated, which primarily affects excretion (see Table 4.10 and Fig. 4.56).

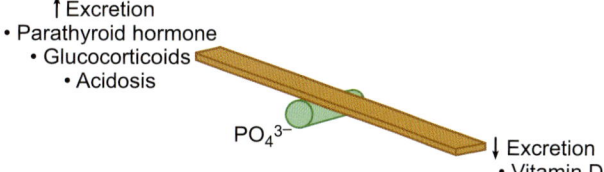

↑ Excretion
• Parathyroid hormone
  • Glucocorticoids
    • Acidosis

PO_4^{3-}

↓ Excretion
• Vitamin D

Fig. 4.56 Hormones affecting phosphate transport.

Normally, <20% filtered PO_4^{3-} is excreted, functioning as an important urinary buffer for H^+. Excretion is increased when plasma concentration exceeds 1.2 mmol/L. A fall in GFR will also cause plasma values to rise. Importantly, the normal amount of filtered PO_4^{3-} (dictated by plasma concentration) is very close to the absorption capacity. Hence, plasma PO_4^{3-} is regulated by the reabsorptive process.

See later for the role of phosphate in acid–base buffering.

Urea

Urea is continuously produced by the liver as a byproduct of protein metabolism, with a normal plasma concentration of 2.5 to 7.5 mmol/L. Production is increased with high-protein diets and decreased during starvation.

Urea is a small molecule and is therefore freely filtered; 40% to 50% is reabsorbed by passive diffusion and the remainder is excreted. Its concentration increases in the filtrate passing down the PT because of H_2O reabsorption.

In addition to its role as a waste product, urea is useful in the control of water balance. Its presence in the later segments of the nephron is important in concentrating the urine, especially when under the influence of ADH. ADH stimulates UT1 (a member of a family of urea transporters (UT1–4) found in renal tissue) in the apical membrane of inner medullary CDs transporting urea into the cell, and the exit from the cell across the basolateral membrane is via a different transport protein, UT4. The DT and outer medullary CDs are impermeable to urea. Water follows the movement of urea in the CDs. During dehydration, the plasma urea will rise owing to reduced filtration as RBF falls and reduced reabsorption in the CDs.

Bicarbonate

HCO_3^- plays a key role in acid–base balance and, by regulating this substance, the kidneys contribute to the regulation of body pH. Normal plasma values are maintained at 20 to 30 mmol/L.

HCO_3^- is freely filtered and it is essential that virtually all is reabsorbed, otherwise the body fluids would become very acidic. The PT reabsorbs about 80%. The process of cellular bicarbonate handling is shown in Fig. 4.57.

- Na^+/K^+-ATPase sets up an ionic gradient driving Na^+ into cells.
- Most Na^+ entry is coupled with H^+ secretion into the lumen via an Na^+/H^+ antiporter in the apical membrane.
- Filtered HCO_3^- combines with this secreted H^+ in the lumen, forming H_2CO_3 (carbonic acid).
- On the brush border, the enzyme carbonic anhydrase (CA) catalyzes the dissociation of $H_2CO_3 \rightarrow CO_2$ and H_2O.
- Both the CO_2 and H_2O diffuse readily into the cell, where intracellular CA catalyzes the reformation of H_2CO_3.
- Intracellular H_2CO_3 then dissociates into:
  - H^+, which is secreted by antiport into the lumen and starts the cycle again.
  - HCO_3^-, some of which moves across the basolateral membrane into the ISF either in exchange for Cl^- or by cotransport with Na^+. Some ICF HCO_3^- exchanges with luminal Cl^-.

When there is an increased load of HCO_3^-, the PT automatically reabsorbs more.

The remainder of HCO_3^- is reabsorbed in the thick ascending limb of Henle, the DT and the CD. In addition to the primary active H^+-ATPase in all H^+-secreting DT segments, type A intercalated cells have a primary active H^+/K^+-ATPase that moves H^+ into the lumen while reabsorbing K^+.

Sulphate

Sulphate reabsorption is an active process that readily reaches its maximal transport capacity. Plasma levels are maintained at 1 to 1.5 mmol/L.

Potassium

Normal plasma values are 3.5 to 5 mmol/L. K^+ is freely filtered with the PT reabsorbing 80% to 90%. This occurs predominantly by passive diffusion through the tight junctions (paracellular route), although there appears to be a small active component as the PT can reabsorb K^+ against a concentration gradient. In the nephron K^+ can be:

- Reabsorbed: In the thick, ascending limb of LoH (cotransported with Na^+ and Cl^-) and the DT (only in severe dietary depletion).
- Secreted: In the thin limb of LoH/DT (generally, Na^+ is reabsorbed and K^+ secreted). K^+ secretion is proportional to the rate of tubular fluid flow and the delivery of Na^+ to distal parts of the nephron. Aldosterone, secreted in response to increased plasma K^+, increases K+ secretion by enhancing Na^+ reabsorption from the cortical CD.

In healthy people, the K^+ balance is maintained so that secretion = K^+ intake. Excretion of filtered K^+ can vary from 1% to 110%. It will be decreased when small amounts of Na^+ reach the DT and when the amounts of H^+ are increased. Thus the following factors affect the amount of K^+ excreted:

- Dietary K^+
- Acid–base balance
- Delivery of Na^+ to the cortical CD
- Aldosterone

Secretion by the proximal tubule

The PT actively secretes a large number of substances (Table 4.11), including many drugs, in addition to its reabsorptive capacity. Some of these substances are filtered freely whereas others are bound to plasma proteins and therefore have a limited filtration, so secretion is vital for their excretion. Substances can be secreted both passively and actively, which can be limited by maximal transport capacity for that substance (carrier saturation) or concentration gradient (time) limited (e.g. PT secretion of H^+). Three transport capacity-limited PT secretory mechanisms exist for:

1. Strong organic acids: Secreted by the pars recta, as substances move out from peritubular capillaries (e.g. PAH).

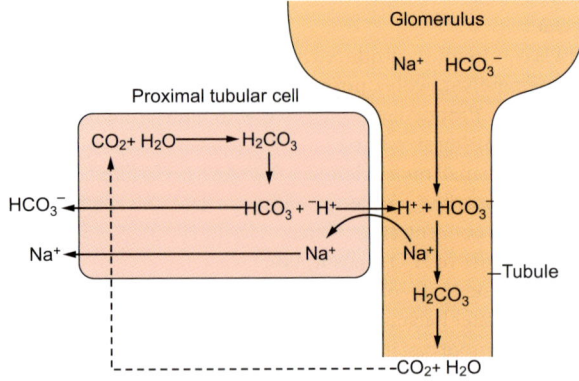

Fig. 4.57 Bicarbonate handling in the tubule.

Table 4.11 Acidic and basic substances secreted by the proximal tubule

	Acidic	Basic
Drugs	Penicillin Salicylates Furosemide Sulphonamide	Atropine Cimetidine Morphine Quinine
Endogenous substances	Bile salts Fatty acids Prostaglandins Urate	Acetylcholine Creatinine Dopamine Epinephrine

2. Strong organic bases: secreted in the pars convoluta (e.g. histamine, thiamine).
3. Ethylenediaminetetraacetic acid.

Gradient-time-limited mechanisms handle H^+ and K^+ secretion:

- H^+: Na^+/H^+ antiporter on the apical membrane is responsible for H secretion, which also depends on HCO_3^- reabsorption.
- K^+: Secretion is variable and dependent on a number of factors (tubular fluid flow, diet, acid–base balance, aldosterone).

Role of the vasa recta

The vasa recta are vessels that originate from the efferent arterioles in juxtamedullary nephrons. Their hairpin arrangement and close association with the LoH enables them to function as a countercurrent exchanger. Hence, the descending and ascending vasa recta run in parallel near each other. The result of this is that H_2O and waste products are removed, aided by high permeability to these substances.

The vasa recta vessels have a relatively low blood flow (1–2% total RBF), which, although not required for the creation of a hyperosmolar medulla, is important in maintaining it. It means that solute can accumulate in the medullary interstitium at a level that is grossly higher than that in the entering blood.

Like other capillaries, the vasa recta are permeable to solute and water. Therefore as the vessels descend progressively further into the medulla, solutes (NaCl and urea) enter the vasa recta while more H_2O diffuses out into the interstitium.

At the tip of the loop, the plasma osmolality approaches that of the interstitium (very high). In addition, the blood is very viscous, with a high plasma protein concentration (high oncotic pressure) secondary to H_2O loss. Therefore in the ascending vasa recta, H_2O diffuses back with loss of most of the solutes, as it tends to equilibrate with the decreasing medullary ISF osmolality.

The vasa recta also reabsorb 5% of the filtered H_2O load from the parts of the CDs and thin descending limb of LoH within the medulla, preventing dilution of the medullary interstitium. This is crucial to the concentration of urine.

Role of urea

Urea contributes to the interstitial osmotic pressure in the medullary pyramids:

- Half of freely filtered urea is reabsorbed in the PT.
- Urea is secreted in the thin segment of the LoH, diffusing into the tubule and restoring the urea to ~100% of that which was filtered.
- When tubular fluid reaches the inner medullary CDs, the luminal urea has risen to 500 mmol/L or greater (100 times plasma concentration). This is because of the different permeability of the cortical CD to urea and H_2O (permeable to H_2O and not permeable to urea) so that the urea becomes even more concentrated as water is reabsorbed.
- This high urea in the medullary CD lumen results in diffusion of urea out into the interstitium via specialized urea transporters (UT1 and UT4).
- There is low blood flow in the medulla, so the urea that has diffused into the interstitium is essentially trapped but the luminal urea is always higher than that in the ISF because of concomitant H_2O reabsorption.
- Approximately half of the filtered load stays in the lumen, which is then excreted.

This recycling of urea into the interstitium greatly contributes to its hyperosmolality.

ADH is required for the permeability of medullary collecting tubules to urea and hence for its diffusion into the medulla, with consequent diffusion into the thin limbs of the LoH. ADH thus results in increased medullary osmolality. In addition, ADH acts to increase H_2O permeability in medullary collecting tubules, causing H_2O reabsorption from the cortical components, both of which result in a more concentrated urine.

Maximum urine osmolality is influenced by dietary protein: low protein diets result in a reduced capacity to elaborate concentrated urine because of the reduced availability of urea for sequestration in the medullary interstitium, that is reduced medullary urea = reduced medullary osmolality = reduced urine osmolality.

Regulation of urine concentration

Daily urine volume can range from 400 mL to 23 L, with an average value of 1 to 1.5 L. Osmolality can similarly vary from 60 to 1200 to 1400 mmol/kg H_2O, with an average value of 600 mmol/kg H_2O.

The obligatory volume of urine excreted per day is dictated by the maximal urine osmolality and the amount of solute to be excreted over that period. Thus if the maximum urine osmolality is 1400 mosmol/kg H_2O and the solute load to be excreted is 800 mosmol/24 h, the obligatory urine volume is 800/1400 ~570 mL/24 h.

Both the concentration and volume of urine are determined by plasma ADH concentration. High ADH conserves body water and increases the concentration of urine by increasing water permeability of the DTs and CDs. As mentioned earlier, the high osmolality of the medullary interstitium provides the gradient for H_2O reabsorption, in the presence of ADH.

Aldosterone—An adrenal steroid—acts on the cortical collecting tubule via the P cells, increasing absorption of NaCl, and also water, which follows by diffusion. This produces a smaller volume of fluid of unchanged osmolality for delivery to inner medullary CDs where water reabsorption (hence urine osmolality) is determined by plasma ADH and the magnitude of the transepithelial osmotic gradient.

RENAL FUNCTIONS AND HOMOEOSTASIS

Body fluid osmolality

Concepts of osmolality

Body fluid volume, manifested as body weight, remains relatively stable on a daily basis. Therefore intake of water over 24 hours (via thirst mechanisms) is balanced by kidney excretion (output). A minimal volume 400 mL/day of urine permits the maintenance of body fluid homoeostasis. Osmolality refers to the ratio of solute to water.

Normal plasma osmolality is strictly maintained at levels of 285 to 295 mosmol/kg H_2O. If a change in either H_2O balance or that of Na^+ causes osmolality to vary by 3 mosmol/kg H_2O, the body's regulatory mechanisms will be stimulated. These are:

- Osmoreceptors: Triggered by a change in osmolality.
- Baroreceptors: Triggered by ↓ in plasma volume that causes ↓ blood pressure.

If both plasma volume and osmolality are reduced simultaneously, osmoreceptors exert more influence. However, a large drop in plasma volume takes priority (plasma becomes hypoosmolar).

Osmoreceptors

Osmoreceptors in the supraoptic and paraventricular areas of the anterior hypothalamus are responsive to changes in plasma osmolality. Their function is to regulate thirst and H_2O excretion:

- ↑ Plasma osmolality → ↑ Stimulation of osmoreceptors → ↑ rate of ADH secretion → ↓ renal H_2O excretion → ↓ plasma osmolality.
- Conversely, ↓ plasma osmolality causes ↓ ADH secretion.
- Plasma osmolality also stimulates thirst centres in the lateral preoptic area which, together with the osmoreceptors, cause the person to feel thirsty and drink H_2O.

Synaptic input to ADH secreting cells from many other areas in the brain also exist. Therefore although to a much lesser degree, pain, fear and nausea can also alter ADH secretion.

Effect of other solutes

Plasma osmolality is dictated mainly by total body Na^+ with its associated anions. However, other solutes can alter osmolality without altering water balance. These solutes vary in their effectiveness to stimulate osmoreceptors, depending on their ability to cause cellular dehydration; that is more effective stimulants will be substances that have more difficulty crossing the membrane.

Antidiuretic hormone

ADH is synthesized as part of a large precursor molecule by cells of the supraoptic and paraventricular nuclei in the hypothalamus (Fig. 4.58). Synthesis is completed after transportation to the posterior lobe of the pituitary gland, where it is thought to undergo progressive cleavage as it moves down the axons. ADH is stored in nerve terminals in the posterior pituitary, associated with neurophysin, until its release is triggered by a rise in plasma osmolality.

Membrane depolarization by action potentials in the neurons causes Ca^{2+} influx. This leads to the membranes of vesicles that store ADH fusing with the cell membrane and the subsequent release of ADH and neurophysin into the bloodstream.

Cellular actions

There are three types of ADH receptor (known as V receptors), all of which are G-protein-coupled receptors. Their functions are as follows:

- V_1 receptors: Stimulate vasoconstriction by increasing intracellular Ca^{2+} in smooth muscle in the walls of blood vessels.
- V_2 receptors: Reduce kidney excretion of H_2O. V_2 receptors are located in the basal membrane of renal tubules.
- V_3 receptors: Appear to mediate the effect of ADH on the pituitary gland, facilitating the release of adrenocorticotrophic hormone (ACTH).

ADH enhances H_2O reabsorption in the cortical collecting tubule by causing fusion of aquaporins (water channels; AQP2) with the luminal membrane. This is particularly important in cortical and outer medullary portion of the CD as they have a negligible H_2O permeability in the absence of ADH.

Plasma ADH concentrations dictate the permeability of the CD system. Therefore with very low ADH, the hypoosmotic urine from the ascending LoH will pass through the DT and proximal

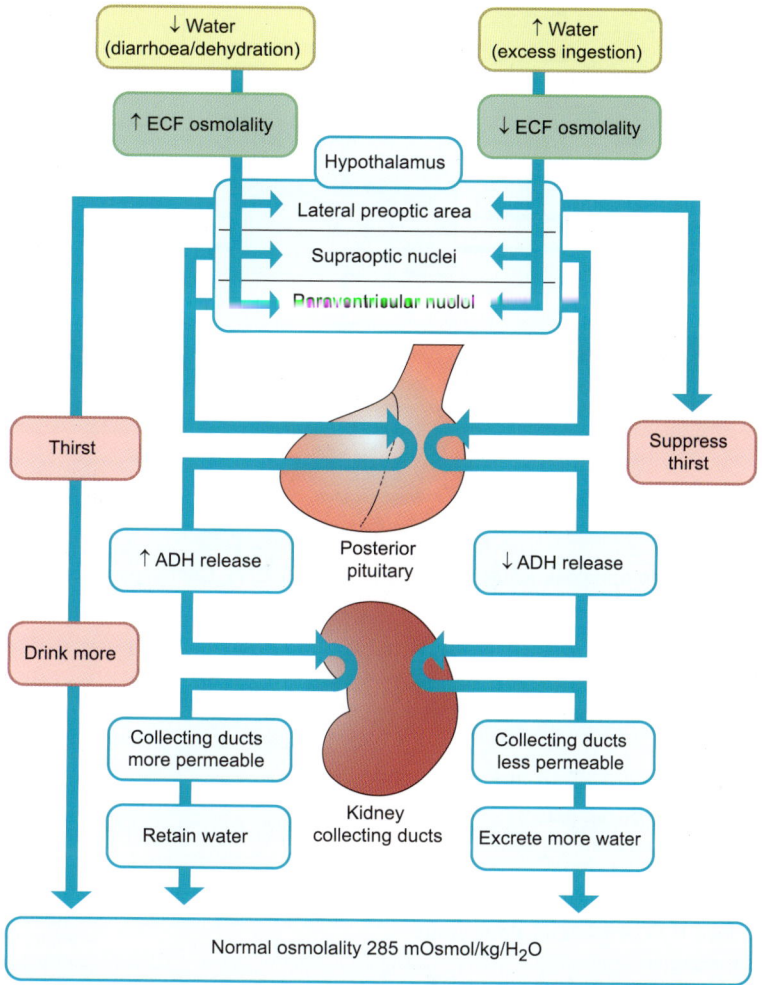

Fig. 4.58 Antidiuretic hormone and its control over plasma osmolality. ADH, *Antidiuretic hormone*; ECF, *extracellular fluid*.

parts of the CD. When it enters the inner medullary portion, there is a massive osmotic gradient between tubular fluid and the interstitium, and so there is some H_2O reabsorption by osmosis, the amount being limited by the finite H_2O permeability of the tubule cells. Hence, the high tubular volume containing a lot of water (therefore hypoosmotic) will be excreted (diuresis).

Features of antidiuretic hormone

Certain metabolic features of ADH ensure plasma osmolality is controlled precisely:

- Rapid release.
- Short half-life (time taken for plasma levels to halve): 10 to 15 minutes.
- Rapid cessation of release.
- Rapid removal from the blood:
  - 50% is removed by the liver and kidney.

- 40% is metabolized.
- 10% is excreted in urine.

Drugs and antidiuretic hormone

Osmoregulation can be disturbed by the actions of certain drugs affecting ADH release, which can be:

- Increased: with nicotine, morphine or barbiturates.
- Decreased: with alcohol or angiotensin-converting enzyme (ACE) inhibitors (by inhibiting angiotensin II, which is a promoter of ADH secretion).

Diseases due to disruption of antidiuretic hormone regulation

Syndrome of inappropriate antidiuretic hormone

An inappropriate secretion of ADH can occur from the pituitary or elsewhere (Fig. 4.59). ADH secretion fails to be suppressed

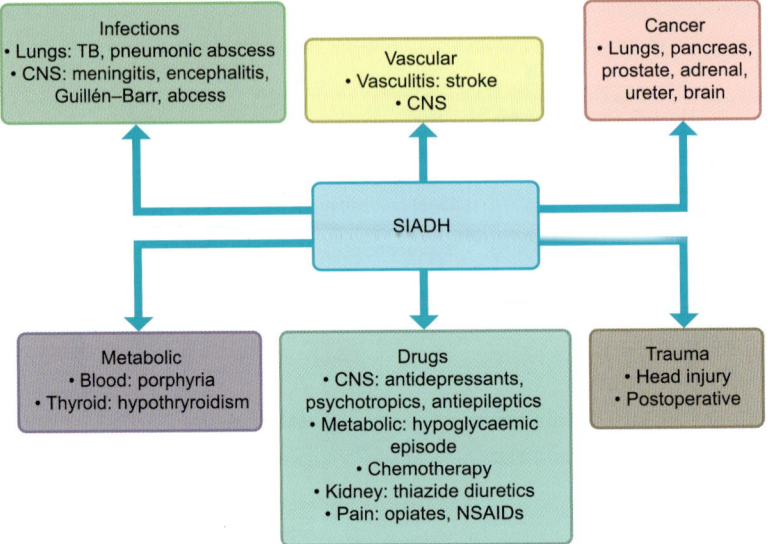

Fig. 4.59 Causes of syndrome of inappropriate antidiuretic hormone (*SIADH*). CNS, *Central nervous system*; NSAID, *nonsteroidal antiinflammatory drug*; TB, *tuberculosis*.

even with low Na⁺, low plasma osmolality and H_2O overload. Clinical features are:

- Inappropriately high urine osmolality (typically >400 mosmol/kg H_2O) in the face of reduced plasma osmolality (i.e. concentrated urine despite plasma fluid overload).
- Inappropriately high urine Na⁺ >20 mmol/L: high plasma volume secondary to retained H_2O switches off aldosterone production so more Na⁺ is excreted.
- Decreased plasma Na⁺ (typically 125 mmol/L (normal values 135–145 mmol/L)) and reduced plasma osmolality ≤260 mosmol/kg H_2O.

Diabetes insipidus

This syndrome is caused by ADH deficiency (central diabetes insipidus (DI)) or when the kidney fails to respond to ADH (peripheral DI) (Fig. 4.60). Without water reabsorption, there is continual H_2O diuresis with a urine output of approximately 25 L/day because ADH-dependent H_2O reabsorption in the kidney is about 23 L. The clinical features are:

- Polyuria (production of large amounts of dilute urine).
- Polydipsia (consumption of large quantities of water with thirst driven by hyperosmolar blood).
- Hypoosmolar dilute urine.
- High plasma sodium (concentrated plasma due to water loss).

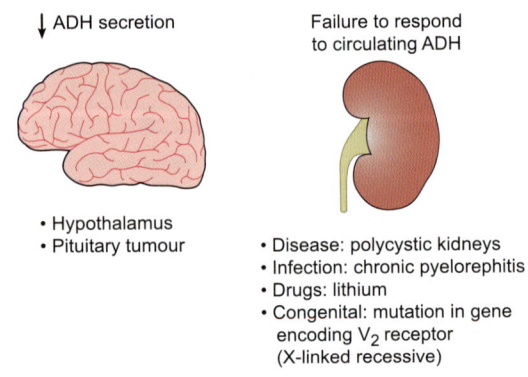

↓ ADH secretion

Failure to respond to circulating ADH

- Hypothalamus
- Pituitary tumour

- Disease: polycystic kidneys
- Infection: chronic pyelorephitis
- Drugs: lithium
- Congenital: mutation in gene encoding V_2 receptor (X-linked recessive)

Fig. 4.60 Causes of diabetes insipidus. ADH, *Antidiuretic hormone*.

CLINICAL NOTES

DIABETES INSIPIDUS

Diabetes insipidus is most frequently seen after pituitary surgery, owing to disruption of antidiuretic hormone release. Plasma sodium, osmolality and urine output should be monitored closely postoperatively.

Water clearance and reabsorption

Plasma osmolality (altered by water balance) affects urine production in the following ways:

- Dehydration: ↑ plasma osmolality → ↑ free H_2O reabsorption by the kidneys resulting in:
  - Plasma dilution.
  - A more concentrated urine with an osmolality higher than that of plasma.
- Too much water: ↓ plasma osmolality → ↑ osmotically free H_2O excretion by the kidneys → dilute urine (osmolality lower than that of plasma).

Effect of solute output on urine volume

The limit of the kidney's concentrating ability restricts the maximum urinary osmolality to about 1400 mosmol/kg H_2O with the volume dependent on the balance between:

- Plasma ADH concentration.
- Amount of excreted solute.

$$\text{Volume of urine produced} = \frac{\text{Amount of excreted solute}}{\text{Maximal urine osmolality (fixed)}}$$

When the kidney's concentrating limit is reached, an increase in solute will lead to an increase in urine volume; therefore more excretory solute, even with maximal ADH concentration, will still result in a degree of diuresis. This can be illustrated by the nonreabsorbable solute, mannitol, which decreases the kidney's ability to concentrate urine and is thus termed an osmotic diuretic.

Adrenal steroids and urinary dilution

The normal renal response to H_2O loading, that is very dilute urine production, is impaired with adrenal insufficiency and/or ↓ adrenal steroids. Corticotropin-releasing hormone (CRH) is released from the hypothalamus during adrenal insufficiency as part of the homoeostatic feedback loop and CRH has an additional action of promoting ADH release. Thus during adrenal insufficiency, the kidneys inappropriately reabsorb water and plasma sodium concentration falls.

Body fluid volume

The portion of extracellular fluid (ECF) that perfuses tissue is known as the effective circulating volume (ECV). Na^+ content, which can be altered by changes in either filtration or reabsorption, will affect ECF volume and hence ECV. This is because, in the ECF, Na^+ is the main osmotically active solute and therefore largely dictates osmolality. This affects the osmoregulatory mechanism, resulting in a change of the ECF volume and osmolality. However, osmolality is corrected within minutes, whereas disturbances in body volume (with altered Na^+ body content) can take days to correct.

If there is a sufficient drop in ECF volume, GFR can be lowered by tubuloglomerular feedback to prevent further volume loss. Maximal Na^+ reabsorption results in a urinary excretion of <1 mM per day with possible consequences on acid–base balance through K^+ and H^+ excretion.

Renin and angiotensin
Renin

The enzyme renin is both synthesized and stored in the juxtaglomerular apparatus (JGA). Its release is stimulated by:

1. ↑ Activity of sympathetic nerves due to ↓ systemic blood pressure (BP) detected by carotid artery baroreceptors.
2. ↓ Afferent arteriole wall tension: ↓ ECF volume → ↓ systemic BP → ↓ renal perfusion pressure → ↓ wall tension at granular cells → renin release.
3. ↓ Na^+ detection by macula densa: Leads to inhibition of synthesis of substances inhibitory to renin release *and* secretion of PGs → renin release.

In addition, renin secretion is increased by diuretics, haemorrhage, upright posture, heart failure and stenosis of the renal artery.

Angiotensin substances

Once it is released from the JGA into the blood, renin acts on angiotensinogen (an α_2-globulin) produced in the liver to yield the physiologically inactive decapeptide angiotensin I. Angiotensin I undergoes removal of two amino acids by angiotensin-converting enzyme (ACE) in the lungs, to form angiotensin II (octapeptide). Angiotensin II acts via two classes of receptors: A_{T1} and A_{T2} to:

- Release aldosterone: By acting directly on the zona glomerulosa of the adrenal cortex.
- Directly vasoconstricts renal arterioles: Affecting efferent more than afferent arterioles—increases glomerular capillary pressure and thus glomerular filtration (to prevent excessive decreases in GFR).
- ↑ Na^+ reabsorption in the PT.
- Release ADH.
- Stimulate thirst.
- Inhibit renin release by negative feedback on JGA cells.

In addition, angiotensin II decreases baroreceptor reflex sensitivity by acting on the brain. Hence, its effects in raising BP can be sustained by this 'faulty' reflex mechanism. Inhibitors of ACE (e.g. ramipril) are used to treat hypertension (high BP) by ↓ angiotensin II production with consequential:

- ↓ Vasoconstriction.
- ↓ Aldosterone secretion (with its subsequent ↓ ECF volume).

Aldosterone

Aldosterone is an adrenal mineralocorticoid hormone. Its release is mediated by:

- ***Direct stimulation of the adrenal gland***
  - Plasma K^+: Very small rises can cause large increases in aldosterone release resulting in increased DT K^+ secretion, returning plasma K^+ to normal.

- ↓ Plasma Na^+: Low Na^+ stimulates aldosterone, although this is not an important mechanism.
- ACTH: Causes transient stimulation of aldosterone secretion even if high ACTH is maintained.
- *Activation of the renin–angiotensin–aldosterone (RAA) system*
  - Angiotensin II.
  - ↓ ECF.
  - ↓ Body Na^+ content stimulates renin release.

Secondary hyperaldosteronism, which can result from heart, liver and kidney failure, can occur by chronic stimulation of the RAA system.

Aldosterone stimulates Na^+ reabsorption by entering P cells and increases transcription of basolateral Na^+/K^+-ATPase and expression of distal nephron Na^+ channels and $Na^+/K^+/2Cl^-$ transporters in the apical membrane to Na^+ reabsorption. Two per cent of the filtered Na^+ load is under the control of aldosterone, which translates as a large amount (~520 mmol/24 h) considering the volume filtered per day (180 L/day).

Its intracellular actions involve increasing Na^+ reabsorption within the kidney as well as other sites: the colon, salivary glands, gastric glands and sweat glands. It further encourages the secretion of K^+ and H^+ in the kidney.

Regulation of erythropoiesis

Cells of the inner cortex and peritubular interstitium of the kidney produce >80% of the body's erythropoietin (EPO). EPO synthesis, which is mediated by prostaglandins, occurs in response to a reduction in PO_2 in the kidneys as a result of hypoxia—most importantly, hypoxic anaemia and renal ischaemia. EPO acts on erythrocyte stem cells of the bone marrow, stimulating an increased production of red blood cells (RBC) and thus improving the blood's oxygen-carrying capacity. EPO has a half-life of 5 hours.

Abnormal EPO secretion is seen in a number of renal diseases. Its secretion can be high or low, depending on the type of disease:

- High secretion, resulting in polycythaemia (high RBC), is a feature in polycystic kidney disease and renal cell carcinoma.
- Low secretion is seen in chronic renal failure.

The decrease in EPO production in chronic renal failure cannot be compensated for by the rest of the body and intravenous or subcutaneous recombinant EPO is administered to rescue the anaemia, providing that is the sole reason for the anaemia.

Failure with EPO treatment can occur, most commonly with iron-deficient anaemia, which requires oral or intravenous ferrous sulphate. In addition, active bleeding or malignancy (anaemia of chronic disease) can cause EPO treatment 'apparently' not to work.

EPO treatment-related complications are usually precipitated by rapid increases in haemoglobin concentration and haematocrit. These include hypertension, thrombotic events and fitting.

Factors affecting Na reabsorption

Sodium (Na^+) is the main osmotically active solute in the ECF, and it must therefore be tightly regulated. Factors that affect the amount of Na^+ reabsorbed by the kidney include:

Starling factors

Na^+ reabsorption in the PT is automatically adjusted to correct disturbances of body Na^+ content and hence that of ECV. This involves altered Starling forces—hydrostatic (P) and oncotic (π) pressures. The rate of reabsorption of NaCl and H_2O in the PT is related to the amount and rate of uptake from the lateral intercellular spaces into the capillaries, which depend on these forces:

Forces favouring capillary uptake

- π_{CAP}: Oncotic pressure of the capillary.
- P_{ISF}: ISF hydrostatic pressure.

Forces opposing capillary uptake

- π_{ISF}: ISF oncotic pressure.
- P_{CAP}: Hydrostatic pressure of the capillary.

For example, ↓ NaCl intake causes ↓ ECF volume with resultant ↓ P_{CAP} but ↑ π_{CAP}. Hence, PT reabsorption of NaCl by tubule cells will increase.

A rise in P_{CAP} or P_{ISF} results in the leaking back of fluid reabsorbed from ISF across tight junctions, the usual cause of the former being venous pressure.

Sympathetic drive from the renal nerves

Renal sympathetic activity is controlled by arterial baroreceptors, which detect changes in plasma/ECF volume that correspond with BP. Na^+ reabsorption will then be altered to correct values of ECF volume and BP. The effects of renal nerve stimulation are:

- Renin secretion: By direct action on β_1-adrenergic receptors of granular cells.
- Vasoconstriction of afferent and efferent arterioles: Activating JGA.
- Na^+ reabsorption: By nerve endings containing catecholamines directly acting on tubular cells.

Prostaglandins

PG synthesis from arachidonic acid is stimulated by a reduced ECV. There are at least three sites for renal PG synthesis; these differ in the type of PG that predominates:

1. Cortex (including glomeruli and arterioles): Prostacyclin or PGI_2 (vasodilator).
2. Medullary interstitial cells: PGE_2 (vasodilator).
3. CD epithelial cells.

PGI_2

The most important afferent arteriole vasodilator which is particularly important when there is a reduction in renal perfusion pressure. It also mediates renin release.

PGE_2

- A vasodilator.

- Mainly affects the CD:
  - Natriuretic: Limits stimulation of ATP-dependent Na$^+$ reabsorption. It is therefore useful in the prevention of medullary tubule cell hypoxia secondary to hypoperfusion (with ↓ ECF) by decreasing the energy requirements of the cell.
  - Diuretic: Impairs the action of ADH thus promoting H$_2$O excretion.

CLINICAL NOTES

NON-STEROIDAL ANTI-INFLAMMATORIES

In healthy people, nonsteroidal antiinflammatory drugs (NSAIDs), such as ibuprofen and diclofenac, inhibit renal prostaglandin (PG) synthesis without altering renal blood flow (RBF) or glomerular filtration rate (GFR). However, when compensatory mechanisms are already maximized to maintain perfusion and filtration in patients with chronically impaired renal function, the vasodilator effects of PGs are required. NSAIDs can then cause drastic impairment of RBF and GFR. This effect is exacerbated by hypovolaemia in the postoperative patient.

Thromboxane A$_2$

Thromboxane A$_2$ (TXA$_2$) is a vasoconstrictor: small amounts are produced after renal damage, which typically results from obstruction of the ureter. The consequence is that less blood goes through a kidney that is not filtering properly.

Atrial natriuretic peptide

Cardiac atrial cells produce the hormone atrial natriuretic peptide (ANP) when atrial fibres stretch in response to high venous return as a consequence of ↑ blood volume. The various vascular and tubular effects of ANP act to promote Na$^+$ excretion through an increase in intracellular cyclic guanine monophosphate, with the following actions:

- Afferent arterial vasodilation: Promoting GFR.
- Inhibition of granular cell release of renin: Will itself ↓ secretion of aldosterone while ↑ dopamine release.
- Inhibition of Na$^+$/K$^+$-ATPase with additional closure of Na$^+$ channels: Acting on various tubular sites, especially the inner medullary CD. Na$^+$ reabsorption is reduced with subsequent Na$^+$ and H$_2$O excretion.

Dopamine

In the kidneys, mostly PT cells synthesize dopamine with the following actions:

- ↓ Tubular Na$^+$ transport by:
  - Inhibition of Na$^+$/K$^+$-ATPase
  - ↓ Na$^+$/H$^+$ antiport activity

- Natriuresis (Na$^+$ excretion): Even when RBF and GFR are unchanged.
- Vasodilatation.

Kinins

Kinins are vasodilator proteins that are cleaved off kininogens by the enzyme kallikrein. Renal-produced kinins have similar functions to PGs:

- Vasodilatation.
- Natriuresis.
- Inhibition of ADH release.

Regulation of body fluid pH

Precise H$^+$ balance, which is the basis of pH, is imperative because it influences almost all the activity of the body's enzymes. The normal arterial blood pH is 7.4, although variations up to 0.05 pH units have no associated negative effects. The range is therefore 7.35 to 7.45, with a corresponding H$^+$ of 45 to 35 nmol/L (H$^+$ is inversely related to pH, on a log scale). A range of pH 7.0 to 7.8 is compatible with life; if pH decreases to 6.8, life can be sustained for only a few hours.

Key to the functions of acid–base balance are:

- Balance of input and output of acids and bases.
- The control of substances involved in minimizing disturbances of H$^+$. These are known as buffer systems.

Input and output

- The output of acids and bases normally matches input on a daily basis. It occurs in the form of respiratory elimination and by kidney excretion.
- Input involves the addition of H$^+$ by many physiological processes:
  - Metabolic generation.
  - Addition by GI activity.
  - Ingestion or products of ingested materials.

Buffer systems

The purpose of a buffer is to minimize pH change given the addition of acid or base. Buffer systems either contain:

- A weak acid and its conjugate base:

$$\underset{\text{Weak acid}}{HA} \quad \leftrightarrow \quad \underset{\text{Proton}}{H^+} \quad + \quad \underset{\text{Conjugate base}}{A^-}$$

- A weak base and its conjugate acid:

$$\underset{\text{Conjugate acid}}{BH} \quad \leftrightarrow \quad \underset{\text{Proton}}{H^+} \quad + \quad \underset{\text{Weak base}}{B^-}$$

Extra H$^+$ added to the system will cause the reaction to swing to the left of the equation, combining with the conjugate base or weak base. Buffers do not eliminate or create H$^+$ de novo, but instead lock them away or release them (if H$^+$ is removed or a strong alkali added).

Importantly, amphoteric substances such as amino acids and PO_4^{3-} can both donate and accept H^+.

Different reactions have different equilibrium values (K) depending on whether the reaction is shifted more to the left or the right.

$$K = [H^+]\,[A^-]/[HA] = [H^+]\,[base]/[acid]$$

Owing to the small value of K, the equation can be reexpressed using the term pK, which is the inverse log of K:

$$pK = \log\lfloor 1/K \rfloor$$

Similarly:

$$pH = \log(1/H^+)$$

Combining these equations results in the Henderson–Hasselbach equation:

$$pH = pK + \log([base]/[acid])$$

Physiological buffers

The key physiological buffers are:

- Bicarbonate.
- Phosphate.
- Proteins.
- Haemoglobin.

Bicarbonate buffer system

The bicarbonate buffer system is the most important of all body compartments. The reaction concerned is:

$$CO_2 + H_2O \leftrightarrow H_2CO_3 \leftrightarrow H^+ + HCO^{3-}$$

where H_2CO_3 = carbonic acid, a weak acid.

CO_2 and HCO_3^- are tightly controlled by the lungs and kidneys, respectively, both of which therefore regulate pH. Carbonic anyhdrase, an enzyme richly distributed within the alveoli of the lungs and renal tubule epithelium, catalyzes the bidirectional conversion of water (H_2O) and carbon dioxide (CO_2) into carbonic acid (H_2CO_3).

The Henderson–Hasselbach equation for this system can be written as:

$$pH = pK + \log\left(\frac{[HCO_3^-]}{0.23 \times PCO_2}\right)$$

As HCO_3 acts as a base, H_2CO_3 (the acid) is determined by the amount of CO_2 dissolved per unit plasma, and the solubility coefficient of CO_2 at 37°C = 0.23.

Normal values for this system are: HCO_3 = 20 to 30 mmol/L, PCO_2 = 4.4 to 5.3 kPa and pK = 6.1. Substituting these values into this final equation gives a calculated pH of 7.4.

Renal handling of acids and bases

HCO_3^- handling by the kidney is essential to acid–base balance. The kidney can produce urine with a pH ranging from 4.5 to 8.0, depending on the pH of the ECF and the consequent balance between the renal excretion of H^+ and HCO_3^-. PO_4^{3-} and ammonium (NH_4^+) processing by the kidney further aids its maintenance of body pH.

HCO_3^- reabsorption

Metabolic processes produce H^+, which reacts with HCO_3^- to form CO_2. This is exhaled by the lungs and is an effective and rapid mechanism by which HCO_3^- is removed from the body.

The kidney is involved in HCO_3^- handling—primarily its reabsorption—regulating ECF HCO_3^- and therefore pH in a less rapid and more chronic manner than the lungs. HCO_3^- is freely filtered and 25 mmol/L enters the PT, where approximately 80% is reabsorbed.

The maximum rate of reabsorption lies very close to normal plasma values. However, this maximal rate can be changed, according to the rate of H^+ secretion.

The process of HCO_3^- reabsorption is secondary active, involving tubular secretion of H^+, and there is no direct transport of HCO_3^-.

H^+ is secreted into the lumen of the PT by Na^+/H^+ exchanger and/or H^+-ATPase. It reacts with luminal HCO_3^-, forming H_2CO_3.

- Carbonic anhydrase (CA): Catalyzes the breakdown of $H_2CO_3 \rightarrow CO_2$ and H_2O.
- CO_2 and H_2O diffuse into epithelial cells.
- Intracellular CA catalyzes the reformation of H_2CO_3.
- H_2CO_3 dissociates into:
  - H^+: Secreted back into the lumen.
  - HCO_3^-: Most of which enters plasma on a 3 Na^+/HCO_3^- cotransporter in the basolateral membrane, and a small amount is secreted back into the lumen on the Cl^-/HCO_3^- exchanger.

In the thick ascending limb of the LoH and DT, H^+ secretion is also vital for the reabsorption of 10% of the HCO_3^-. In the DT:

- Intercalated cells: They involve specifically in this reabsorption, and they secrete H^+ by H^+-ATPase and H^+/K^+-ATPase.
- CA: It is limited and so less CO_2 and H_2O are formed.

Conversion of alkaline PO_4^{3-} to acidic PO_4^{3-}

Acidic (HPO_4^{2-}) and basic ($H_2PO_4^-$ forms of inorganic PO_4^{3-}) exist in plasma, with a predominance of the basic type ($H_2PO_4^-$).

PO_4^{3-} is filtered through to the PT, where acidic conversion of basic PO_4^{3-} occurs as a result of H^+ secretion by this portion of the nephron. This conversion occurs at all nephron segments where H^+ is secreted. H^+ excretion associated with PO_4^{3-} is ~40 mmol/day. Equally important is that for each H^+ secreted (from the dissociation of H_2CO_3 in the renal tubular cells) 1 molecule of HCO_3^- is formed and returned to the blood.

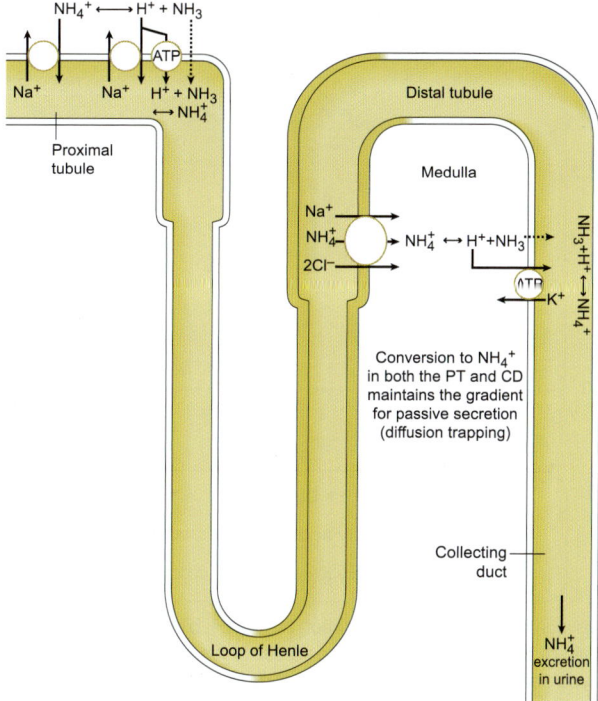

Fig. 4.61 Ammonium handling by the kidney. CD, *Collecting duct*; PT, *proximal tubule*.

Ammonium (NH$_4$$^+$) secretion

The liver generates ammonia (NH$_4$$^+$) and HCO$_3$$^-$ from the products of protein catabolism. The NH$_4$$^+$ and HCO$_3$$^-$ are further processed to urea or glutamine, the latter of which is taken up by PT cells (Fig. 4.61), which convert glutamine back into HCO$_3$$^-$ and NH$_4$$^+$ (dissociates into NH$_3$ and H$^+$).

Cell membranes are freely permeable to NH$_3$, and diffusion into the lumen occurs where it forms NH$_4$$^+$ with secreted H$^+$. In addition, NH$_4$$^+$ can masquerade as other ions so some is secreted into the lumen of the PT by the Na$^+$/H$^+$ exchanger (in place of H$^+$). Approximately 50% of NH$_4$$^+$ delivered to the LoH is reabsorbed in the thick ascending limb by the Na$^+$/K$^+$/2Cl$^-$ transporter (replaces K$^+$). Dissociation of the NH$_4$$^+$ to NH$_3$ and H$^+$ in the medullary ISF occurs, and NH$_3$ diffuses into the CD lumen where it combines with secreted H$^+$ (from H$_2$CO$_3$; apical H$^+$/K$^+$-ATPase) and is excreted as NH$_4$$^+$ (diffusion trapping; Fig. 4.62).

Hence, the purpose of NH$_4$$^+$ secretion is to facilitate the regeneration of HCO$_3$$^-$. Excretion of NH$_4$$^+$ removes 1 H$^+$ and returns 1 HCO$_3$$^-$ to the blood due to overall glutamine handling by the nephron.

NH$_4$$^+$ excretion is increased by acidosis, as ↓ ECF pH increases the generation of glutamine by the liver. In the kidney, ↓ ECF pH also stimulates the oxidation of glutamine in the PT cells (the opposite happens with ↑ ECF pH). Hence, renal synthesis and excretion of NH$_4$$^+$ are massively increased and more HCO$_3$$^-$ is produced, returning ECF pH to normal.

Hence the NH$_3$/NH$_4$ secretion/excretion allows:

- Toxic NH$_3$ to be removed.
- The excretion of H$^+$.
- The generation of HCO$_3$$^-$.

Acid–base disturbances

Disturbances of acid–base can be categorized according to:

- pH change:
  - Acidosis if pH <7.35.
  - Alkalosis if pH >7.45.
- System responsible:
  - Respiratory: If PaCO$_2$ is affected.
  - Metabolic: If HCO$_3$$^-$ is affected.

Four types of disturbance are therefore recognized, as classified using the Davenport diagram (see Fig. 4.62):

1. Respiratory acidosis.
2. Respiratory alkalosis.
3. Metabolic acidosis.
4. Metabolic alkalosis.

Arterial blood gas (ABG) measurements of pH, PaCO$_2$ and PaO$_2$ are useful for identifying the type of acid–base imbalance.

Compensation—Compensation is the restoration of pH by HCO$_3$$^-$ and/or PaCO$_2$. For example, if the primary cause of an

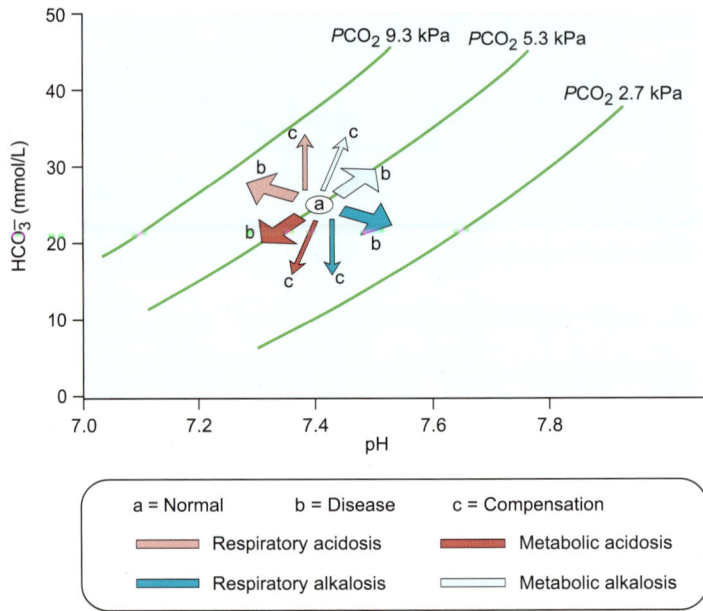

Fig. 4.62 The Davenport diagram explains the relationships between blood pH, bicarbonate and partial pressure of carbon dioxide. Starting at the physiological normal represented by 'a,' the graph shows the values of the above at different pathological states. For example, in uncompensated metabolic acidosis you see the pH and the bicarb level drop represented by 'b.' If then, the body compensates, you see a lowering in carbon dioxide which can either partially or completely correct the pH back to normal value as seen by 'c.'

acid–base disturbance is caused by a metabolic process, respiratory compensation by altering minute volume (and therefore changing $PaCO_2$) can provide rapid compensation. In a compensated state, the changes in HCO_3^- and $PaCO_2$ will mirror each other—both high or both low.

Correction—In correction, there is restoration of pH and of HCO_3^- and $PaCO_2$ values. Correction involves rectification by the system at fault and is typically slower to achieve than compensation.

Examples of acid–base disturbances
Respiratory acidosis
Anything resulting in inadequate removal of CO_2 from the body by the respiratory system will cause respiratory acidosis where an ABG will show: ↓ pH and $PaCO_2 \geq 6\,kPa$. The higher $PaCO_2$ combines with water to form more carbonic acid which is responsible for the lower pH.

The kidney responds to the PCO_2 in body fluids by increasing its secretion of H^+ and by increasing HCO_3^- reabsorption and generation. This renal compensatory response normally corrects pH although it takes several days to fully compensate. Only when the primary disturbance is removed will full correction be achieved.

Causes include:

Factors affecting the respiratory centres
- Drugs: General anaesthesia, morphine, barbiturates (these depress the respiratory centre).

- Injury, for example traumatic brain injury to the brainstem respiratory centre.

Conditions decreasing elimination of CO_2 by the lungs
- Conditions affecting work of breathing to expand the chest wall:
  - Burns (scarring restricts chest expansion and chest wall movement).
  - Obesity (if severe enough, often acting in conjunction with another factor).
  - Mechanical chest injuries, for example flail chest.
  - Muscular dystrophies: Eaton–Lambert syndrome and Duchenne disease.
  - Infections: poliomyelitis.
  - Autoimmune: Guillain–Barré syndrome.
  - Chest wall deformities.
  - Spinal defects: scoliosis/kyphosis.
- Conditions affecting work of breathing due to airway resistance:
  - Severe asthma (smaller airways constitute 20% total airway resistance).
  - Chronic obstructive pulmonary disease (large airways constitute 40% total airway resistance).
  - Obstruction of airway (e.g. foreign body, tumour, mucous plug).

- Conditions affecting the gas exchange:
  - Increased diffusion distance (pulmonary oedema, pulmonary fibrosis).

Respiratory alkalosis

Respiratory alkalosis is caused by lung overventilation and the consequent loss of CO_2, and it is infrequently due to pathological lung conditions. An ABG sample would show ↑ pH and PCO_2 <4.5 kPa. The stimulation of respiratory centres can be the result of:

- Hypoxia: Hypoxic respiratory drive induces hyperventilation:
  - High altitude (uncommon in the United Kingdom).
  - Pulmonary conditions: pulmonary embolus, infection.
- Higher centres: Hysteria, anxiety, pain.

Renal compensation involves ↓ H^+ secretion with ↓ HCO_3^- reabsorption and consequent HCO_3^- excretion in alkaline urine. As with all forms of respiratory acid–base disturbance, correction comes from the respiratory system itself.

Metabolic acidosis

Metabolic acidosis refers to all other causes of acidosis not due to $PaCO_2$. An ABG would show ↓ pH, ↓ HCO_3^- and a normal $PaCO_2$ (if no compensation has occurred). Causes include:

H^+ addition

- Excessive metabolic acid production: Lactic acidosis and diabetic ketoacidosis (DKA).
- Drugs: Methyl alcohol and aspirin.
- Tubular acidosis: Insufficient H^+ secreted, if any at all.

HCO_3^- loss

- Loss of alkaline intestinal fluid:
  - Vomiting of intestinal contents.
  - Severe diarrhoea.
  - Fistula drainage.
- Proximal renal tubular acidosis: The PT is the primary site of HCO_3^- reabsorption.

  With a metabolic acidosis, the respiratory system will compensate through hyperventilation (Kussmaul breathing) to create ↓ $PaCO_2$.

  Resolution of pH permits a further decrease in HCO_3^-. The kidneys respond to increasingly acidic plasma by increasing HCO_3^- reabsorption and excreting H^+ as titratable acid and NH_4^+ to generate new HCO_3^-. If plasma pH is normal, these renal mechanisms are not activated.

Anion gap and metabolic acidosis

Changes in the anion gap are important in ascertaining the causes of metabolic acidosis. The anion gap = plasma cations (Na and K)—plasma anions (Cl and HCO_3) and thus is a measure of the amount of organic anion, for example lactate, that exists. It is predicated on the assumption that every anion has either Na or K as its cation.

> **HINTS AND TIPS**
>
> The causes of a raised anion gap metabolic acidosis can be remembered with the mnemonic 'MUDPILES':
> M—*m*ethanol
> U—*u*raemia
> D—*D*KA
> P—*p*araldehyde
> I—*i*soniazid
> L –*l*actic acidosis
> E—*e*thylene glycol
> S—*s*alicylates (aspirin)

Metabolic alkalosis

A metabolic alkalosis refers to an alkalosis that is not due to a disturbance in $PaCO_2$. An ABG would show ↑pH and a normal PCO_2. Causes include:

- Loss of H^+: Vomiting of gastric contents.
- Ingestion of alkali:
  - Excessive antacid ingestion.
  - Antacid taken with milk: milk–alkali syndrome.
  - Citrate from transfused blood.
- ECF depletion (strong stimulation to reabsorb Na^+ at the expense of H^+):
  - Shock.
  - Diuretics (↑Na^+ delivery to distal nephron → ↑H^+ secretion).
- Excessive mineralocorticoid activity:
  - Cushing syndrome, primary and secondary hyperaldosteronism.
- K^+ depletion in plasma and subsequently tubular fluid:
  - Na^+ reabsorption will occur by exchange preferentially with H^+ rather than K^+ due to the low amount of K^+ in cortical CD.
  - Decreased dietary intake.
  - GI: Vomiting, diarrhoea and intestinal obstruction.
  - Liddle syndrome.

Regulation of calcium and phosphate

Calcium

Calcium (Ca^{2+}) is the most abundant cation in the body and is essential for many bodily functions. Of the body's Ca^{2+}, 99% is stored with PO_4^{3-} as complex salts in bone, which functions as a large reservoir or buffer system. Approximately 1% of Ca is in the ECF (normal plasma values 2.2–2.6 mmol/L). Plasma Ca^{2+} regulates the threshold for excitation in the nerves and muscles. The difference between the resting membrane potential and the threshold potential, which is inversely proportional to plasma Ca^{2+}, dictates the excitability of the membranes of these cells. Therefore concentration should be kept within a fine limit otherwise, over or under-excitability of cell membranes create symptoms experienced by patients (see Fig. 4.64).

Calcium is present in three forms in the plasma:

1. Ionized Ca^{2+} (normal plasma value 1.25 mmol/L), which is the only biologically active form (50%).
2. Reversibly bound to plasma proteins (especially albumin) (40%).
3. Complexed to relatively LMW anions (PO_4^{3-} and citrate) ($\approx$10%).

Approximately 0.1% of the body's Ca^{2+} is found in the ICF (normal concentration 1×10^{-4} mmol/L). Ca^{2+} is:

- Sequestered in smooth endoplasmic reticulum and mitochondria.
- Complexed with specific Ca^{2+}-binding proteins such as calmodulin.

Low ICF Ca^{2+} is maintained by active transport mechanisms.

Plasma pH is an important regulator of the degree of Ca^{2+} binding to nerve membranes. H^+ and Ca^{2+} compete for binding sites on albumin. A high pH lowers free Ca^{2+}, which explains the presence of features of hypocalcaemia, such as tetany, in alkalotic patients.

Calcium handling by the kidney

Normally, urinary loss of calcium per day = net intestinal absorption for homoeostasis of body Ca^{2+} in health. Proportionally less Ca^{2+} will enter the blood than is consumed. Hence, changing dietary input has little effect on renal excretion of Ca^{2+}.

Approximately 60% of plasma Ca^{2+} (i.e. not bound to proteins) is filtered. Subsequently:

In the PT:

- 65% of reabsorption occurs mostly in the pars convoluta.
- The membrane Ca^{2+} permeability is very low.
- Ca^{2+} transport is largely passive and paracellular, driven by the small lumen-positive potential difference (PD).
- Small component of transcellular movement involves passive entry via Ca^{2+} specific channels in the apical membrane and exit across the basolateral membrane via Na^+/Ca^{2+} exchanger and Ca^{2+}-ATPase.

In the thick ascending LoH:

- 20% to 25% of reabsorption occurs by both paracellular movement driven by the lumen-positive PD and transcellular movement by mechanisms described for the PT.
- Furosemide: A diuretic inhibiting $Na^+/K^+/2Cl^-$ transporters reduces lumen-positive PD in the LoH which inhibits paracellular Ca^{2+} reabsorption.

In the DT:

- 5% to 10% reabsorption via transcellular pathway by mechanisms described for the PT.

- Renal Ca^{2+} handling is controlled.
- Thiazide diuretics inhibit apical NaCl symport, promoting Ca^{2+} reabsorption, possibly by the Na^+ gradient across the basolateral membrane and enhancing Na^+–Ca^{2+} exchange.

In the CD: <0.5% of Ca^{2+} is reabsorbed against an electrochemical gradient. Ca^{2+} reabsorption through apical channels is also controlled by parathyroid hormone in PT, LoH and DT.

Phosphate

Inorganic PO_4^{3-} exists in plasma in both acid and alkali forms:

$$H_2PO_4^-: acid$$
$$HPO_4^{2-}: alkali$$

The relative proportions are controlled by pH:

$$H_2PO_4^- \leftrightarrow H^+ + HPO_4^{2-}$$

At plasma pH 7.4, these two exist in the ratio 4 HPO_4^{2-}:1 $H_2PO_4^-$.

Organic PO_4^{3-} is also present inside the cell, incorporated into organic molecules such as cyclic AMP, ADP and ATP. In the kidney, 90% to 95% of PO_4^{3-} is filtered ($\approx$5% is protein bound) with the same ratio of inorganic PO_4^{3-} as in the plasma. In the DT and the PT, H^+ secretion converts alkali PO_4^{3-} into the acid form.

Reabsorption mainly occurs in the PT, and $\approx$75% occurs by symport with Na^+.

Renal tubules have a transport maximum limited mechanism for PO_4^{3-} (reabsorption of 0.1 mM/min). If more than this is present in glomerular filtrate, the excess is excreted. This is normal, as many people consume large amounts of PO_4^{3-} in milk products and meat.

Renal excretion of PO_4^{3-} is:

- Increased by PTH, calcitonin and glucagon.
- Decreased by insulin.

PTH is the only hormone known to regulate tubular PO_4^{3-} transport.

Calcium and phosphate homoeostasis

The regulation of calcium and phosphate are closely linked. Both calcium and phosphate enter the ECF orally via the intestines and from bones. They leave via the kidneys and are taken up again by the bones (Fig. 4.63).

Increasing one will decrease the other making their concentrations inversely proportional. However, small changes in plasma Ca^{2+} can be mimicked by changes in plasma PO_4^{3-}. Regulation of these two substances is by:

1. PTH: Dissolves bone and mobilizes Ca^{2+}.
2. Active vitamin D (1,25 [OH]2 D3): Acts mainly to stimulate intestinal absorption of Ca^{2+} and PO_4^{3-}.
3. Calcitonin.

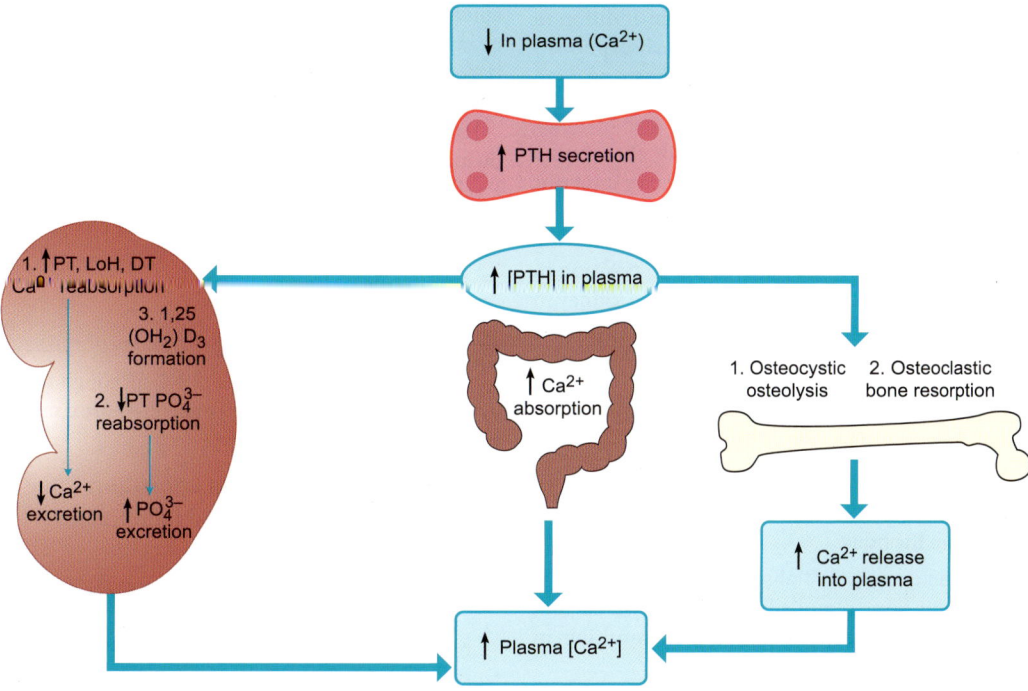

Fig. 4.63 Mechanisms of calcium and phosphate homoeostasis. DT, *Distal tubule*; LoH, *loop of Henle*; PTH, *parathyroid hormone*.

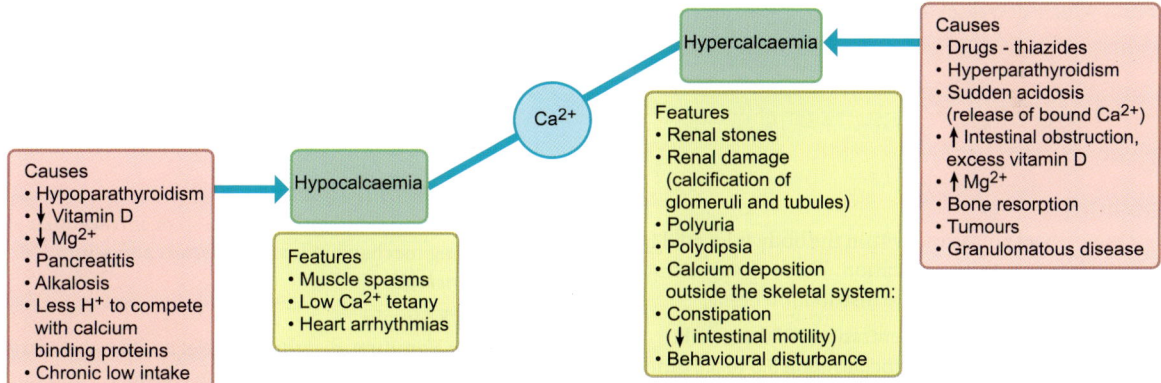

Fig. 4.64 Causes and features of calcium imbalance.

The symptoms of calcium disturbance can be seen in Fig. 4.64.

Parathyroid hormone

Parathyroid hormone is a polypeptide that directly or indirectly exerts an effect on the GI tract, kidneys and bone. Its secretion by the parathyroid gland is mainly stimulated by low Ca^{2+}, but high PO_4^{3-} will also stimulate secretion. Finally, vitamin D alters the sensitivity of the parathyroid gland to Ca^{2+}, and exerts slow, inhibitory effects.

In summary, PTH has four effects on Ca^{2+} homoeostasis:

- ↑ Movement of Ca^{2+} from bone into plasma by stimulating:
  - Rapid Ca^{2+} retrieval produced by osteocytic osteolysis.
  - Osteoclast resorption.
- Activation of vitamin D by stimulating the enzyme which converts inactive to active vitamin D (see below), which then promotes intestinal absorption of Ca^{2+}.
- ↑ Ca^{2+} reabsorption in the PT, LoH and DT of the kidney through apical membrane Ca^{2+} channels.
- Decreased PO_4^{3-} reabsorption in the PT.

Although more PO_4^{3-} is absorbed intestinally, in addition to calcium, by the action of vitamin D, inhibition of reabsorption in the PT caused by PTH means more is excreted in the urine.

Vitamin D

Vitamin D refers to a closely related sterol family that can be derived from provitamins that form part of the dietary intake or produced from ultraviolet light on the skin. These must undergo a series of metabolic steps in the liver and kidney before having any effect. Cholecalciferol is hydroxylated at the 25 position in the liver and then hydroxylated in the 1 position in the kidney to give the active 1,25 hydroxycholecalciferol. The main function of vitamin D is to ↑ serum Ca^{2+} and PO_4^{3-} by:

Enhancing active reabsorption of Ca^{2+} and PO_4^{3-} in the intestine by stimulating the synthesis of proteins involved in their transport.

- Decreased excretion by enhancing movement across the basolateral membrane.
- ↑ Ca^{2+} release from the bone.

In vitamin D deficiency, ↓ Ca^{2+} absorption means that less calcium is available for bone remodelling. In children, osteoid (bone matrix) fails to be mineralized properly, resulting in rickets.

Calcitonin

The parafollicular cells in the thyroid gland produce the peptide calcitonin, which decreases ECF Ca^{2+} by ↓ Ca^{2+} release from bone.

Regulation of potassium and magnesium

Potassium

The vast majority of potassium within the body is located intracellularly where it is the main cation. There is approximately 150 g K^+ (3–4 mol) in the body, the distribution being:

- 98% in ICF: Normal cell concentration ~150 mmol/L.
- 2% in ECF: Normal plasma concentration 3.5 to 5.0 mmol/L.

The ratio of intracellular to extracellular K^+ is crucial when determining membrane excitability making K^+ homoeostasis essential to life.

Renal handling of potassium

After free filtration at the glomerulus, 80% is reabsorbed by the PT. This reabsorption is by passive diffusion down the concentration gradient via the paracellular route aided by H_2O reabsorption (solvent drag).

Some recycling occurs in the LoH, and the descending limb secretes some K^+ and the ascending limb reabsorbs. The thick ascending LoH reabsorbs 10% to 15% K^+, 50% of which is via the paracellular route (as for Na^+) and 50% transcellular via the apical $Na^+/K^+/2Cl^-$ transporter and Na^+/K^+-ATPase and K^+-channel in the basolateral membrane. Hence, reabsorption here is dependent on that of Na^+. Less than 10% of the filtered K^+ reaches the distal nephron.

In the early DT, there is minimal change in tubular fluid K^+, owing to leakage back similar in magnitude to that reabsorbed. P cells in the late DT and CD secrete K^+ passively into the lumen after active transport via the Na^+/K^+-ATPase pump from the interstitium. Secretion is increased by:

- ↑ Intracellular K^+.
- ↑ Tubular flow rate.
- ↑ Na^+ delivery from more proximal nephron segments.

The medullary CDs reabsorb K^+, although the amounts will be small if large amounts were secreted proximally to this portion of the nephron.

Regulation of potassium secretion

$K+$ secretion and thus excretion is affected by:

- Plasma K^+:
  - Affects Na^+/K^+-ATPase in the P cells of the cortical CD, which increase in activity.
  - Stimulates aldosterone production.
- Aldosterone: Activates apical K^+ channels (ROMK) in the P cells, thereby promoting K^+ secretion and hence excretion.
- Amount of Na^+ reaching distal nephron: Na^+ delivery to cortical CD results in greater Na^+ reabsorption and more K^+ secreted.
- Tubular flow rate: A high rate would maintain the steep diffusion gradient favouring secretion.
- ADH: Enhances Na^+ permeability of epithelial cells, making the lumen more negative, which favours K^+ secretion.

Disturbances of potassium

Hypokalaemia—Either K^+ depletion or intracellular shift is the underlying mechanism for a low serum potassium.

Causes include:

- Reduced K^+ intake.
- GI losses: Vomiting, diarrhoea, bowel ileus or obstruction.
- Drugs: Excess insulin, steroid (drive plasma K^+ into the cells).
- Diuretic abuse (increases urinary losses).
- Metabolic alkalosis.
- Hyperaldosteronism: It can be primary or secondary, resulting in ECF depletion, organ failure of heart, kidney or liver.
- Renal tubular acidosis.

The following events can occur in hypokalaemia:

- Decreased membrane excitability: They are hyperpolarized. This presents as fatigue, muscle weakness and cramps that progress upwards from the lower extremities. In prolonged, severe cases, death occurs by respiratory muscle paralysis.

- Decreased conversion of glucose to glycogen by the liver: This normally requires K^+ and might manifest as impaired glucose tolerance.
- Cardiac arrhythmias, including asystole: With hypokalaemia, it takes longer for cardiac muscles to repolarize. Characteristic electroencephalogram (ECG) changes include ST depression, flattened or inverted T waves and U waves.
- Metabolic alkalosis from decreased K^+ delivery to the distal nephron: Normally, Na^+ reabsorption in this portion occurs by exchange with either K^+ or H^+. If K^+ is low then exchange will occur preferentially with H^+, which is then excreted, that is H^+ is lost.
- Impaired response to ADH: Creates thirst and polyuria because the patient is unable to concentrate their urine.

Generally, no clinical features occur with K^+ >2 to 2.5 mmol/L. However, treatment should always involve identification and treatment of the underlying cause, with care to avoid rebound hyperkalaemia. Potassium might need to be administered, either orally or intravenously, with ECG monitoring.

Hyperkalaemia—A high serum potassium, known as hyperkalaemia, is due to either extracellular shift of K^+ or reduced renal excretion. Causes include:

- Increased intake of K^+.
- Cell death or hypoxia: GI bleeding, catabolism, rhabdomyolysis.
- Metabolic acidosis: DKA, lactic acidosis.
- Insulin deficiency: Addison disease, diabetes.
- Drugs causing a release of intracellular K^+: Beta-blockers, excessive digoxin.
- Drugs impairing renal K^+ excretion:
  - Impaired K^+ secretion: ACE inhibitors, NSAIDs, heparin.
  - Render nephron insensitive to aldosterone: Spironolactone, amiloride.
- Decreased plasma aldosterone.
- Renal failure.

Clinical features are generally not seen with concentrations <7 mmol/L. The following events can happen:

- Increased excitability and decreased threshold for depolarization: Symptoms range from slight paraesthesia to severe muscle weakness with loss of tendon jerks. If the threshold is lowered so that it is less than the resting potential, repolarization is prevented, with flaccid paralysis.
- Cardiac arrhythmias: They may be the first presentation of hyperkalaemia and are likely to occur with values >7 mmol/L. Characteristic ECG changes include prolonged PR interval, broad QRS complexes and tall-tented T waves.

Treatment includes rectification of the underlying cause while correcting the K^+ levels with ECG monitoring. This normally includes intravenous insulin with dextrose (to drive K^+ intracellularly) and intravenous calcium gluconate (to protect against membrane hyperexcitability). If the above measures fail, urgent renal replacement therapy can be considered.

CLINICAL NOTES

RENAL REPLACEMENT THERAPY

Renal replacement therapy (RRT), which includes haemodialysis, haemofiltration, haemodiafiltration or peritoneal dialysis, is the mainstay of treatment for people with end-stage renal failure. It may also be required as an emergency measure for acute or acute on chronic renal injury, most frequently done in intensive care unit (ICU). Absolute indications for initiating RRT on ICU include:

- Refractory hyperkalaemia, not responsive to medical therapy.
- Symptomatic uraemia (uraemic encephalopathy or pericarditis).
- Fluid overload secondary to oliguria/anuria and nonresponsive to medical therapy.
- Certain drugs/toxins.
- Refractory metabolic acidosis.

Other indications such as severe sepsis or temperature management, for example severe hypothermia, may also be considered for starting a patient on RRT.

Magnesium

Magnesium is the second most important cation within the cells of the body. It has the following roles:

- Mitochondrial energy production: regulated by Mg^{2+} ATP.
- Protein synthesis.
- Cell membrane K^+ and Ca^{2+} channel regulation.
- Dietary intake is normally 300 mg, of which only half is absorbed. Plasma concentration is 0.7 to 1.0 mmol/L. Body Mg^{2+} totals 28 g, which is widely distributed:
  - Bone: stores >50%.
  - ICF: approximately 45%.
  - ECF: <1%.

Hypermagnesaemia

Hypermagnesaemia is rare due to renal handling of magnesium. Only really seen in renal failure.

Hypomagnesaemia—Magnesium derangements are usually accompanied by K^+, Ca^{2+} or acid–base disturbances. Causes include:

- Reduced intake: Especially protein–energy malnutrition.
- GI tract loss: Including vomiting and diarrhoea.
- Drugs affecting the kidney: Loop diuretics and gentamicin.
- Other metabolic conditions: Acute pancreatitis, hyperparathyroidism, primary or secondary hyperaldosteronism.
- Renal disease: Renal tubular acidosis, Gitelman syndrome.

Clinical features:

- Neuromuscular: Tremor.

- Behavioural: Agitation.
- Neuropsychiatric symptoms: Confusion.
- Cardiac arrhythmias: Especially torsade de pointes.

Renal handling—Approximately 75% of magnesium is filtered (25% bound to plasma proteins), most of which is ionized, although a small amount is complexed with anions (including citrate and PO_4^{3-}).

- PT: Passive paracellular reabsorption of ~15% filtered load, permeability of epithelial cells is lower for Mg^{2+} than either Na^+ or Ca^{2+}.
- Thick ascending limb of LoH: It is the main site for absorption; $\approx$65% of Mg^{2+} is reabsorbed here, mainly paracellular driven by the lumen-positive PD. Additionally, reabsorption is aided by Na^+/Mg^{2+} antiport and basolateral Mg^{2+}-ATPase.
- DT: Reabsorbs 5% to 10%.

Regulation of magnesium reabsorption—A reabsoprtion maximum dependent mechanism applies with any excess staying in the tubular filtrate, thus maintaining plasma values and preventing hypermagnesaemia. Intrinsic regulation is by the cells of the thick ascending limb of LoH: if cells encounter tubular fluid with low Mg^{2+} (secondary to ↓ filtered loads), they transport more Mg^{2+}.

PTH acts on the thick ascending limb to increase reabsorption and therefore decrease excretion.

Ureters

The ureters are muscular tubes that connect the renal pelvis to the bladder. They descend retroperitoneally at the medial border of the psoas muscle and cross the pelvic brim at the level of the common iliac artery bifurcation (Fig. 4.65). At the level of the ischial spine, the ureters move anteriorly and enter the bladder at an oblique angle. This oblique angle prevents reflux of urine back into the ureter.

There are three points of narrowing in the ureter:

1. Ureteropelvic junction.
2. Where the ureters cross the pelvic brim.
3. Vesicoureteric junction.

CLINICAL NOTES

RENAL CALCULI

Calculi of the renal tract, more commonly known as 'kidney stones', affect approximately 3% of the Western population, forming when solutes in the urine crystalise. These stones are typically made of calcium (80%), struvite, urate or cystine. Should a stone grow large enough or migrate to a narrow point of the urinary tract, it can cause impaction with subsequent pain and the risk of renal injury due to postrenal obstruction. The three most

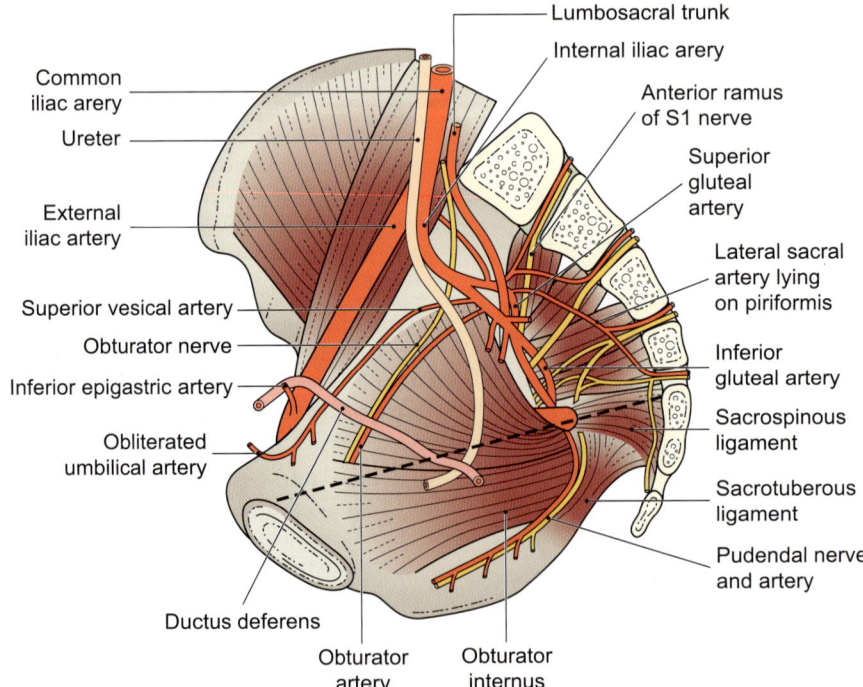

Fig. 4.65 Course of the ureter in the male pelvis.

narrow and therefore most common points of stone impaction are the uteropelvic junction, where the ureters cross the pelvic brim and the vesicoureteric junction.

Blood supply to the ureters is segmental, arising directly from the aorta and the renal, gonadal and iliac arteries. The sympathetic supply is from the coeliac, mesenteric and hypogastric plexus, which also carries the pain sensation. Parasympathetic supply is from the pelvic splanchnic nerves.

CLINICAL NOTES

ABNORMAL INSERTION OF URETERS

The ureters normally enter the bladder at an oblique angle, which creates a valve-like flap to prevent reflex of urine back into the ureter. If the ureters insert perpendicular to the bladder then urine refluxes and the patient, usually a child, is prone to recurrent urinary tract infections.

CLINICAL NOTES

HYSTERECTOMY

The close proximity of the ureter and uterine artery may result in damage to the ureter during hysterectomy as the uterine artery is ligated.

Bladder

In adults, the distended bladder lies in the pelvis, whereas in neonates, it is an abdominal organ that descends with age. It has a pyramidal shape with a base (trigone), apex, two inferolateral surfaces and a superior surface. The apex directs anteriorly and is attached to the umbilicus by the medial umbilical ligament (a remnant of the urachus).

The trigone is the triangular surface formed by the ureters and urethra at its three corners (Fig. 4.66). In males, the ductus deferens and seminal vesicles are attached to the base. In females, the trigone lies against the vagina and cervix. The interureteric fold (a continuation of the longitudinal muscles of the ureter) connects the two ureteric openings.

The neck of the bladder surrounds the beginning of the urethra. In males, it lies on top of the prostate, and in females, it lies on the pelvic floor.

CLINICAL NOTES

SUPRAPUBIC CYSTOSTOMY

When the bladder is distended, it rises above the pubic symphysis. If it is not possible to insert a urethral catheter, the bladder can be drained in an emergency by inserting a needle just above the pubic symphysis.

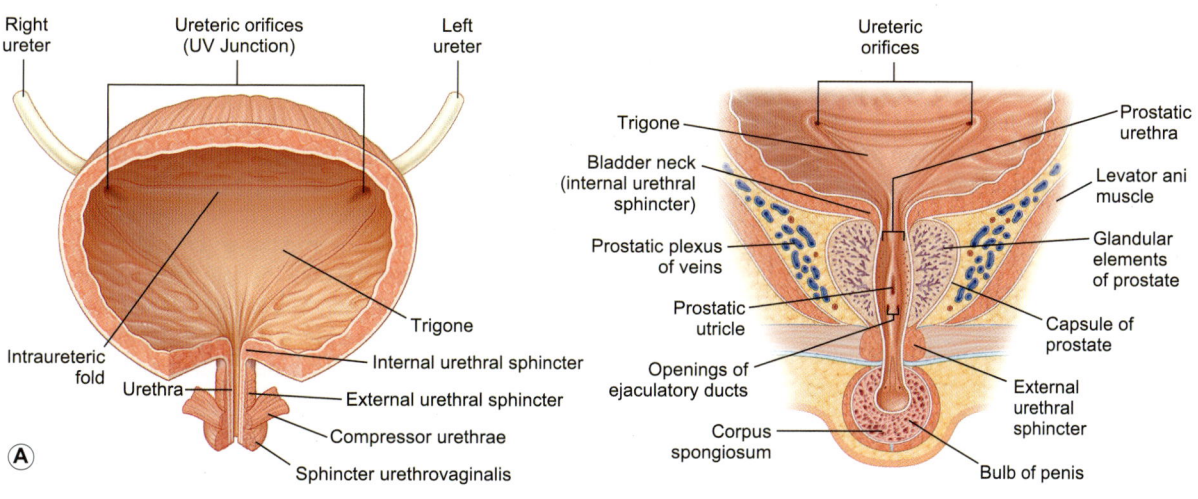

Fig. 4.66 Trigone of the bladder. A) coronal section of the female bladder. B) coronal section of the male bladder to include prostate anatomy. (From Drake, R. L., et al. (2021). *Gray's atlas of anatomy* (3rd ed.). Elsevier.)

Bladder wall

The bladder wall is composed of three layers. The layers are an outer layer (serosa), a middle layer of smooth muscle (detrusor) and an inner layer of transitional epithelium (urothelium).

The detrusor muscle contracts under stimulation of the parasympathetic nervous system in response to stretch receptors signalling a distended bladder. In males, the smooth muscles are arranged circularly around the urethral opening as the internal urethral sphincter. The detrusor muscle is relaxed during filling of the bladder to keep the pressure at a minimum.

The epithelium is able to stretch with bladder filling. In the trigone, the epithelium is smooth, but in the rest of the bladder wall, it is loosely attached to the detrusor muscle, creating the trabeculated appearance.

Vessels and nerves of the bladder

In males, the arterial supply of the bladder is from the superior and inferior vesical arteries, whereas in females, it is from the superior vesical and vaginal arteries. In both sexes, venous drainage is via a plexus that drains into the internal iliac vein. Lymph drains into the internal and external iliac nodes. The nervous supply to the bladder is as follows:

- Parasympathetic: Pelvic splanchnic nerves—detrusor contraction and sphincter relaxation.
- Sympathetic: Superior hypogastric and pelvic plexuses—relaxes the detrusor and contracts the sphincters.
- Pudendal nerve: Supplies the external urethral sphincter.

CLINICAL NOTES

SUPRAPUBIC CYSTOSTOMY

When the bladder is distended, it rises above the pubic symphysis. If it is not possible to insert a urethral catheter, the bladder can be drained in an emergency by inserting a needle just above the pubic symphysis.

Urethra

Urethral anatomy is dependent on sex with males having longer urethras that pass through several structures, making them more complex than female urethras.

Female urethra

The female urethra is only 4 cm long and begins at the bladder neck. It runs through the pelvic floor and perineal membrane and opens in the vestibule anterior to the vaginal opening. The shorter length of the urethra makes females more prone to urinary tract infections.

CLINICAL NOTES

URETHRA LENGTH

The shorter length of the female urethra and its proximity to the anus mean that urinary tract infections, most commonly caused by gut flora (particularly *Escherichia coli*), are more common in females.

Male urethra

The male urethra is 20 cm long and commences at the bladder and ends at the external urethral meatus (Fig. 4.67). It has four sections:

1. Preprostatic: Passes through the bladder wall and ends before the prostate.
2. Prostatic: The section enclosed by the prostate. A central ridge called the urethral crest lies on the posterior wall. On the sides of the ridge lie the openings of the ejaculatory ducts.
3. Membranous: Initially surrounded by the external urethral sphincter before passing through the perineal membrane and ends at the bulb of the penis.
4. Spongy: Passes through the corpus spongiosum and the glans of the penis. The bulbourethral glands drain into the spongy urethra. Numerous urethral glands secrete mucous into the spongy urethra along its length.

CLINICAL NOTES

RUPTURE OF URETHRA

Rupture of the proximal spongy urethra, inferior to the perineal membrane (often secondary to straddle injuries), leads to extravasation of urine into the superficial perineal pouch and the fascia around the penis, the scrotum and superiorly into the anterior abdominal wall. Urine will not enter the anal triangle because the superficial perineal fascia adheres to the perineal membrane along its posterior margin. It will not enter the thigh because the superficial perineal fascia is attached to the fascia lata of the thigh.

Prostate: anatomy and function

The prostate lies inferior to the male bladder and above the perineal membrane. Anatomically, the prostate has five lobes—a

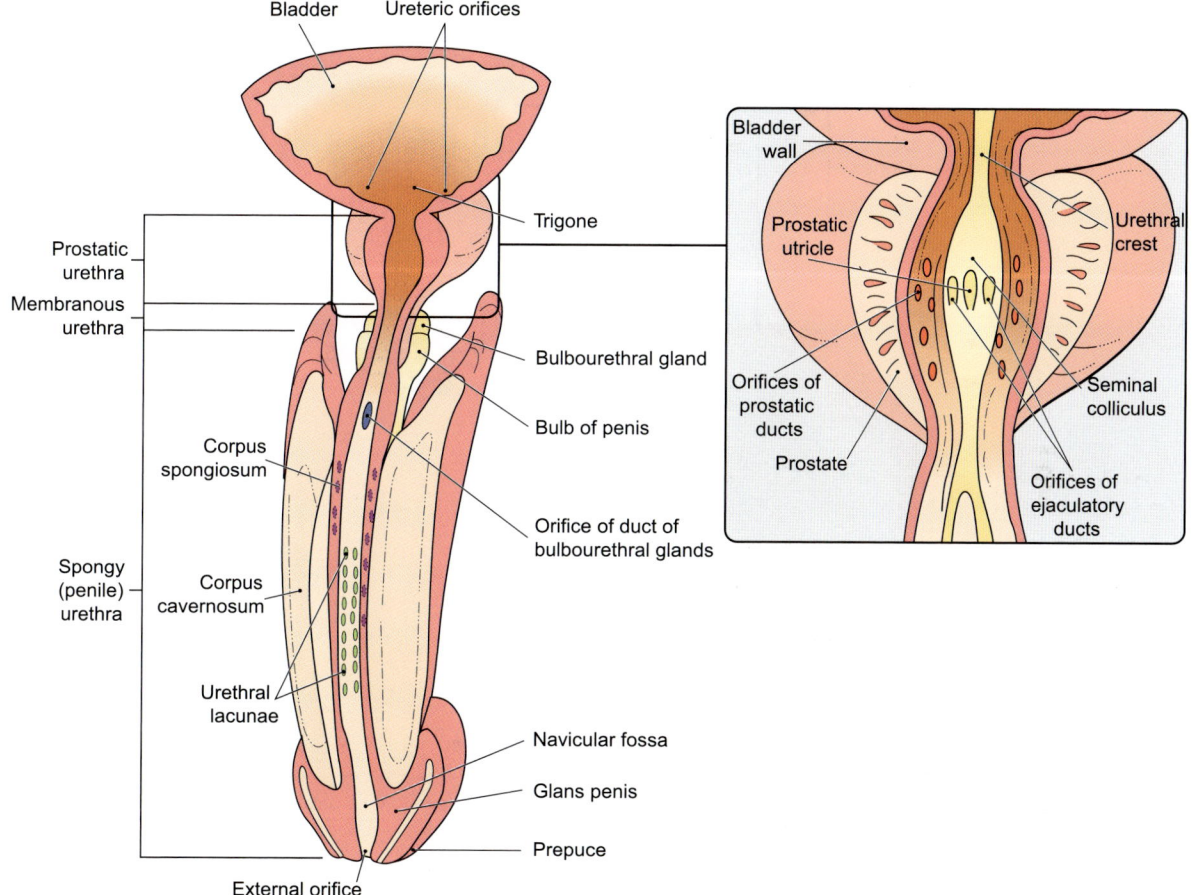

Fig. 4.67 The male urethra.

anterior, median and posterior, and two lateral lobes. The lateral lobes are joined by the isthmus anteriorly and the median lobe posteriorly. For pathological descriptions, the prostate is divided into central, transitional and peripheral zones.

The prostate is surrounded by a fibrous capsule and then a fibrous sheath. Between these two layers is the prostatic plexus of veins.

The blood supply to the prostate is from the inferior vesical and middle rectal arteries. The prostatic venous plexus drains into the internal iliac veins.

The function of the prostate is to secrete an alkali fluid into the ejaculate, which helps neutralize the acidity of the vaginal tract. Secretion from the prostate is under the control of the sympathetic nervous system.

ORGANIZATION OF THE SUPRARENAL GLANDS

The adrenal (suprarenal) glands lie on the superior pole of each kidney. The left adrenal gland lies posterior to the stomach with the lesser sac between them and the right adrenal gland lies posterior to the liver and inferior vena cava. Each gland consists of an outer cortex and an inner medulla (Fig. 4.68).

The adrenal gland is supplied by three main arteries:

1. Superior adrenal: Branch of the inferior phrenic artery.
2. Middle adrenal: Branch of the aorta.
3. Inferior adrenal: Branch of the renal artery.

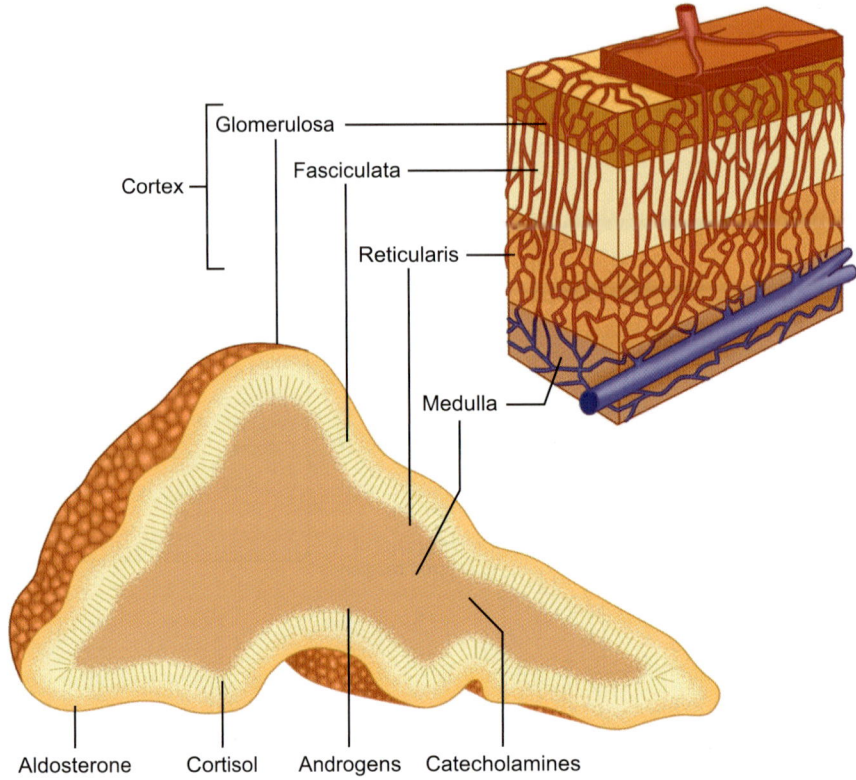

Fig. 4.68 Anatomy of the adrenal glands.

Adrenal hormones

The adrenal cortex is divided into three layers:

1. Zona glomerulus: Produces aldosterone in response to angiotensin II.
2. Zona fasciculata: Produces cortisol in response to stimulation by ACTH.
3. Zona reticularis: Produces dihydroepiandrosterone (androgen).

The adrenal medulla produces and secretes catecholamines such as adrenaline and noradrenaline, and small quantities of dopamine, under the control of the sympathetic nervous system.

OVERVIEW OF THE PELVIS

This chapter will cover the anatomy of the pelvis and the organs within it and explore the physiology of the male and female reproductive systems.

STRUCTURE OF THE PELVIS

The pelvis is a bony structure connecting the spine to the lower limbs. It comprises the sacrum and coccyx posteriorly and the paired hip bones laterally. The hip bones consist of the ilium, ischium and pubis, which fuse at the acetabulum, forming the hip joint. The pelvic cavity houses the male and female reproductive organs and the lower parts of the digestive and urinary tracts. The pelvic brim delineates the division between the greater (false) and lesser (true) pelvis. The pelvis bones and ligaments provide support for abdominal organs, provide stability for posture and serve as a conduit for childbirth in females.

FUNCTIONS OF THE REPRODUCTIVE SYSTEM

The primary purpose of both the male and female reproductive systems is to facilitate the process of reproduction by amalgamating male and female gametes for fertilization, ultimately resulting in the creation of offspring.

The male reproductive system produces and delivers sperm from the testes. Sperm is created by spermatogenesis and travels through the epididymis, vas deferens and ejaculatory ducts during ejaculation. The prostate and seminal vesicles contribute seminal fluid.

The female reproductive system initiates oogenesis in the ovaries, releasing an egg during ovulation. The egg is transported along the fallopian tubes to the uterus, where fertilization may occur. Cyclical changes in the endometrium prepare for embryo implantation or menstruation. Hormonal regulation by the hypothalamus, pituitary and ovaries governs menstrual cycles and maintains reproductive health.

In addition, testosterone influences secondary sexual characteristics in males, whereas oestrogen and progesterone influence secondary sexual characteristics in females.

PELVIC WALL AND BONY PELVIS

The pelvic and abdominal cavities are continuous with each other, as is the peritoneum lining both cavities. The pelvic walls are composed of bones, muscles and ligaments. The bony pelvis is formed by the ilia, the sacrum and the coccyx. It is open superiorly (pelvic inlet) and inferiorly (pelvic outlet) (Fig. 5.1B). The pelvis is described in two parts: the false pelvis and the true pelvis. The false pelvis (the greater pelvis) is located superior to the pelvic brim (pelvic inlet) and consists of the ilia, sacrum and coccyx. The true pelvis (lower pelvis) lies inferior to the pelvic brim, between the inlet and outlet (Fig. 5.2; also see Figs 5.1 and 6.5). The pelvic inlet lies at an angle of approximately 45 degrees to the pelvic outlet. The pelvic cavity is limited inferiorly by the pelvic diaphragm. The perineum lies inferior to the pelvic diaphragm.

Bony pelvis

The bones of the pelvis consist of two hip bones which articulate with the sacrum and coccyx at the sacroiliac joint (a modified synovial joint) and with each other at the pubic symphysis (a secondary cartilaginous joint) (see Fig. 5.1), thus forming a bony ring that protects the contents of the pelvis. Each hip bone develops from three bones, the ilium, ischium and pubis, which fuse at the acetabulum (Fig. 5.3).

The ilia protect underlying structures and provide a site for muscle attachment. The superior border of the ilium—the iliac crest—runs from the anterior superior iliac spine (ASIS) to the posterior superior iliac spine (PSIS). The iliac tubercle is the highest point of the crest. The three muscle layers of the anterolateral abdominal wall originate from the iliac crest, as do latissimus dorsi, quadratus lumborum and the thoracolumbar fascia.

CLINICAL NOTES

NECK OF FEMUR FRACTURE

Although medically and colloquially we often refer to 'hip fractures', usually we are actually referring to a fracture of the femur, typically the neck of the femur. Fractured necks of femurs are common in elderly patients with osteoporosis following falls and rarely involve fractures of the pelvic bones.

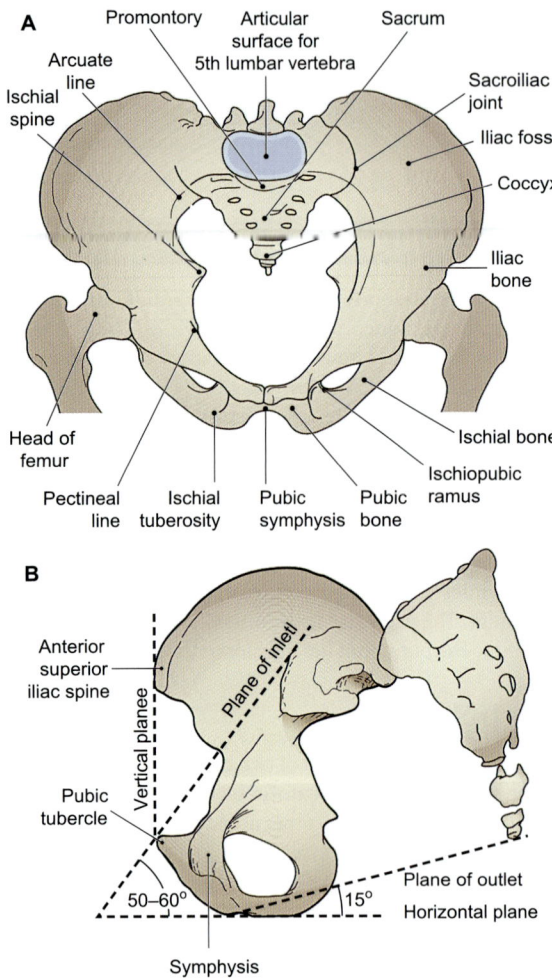

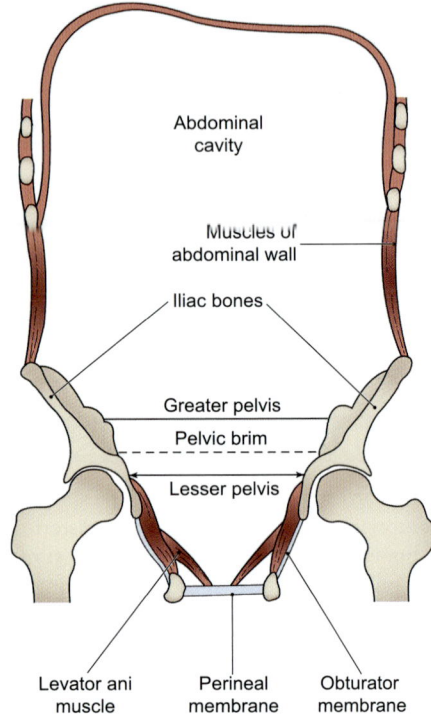

Fig. 5.2 Skeleton of the abdomen and pelvis.

Fig. 5.1 (A) The pelvic girdle. (B) Pelvic inlet and outlet.

Bony pelvic landmarks

The iliac crest can be palpated along its entire length. It stretches from the ASIS to the PSIS. The ASIS lies at the anterior border of the iliac crest, in the fold of the groin superiorly. The PSIS lies at the posterior border of the iliac crest, deep to a dimple visible on the skin of the back, at the level of the S2 vertebra.

The pubic tubercle is palpable on the upper border of the pubic bone. The pubic symphysis joins the two pubic bones and is also palpable. The pubic crest is a ridge of bone on the superior surface of the pubic bone, medial to the pubic tubercle. The ischiopubic ramus runs from the pubic symphysis to the ischial tuberosity (see Fig. 5.1A).

The spinous processes of the sacrum fuse to form the median sacral crest (Fig. 5.4). The crest can be felt deep to the skin in the

buttock cleft. The sacral hiatus is found at the lower end of the sacrum, about 5 cm above the coccyx. The coccyx is palpable approximately 2.5 cm posterior to the anus in the natal cleft (intergluteal).

Sacrum and coccyx

The sacrum consists of the five fused sacral vertebrae (see Fig. 5.4). There are four anterior and four posterior sacral foramina for the passage of the anterior and posterior rami of the sacral spinal nerves. The median sacral crest represents the fused spinal processes of the sacral vertebrae.

The sacrum articulates with the ilium at the sacroiliac joints. The coccyx lies inferior to the sacrum, attached together by the sacrococcygeal symphysis, a fibrocartilaginous joint.

Ilium

The superior border of the ilium is the iliac crest. The ASIS and PSIS lie on the anterior and posterior extremities of the iliac crest, with the anterior and posterior inferior iliac spines lying below (Fig. 5.5). The iliac fossa lies on the internal surface of the ilium and is the origin of the iliacus muscle. The articular surfaces of the ilium and sacrum form the sacroiliac joint. The ilium forms part of the acetabulum and the bony margin of the greater sciatic notch.

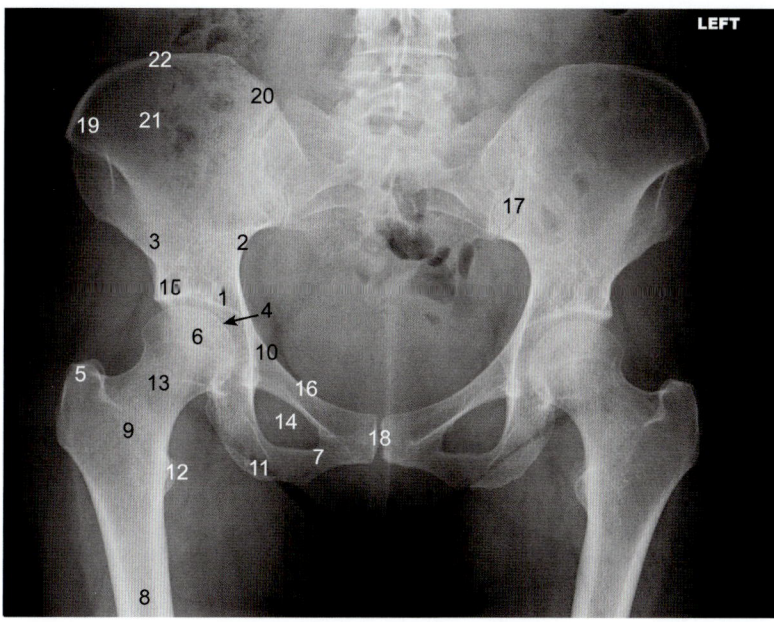

1. Acetabulum
2. Arcuate line
3. Ilium
4. Fovea
5. Greater trochanter of femur
6. Head of femur
7. Inferior ramus of pubis
8. Shaft of the femur
9. Intertrochanteric line
10. Ischial spine
11. Ischial tuberosity
12. Lesser trochanter
13. Neck of femur
14. Obturator foramen
15. Rim of the acetabulum
16. Superior ramus of pubis
17. Sacroiliac joint
18. Pubic symphysis
19. Anterior superior iliac spine
20. Posterior superior iliac spine
21. Ala of ilium
22. Iliac crest

Fig. 5.3 An anteroposterior x-ray of the right hip and pelvis.

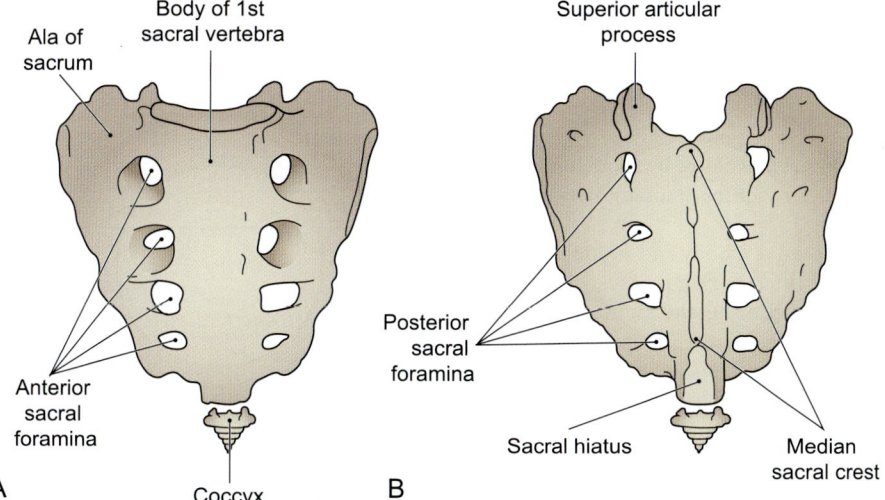

Fig. 5.4 The sacrum and coccyx bones.

Pubis and ischium

The pubic bones articulate in the midline at the pubic symphysis (see Fig. 5.5). Each pubic bone has a body, a superior ramus and an inferior ramus. The superior ramus consists of the pubic symphysis, pubic crest, pubic tubercle and pecten pubis. It joins with the arcuate line of the ischium to form the pelvic brim. The obturator foramen is surrounded by the rami of the pubis and the

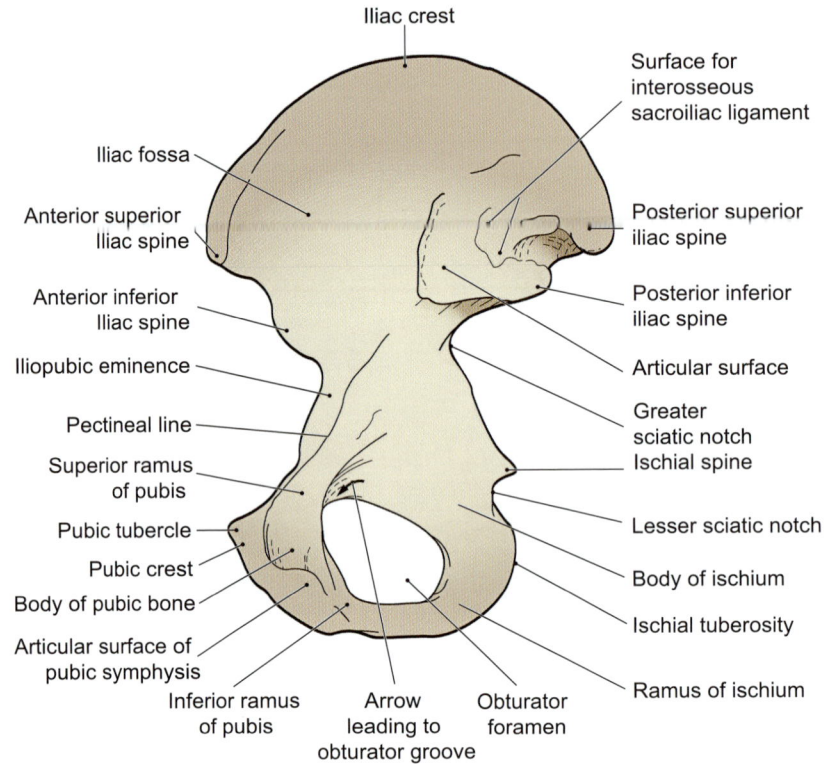

Fig. 5.5 Medial view of the hip bone.

ischium. The obturator foramen is closed by the obturator membrane, in which there is a canal for the obturator nerves and vessels to exit the pelvis.

The ischium is composed of a body and superior and inferior rami. Anteriorly the inferior ramus fuses with the inferior ramus of the pubis, forming the ischiopubic ramus. Posteriorly it fuses with the ilium. The ischial tuberosity, which bears the weight of the body when sitting, projects posteroinferiorly from the body of the ischium. The posterior border of the ischium contributes to the formation of the greater and lesser sciatic notches. The two notches are separated by the ischial spine. The sacrotuberous and sacrospinous ligaments transform the notches into the greater and lesser sciatic foramina.

The position of the pelvis

When standing, the pelvis lies obliquely in relation to the trunk, with the ASIS and the superior border of the pubic symphysis lying in the same vertical plane. The horizontal plane from the superior border of the pubic symphysis passes through the ischial spine and coccyx.

Table 5.1 Differences between the male and female pelves

	Male	Female
Acetabulum	Large	Small
Bones	Robust/heavier	Lighter/smoother
Inferior pelvic aperture	Relatively small	Relatively large
Obturator foramen	Round	Oval
Pubic arch	Narrow	Wide
Superior pelvic aperture	Usually heart shaped	Usually oval or rounded

Male and female pelvises

The male and female pelves exhibit sexual dimorphism owing to their respective functions. These differences are explored in Table 5.1 and Fig. 5.6.

Pelvic joints

Pubic symphysis

The pubic symphysis is a secondary cartilaginous joint between the two pubic bones (see Fig. 5.5). It is usually immobile,

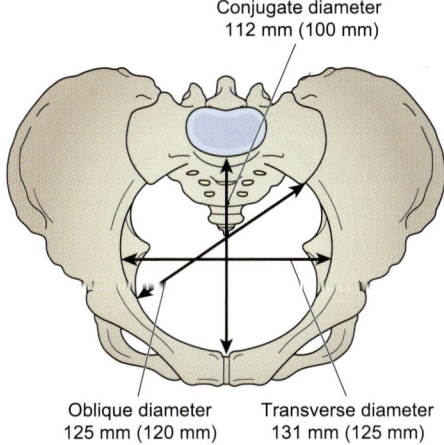

Fig. 5.6 Female pelvic inlet and its average diameters compared with male average diameters in brackets.

Conjugate diameter
112 mm (100 mm)

Oblique diameter
125 mm (120 mm)

Transverse diameter
131 mm (125 mm)

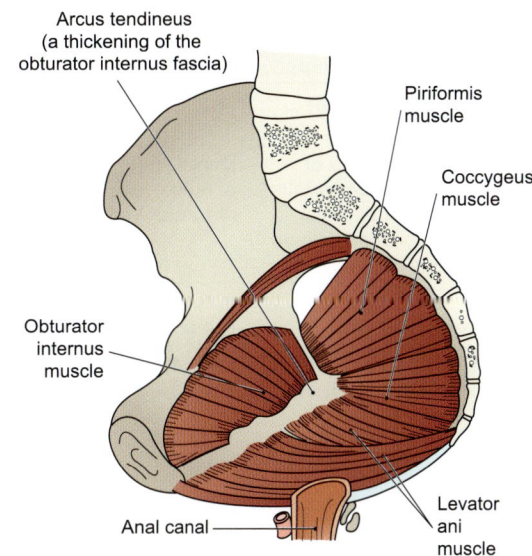

Fig. 5.7 Muscles of the pelvic wall.

Arcus tendineus
(a thickening of the
obturator internus fascia)

Piriformis
muscle

Coccygeus
muscle

Obturator
internus
muscle

Anal canal

Levator
ani
muscle

reinforced by the superior pubic ligament and the inferior arcuate pubic ligament.

Sacroiliac joint

This is a specialized synovial joint, which allows only minimal movement. It is strengthened by interosseous and anterior and posterior sacroiliac ligaments. The sacrospinous and sacrotuberous ligaments prevent rotation at the joint. The joint transmits all the body weight to the hip bones.

Pelvic walls and floor

The lateral walls of the pelvis are formed by the hip bones with obturator internus muscles lying deep to the obturator membrane (Fig. 5.7). The posterior wall is formed by the sacrum and coccyx, with piriformis lying on the internal surface of the sacrum. Table 5.2 outlines the muscles of the pelvic wall and floor.

The levator ani takes its origin from the tendinous arch (a thickening of the fascia over obturator internus running from the body of the pubis to the ischial spine). The levator ani and coccygeus form a continuous section of muscle known as the pelvic diaphragm, inserting into a series of midline structures. This forms a bowl of muscle around the terminal parts of the rectum, prostate and urethra in the male, and the rectum, vagina and urethra in the female (Fig. 5.8).

Perineal body

The perineal body is a midline knot of fibromuscular tissue that lies at the centre of the line dividing the anal and urogenital triangles. It lies posterior to the prostate or vagina. Parts of the levator ani, bulbospongiosus, the external anal sphincter and the superficial and deep transverse perineal muscles are attached to and

comprise part of the perineal body; thus it has an essential role in supporting pelvic and perineal structures.

Anococcygeal body

The anococcygeal body is a midline raphe running from the anorectal junction to the tip of the coccyx, into which the levator ani inserts. It separates the two ischioanal fossae posterior to the anal canal.

Pelvic fascia

Over the internal surface of the pelvic wall, the fascia forms a strong covering over obturator internus and piriformis muscles, continuous with that of the abdomen. The spinal nerves lie external to the fascia and vessels lie internal to it. The sacral plexus lies between the fascia and piriformis.

Over the pelvic floor, the fascia consists of loose areolar tissue. This condenses around neurovascular bundles to form ligaments and gives rise to the puboprostatic and pubovesical ligaments in the male and female, respectively. These fibromuscular bands, on either side of the median plane, run from the pubic bone to the bladder neck—immobilizing it and supporting the bladder. The deep dorsal vein of the penis or clitoris passes between the ligaments. The fascia varies in thickness over the pelvic viscera.

Pelvic peritoneum

In the male, the peritoneum lines the pelvic walls and the pelvic cavity inferiorly. From the anterior abdominal wall, the

215

Table 5.2 Muscles of the pelvic wall and floor

Name of muscle (nerve supply)	Origin	Insertion	Action
Coccygeus (fourth and fifth sacral nerves)	Ischial spine	Inferior aspect of sacrum and coccyx	Supports pelvic viscera, flexes coccyx
Levator ani—composed of pubococcygeus, puborectalis and iliococcygeus (perineal branches of the pudendal nerve and fourth sacral nerve)	Ischial spine, body of pubis, fascia of obturator internus	Perineal body, anococcygeal body, walls of prostate, vagina, rectum and anal canal	Supports pelvic viscera; sphincter to anorectal junction and vagina Counteracts increased abdominal pressure, e.g. defaecation, parturition
Piriformis (first and second sacral nerves)	Anterior aspect of sacrum	Greater trochanter of femur	Rotates femur laterally at hip and stabilizes hip joint
Obturator internus (nerve to obturator internus; L5, S1, S2)	Obturator membrane and adjacent hip bone	Greater trochanter of femur	Rotates femur laterally at hip and stabilizes hip joint

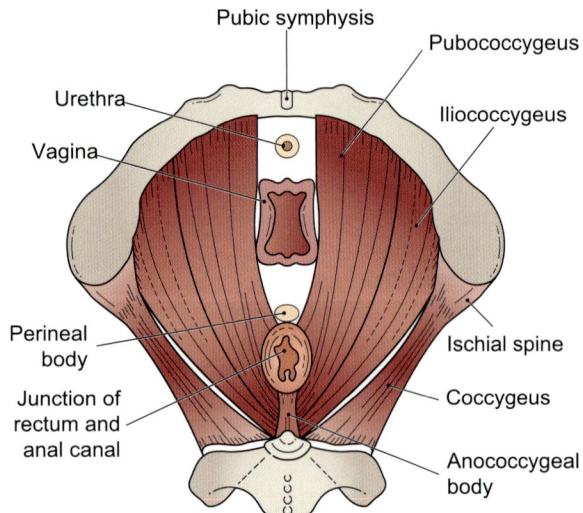

Fig. 5.8 Pelvic floor viewed from below.

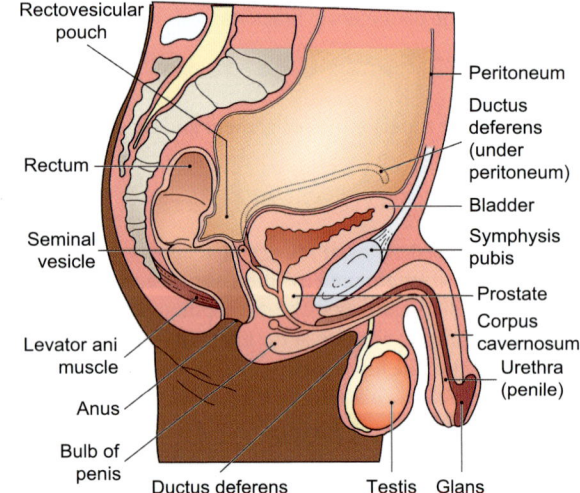

Fig. 5.9 A section through the male pelvis, illustrating the rectum and rectovesical pouch.

peritoneum is reflected onto and attaches to the superior surface of the bladder. This means that as the bladdwer fills and enlarges, it peels the peritoneum away from the anterior abdominal wall. The peritoneum descends on the base of the bladder before ascending onto the rectum, forming the rectovesical pouch (Fig. 5.9).

In females, the peritoneum leaves the base of the bladder to pass over the uterus, forming the uterovesical pouch. From the superior aspect of the uterus and upper vagina, the peritoneum ascends to cover the rectum, forming the rectouterine pouch (pouch of Douglas) (Fig. 5.10). The fold of peritoneum containing the uterus passes to the lateral walls of the pelvic cavity and is known as the broad ligament of the uterus.

CLINICAL NOTES

THE RECTOVESICULAR AND RECTOUTERINE POUCHES

The rectovesicular and rectouterine pouches are the most inferior sections of the peritoneum within the abdominopelvic cavity in males and females, respectively. Therefore fluids released into the abdominopelvic cavity are likely to collect in these pouches which can occur in pathologies such as ectopic pregnancy. Furthermore, drains are often placed in these pouches during abdominopelvic surgery to collect any residual fluid postoperatively.

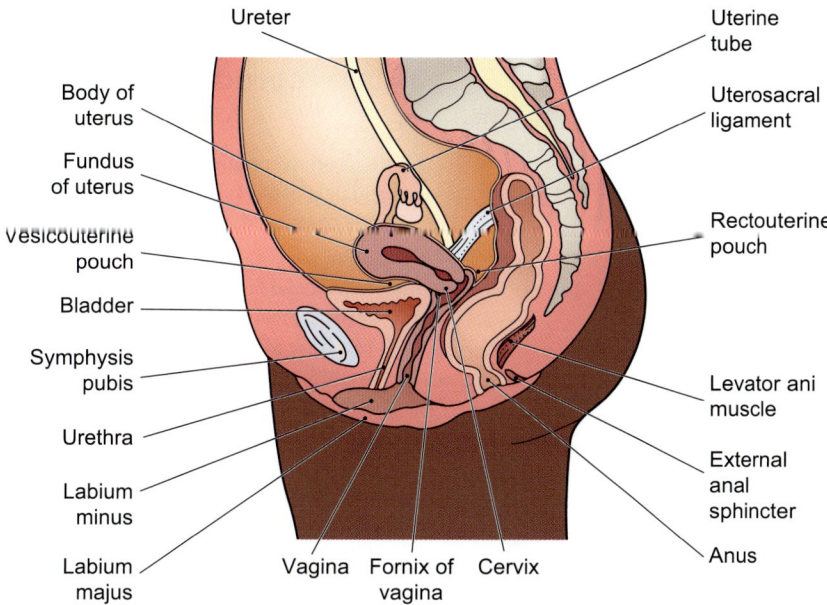

Fig. 5.10 Sagittal section through the female pelvis.

PELVIC CONTENTS

The contents of the pelvis include:

- Small intestine
- Sigmoid colon and rectum
- Ureters and bladder
- Urethra
- Ovaries, fallopian tubes, uterus and vagina in females
- Cervix
- Ductus deferens, seminal vesicles and prostate in males
- Lumbosacral trunk, obturator nerve, sympathetic trunks and sacral plexus
- Common iliac arteries, gonadal arteries and superior rectal arteries

Pelvic organs

Ureters, bladder and urethra

The ureters, bladder and urethra are all discussed in detail in Chapter 4, Page 206–208.

Rectum

The rectum commences as a continuation of the sigmoid colon at the level of the S3 vertebra (where the sigmoid mesocolon ends). It is approximately 12 cm long and ends at the anorectal junction, piercing the pelvic floor at the border of puborectalis to become the anal canal. The rectum can be distinguished from the colon by a lack of appendices epiploicae, taeniae coli and haustra.

The rectum is concave anteriorly, following the curve of the sacrum—it also has three lateral curves (right, left and right). It contains three to four transverse folds containing mucous membranes and circular muscle, which project into the lumen of the rectum. These provide support for faecal material. The most inferior part of the rectum dilates as the rectal ampulla.

The rectum has no mesentery. The upper third is covered by peritoneum on its anterior and lateral surfaces. The middle third is covered by peritoneum on its anterior surface, which reflects onto the posterior surface of the bladder in males (forming the rectovesical pouch) and the superior aspect of the uterus and upper vagina in females (forming the rectouterine pouch—the pouch of Douglas). The peritoneum is absent from the lower third of the rectum (see Fig. 5.9). Posteriorly, the rectum is related to the sacrum, coccyx and pelvic floor.

CLINICAL NOTES

RECTAL EXAMINATION

A rectal examination is performed for various reasons, for example as part of an examination for prostate or colorectal cancer, in cases of rectal bleeding or as part of an abdominal examination. The patient is asked to lie on their left side, in the foetal position, with their knees drawn up to their chest. The perineum and perianal

(Continued)

CLINICAL NOTES — *Contd.*

areas are inspected looking for ulceration, warts, bleeding, discharge, and so forth. A gloved, lubricated finger is inserted, facing posteriorly, into the anus. A brief assessment can be made of anal tone at this point. The walls of the rectum can be examined by rotating the finger 180 degrees clockwise and anticlockwise. The following structures can be palpated:

- Anteriorly: Males—the bulb of the penis, the membranous urethra, the prostate; females—the body of the uterus and the cervix.
- Posteriorly: the sacrum, the coccyx.
- Posterolaterally: The ischial spines.

Vessels and nerves of the rectum

Blood supply to the rectum arises from the superior, middle and inferior rectal arteries. The superior rectal artery is a continuation of the inferior mesenteric artery. The middle and inferior rectal arteries are discussed in the section describing the blood supply to the pelvis.

The rectum drains to the superior rectal vein (into the inferior mesenteric vein, which drains into the portal venous system), and the middle and inferior rectal veins drain to the internal iliac vein (part of the systemic venous system). The superior rectal vein anastomoses with the middle and inferior rectal veins, forming one of the important sites of portosystemic anastomosis. Lymphatics accompany branches of the superior and middle rectal arteries and eventually drain to the preaortic nodes at the origin of the inferior mesenteric vessels.

The nerve supply of the rectum arises from the hypogastric plexus (sympathetic) and pelvic splanchnic nerves (parasympathetic).

Male reproductive organs in the pelvis

Scrotum

The scrotum contains the testes, epididymis, vas deferens and the distal part of the spermatic cord (Fig. 5.11). The wall of the scrotum is composed of several layers (from superficial to deep):

- Skin.
- Superficial fascia containing the dartos muscle. The dartos muscle receives sympathetic innervation and contracts in response to cold, pulling the testes closer to the body and wrinkling the skin. The scrotum is divided into two compartments by the median raphe (composed of superficial fascia), separating the testes. Deep to the dartos muscle lies Colles fascia—a continuation of the Scarpa fascia of the abdomen.
- External spermatic fascia.
- Cremasteric fascia.
- Internal spermatic fascia.
- Parietal layer of the tunica vaginalis.

Blood and nerve supply of the scrotum

The arterial supply of the scrotum arises from anterior and posterior scrotal arteries (branches of the external pudendal artery and internal pudendal artery, respectively). Venous drainage occurs via scrotal veins, which drain into the external pudendal vein and, eventually, into the great saphenous vein. Innervation of the scrotum occurs via the genitofemoral nerve, ilioinguinal nerve, pudendal nerve and the posterior cutaneous nerve of the thigh. The ilioinguinal nerve supplies the anterior third of the

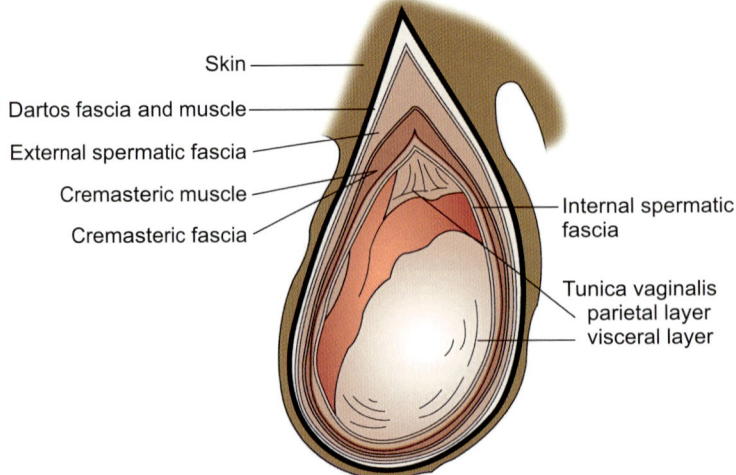

Skin

Dartos fascia and muscle

External spermatic fascia

Cremasteric muscle

Cremasteric fascia

Internal spermatic fascia

Tunica vaginalis
parietal layer
visceral layer

Fig. 5.11 Cross section through the scrotum.

scrotum. The posterior two-thirds is innervated by the posterior scrotal branch of the perineal nerve (medially) and the perineal branch of the posterior cutaneous nerve of the thigh (laterally). Lymph vessels drain to the medial superficial inguinal lymph nodes of the thigh.

CLINICAL NOTES

CREMASTER REFLEX

In the male, the genital branch of the genitofemoral nerve supplies the cremaster muscle. Its femoral branch supplies a small area of skin on the thigh. Stimulation of this skin causes the cremaster muscle to contract, raising the testis towards the inguinal canal—testing L1. This reflex is very active in children, often leading to a misdiagnosis of undescended testes. The absence of the cremasteric reflex in the context of testicular pain is often suggestive of testicular torsion.

Spermatic cord

The structures entering the deep inguinal ring pick up a covering from each layer of the abdominal wall as they pass through the canal to form the spermatic cord (Fig. 5.12). The spermatic cord is not complete until it emerges from the superficial inguinal ring with all of its coverings.

The coverings from superficial to deep are:

- External spermatic fascia: Derived from the aponeurosis of external oblique muscle.
- Cremasteric fascia: Derived from the internal oblique and the transversus abdominis muscles.
- Internal spermatic fascia: Derived from the transversalis fascia.

The contents of the spermatic cord are:

- The ductus deferens.
- Arteries: Testicular artery (from the abdominal aorta), the artery to the ductus deferens (from inferior vesical arteries) and the cremasteric artery (from the inferior epigastric artery).
- Veins: The pampiniform plexus of veins.
- Lymphatics: Accompany the veins from the testis to the paraaortic nodes.
- Nerves: The genital branch of the genitofemoral nerve supplies the cremaster muscle, and sympathetic nerves supply arteries and smooth muscle of the ductus deferens.
- The processus vaginalis: The obliterated remains of the peritoneal connection with the tunica vaginalis of the testis.

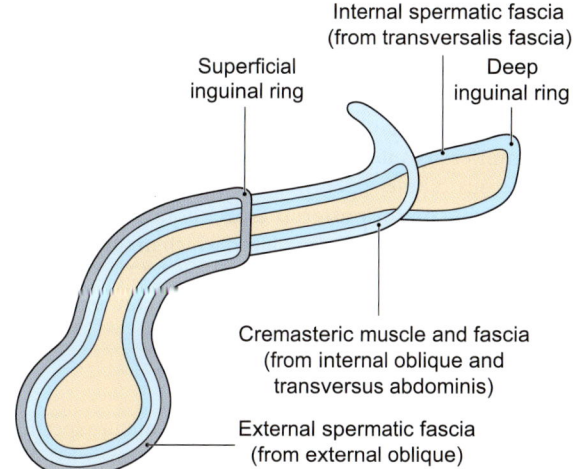

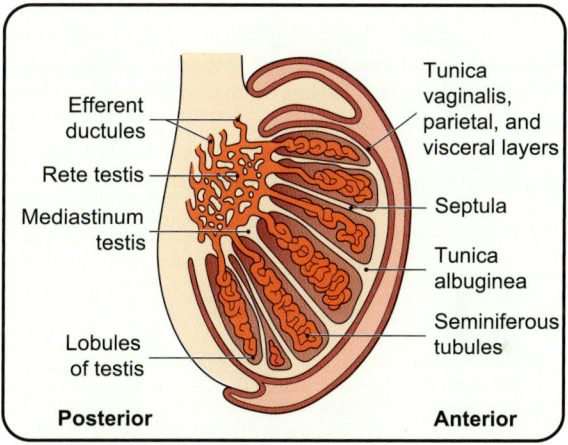

Fig. 5.12 Left testis and coverings of the spermatic cord.

Testis

The testis is suspended in the scrotum by the spermatic cord (see Fig. 5.12) and is surrounded by three layers (tunics): the tunica vaginalis, tunica albuginea and tunica vasculosa. The outermost layer is the tunica vaginalis, composed of a parietal and visceral layer. Testicular development begins at approximately 6 weeks' gestation, on the posterior abdominal wall. In the third month of foetal development, a sock-like evagination of the foetal peritoneum (processus vaginalis) passes through the abdominal wall, into the developing scrotum. At 7 to 9 months' gestation, the testis descends retroperitoneally into the scrotum (preceded by the gubernaculum) coming to lie posterior to the processus vaginalis. After testicular descent is complete, the proximal part of the processus vaginalis is obliterated, leaving a double-layered, serous sac at the distal end—the tunica vaginalis. The tunica vaginalis covers the epididymis and the testis except for its posterior surface, where it reflects onto the wall of the scrotum.

Deep to the tunica vaginalis lies the tunica albuginea, a tough fibrous capsule, which gives rise to numerous septa, dividing the testis into 200 to 300 lobules. Within the lobules lie the seminiferous tubules (the site of spermatogenesis). The seminiferous tubules open into the rete testis (a network of channels lying on the posterior aspect of the testis). The rete testis converges on the efferent ducts, which in turn connect to the first part of the epididymis (see Fig. 5.12). Deep to the tunica albuginea lies the tunica vasculosa, containing blood vessels and areolar tissue.

Spermatogenesis

Spermatogenesis is the production process of mature sperm (the male gamete) by way of mitosis and meiosis (Fig. 5.13). Daily, healthy males will produce roughly 200 to 300 million sperm. Approximately 100 to 150 million become fully viable after maturation in the epididymis. During spermatogenesis, germ cells move from the basal layer of the wall of the seminiferous tubules towards the inner lumen, passing through various stages to form spermatids (immature sperm).

The process of spermatogenesis can be divided into two phases: spermatocytogenesis and spermiogenesis.

Spermatocytogenesis—Spermatocytogenesis describes the process of a single germ cell dividing into four spermatids. Starting in the wall of the seminiferous tubule with germ cells known as primary spermatogonium type A, mitosis produces two new cell types. Firstly, primary spermatogonium type B cells are produced which, through autoreproduction, have a vital role in maintaining the number of primary spermatogonium type A cells. The other products of spermatogonium mitosis are primary spermatocytes. These are diploid cells maintaining their number of chromosomes. The second stage of division produces secondary spermatocytes through meiosis I, thus halving the chromosomal material. Therefore secondary spermatocytes are haploid cells. Secondary spermatocytes then undergo meiosis II to form four immature haploid spermatids.

During these stages of division, support and nutrition of the developing gametes are provided by Sertoli cells.

Spermiogenesis—During spermiogenesis, no further cell division occurs but maturation and differentiation produce mature sperm from the spermatids. The spermatids produced from spermatocytogenesis are immature and are incapable of fertilization. They contain organelles including the Golgi apparatus, centrioles and mitochondria. Spermiogenesis occurs through four phases:

1. Golgi phase: The enzymes of the Golgi body form the enzymes of the acrosome.

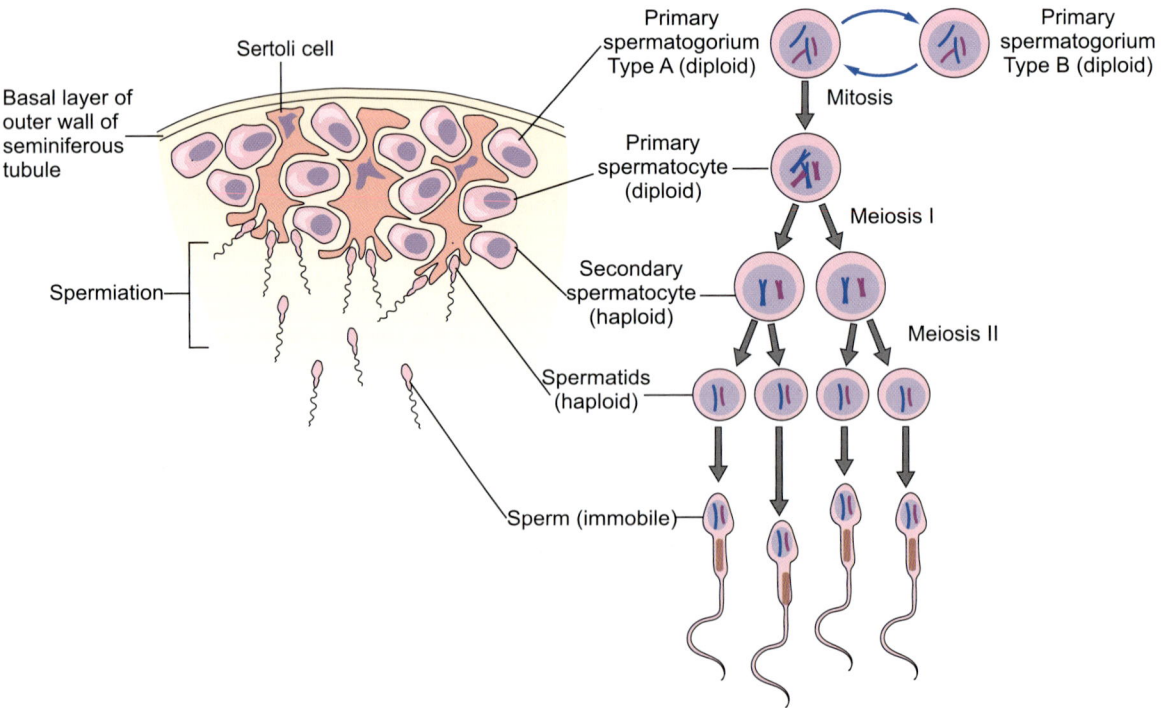

Fig. 5.13 Spermatogenesis.

2. Acrosomal phase: The formed acrosome condenses around the nucleus forming the acrosomal cap of the sperm. The enzymes of the acrosome break down the zona pellucida of the ovum to allow the nucleus of the sperm to join the nucleus of the ovum to instigate fertilization.
3. Tail phase: The centriole present in the spermatid elongates to form the tail of the sperm.
4. Maturation phase: Maturation occurs under the influence of testosterone. Sertoli cells phagocytose excessive and unnecessary cytoplasm and organelles.

At this stage, the sperm are mature yet remain immobile. Through a process called spermiation, mature sperm are released into the lumen of the seminiferous tubules. The mature sperm are then transferred to the epididymis in testicular fluid secreted by Sertoli cells with the aid of peristaltic contractions. In the epididymis, sperm gain motility rendering them capable of fertilization.

Blood supply to the testes

The testicular artery (a branch of the abdominal aorta at the level of the L2 vertebra) enters the spermatic cord and supplies the testis and epididymis. The pampiniform plexus of veins drains these structures. In the inguinal canal, the plexus forms four veins. As they emerge through the deep inguinal ring, they merge to form two veins, which subsequently join to form a single testicular vein. The left testicular vein drains into the left renal vein and the right directly into the inferior vena cava. The plexus surrounds the testicular artery and cools the arterial blood, thereby providing the cooler environment required for spermatogenesis in the testis. Lymphatic drainage of the testes is to the paraaortic nodes in the abdomen.

HINTS AND TIPS

BLOOD SUPPLY TO THE SCROTUM

It is important to remember that the scrotum is part of the body wall and receives a local arterial and nerve supply, while the testes develop in the abdomen during foetal life and retain their vascular supply and abdominal lymphatic drainage. In the female, the ovaries are retained within the abdominal cavity.

CLINICAL NOTES

SEMEN ANALYSIS

During ejaculation, sperm is mixed with fluids produced from the following locations:

- Seminal vesicles of the testes: A yellowish fructose-rich fluid comprising approximately 70% of semen.
- The prostate: A whitish fluid that contains proteolytic enzymes, lipids and acids under the influence of testosterone.
- Bulbourethral glands of the penis: A clear fluid that acts as a lubricant.

Semen analysis is performed clinically to evaluate male fertility. Male fertility is multifactorial, and depending on the exact method used, a number of characteristics are evaluated including:

- Sperm concentration: A concentration of over 15 million sperm per millilitre of semen is considered normal.
- Motility: An assessment of how mobile a male's sperm is can be divided into four grades, grade A (progressive and motile) to grade D (immotile and fail to move).
- Morphology: A sample is described as 'normal' where 4% or more of observed sperm have normal morphology.
- Volume: Greater than 1.5 mL of semen per ejaculation is considered normal.
- pH: A pH range of between 7.2 and 7.8 is considered normal.

Poor male fertility may be the result of an individually poor semen characteristic despite others being normal.

CLINICAL NOTES

CONDITIONS AFFECTING THE TESTES

Undescended testis:

- The testis may not descend completely, stopping at any point along its descent.

Testicular torsion:

- Testicular torsion occurs when the spermatic cord becomes twisted. This compromises the blood supply to the testicle resulting in a surgical emergency.

Testicular swellings:

- A hydrocele is an accumulation of serous fluid within the tunica vaginalis, usually secondary to a persistent processus vaginalis.
- A varicocele is an abnormal dilatation of the veins of the pampiniform plexus, usually secondary to failures of valves in the testicular vein or due to the compression of the venous drainage of the testicle.
- A spermatocele is a cystic structure which arises from the epididymis and contains spermatozoa.

The cause of most testicular swellings can be diagnosed by ultrasound examination.

Epididymis

The epididymis lies on the posterolateral border of the testis. It is a tightly coiled single tube, the site of sperm storage and maturation. It is composed of a head (lying at the upper poles of the testis), a body and a tail. The efferent ducts drain into the head of the epididymis. At its tail, the epididymis becomes less coiled and wider and becomes known as the ductus (vas) deferens.

Ductus deferens

The ductus deferens passes from the epididymis to the pelvic cavity via the inguinal canal. At the deep inagural ring, the ductus deferens hooks around the inferior epigastric artery, crossing the external iliac vessels to enter the pelvic cavity. The ductus deferens crosses the ureter and the base of the bladder. The terminal part dilates, forming the ampulla. The ductus deferens joins the duct of the seminal vesicle to form the ejaculatory duct, which opens into the prostatic urethra on the colliculus.

Muscular contractions of the ductus transmit sperm from the epididymis to the prostatic urethra during ejaculation (sympathetic innervation). The arterial supply to the ductus arises from a small branch of the superior vesical artery.

Seminal vesicles

The seminal vesicles are two elongated lobular sacs lying lateral to the ampulla of the ductus deferens. They produce seminal fluid.

Prostate

The prostate is a walnut-shaped organ lying inferior to the bladder and superior to the perineal membrane. The prostatic urethra passes through it (see Fig. 4.67). The base of the prostate is attached to the bladder neck and its apex points inferiorly.

Anatomically, the prostate is described in terms of lobes (Fig. 5.14). The prostate has five lobes—two lateral lobes, an anterior lobe, a median lobe and a posterior lobe. The lateral lobes are joined by the

isthmus anteriorly and the median lobe posteriorly. In pathological terms, the prostate is divided into zones—a central zone, a peripheral zone and a transitional zone.

The fibrous capsule of the prostate completely surrounds the gland. This is surrounded by a fibrous sheath. The capsule and sheath are separated by the prostatic plexus of veins.

Blood supply arises from the inferior vesical and middle rectal arteries. Veins drain to the prostatic plexus, which eventually drains into the internal iliac veins. Lymph drains to the internal iliac and sacral nodes. Parasympathetic innervation of the prostate occurs via the pelvic splanchnic nerves, and sympathetic innervation (stimulates the smooth muscle during ejaculation) occurs via the inferior hypogastric plexus.

CLINICAL NOTES

PROSTATIC HYPERTENSION

Enlargement of the prostate may be because of benign or malignant disease. Benign enlargement (benign prostatic hypertrophy (BPH)) commonly begins after the age of 30, although it may not produce symptoms until 45 to 50 years of age. BPH commonly affects the lateral lobes or transitional zone. Outward enlargement of the gland is limited by the capsule; therefore the gland enlarges inwards, leading to compression of the urethra, resulting in urinary obstruction. It is detectable on rectal examination, producing an enlarged but smooth prostate.

Malignant disease commonly affects the posterior lobe or peripheral zone, resulting in an enlarged, hard and craggy prostate. Prostate cancer may metastasize to the lumbar vertebrae, owing to the communication between prostatic veins and the internal vertebral venous plexus in the vertebral canal.

Female reproductive organs in the pelvis

Vagina

The vagina extends from the vaginal orifice (introitus) in the vestibule, passing superiorly and posteriorly to reach the cervix of the uterus (see Fig. 5.10). The fornices of the vagina surround the vaginal portion of the cervix. There are four fornices, namely the anterior, right and left lateral and posterior fornices. The largest is the posterior fornix. The wall of the vagina is composed of three layers. An outer fibrous layer attaches the vagina to other pelvic viscera. Deep to this lies a muscular layer composed of an external longitudinal layer and an inner circular layer. The internal surface of the vagina is lined by stratified squamous epithelium. Rugae are visible on its surface, which allows distension of the vagina during

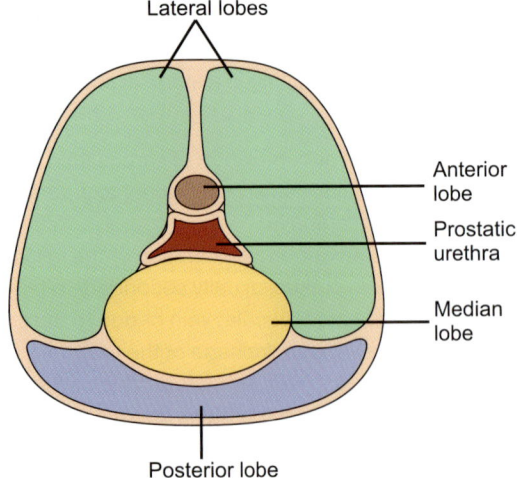

Lateral lobes

Anterior lobe

Prostatic urethra

Median lobe

Posterior lobe

Fig. 5.14 The prostate gland.

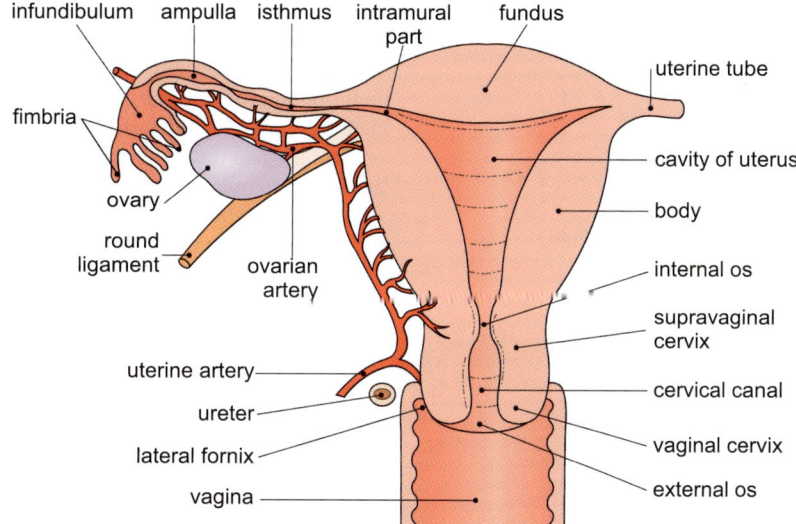

Fig. 5.15 Female reproductive system and its blood supply.

intercourse. The vagina is related to the bladder and urethra anteriorly and the rectum and anal canal posteriorly.

The superior part of the vagina is supplied by the uterine artery. The middle and inferior parts are supplied by the vaginal branches of the internal iliac and internal pudendal arteries. Veins drain into the uterine and vaginal plexuses and then into the internal iliac veins. Lymph from the upper vagina drains to the internal iliac nodes and from the lower vagina to the superficial inguinal nodes.

The upper vagina is innervated by the hypogastric plexus. The lower vagina is innervated by the pudendal and ilioinguinal nerves.

Uterus

The uterus is a muscular organ that accommodates the developing embryo. The wall is composed of an outer serosal layer, myometrium (a thick, smooth muscle layer) and a lining of endometrium. The thickness of the endometrium varies throughout the menstrual cycle and is shed during menstruation (see later).

The uterus is composed of the following regions (Fig. 5.15):

- The body: This includes the fundus, which lies superior to the openings of the fallopian tubes. The cavity of the uterus occupies the body: slitlike in transverse section, triangular in longitudinal section.
- The cervix: This is the narrowest region of the uterus and is separated from the body by the narrow isthmus. It has a supravaginal part and a vaginal part. The vaginal part is surrounded by the vaginal fornices. The endocervical canal is continuous with the uterine cavity at the internal os. The endocervical canal opens into the vagina at the external os.

The nonpregnant uterus is not usually palpable. In pregnancy, the fundus becomes palpable from about week 12 and at term will lie at the level of the xiphisternum.

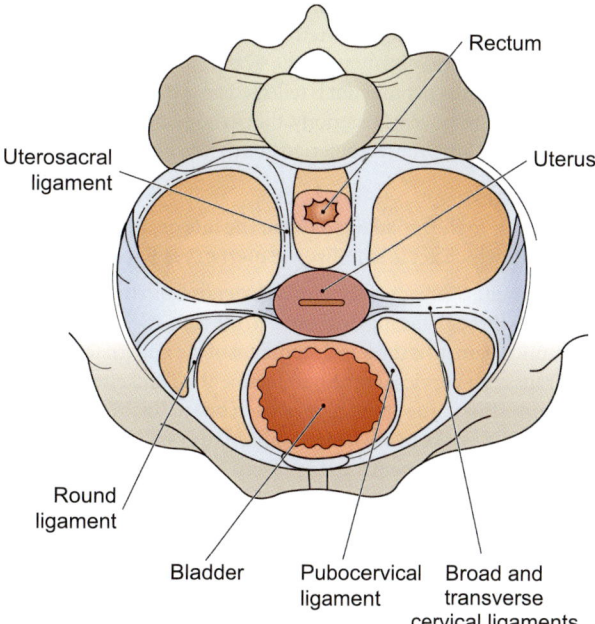

Fig. 5.16 Ligaments of the uterus, viewed from above.

The upper anterior, superior and posterior surfaces of the uterus are covered by a sheet of peritoneum. Laterally, the two layers of the peritoneum come into contact with each other, forming the broad ligament, which connects the uterus to the pelvic walls (see Fig. 5.17). The broad ligament has three divisions (Fig. 5.16):

- The mesometrium: A mesentery containing the uterus.
- The mesosalpinx: A mesentery containing the fallopian tubes.

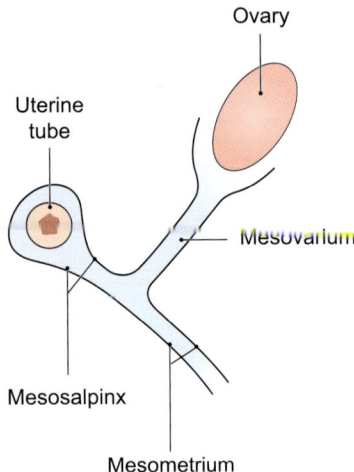

Fig. 5.17 The three sections of the broad ligament.

- The mesovarium: A mesentery containing the ovaries.

The broad ligament also contains the ovarian and uterine arteries, the ovarian ligament, the round ligament of the uterus and the suspensory ligament of the ovary.

Anteriorly, the peritoneum is reflected onto the bladder, forming the uterovesical pouch. Posteriorly, the peritoneum is reflected onto the rectum to form the rectouterine pouch (see Fig. 5.10).

Ligaments

In addition to the broad ligament of the uterus, there are several ligaments which act to stabilize the uterus (see Fig. 5.15):

- The round ligament of the uterus: Extends from the body of the uterus through the inguinal canal to the labia majora. The round ligament is the female remnant of the gubernaculum.
- Transverse cervical (cardinal) ligaments: Thickened connective tissue at the base of each broad ligament; extends from the cervix to the lateral walls of the pelvis.
- Uterosacral ligaments: Extend from the posterior aspect of the cervix to the sacrum.
- Pubocervical ligaments: Extend from the cervix and upper vagina to the posterior aspect of the pubic bones.

CLINICAL NOTES

POSITIONS OF THE UTERUS

The normal position of the uterus is anteflexed (the fundus and body point forward relative to the cervix) and anteverted (the uterus is angled forward relative to the vagina) as seen in Fig. 5.10. In approximately 20% of females, the uterus is retroverted (angled backwards)—this may cause discomfort during intercourse but has no effect on fertility.

Fallopian tubes

The fallopian tubes extend from the peritoneal cavity close to the ovaries, to the lateral horns of the uterus, at the junction of the body and fundus. They lie in the superior edge of the broad ligament (see Fig. 5.16) supported by the mesosalpinx.

The fallopian tube is composed of the conical infundibulum, the dilated ampulla (usually the site of fertilization) and the isthmus. The infundibulum, which is open to the peritoneal cavity, bears fimbriae that lie over the medial aspect of the ovary. One fimbria, the ovarian fimbria, is attached to the ovary. When the ovum is shed, it is captured by the fimbriae, enters the infundibulum and travels to the uterus.

CLINICAL NOTES

ECTOPIC PREGNANCY

A fertilized ovum, which normally implants in the uterus, may implant elsewhere, most commonly in the fallopian tube. This is known as an ectopic pregnancy. It may result in rupture of the fallopian tube and haemorrhage into the peritoneal cavity. Ectopic pregnancy is a differential diagnosis of right iliac fossa pain and may be mistaken for appendicitis. Therefore it is important to perform a pregnancy test in all females of childbearing age who present with pain in the right iliac fossa.

Vessels of the uterus and fallopian tubes

The uterine artery, a branch of the internal iliac artery, runs in the broad ligament. It anastomoses with branches of the ovarian artery. Each artery gives rise to tubal branches, which anastomose and supply the fallopian tubes (see Fig. 5.15). Veins of the uterus form a uterine plexus on either side of the cervix. The plexus empties into the uterine vein, which drains into the internal iliac vein.

Lymphatic drainage of the uterus occurs via the lumbar, superficial inguinal, internal and external iliac and sacral nodes. Lymphatic drainage of the fallopian tubes is to the aortic nodes. Innervation of the uterus arises from the inferior hypogastric plexus. Many postganglionic parasympathetic fibres arise in large pelvic ganglia close to the cervix.

Placenta

The placenta is a temporary organ that develops from the blastocyst after implantation within the uterus at around week 4 of pregnancy. It facilitates essential nutrient, gas and waste exchange between the foetal and maternal circulations. The placenta also functions as an endocrine organ producing hormones that control foetal and maternal physiology throughout pregnancy and acts as an immunological barrier.

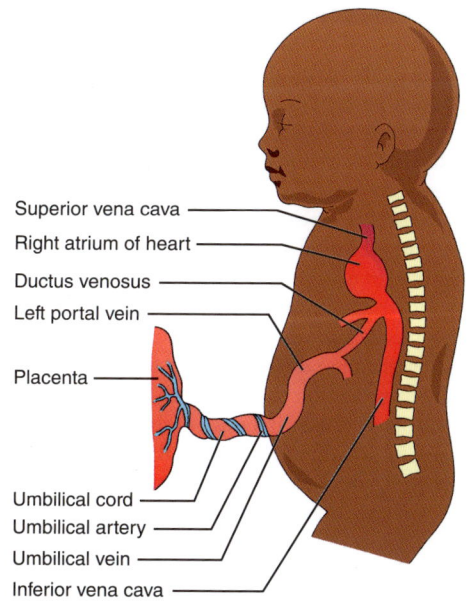

Superior vena cava
Right atrium of heart
Ductus venosus
Left portal vein
Placenta
Umbilical cord
Umbilical artery
Umbilical vein
Inferior vena cava

Fig. 5.18 The umbilical cord acts as a conduit between the placenta and the embryo or foetus.

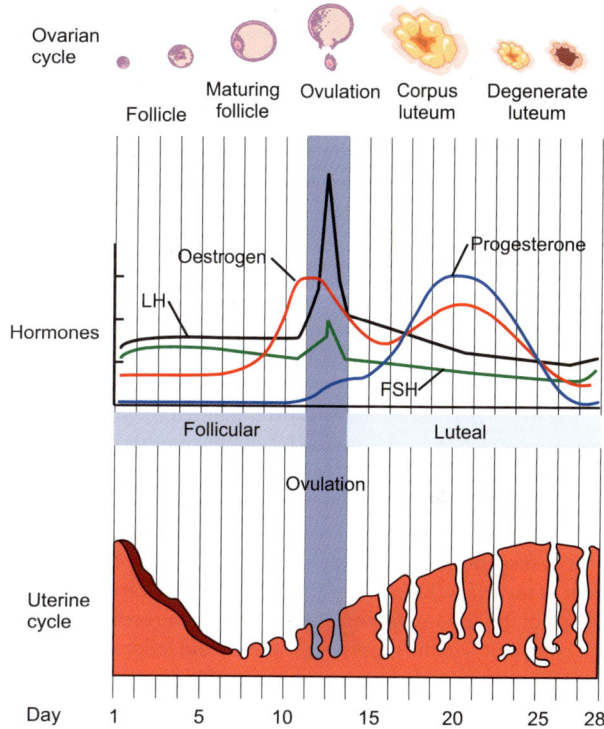

Fig. 5.19 The uterine and ovarian cycle. FSH, *Follicle-stimulating hormone*; LH, *luteinizing hormone*.

At term, the placenta is a crimson-coloured discoid shape and typically sits on the anterior or posterior wall of the uterus. It weighs approximately 470 g with a diameter of 22 cm and a thickness of 2 to 2.5 cm.

The umbilical cord acts as a conduit between the placenta and the embryo or foetus (Fig. 5.18). The umbilical cord carries two umbilical arteries and one umbilical vein; the umbilical vein carries oxygenated, nutrient-rich blood from the placenta to the foetus and the umbilical arteries return deoxygenated, nutrient-deplete blood from the foetus to the placenta.

Overview of uterine physiology including menstrual cycle

The innermost layer of the uterus, the endometrium, is highly responsive to endocrine influence. Throughout each monthly menstrual cycle, the endometrium goes through three phases: menses, proliferative and secretory (Fig. 5.19).

Menses typically lasts for 3 to 5 days (although 2–7 days is considered normal) and occurs as the result of a female not becoming pregnant during the previous menstrual cycle. During this stage, the thickened endometrial wall breaks down and is noticed as passing blood from the vagina. During this stage, a female may lose 10 to 80 mL in this manner; excessive blood loss, menorrhagia, may lead to an iron deficiency anaemia. Menses can also be accompanied by lower abdominal/back cramping pain and mood changes.

The proliferative phase follows in response to an increase in oestrogen, released by maturing follicles in the ovary. The oestrogen initiates a new layer of endometrium to form – proliferative endometrium. Fertile cervical mucus is also produced from cervical crypts.

The final stage of the uterine cycle is the secretory phase. It typically occurs in collaboration with the luteal phase of the ovarian cycle where progesterone is produced from the corpus luteum. These progesterones act in a 'pro-pregnancy' manner and make the endometrium receptive to a blastocyst to implant. It does this by increasing uterine blood flow and secretions, as well as reducing myometrial contractions.

If at the end of the secretory stage, pregnancy has not been achieved, menses will begin with the above cycle repeated.

Ovaries

The ovary lies in the ovarian fossa (between the internal and external iliac vessels), closely related to the obturator nerve. It contains ova and produces oestrogen and progesterone.

The ovary is attached to the broad ligament by the mesovarium. It is attached to the uterus by the ligament of the ovary, which runs between the two layers of the broad ligament, and is continuous with the round ligament, both being remnants of the gubernaculum (see Fig. 5.17).

It is suspended from the pelvic wall by the suspensory ligament of the ovary. Blood supply arises from the ovarian artery, a branch of the abdominal aorta which runs in the broad ligament and contributes to the supply of the uterus and fallopian tubes by anastomosing with the uterine artery. An ovarian venous plexus communicates with the uterine venous plexus. Two ovarian veins follow the artery: the right ovarian vein drains into the inferior vena cava and the left vein drains into the left renal vein. Innervation of the ovary arises from the ovarian plexus. Lymphatic drainage is to aortic nodes.

Overview of ovarian physiology including hormonal control

Each ovary is responsible for producing egg cells, the female gamete. On starting puberty, a female has around 400,000 eggs; however, only a small fraction (<1%) of these progress to maturation and subsequent ovulation. Within each ovarian cortex lie follicles. Within each follicle lies a primary oocyte as well as support cells and hormone-producing cells. It is within these follicles that the oocytes mature before being released for potential fertilization. During each menstrual cycle (see Fig. 5.19), a single mature egg is released from either the left or right ovary (rarely, both may release an egg). It is poorly understood which ovary releases an egg each month, although it appears entirely random.

The ovarian cycle is divided into three phases:

- The follicular phase.
- Ovulation.
- The luteal phase.

During the follicular stage, a few ovarian follicles that have been developing for approximately a year already are stimulated to develop further. This occurs through the influence of follicle-stimulating hormone (FSH), which is released from the anterior pituitary gland. Under the control of a variety of hormones, one follicle will become dominant and continue to full maturation; the other follicles will shrink and die.

As the egg nears maturation, oestradiol levels increase to a level that exceeds a certain threshold. Above this threshold, the previously suppressed luteinizing hormone (LH) spikes; this is known as the LH surge and may last 48 hours. This level of LH matures the egg further before weakening the follicle wall, causing the developed follicle to release a secondary oocyte, which subsequently becomes an ootid and then a mature ovum. This occurs from either the left or right ovary, randomly. The released egg is then swept into the fallopian tube by the fimbria. If fertilization is to occur, it typically happens in the ampulla of the fallopian tube. However, if fertilization does not occur, the unfertilized egg will break up and dissolve after approximately 24 hours.

The luteal phase is the final stage of the cycle. The remains of the dominant follicle that has released the egg becomes the corpus luteum, which develops in the presence of LH and FSH from the pituitary gland. The corpus luteum produces high levels of progesterone, a key controlling factor of the secretory phase of the uterine cycle. The level of progesterone also induces the production of oestrogen. Both oestrogen and progesterone subsequently suppress the production of FSH and LH. This reduced level of FSH and LH causes the atrophy of the corpus luteum, reducing progesterone levels and triggering menstruation. If the egg becomes fertilized, the syncytiotrophoblast (part of the embryo-containing structure) releases human chorionic gonadotropin (hCG). hCG supports the existence of the corpus luteum which continues to produce progesterone and support the pregnancy.

Pregnancy

Pregnancy is the physiological process that occurs in females, starting with fertilization and concluding with childbirth. Typically, pregnancy lasts for 40 weeks from the beginning of the last menstrual period and is divided into three trimesters (weeks 1–12, 13–26 and 27–40).

During pregnancy, body systems within the mother are required to adapt to meet the physiological demands of pregnancy. These physiological adaptations are required to support and protect the foetus while also preparing maternal physiology and anatomy for labour. These changes are briefly summarized below:

- Endocrine: Changing levels of hormones such as hCG, oestrogen and progesterone, which are essential for maintaining the pregnancy, supporting foetal growth and preparing the mother for labour.
- Cardiovascular: To increase the supply of nutrients and oxygen to the foetus, blood volume and cardiac output increase during pregnancy. Mean arterial blood pressure remains largely unchanged.
- Respiratory: The developing foetus puts a greater oxygen demand on the mother and the growing uterus causes the diaphragm to rise. As pregnancy progresses, ribs flare outwards, and both tidal volume and vital capacity increase in response.
- Gastrointestinal: Hormonal changes cause slower digestion and delayed gastric emptying. Coupled with pressure on the stomach from the growing uterus, this can result in symptoms of reflux and nausea.
- Haematological: Pregnancy results in a hypercoagulable state. This helps to protect the mother from significant blood loss during labour but increases the risks of thromboembolic diseases.
- Musculoskeletal: The growing uterus changes the centre of gravity and causes an exaggerated lumbar lordosis. In addition, hormonal changes cause the loosening of ligaments, preparing the pelvis for delivery.

> ### CLINICAL NOTES
>
> #### SHORTNESS OF BREATH IN PREGNANCY
>
> Shortness of breath (dyspnoea) is a common symptom for pregnant mothers. Although it is essential to consider pathologies such as pulmonary embolus and anaemia, the sensation of dyspnoea can be normal during pregnancy, especially during the third trimester of pregnancy.

Labour

Labour refers to the process by which the female body facilitates the delivery of a baby and is divided into three stages:

- First stage: From the onset of established labour until full cervical dilation.
- Second stage: From full cervical dilation until the birth of the baby.
- Third stage: From the birth of the baby until the delivery of the placenta and membranes.

The mechanism of normal labour allows the foetus to negotiate the pelvic anatomy and is determined by the interaction of three factors: passage, passenger and power.

- Passage refers to the structure of the bony pelvis and soft tissues and the suitability of the pelvis to facilitate the delivery of a foetus through it.

- Passenger refers to the size, position and attitude of the foetus as it travels through the pelvis.
- Power refers to the strength of contractions and maternal efforts during the second stage of labour.

In addition to the passage, passenger and power, clinicians also refer to psyche, which takes into consideration the emotional state of the mother during the progression of labour. Relevant considerations include stress levels, exhaustion, anxiety about the process and an adequate supportive environment.

The cardinal movements are the innate specific movements of the foetus to ensure passage through the birth canal. The seven cardinal movements are engagement, descent, flexion, internal rotation, extension, external rotation (restitution) and expulsion (Fig. 5.20).

> ### CLINICAL NOTES
>
> #### CARDIOTOCOGRAM
>
> During labour a cardiotocogram can be used to assess the response of the baby to uterine contractions and help guide medical decisions regarding the delivery. It involves measuring foetal heart rate alongside uterine contractions over time.

Menopause

Menopause is a natural biological process and refers to the permanent cessation of menstrual periods. Menopause can be diagnosed after greater than 12 months of absent menstruation with perimenopause referring to the preceding ill-defined period of time that surrounds the final years of a female's fertility. In the United Kingdom, the average age of menopause is 51, and it generally occurs between the ages of 45 and 55 years. Premature menopause occurs before the age of 40 and is often induced by medical interventions such as chemoradiotherapy or surgery.

Menopause can present with a variety of symptoms, commonly including hot flushes, muscle aches, mood disturbance, decreased libido and vaginal dryness. Hormone replacement therapy (HRT) is used to address these symptoms and can contain oestrogen and progesterone or oestrogen alone, depending on whether the patient has had a hysterectomy.

> ### CLINICAL NOTES
>
> #### MENOPAUSE MANAGEMENT
>
> HRT is a successful treatment for many patients; however, as with all drugs, it is not without risks. It is therefore important to also discuss with patients the benefits of conservative options that can include lifestyle changes and cognitive behavioural therapy.

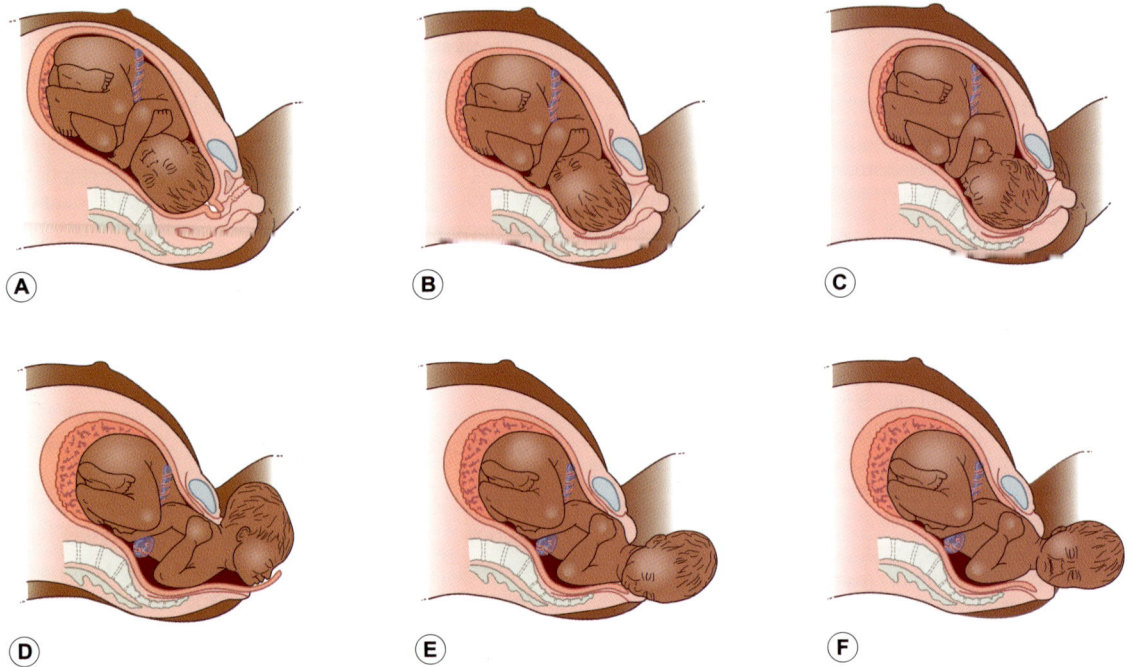

Fig. 5.20 The mechanisms of normal labour involve (A) engagement and descent of the presenting part; (B) flexion of the head; (C) internal rotation; (D) extension of the foetal head; (E) external rotation; (F) expulsion.

Vessels of the pelvis

The pelvis is mainly supplied by the internal iliac arteries and the internal iliac veins.

Internal iliac artery

The common iliac artery bifurcates at L4/5, typically at the pelvic brim near the sacroiliac joint. It separates into the internal and external arteries (Fig. 5.21). The internal iliac artery passes inferiorly and branches into anterior and posterior divisions. The branches may be divided into:

- Those supplying the body wall (iliolumbar, lateral sacral).
- Those leaving the pelvis to supply the lower limb and gluteal region (obturator, superior and inferior gluteal).
- The visceral branches (superior and inferior vesical, uterine, vaginal, middle rectal, etc.).

Internal iliac vein

The internal iliac vein commences at the greater sciatic notch and passes superiorly out of the pelvis, posterior to the artery, on the medial surface of psoas major. At the pelvic brim, it joins the external iliac vein to form the common iliac vein. Tributaries include:

- Veins corresponding to the arteries.
- The uterine and vesicoprostatic venous plexuses.

- The rectal venous plexuses.
- The lateral sacral veins (the internal iliac vein communicates with the vertebral venous plexus via the veins).
- The obturator vein.

Nerves of the pelvis

Obturator nerve

The obturator nerve supplies the adductor compartment of the thigh by piercing the medial border of psoas muscle and passing on the lateral wall of the pelvis to the obturator foramen. The obturator nerve passes through the obturator foramen into the thigh. It supplies the adductor compartment of the thigh and skin on the medial surface of the thigh.

CLINICAL NOTES

OOPHORECTOMY COMPLICATIONS

The obturator nerve may be damaged during removal of the ovaries (oophorectomy). This results in spasm of adductor muscles of the thigh and cutaneous sensory loss over the medial thigh and knee.

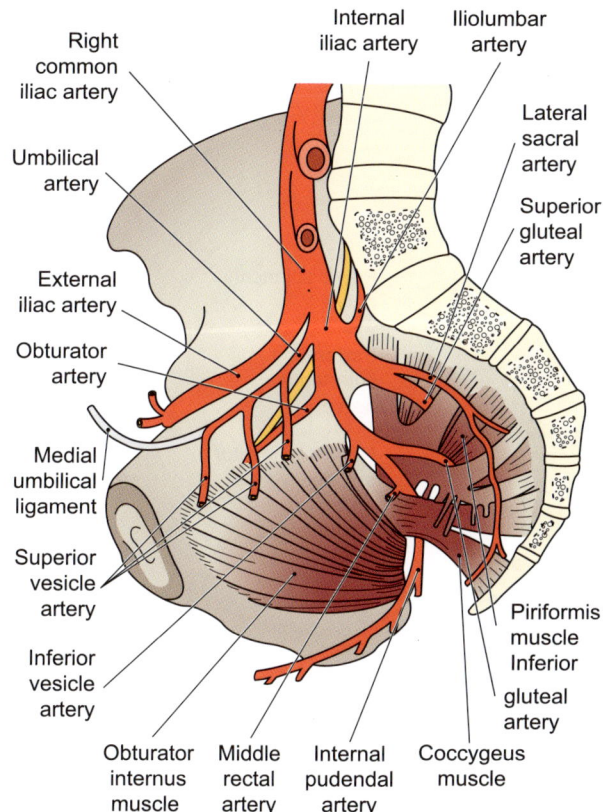

Fig. 5.21 Branches of the internal iliac artery.

Labels (clockwise):
Right common iliac artery · Umbilical artery · External iliac artery · Obturator artery · Medial umbilical ligament · Superior vesicle artery · Inferior vesicle artery · Obturator internus muscle · Middle rectal artery · Internal pudendal artery · Coccygeus muscle · Inferior gluteal artery · Piriformis muscle · Superior gluteal artery · Lateral sacral artery · Iliolumbar artery · Internal iliac artery

---

HINTS AND TIPS

LOWER LIMB VENOUS DRAINAGE

If venous drainage of the lower limb becomes obstructed, the pelvic veins enlarge and provide an alternative route for venous return.

Sacral plexus

The sacral plexus lies on piriformis muscle, covered by pelvic fascia. The lateral sacral arteries and veins lie anterior to the plexus. The plexus is formed by the anterior rami of L4 and L5 spinal nerves (the lumbosacral trunk) and the anterior rami of S1 to S4 spinal nerves (Fig. 5.22). The sacral nerves and lumbosacral trunk give off branches and then divide into the anterior and posterior divisions.

Sacral sympathetic trunk

The sacral sympathetic trunk crosses the pelvic brim behind the common iliac vessels. There are four ganglia along each trunk which unite in front of the coccyx at the ganglion impar. The sacral sympathetic trunk gives somatic branches to all the sacral nerves and visceral branches to the inferior hypogastric plexus.

Inferior hypogastric plexus

The right and left inferior hypogastric plexuses comprise the pelvic plexuses (Fig. 5.23). They lie on the side wall of the pelvis, lateral to the rectum. They receive the right and left hypogastric nerves from the superior hypogastricplexus.

Branches of the plexus are visceral. Functions include the control of micturition, defecation, emission, erection, ejaculation and orgasm.

PERINEUM

The perineum describes the area between the superior medial aspects of the thighs. The superior boundary is the pelvic diaphragm, and the inferior boundary is the skin and superficial fascia. The perineum is a diamond-shaped region, divided into an anterior urogenital triangle and a posterior anal triangle by an imaginary line drawn between the two ischial tuberosities. The boundaries of the perineum are illustrated in Fig. 5.24.

The blood and nerve supply to the perineum arises from the pudendal artery and nerve (S2–S4).

Anal triangle

The boundaries of the anal triangle are (see Fig. 5.24):

- Anteriorly: an imaginary transverse line between the ischial tuberosities.
- Laterally: the sacrotuberous ligaments.
- Apex: tip of the coccyx.
- Base: superficial transverse perineal muscles.

It contains the two ischioanal fossae separated in the midline by the anal canal, the internal and external anal sphincters, the anococcygeal ligament and the perineal body. The triangle slopes anteriorly and inferiorly from its apex. Muscles of the anal triangle are outlined in Table 5.3.

CLINICAL NOTES

PERINEAL TEAR

Perineal tear refers to trauma that occurs between the vaginal opening and anus during vaginal childbirth. There are four degrees of perineal tear depending on how far the tear extends towards or into the anus. An episiotomy is a preemptive surgical incision through the pelvic floor muscles in a mediolateral direction away from the anus. This is performed to prevent perineal tears during childbirth which can ultimately threaten the integrity of the anus.

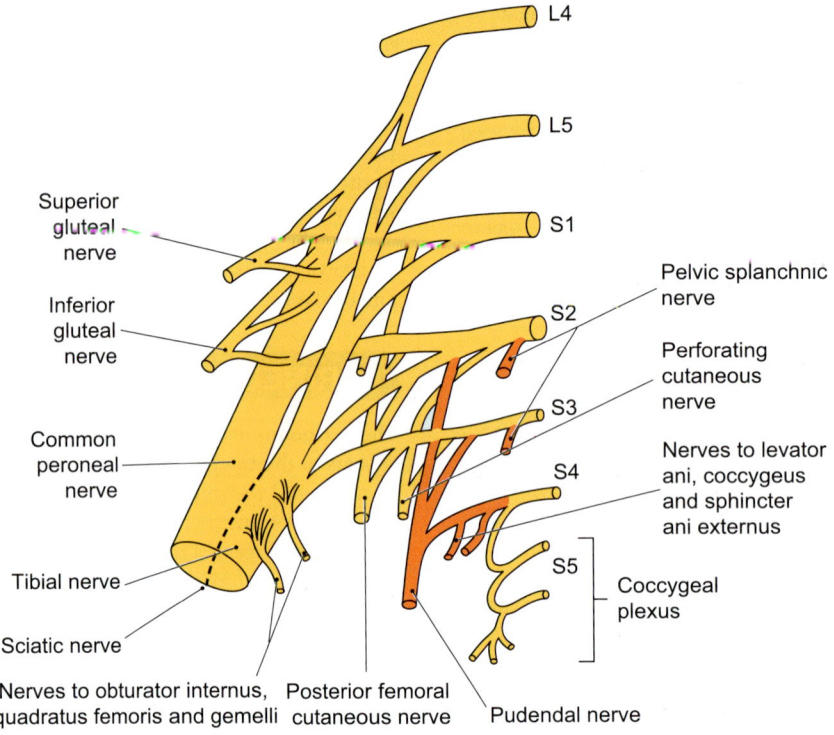

Fig. 5.22 Sacral plexus.

Anal canal

The anal canal is approximately 4 cm long. It commences at the anorectal junction, where it forms a sharp angle with the rectum, owing to traction of the puborectalis muscle at the level of the pelvic floor. The anal canal ends at the anus.

Lining of the anal canal

The anal canal is divided into an upper two-thirds and a lower one-third by the dentate line. The upper part is lined by columnar epithelium. The anal canal features longitudinal folds known as anal columns. Inferiorly, the columns are linked by horizontal folds, forming the anal valves. The recesses between the columns and valves are known as the anal sinuses, into which the anal glands open. The lower margins of the anal valves lie at the dentate line. The lower one-third of the canal is lined by stratified squamous epithelium, as is the skin around the anus (Table 5.4).

Muscular wall of the anal canal

The anal canal is lined by mucous membrane, which is surrounded by the muscular internal and external anal sphincters (Fig. 5.25).

The internal anal sphincter is a continuation of the circular smooth muscle of the rectum. It surrounds the upper part of the anal canal. The internal anal sphincter is innervated by the hypogastric and pelvic plexuses (sympathetic) and the pelvic plexus (parasympathetic).

The external anal sphincter is striated and under voluntary control via the perineal branch of S4 spinal nerve and the inferior rectal nerve (a branch of the pudendal nerve). The external anal sphincter is connected to the coccyx via the anococcygeal body. Superiorly, the external anal sphincter blends with puborectalis muscle. In combination with the internal anal sphincter, this forms the anorectal ring. The anorectal ring is the chief muscle of continence.

Table 5.4 shows the blood supply and lymphatic drainage of the anal canal. Veins anastomose, forming an internal rectal plexus inside the submucosa and an external rectal plexus outside the muscular wall.

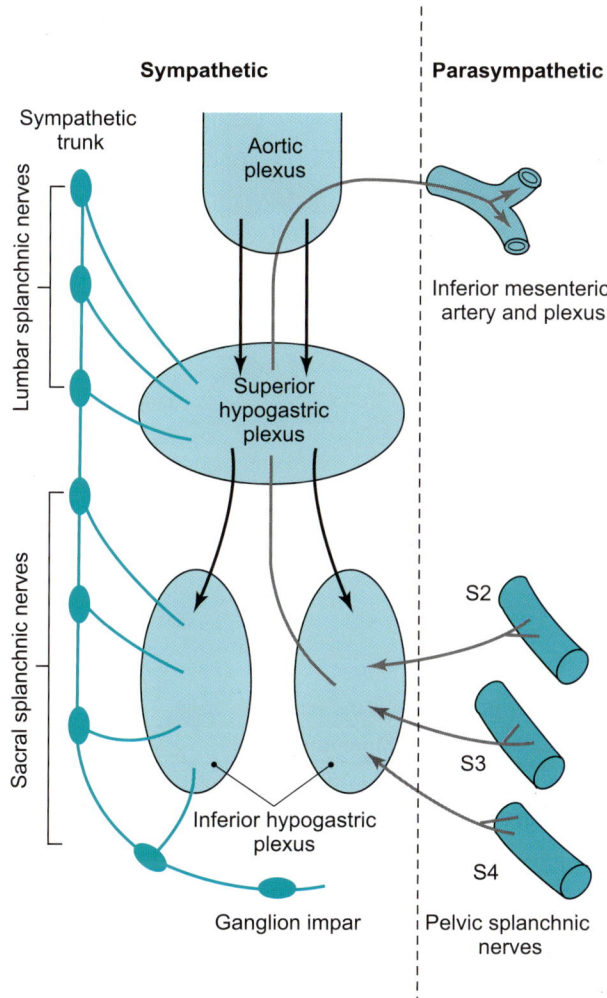

Fig. 5.23 Autonomic plexuses in the pelvis.

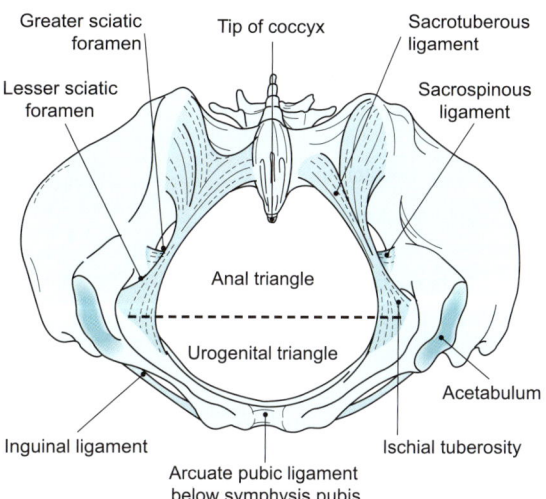

Fig. 5.24 Boundaries of the perineum.

Table 5.3 Muscles of the anal triangle

Name of muscle (nerve supply)	Origin	Insertion	Action
External anal sphincter—subcutaneous part (inferior rectal nerve and perineal branch of fourth sacral nerve)	Encircles anal canal, no bony attachments	Anococcygeal ligament	Voluntary sphincter of anal canal
External anal sphincter—superficial part (inferior rectal nerve and perineal branch of fourth sacral nerve)	Perineal body	Coccyx	
External anal sphincter—deep part (inferior rectal nerve and perineal branch of fourth sacral nerve)	Encircles anal canal	Coccyx	

Adapted from Moore, K. L. (1996). Essential clinical anatomy. Williams & Wilkins.

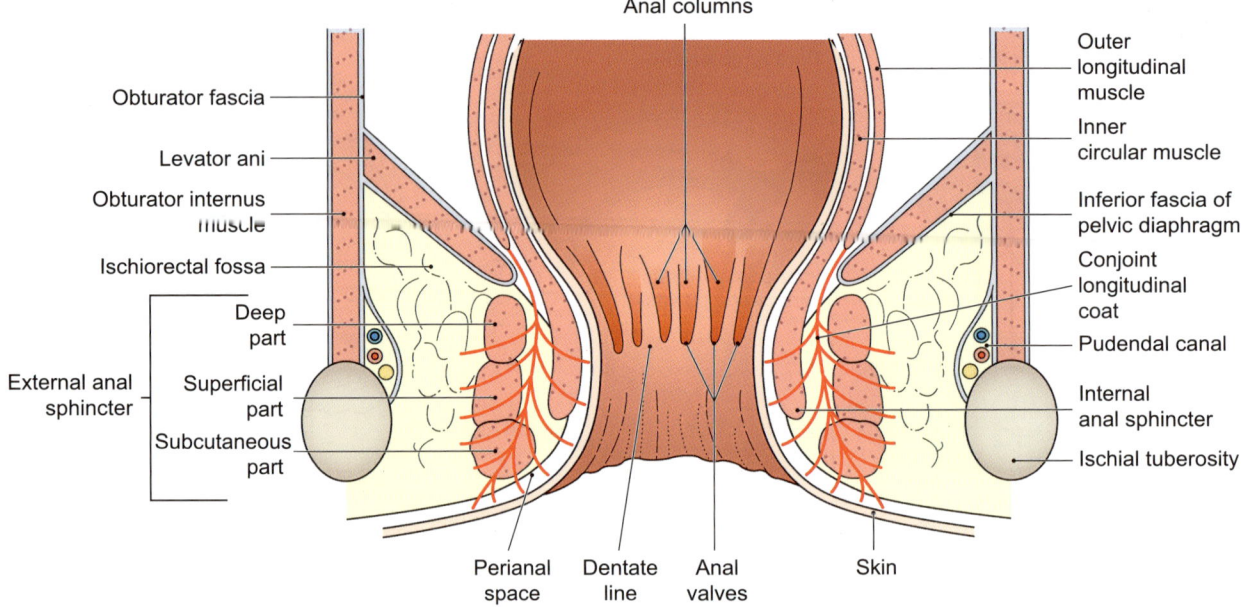

Fig. 5.25 Anal canal and ischioanal fossa.

Table 5.4 Blood supply, lymphatic drainage and nerve supply of the anal canal

	Above dentate line	Below dentate line
Epithelium	Columnar (mucosa)	Stratified squamous
Arteries	Superior rectal (from inferior mesenteric)	Middle and inferior rectal (from internal iliac)
Venous drainage	Superior rectal vein	Middle and inferior rectal veins
Lymphatic drainage	Internal iliac nodes	Superficial inguinal nodes
Nerve supply	Visceral–inferior hypogastric plexus Sensitive to stretch	Somatic–inferior rectal from pudendal (S2–S4) Sensitive to pain, touch, etc.

Table 5.5 Boundaries of the ischioanal fossa

Boundary	Components
Base	Skin over anal region of perineum
Medial wall	Anal canal and levator ani
Lateral wall	Ischial tuberosity and obturator internus
Apex	Where levator ani is attached to its tendinous origins over obturator fascia
Anterior extension	Superior to deep perineal pouch

CLINICAL NOTES

ISCHIOANAL FOSSA

The adipose tissue of the ischioanal fossa has a poor blood supply. Therefore it is vulnerable to infection and abscess formation.

Ischioanal fossa and pudendal canal

The ischioanal fossa lies lateral to the anal canal, is filled with adipose tissue and contains the pudendal canal. The pudendal canal is roofed by fascia that is continuous with the obturator internus fascia above and which fuses with the ischial tuberosity below. The canal contains the internal pudendal vessels and the pudendal nerve, which pass from the lesser sciatic foramen to the deep perineal pouch. The fossa also contains the inferior rectal arteries and nerves (see Fig. 5.25). Its boundaries are detailed in Table 5.5.

The male urogenital triangle

The male urogenital triangle is bounded posteriorly by an imaginary transverse line between the two ischial tuberosities. Its lateral boundaries are the ischiopubic rami, which meet anteriorly at the pubic symphysis (see Fig. 5.24).

Within the urogenital triangle lies the deep perineal space, lying inferior to the anterior part of the levator ani muscle, and superior to the perineal membrane. The deep perineal space contains the following structures 'sandwiched' between superior and inferior layers of fascia:

- Deep transverse perineal muscles.
- Sphincter urethrae.
- Membranous urethra.
- Bulbourethral glands.
- Pudendal vessels (continuing forward from the pudendal canal).
- Dorsal nerve of the penis.

Loose pelvic fascia forms the superior fascial layer of the deep space. The inferior fascial layer forms the inferior boundary of the deep perineal space. This layer is known as the perineal membrane. It is attached to the ischiopubic rami, from immediately posterior to the pubic symphysis to the ischial tuberosities. In the anatomical position, it lies horizontally. The urethra penetrates the deep perineal space and perineal membrane (Fig. 5.26).

The perineal membrane, sphincter urethrae and pelvic fascia together constitute the urogenital diaphragm. The bulbourethral glands are two small glands lying on either side of the membranous urethra (see Fig. 5.26)—their ducts pierce the perineal membrane to enter the spongy part of the urethra and their secretions contribute to seminal fluid.

Between the perineal membrane and the superficial perineal fascia (of Colles) lies the superficial perineal space. Table 5.6 outlines the muscles of the urogenital triangle. These muscles are involved in micturition, copulation and support of the pelvic viscera.

> **HINTS AND TIPS**
>
> **PUDENDAL NERVE**
>
> The pudendal nerve supplies levator ani (S2–S4)—so remember: S2, 3, 4, keep your guts off the floor.

Superficial perineal space

The superficial perineal space is lined inferiorly by Colles fascia, a continuation of the membranous superficial fascia (Scarpa fascia) of the anterior abdominal wall, which descends to line the scrotum. Superiorly, the space is limited by the perineal membrane. The contents of the space include the root of the penis, the superficial transverse perineal, bulbospongiosus and ischiocavernosus muscles, and the perineal branches of the internal pudendal artery and pudendal nerve.

The male external genitalia

The male external genitalia consist of the penis and the scrotum.

Penis

The penis is suspended from the pubic symphysis by its suspensory ligament. The penis consists of the root, the shaft and the glans (Fig. 5.27).

The root of the penis is composed of three masses of erectile tissue: the bulb of the penis and the right and left crura. The bulb

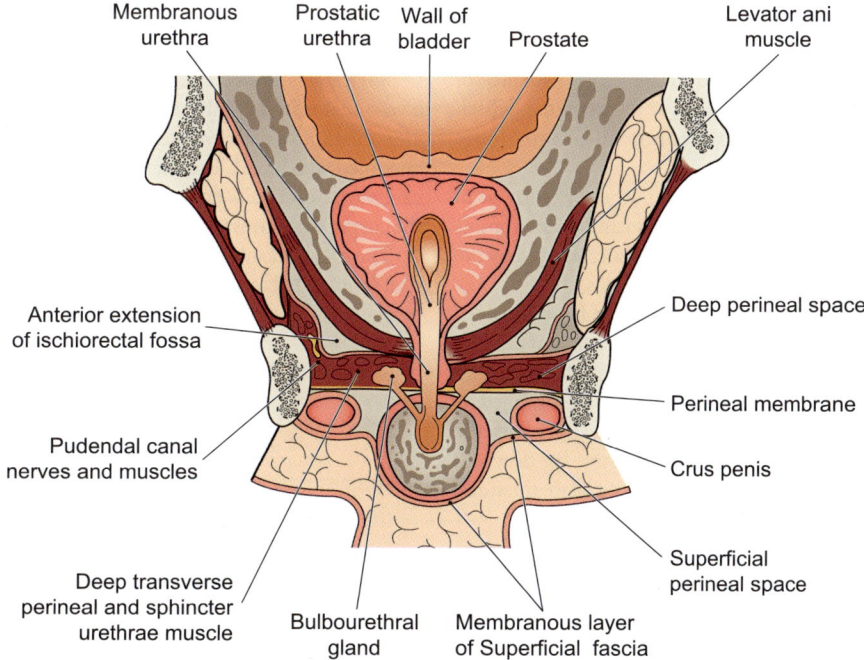

Fig. 5.26 Coronal section of the male perineum.

Table 5.6 Muscles of the urogenital triangle

Name of muscle (nerve supply)	Origin	Insertion	Action
Superficial transverse perineal muscle (perineal branch of pudendal nerve)	Ischial tuberosity	Perineal body	Fixes perineal body
Bulbospongiosus (perineal branch of pudendal nerve)	Perineal body and median raphe in male, perineal body in female	Fascia of bulb of penis and corpora spongiosum and cavernosum in male, fascia of bulbs of vestibule in female	In males, empties urethra after micturition and ejaculation and assists in erection of penis; in females, sphincter of vagina and assists in erection of clitoris
Ischiocavernosus (perineal branch of pudendal nerve)	Ischial tuberosity and ischial ramus in male and female	Fascia covering corpus cavernosum	Erection of penis or clitoris
Deep transverse perineal muscle (perineal branch of pudendal nerve)	Ramus of ischium	Perineal body	Fixes perineal body
Sphincter urethrae (perineal branch of pudendal nerve)	Pubic arch	Surrounds urethra	Voluntary sphincter of urethra, important muscle of urinary incontinence

and crurae are partially surrounded by the bulbospongiosus and ischiocavernosus muscles.

Distally, the crurae become the corpora cavernosa and the bulb becomes the corpus spongiosum. Cavernous spaces are present in the erectile tissue of the corpus cavernosa. The urethra passes through the corpus spongiosum, which passes from the erectile tissue of the bulb to end at the external urethral orifice. The distal end of the corpus spongiosum expands to form the glans penis. At the proximal part of the glans penis, the skin is reflected on itself to form the prepuce (foreskin), which covers the glans. The prepuce is attached to the ventral surface of the glans by a fold of skin, the frenulum of the prepuce, which contains a small artery. The shaft is surrounded by thin, loose skin.

A tough tunica albuginea surrounds the corpora cavernosa of the penis. Superficial to the corpora cavernosa and corpus spongiosum lies the deep fascia of the penis. This is surrounded by the superficial fascia of the penis.

The crura and corpora cavernosa receive blood from the deep arteries of the penis. These vessels allow rapid distension of the cavernous spaces to produce an erection (under the control of parasympathetic nerves). The bulb and corpus spongiosum are supplied by the bulbourethral artery. The dorsal artery supplies the glans, the prepuce and the skin of the penis. Venous drainage is to the deep and superficial dorsal veins. Lymph drains to the superficial inguinal and subinguinal lymph nodes.

Parasympathetic nerves (responsible for erection) and sensory nerves (dorsal nerves supplying the skin) to the penis arise from the pudendal nerves (S2–S4). The dorsal nerve of the penis runs with the dorsal artery of the penis. It passes over the dorsum of the penis lateral to the artery and terminates in the glans.

Physiology of a penile erection

A penile erection describes the phenomenon whereby the penis becomes enlarged and engorged, often a result of sexual arousal, although it also occurs spontaneously. For an erection to occur, a complex interaction of neural, vascular, psychological and endocrine factors is required. For example, the cerebral cortex may initiate a voluntary erection (in response to auditory, visual, tactile stimuli) or the erection may be initiated in the presence of mechanical stimulation and an absence of input from the cortex.

The parasympathetic nervous system of the autonomic nervous system triggers an erection. This causes a rise in nitric oxide, acting as a vasodilator in the trabecular arteries and penile smooth muscle. This dilation of arteries causes the corpora cavernosa to become engorged with blood. These arterial changes are aided by the ischiocavernosus and bulbospongiosus muscles to compress the veins of the corpora cavernosa, preventing blood flow from the penis.

The erection subsides after the cessation of stimulus, ejaculation (controlled by the sympathetic nervous system) or parasympathetic activity reduces to baseline.

HINTS AND TIPS

ERECTION AND EJACULATION

Parasympathetic activity arouses a penis to become erect and 'point' upwards. Sympathetic innervation is involved in the process of ejaculation, causing the 'shooting' of ejaculate from the urethra. Remember, 'point and shoot', due to parasympathetic and sympathetic innervation, respectively.

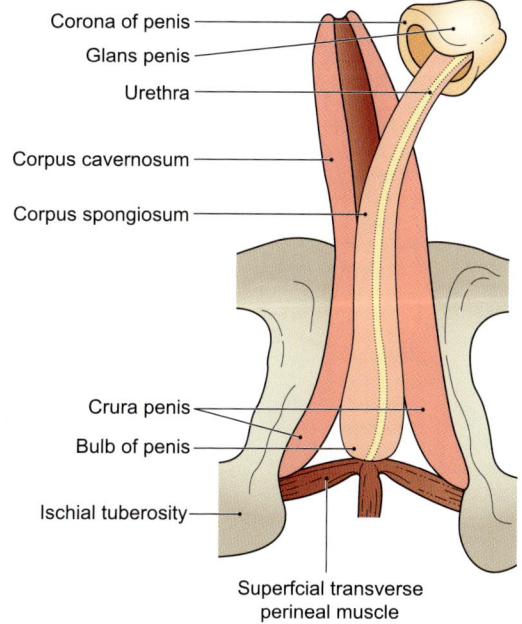

Table 5.7 Branches of the urogenital triangle	
Vessel	**Course and distribution**
Inferior rectal artery	Crosses the ischiorectal fossa to supply the muscles and skin of the anal canal
Perineal branch	Passes to the superficial perineal space to supply its muscles and the scrotum in males or labia in female
Artery to bulb of penis or clitoris	Supplies the erectile tissue of the bulb of the penis and corpus spongiosum in males or the bulb of the vestibule in females
Dorsal artery of penis or clitoris	Passes to the dorsum of the penis or clitoris. It supplies the erectile tissue of the corpus cavernosum and superficial structures in both males and females
Urethral artery	Supplies the urethra

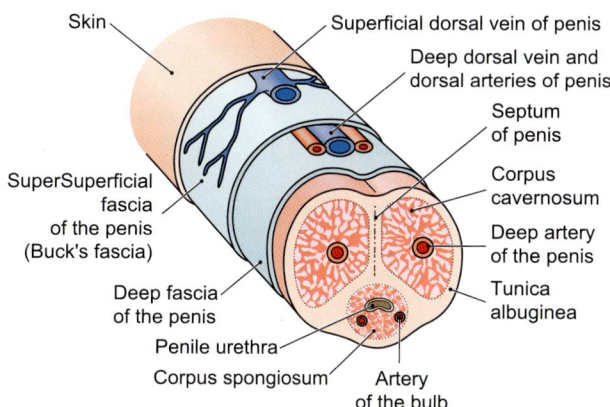

Fig. 5.27 Composition and structure of the penis.

Vessels of the male urogenital triangle

The internal pudendal artery is a branch of the internal iliac artery. It exits the pelvis via the greater sciatic foramen to enter the pudendal canal, entering the perineum via the lesser sciatic foramen at the ischial spine. At the anterior end of the canal, the internal pudendal artery enters the deep perineal pouch and continues forward on the deep surface of the perineal membrane. It terminates by dividing into the dorsal and deep arteries of the penis or clitoris. Branches of the internal pudendal artery are outlined in Table 5.7.

The internal pudendal veins are the venae comitantes of the arteries. The deep dorsal vein of the penis drains into the prostatic plexus. The superficial dorsal vein of the penis drains to the superficial pudendal vein, which drains to the femoral vein.

Nerves of the male urogenital triangle

The pudendal nerve (S2–S4) passes with the internal pudendal artery through the lesser sciatic foramen and the pudendal canal, where it gives rise to the inferior rectal nerve. The inferior rectal nerve supplies the external anal sphincter and the skin around the anus. At the posterior border of the perineal membrane, the nerve divides into the perineal nerve and the dorsal nerve of the penis. The perineal nerve passes superficial to the perineal membrane and supplies the scrotum posteriorly and all the remaining striated muscles of the perineum. Spinal segments S2 to S4 are therefore essential for continence.

The female urogenital triangle

The muscles, fasciae and spaces of the female urogenital triangle are similar to those of the male urogenital triangle. However, certain features differ because of the presence of the vagina and external female genitalia; the vagina pierces both superficial and deep perineal spaces. The deep perineal space also lacks the female equivalent of the bulbourethral gland.

The superficial perineal space again is similar to that of the male. However, it is lined by a less-defined superficial perineal fascia, is full of fat, is smaller and is found within the labia majora.

Perineal membrane

The perineal membrane is wider in the female since the pelvis is wider. It is also weaker than in the male because of the presence of the vagina. As the urethra and vagina pierce the membrane, their outer fascial covering fuses with it.

Perineal body

In the female, the perineal body lies between the vagina and the anal canal. The perineal body lacks support from the perineal membrane because of the presence of the vagina, so the perineal body in the female has greater mobility. The superficial and deep transverse perineal muscles, pubovaginalis and bulbospongiosus muscles and the superficial part of the external anal sphincter are attached to the perineal body.

> **CLINICAL NOTES**
>
> **FEMALE GENITAL MUTILATION (FGM)**
>
> FGM includes all nonmedical procedures involving partial or total removal of the external female genitalia or any other injury to the female genital organs. It is illegal to perform or facilitate FGM in the United Kingdom. There are four types of FGM, which are distinguished by the extent of genital tissue that is removed or altered.

The female external genitalia

The female external genitalia consist of the following structures, which together comprise the vulva (Fig. 5.28):

- Mons pubis: The mound of coarse-haired skin and fat anterior to the pubic symphysis. The mons pubis extends posteriorly as the labia majora.
- Labium majus: Two fatty folds of skin, joined anteriorly to form the anterior commissure, and continuous with the mons pubis. The labia pass posteriorly blending into the skin near the anus, forming the posterior commissure, which overlies the perineal body.
- Labium minus: Skin folds lying within the labia majus, surrounding the vestibule of the vagina. They enclose the clitoris, by forming the prepuce in front and the frenulum behind.
- Clitoris: Consists of two erectile crura attached to the perineal membrane and ischiopubic rami. Anteriorly, the crura become the corpora cavernosa. These are bound together by fascia to form the body of the clitoris. The external part of the clitoris is known as the glans clitoris and is covered by the clitoral hood (Fig. 5.29).

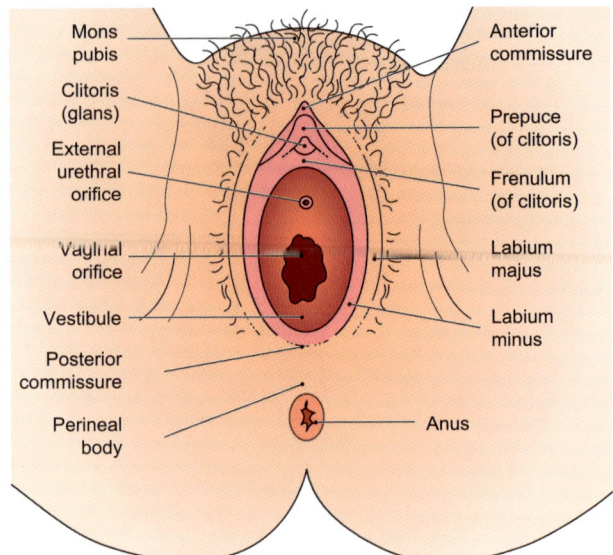

Fig. 5.28 Female external genitalia.

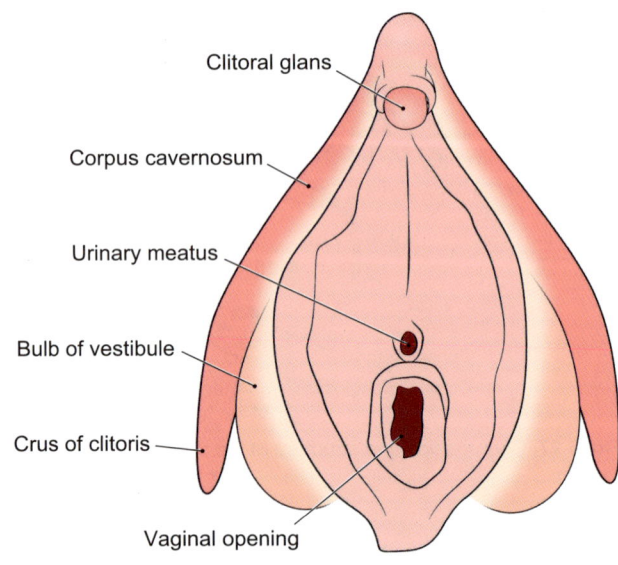

Fig. 5.29 Clitoris.

- Vestibule: Contains the openings of the greater vestibular (Bartholin) glands, the vagina and the external urethral orifice.
- Bulb of the vestibule: These are two erectile masses, either side of the vagina and are attached to the perineal membrane. Anteriorly, they join the glans of the clitoris. Each is covered by the bulbospongiosus muscle.

- Greater vestibular (Bartholin) glands: These are found in the superficial perineal pouch, in contact with the posterior end of the bulb of the vestibule. Their ducts open into the vestibule and lubricate the vagina in sexual arousal.
- Vagina: Superiorly, the vagina passes through the pelvic floor, surrounded by part of the puborectalis. Anteriorly, it is closely related to the urethra; posteriorly, the perineal body separates it from the anal canal; inferiorly it opens into the vestibule at the introitus. This opening is partially occluded by a thin membrane—the hymen—which may be torn by intercourse, internal examination or sporting activity, such as horse riding or cycling.
- External urethral orifice: This lies in the vestibule posterior to the glans of the clitoris and anterior to the vagina.

CLINICAL NOTES

BARTHOLIN CYST

Bartholin cysts are the most common cause of swelling within the labia majora among females of reproductive age. The cyst is noninfectious and caused by occlusion of the duct, causing retention of secretions. It can normally be managed conservatively with warm compresses to aid drainage.

Vessels and nerves of the female urogenital triangle

The internal pudendal artery has a similar course and distribution in the female as in the male, except:

- Posterior labial branches replace scrotal branches.
- The artery to the bulb and vestibule and the dorsal arteries of the clitoris replace the arteries to the penis.
- The blood supply to the external genitalia of the female mirrors that to the scrotum. The external genitalia receive superficial and deep external pudendal arteries (from the femoral artery). Venous drainage occurs via venae comitantes and ends in the great saphenous vein. The pudendal nerve has a similar distribution in both sexes. The only difference is in the naming of the nerves, in which labial replaces scrotal.

The nerve supply to the labia mirrors that of the scrotum:

- The anterior third is supplied by the ilioinguinal nerve.
- The posterior two-thirds are supplied by the posterior labial branch of the pudendal nerve (medially) and by the perineal branch of the posterior femoral cutaneous nerve (laterally).

LYMPHATIC DRAINAGE OF THE PELVIS AND PERINEUM

Pelvis

The lymphatic drainage of the pelvis is different for the various organs/structures in the pelvis. This is summarized in Table 5.8.

Male urogenital triangle

The penis and scrotum drain into the superficial (skin) and deep (glans and corpora) inguinal nodes.

Female urogenital triangle

Lymph drains to the superficial inguinal lymph nodes.

Table 5.8 Lymphatic drainage of the pelvis

Structure	Lymphatic drainage
Anal canal	Superficial inguinal nodes
Bladder	Internal and external iliac nodes
Ovary	Aortic nodes
Rectum	Inferior mesenteric nodes, internal iliac nodes, pararectal nodes, preaortic nodes
Urethra	Internal iliac nodes, superficial inguinal nodes
Uterus/fallopian tubes	Internal and external iliac nodes, sacral nodes
Vagina	Internal and external iliac nodes, superficial inguinal nodes

TRANSGENDER ANATOMY

Individuals may undergo transgender surgery, also known as gender-affirming surgery or as part of their gender transition to align their physical appearance with their identified gender. This is commonly due to gender dysphoria, a condition where a person's assigned gender at birth contradicts their deeply felt sense of gender.

Transgender surgery plays a pivotal role in gender affirmation for many patients and can involve various masculinizing or feminizing procedures, including:

- Facial and aesthetic surgery.
- Vocal cord surgery.
- Chest surgery (mastectomy or breast augmentation).
- Genital surgery (phalloplasty, metoidoplasty or vaginoplasty).

Transgender men undergoing female-to-male interventions may have masculinizing procedures, including the construction of a penis through metoidioplasty or phalloplasty with scrotoplasty to create a scrotum. Further procedures may include breast reconstruction/mastectomy, hysterectomy and oophorectomy.

Transgender women undergoing male-to-female interventions may have feminizing procedures including vaginoplasty to create a neovagina alongside penectomy and orchidectomy. Further operations may include breast augmentation, facial feminizing surgery, voice feminization surgery and tracheal shave to reduce the laryngeal prominence.

The most common genital procedure in the United Kingdom is the vaginoplasty which is performed via the penile inversion technique. In addition to orchidectomy, the procedure involves creating a neovagina within the rectovesicular fascia posterior to

Man to Woman Transgender Anatomy
Preoperative

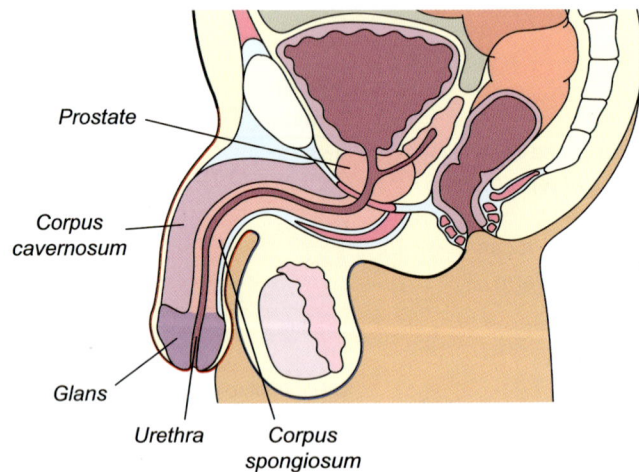

Postoperative

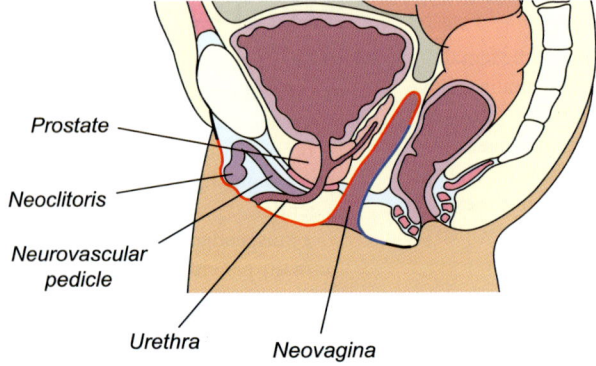

Fig. 5.30 Example of the anatomical changes that occur with vaginoplasty surgery. (Courtesy Dr Joe Yapp.)

the urethra and prostate and anterior to the rectum. Part of the glans of the penis is harvested and remodelled to create a functioning neoclitoris, while the urethra is shortened to fit within the neovulva. This surgery leaves the prostate and seminal vesicles in situ, meaning that the patients will ejaculate when they orgasm; however, the ejaculate will be azoospermic due to the orchidectomy (Fig. 5.30).

As part of the process, patients may also take lifelong hormonal replacement. For transgender men, this consists of androgens and oestrogen antagonists and for transgender women, oestrogens and/or androgen antagonists.

CLINICAL NOTES

NEW ANATOMY

When caring for patients who have had gender-affirming surgery, it is important to understand their new anatomy and to know which organs have been removed, reformed or created. Knowing which organs are in situ will help you distinguish what pathologies a patient may have. For example, the vast majority of transgender women will still have a prostate after a vaginoplasty and remain at risk of prostatic diseases.

Musculoskeletal system

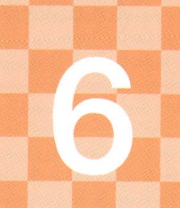

OVERVIEW OF THE MUSCULOSKELETAL SYSTEM

This chapter includes the anatomy of the upper and lower limbs and the vertebral column. The chapter also explores the physiology of bone, muscle, connective tissue and the spinal cord.

Structure

The upper limb is joined to the trunk by the pectoral girdle (scapula and clavicle), which along with the glenohumeral joint forms the shoulder. The upper limb consists of the arm (humerus), forearm (radius and ulnar) and the hand that is connectewd to the forearm by the radiocarpal joint (wrist). The arterial supply to the upper limb is via the subclavian artery, and the nervous supply originates from the brachial plexus, which gives rise to five key terminal nerves (axillary, musculocutaneous, radial, ulnar and median).

The lower limb starts at the hip joint where the head of the femur joins to the acetabulum of the pelvis to form a ball-and-socket joint. Distally, the femur articulates with the patella, tibia and fibula at the knee joint. The lower leg connects with the foot at the ankle joint.

The vertebral column usually consists of 33 vertebrae arranged in five distinct regions (5 cervical, 12 thoracic, 5 lumbar, 5 sacral and 4 coccygeal vertebrae). The sacral and coccygeal vertebrae fuse into one unit. The vertebrae articulate with each other through the intervertebral discs and the facet joints.

Function

The musculoskeletal system has several functions, with the main ones being:

- Support and protection of organs
- Maintain posture
- Facilitate movement
- Mineral storage, for example calcium and phosphate
- Haematopoiesis

The vertebral column has the additional role of protecting the spinal cord, an integral part of the central nervous system (CNS). It has multiple motor and sensory functions, which will be explored towards the end of this chapter.

Muscle types

There are three types of muscle: skeletal, smooth and cardiac.

Skeletal (striated)

- Attached to the skeleton
- Maintain posture and move limbs
- Under voluntary control

Smooth (nonstriated)

- Line blood vessels and hollow organs
- Control the diameter of vessels and other structures
- Under involuntary control

Cardiac

- Only located within the heart
- Contraction of the heart
- Under involuntary control

Skeleton

The skeleton has four components: bone, cartilage, ligaments/tendons and joints.

Bones

Bone is a highly specialized form of connective tissue that provides attachment for muscles.

Cartilage

A semirigid form of connective tissue, present at the mobile parts of bones.

Tendons and ligaments

Both tendons and ligaments are fibrous tissue with many similarities; tendons join muscle to bone and ligaments join bone to bone.

Joints

There are three main types of joints: synovial, fibrous and cartilaginous.

- Synovial: The most common type, where two bone ends articulate within a capsule of lubricated fluid (synovial fluid), for example hip and knee joints.
- Fibrous: Bones are joined by dense connective tissue, for example the sutures between bones of the skull. They tend to be immovable (synarthrosis) or only allow a limited amount of movement (amphiarthrosis).
- Cartilaginous: Bones are connected by the cartilage. They can be primary cartilaginous—where there is a hyaline cartilage between the bones and are synarthrosis, for example at the growth plate of long bones—or secondary cartilaginous where they are amphiarthrosis with dense fibrocartilage in the middle, for example intervertebral discs and the pubic symphysis.

PHYSIOLOGY OF SKELETAL MUSCLE

Microstructure

Muscle fibres are bound together to form a fascicle and multiple fascicles form the muscle. Each muscle fibre is surrounded by a connective tissue called endomysium. Each fascicle is bound by connective tissues and is known as the perimysium. The whole muscle is encased by the epimysium (Fig. 6.1).

Skeletal muscle fibres

Each muscle fibre has a width between 10 and 100 μm and can be up to 30 cm long. Muscle fibres are multinucleated and can be further divided into myofibrils. Myofibrils are formed by thin (actin)

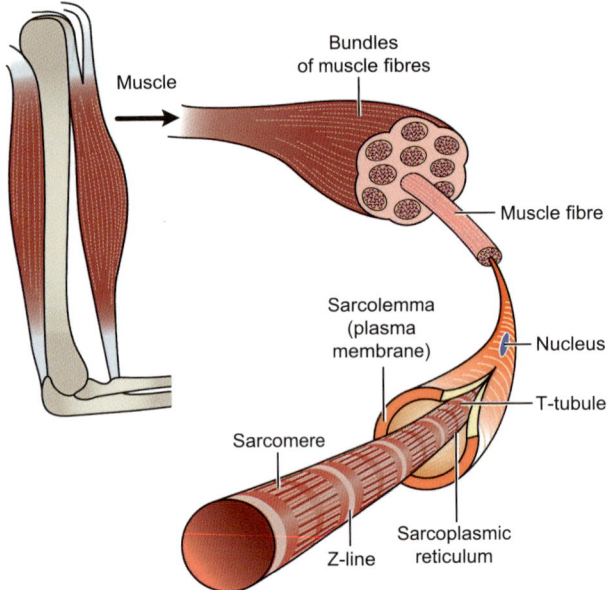

Fig. 6.1 The structure of a skeletal muscle.

and thick (myosin) fibres which run the length of the muscle fibre. Each myosin fibre is surrounded by six actin fibres. The movement of these fibres against each other causes the muscle to contract or relax. The arrangement of fibres is shown in Fig. 6.2. Each actin fibre is surrounded spirally by a tropomyosin fibre, and these have a protein complex of troponin C, I and T at 40-nm intervals. The troponins are key to making the thin and thick fibres move against each other, as will be described later. The sarcomere is the functional unit of the muscle fibre and is measured from one Z-line to another. The Z-line is a fibrous disc running across the muscle fibre. Sarcoplasm is the muscle fibre matrix in which the myofibrils are suspended. The sarcoplasm contains:

- Ions: potassium, magnesium and phosphate
- Enzymes
- Mitochondria

Sarcoplasmic reticulum

- This is the muscle equivalent of the endoplasmic reticulum.

Sarcolemma

- The sarcolemma is the muscle equivalent of a cell membrane that wraps around each muscle fibre and invaginates at each Z-line to form a T-tubule. Each T-tubule is met by two sarcoplasmic reticula and the latter enlarge to form the terminal cisternae. This triad of structures is important for excitation–contraction coupling between the nerve and muscle.

Resting membrane potential and neuromuscular junction

Muscle fibres, like nerves, maintain a membrane potential of −90 mV using Na$^+$/K$^+$-adenosine triphosphatase (ATPase) to transport sodium out of the cell and potassium into it.

Neuromuscular junction

The skeletal muscle fibres are innervated by motor neurones that originate in the anterior horn of the spinal cord. When the nerves

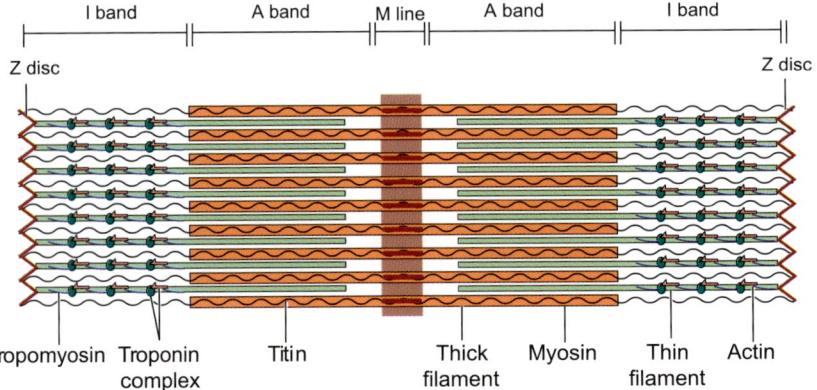

Fig. 6.2 The muscle fibre.

reach the muscle, they lose their myelin coating, branch out and end in a swelling called the terminal bouton. This bouton and the underlying muscle membrane constitute the neuromuscular junction (NMJ). Each muscle fibre has one NMJ.

Transmission at the neuromuscular junction
- Nerve impulses reach the terminal bouton where the action potential opens voltage-gated calcium channels, causing a rapid influx of calcium.
- Calcium causes acetylcholine (ACh)-filled vesicles to bind to the cell membrane at active zones.
- ACh is released into the synaptic cleft.
- When two molecules bind to an ACh receptor on the postsynaptic membrane, the receptor becomes activated and Na^+ flows into the muscle fibre. This electric potential change is called the end-plate potential (EPP).
- The EPP creates an action potential within the muscle fibre membrane.
- The ACh in the synaptic cleft is metabolized by ACh esterase so that the ACh receptors are not constantly activated.

Excitation–contraction coupling
The cell membrane of the muscle fibre is so large that the action potential does not flow into the middle of the fibre. The T-tubules dip into the middle of the fibre and carry the action potential inwards. At the base of the T-tubule, the adjacent sarcoplasmic reticulum is activated to release calcium into the sarcoplasm.

SKELETAL MUSCLE CONTRACTION

Contractile filaments
- Myosin: Each myosin fibre comprises six smaller fibres—four heavy and two light—which are intertwined to form a helix. Part of this helix protrudes as a neck and head which then cross-bridges with the actin fibres (Fig. 6.3).

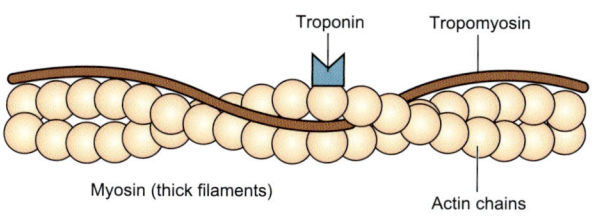

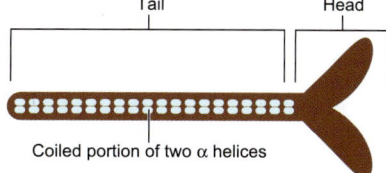

Fig. 6.3 The actin and myosin filaments.

- Actin filament: Each actin filament has three parts: actin, tropomyosin and troponin.
- Actin: A double-stranded F-actin comprises the backbone of the actin filament. Each F-strand is made up of G-actin molecules which have an associated ATP and are the site of myosin cross-bridges.
- Tropomyosin: Tropomyosin covers the actin-binding sites and so stops myosin from binding in the resting state.
- Troponin: Troponin is a complex of C, I and T subunits. Its main function is to bind to tropomyosin and respond to changes in sarcoplasmic calcium concentration.

Mechanism of contraction
The mechanism of contraction is shown in Fig. 6.4. In brief:
1. Calcium ions that have been released from the sarcoplasmic reticulum bind to troponin C which causes it to undergo a conformational change. This displaces tropomyosin from the actin-binding site.
2. Myosin heads form a cross-bridge to the binding site.
3. The ATP is hydrolyzed by ATPase on the myosin head which releases energy and makes the myosin head tilt, dragging the actin fibre with it. This is known as the power stroke. This process generates adenosine diphosphate (ADP) which remains at the binding site and the extra phosphate is released.
4. This movement continues up the actin fibre until the Z-lines have been pulled together or until the force resisting the muscle is too great to be overcome.

Relaxation
When the action potential in the cell membrane stops, calcium re-enters the sarcoplasmic reticulum. The contraction process described in the previous section then happens in reverse, and the fibres slide back over themselves to lengthen the muscle. Energy from ATP is required to reform the original ATP on the binding site.

CLINICAL NOTES

MUSCLES AFTER DEATH
Rigor mortis occurs after death because there is a depletion of ATP, which is necessary to reform ATP at the binding site during muscle relaxation. Later on, actin–myosin complexes are broken down by proteolysis which ends rigor mortis.

Bioenergetics of muscle contraction
The mechanism of contraction requires energy for several stages:
- The power stroke.
- Pumping Ca^{2+} back from the sarcoplasm into the sarcoplasmic reticulum.
- Pumping Na^+ and K^+ to maintain the membrane potential.

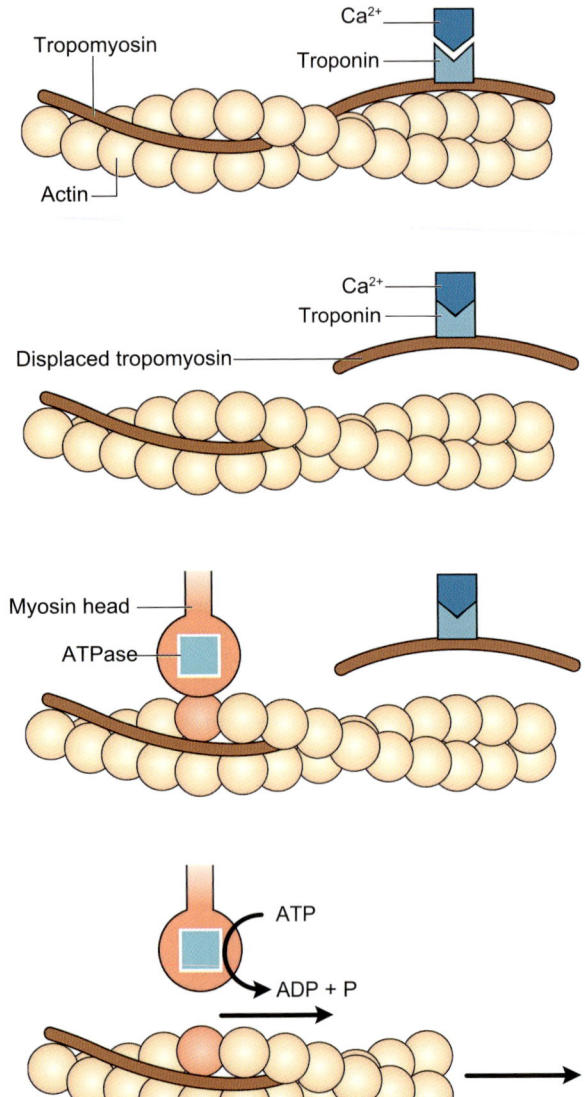

Fig. 6.4 Mechanism of muscle contraction. ATPase, *Adenosine triphosphatase*.

Sources of energy

- Phosphocreatine contains a high-energy phosphate bond that can be used to convert ADP to ATP using the enzyme creatine kinase.
- Anaerobic respiration uses glycogen stored in muscles and rapidly breaks it down into pyruvic acid and lactate. It can occur in the absence of oxygen, but only for short bursts of activity before lactate concentrations become too high.
- Oxidative phosphorylation within aerobic respiration produces 38 ATP molecules for every glucose molecule.

Motor units

A motor unit comprises several muscle fibres and the motor neurone that controls them. All of the muscle fibres innervated by the motor neurone contract together. Muscles requiring fine control have fewer muscle fibres per neurone.

Muscle mechanics

There are two types of contraction:

- Isometric: The muscle contracts but does not change length, for example when holding an object steady in one position. This is important for maintaining body posture.
- Isotonic: The muscle shortens during contraction. Concentric contraction is the act of shortening a muscle, whereas eccentric contraction is a controlled relaxation where the muscle gradually lengthens, that is lowering an object.

Maintaining muscle contraction
Twitch contraction

A twitch contraction is the effect of a single action potential; however, it is insufficient to cause useful movement. Combining twitches is required for purposeful movement.

- Multiple fibre summation: Combining multiple motor units at the same time.
- Frequency summation (tetany): Multiple twitches in a short space of time. If the frequency is high enough for the contractions to overlap, a greater overall contraction is achieved (Fig. 6.5).

Length–tension relationship

The force of contraction is dependent on the length of the fibres before contraction. If the fibres are stretched, the actin and myosin have little overlap, and there will be only a few myosin heads in position to bind the actin for a power stroke.

Types of muscle fibre

Mammals have three types of fibres: fast (divided into fast and very fast) and slow, referring to the speed of their contraction (Table 6.1). Extraocular muscles are the fastest (40 ms) followed by the hand (50 ms). The slowest muscles are the gastrocnemius (100 ms) and the soleus (120 ms). Slow muscles have a higher capillary supply and more myoglobin and so are more resistant to fatigue. Fast muscle is capable of more intense activity but fatigues more quickly.

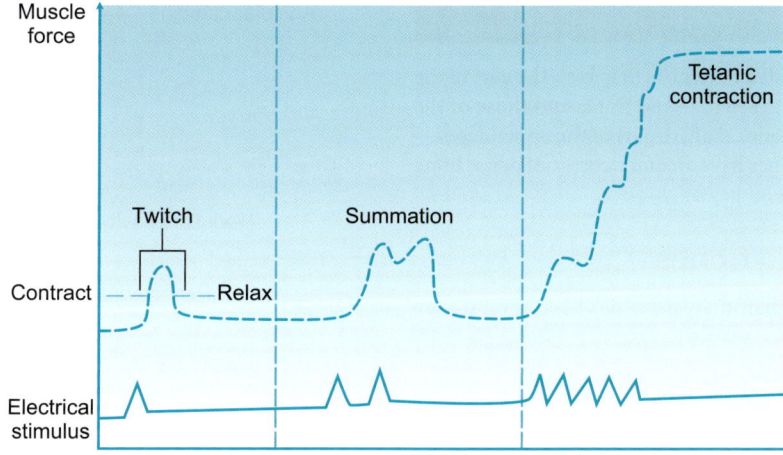

Fig. 6.5 Summative contractions.

Property	Type I fibres	Type II A fibres	Type II B fibres
Contraction time	Slow	Fast	Very fast
Size of motor neurone	Small	Large	Very large
Resistance to fatigue	High	Intermediate	Low
Activity used for	Aerobic	Long-term anaerobic	Short-term anaerobic
Force production	Low	High	Very high
Mitochondrial density	High	High	Low
Capillary density	High	Intermediate	Low
Oxidative capacity	High	High	Low
Glycolytic capacity	Low	High	High
Location	Postural muscles	Leg muscles	Bicep muscles
Colour	Red	Red pink	White/pale
Myoglobin content	High	High	Low

Table 6.1 Characteristics of muscle fibre types

Muscle plasticity

Muscle plasticity refers to changes in muscle relative to its functional requirement. Many characteristics can be altered including muscle length, diameter, vascular supply and strength. The fibre types can be altered by:

- Hypertrophy: The muscle mass increases owing to the thickening of fibres in response to weight training, but the number of fibres remains the same.
- Hyperplasia: Splitting of the muscle fibres so that the number increases; this is less common than hypertrophy.

Peripheral motor control

Proprioception allows the body to sense the position of the muscles and joints to help control the limbs and indicates the extent of contraction. The main types of sensors are the Golgi tendon organs and the muscle spindles.

Muscle spindles

These spindle-shaped structures lie parallel to skeletal muscle fibres and consist of intrafusal muscle fibres surrounded by nerve endings. Spindles are connected by connective tissue to the endomysium and perimysium. They are more concentrated in organs that perform fine movement, such as the extraocular muscles. Muscle spindles measure the amount of muscle stretch, and their fibres are supplied by γ-motor neurones.

Golgi tendon organs

Golgi tendon organs are present at the muscle–tendon interface and are compressive sensory nerve endings wrapped around bundles of collagen. They protect the tendons and muscles from stretching excessively and causing damage. Stretching the Golgi tendon organs by hitting them with a tendon hammer causes a reflex compensatory contraction of the muscle in an effort to reduce the apparent stretch.

BONE

Bones can be broadly divided into those that form the part of the axial skeleton (e.g. pelvis, vertebrae and skull) and those of the appendicular skeleton (bones that are part of the appendages—femur, humerus, etc.). Bones have an outer cortex of dense bone and inner cancellous bone.

Structure of long bones

Long bones (i.e. longer than they are wide) have several core parts (Fig. 6.6):

- Diaphysis: The bone shaft.
- Epiphysis: The end of a long bone.
- Metaphysis: Joins the shaft to the end of the bone.
- Medullary cavity: Contains bone marrow and is lined by endosteum.
- Articular cartilage: Covers the articulating end of the bone at the joints.
- Periosteum: Surrounds the bone, containing bone-forming cells and nourishing the bone.

Histology of bone

Bone is a matrix surrounded by cells. The matrix is composed of:

- 35% organic component (90% collagen type 1).
- 40% inorganic components (hydroxyapatite, i.e. calcium phosphate and calcium carbonate, which are deposited on the collagen).
- 25% water.

Bone cells

- **Osteogenic cells**: Unspecialized stem cells that undergo mitosis and form osteoblasts. They are present in the endosteum and periosteum.
- **Osteoblasts**: Bone-forming cells which synthesize matrix and calcification. Osteoblasts surround and encase themselves with deposited matrix before becoming osteocytes.
- **Osteocytes**: Found in lacunae, which are small cavities in the bone.
- **Osteoclasts**: Giant, multinucleated cells formed by the fusion of monocytes; they release lysosomal enzymes which reabsorb the bone matrix.

Bone formation and remodelling

Bones have mesenchymal origins and then ossify by either intramembranous or endochondral methods. Following ossification, bone undergoes a continuous, lifelong remodelling by osteoblasts and osteoclasts.

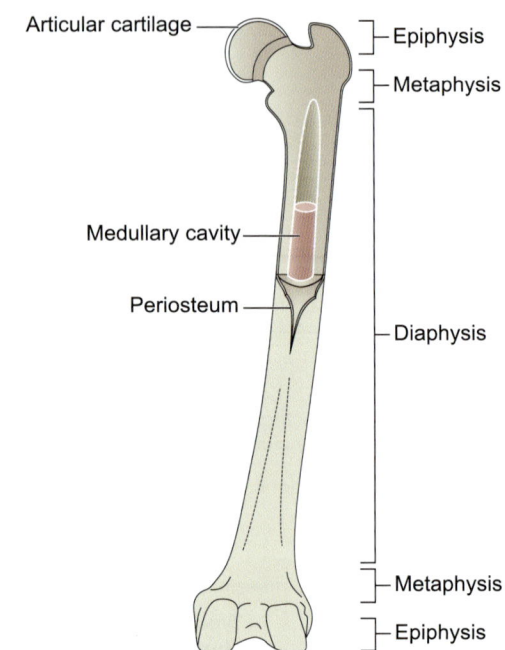

Fig. 6.6 Structure of a typical long bone.

Intramembranous ossification

- Mesenchymal cells migrate to the site of bone formation.
- The cells proliferate, condense, align and secrete an organic framework of extracellular matrix (ECM) onto a pre-bone framework or osteoid.
- Some mesenchymal cells differentiate to become osteoblasts and line the osteoid with collagen–proteoglycan matrix that can bind calcium salts.
- The bone matrix then becomes mineralized organic strands which are termed trabeculae.
- As the trabeculae increase in thickness, consecutive growth rings called lamellae are seen.
- Osteoblasts that become trapped in the matrix they create become osteocytes.
- Cycles of osteoid secretion and mineralization by the mesenchymal cells and osteoblasts add to the lamellae.
- A lattice structure forms when multiple trabeculae within the developing bone contact one another.

Endochondral ossification

- Mesenchymal cells migrate to the site of eventual bone formation and transform into chondrocytes.
- These produce cartilage, which takes the shape of the ensuing bone.
- Chondrocytes secrete a loose ECM comprising collagen and mucopolysaccharides.

- The chondrocytes are prised apart and become encapsulated.
- The cartilage is also surrounded by a layer of connective tissue cells (the perichondrium) that is also derived from mesenchyme.
- Within the body of the cartilage, the encapsulated cells die and the matrix erodes. At this point, the cartilage begins to be replaced by bone.
- Blood vessels invade the cartilage.
- The outer layer of mesenchyme cells is now called the periosteum which is identical to the perichondrium except for its location.
- As the cartilage is degraded, strands of remaining cartilage act as templates for osteoblasts, which secrete more ECM that undergoes calcification.

The main difference between these two types of bone formation is that endochondral ossification forms cartilage before this is then replaced by bone (such as the femur), whereas intramembranous ossification forms bone directly (such as the skull bones). Within both of these formations, both compact bones which are filled in completely and cancellous bones which contain a lattice-type structure within are created. Most bones are a combination of both types.

Functions of bone

Calcium regulation

Calcium is important for blood coagulation, muscle contraction and nervous system stability. Ninety-nine per cent of the body's calcium is stored in the bones as hydroxyapatite. Parathyroid hormone and vitamin D increase osteoclast activity so that more calcium is released into the blood, while calcitonin inhibits osteoclasts.

CLINICAL NOTES

HYPERCALCEMIA

Hypercalcemia is a clinical condition with many cause including hyperparathyroidism and cancer. In cancer, hypercalcaemia may result from bone metastases, ectopic production of parathyroid hormone–related protein by malignant cells (such as in small cell lung cancer) or from conditions like multiple myeloma. Patients may present with symptoms of hypercalcemia which can be remembered as: stones, bones, abdominal groans and psychic moans, meaning patients are at risk of renal stones; bone pain; gastrointestinal upset (nausea/vomiting/constipation); and lethargy, tiredness or depression.

Haematopoiesis

There are two types of bone marrow: yellow which is fatty and inactive, and red (myeloid) which is responsible for the production of blood cells, such as red cells, lymphocytes and platelets.

UPPER LIMB

The upper limb is joined to the trunk by the pectoral girdle (scapula and clavicle), which along with the glenohumeral joint forms the shoulder. The arm (humerus) lies between the shoulder and the elbow, and the forearm (radius and ulna) lies distal to the elbow. At the distal end of the forearm is the radiocarpal joint (wrist), and distal to this is the hand.

The arterial supply to the upper limb is from the subclavian artery, which becomes the axillary artery at the first rib. At the inferior border of teres major, the axillary artery becomes the brachial artery, and then in the cubital fossa, it divides into the radial and ulnar arteries.

The nervous supply to the upper limb originates in the brachial plexus, which gives rise to five key terminal nerves (axillary, musculocutaneous, radial, ulnar and median).

SURFACE ANATOMY OF THE UPPER LIMB

The surface anatomy of the upper limb is shown in Fig. 6.7.

Clavicle

The clavicle is a bicurved bone which can be palpated along its length. The medial two-thirds is convex anteriorly and the lateral one-third is concave anteriorly.

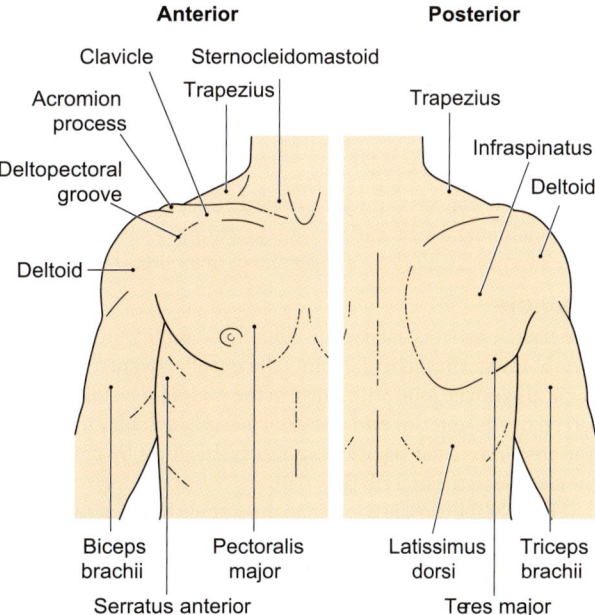

Fig. 6.7 Surface anatomy of the shoulder—anterior and posterior views.

Scapula

The tip of the coracoid process can be palpated in the deltopectoral triangle (bounded by the pectoralis major, the clavicle and the deltoid muscle). The acromion process is palpable superior to the deltoid muscle. The spine of the scapula is palpable along its length on the posterior aspect of the shoulder.

Elbow

The medial and lateral epicondyles of the humerus and the olecranon are clearly palpable. When the elbow is fully extended, the head of the radius can be felt lateral to the olecranon. The tendon of the biceps brachii is felt medially in the cubital fossa and becomes more pronounced as the elbow flexes.

Wrist and hand

The styloid processes of the ulna and radius can be palpated at the wrist. The scaphoid and pisiform bones are felt anteriorly at the base of the hand. The radial artery is felt on the lateral aspect of the anterior forearm, lateral to the flexor tendons, whereas the ulnar artery can be felt on the medial aspect of the forearm. The 'anatomical snuffbox' is located between the extensor pollicis brevis and longus tendons, with the radial styloid on the dorsum of the hand at its apex.

> **CLINICAL NOTES**
>
> **THE ANATOMICAL SNUFFBOX**
>
> If palpating the anatomical snuffbox elicits tenderness, it is a significant indicator of a scaphoid fracture that requires further investigation promptly.

BONES AND JOINTS OF THE UPPER LIMB

Shoulder region

The shoulder consists of the pectoral girdle (scapula and clavicle) and the glenohumeral joint with the clavicle acting as a strut. The limited bony attachments allow for a greater range of motion at the shoulder.

Clavicle

The clavicle articulates medially with the manubrium of the sternum at the sternoclavicular joint. The sternoclavicular joint is an atypical synovial joint with a disc in the middle. The joint is reinforced by the anterior and posterior sternoclavicular ligaments. The costoclavicular ligament supports this joint by connecting the clavicle to the first rib (Fig. 6.8).

Laterally, the clavicle is joined to the scapula by the acromioclavicular joint and coracoclavicular ligaments (trapezoid and conoid).

Scapula

The scapula is a flat, triangular bone with a superior, lateral and medial border. The glenoid cavity is a lateral landmark and articulates with the head of the humerus. The subscapular fossa

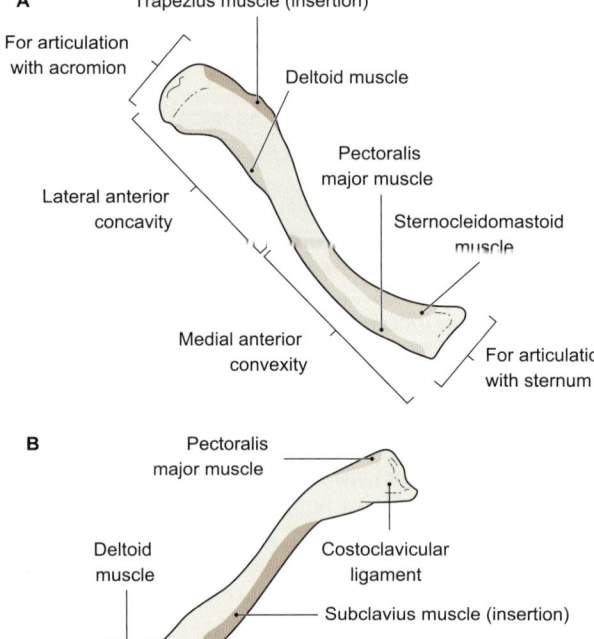

Fig. 6.8 Superior (A) and inferior (B) aspects of the clavicle and its muscular attachments.

forms the anterior surface, and the posterior surface is divided into the infraspinous and supraspinous fossa by the spine of the scapula. The acromion process is the distal enlargement of the scapula spine. Medially the scapula is attached to the spine by trapezius and rhomboid major and minor muscles.

Glenohumeral joint and humerus

The humerus is the bone of the proximal arm and articulates with the scapula at the glenohumeral joint. On the head of the humerus, the greater tubercle lies lateral, and the lesser tubercle lies medial, to the intertubercular sulcus. The anatomical neck is between the head and tubercles, whereas the surgical neck is between the tubercles and the shaft. The surgical neck is related to the axillary nerve and circumflex arteries. The radial groove on the posterior humerus is related to the radial artery.

> **CLINICAL NOTES**
>
> **RADIAL NERVE TRAUMA**
>
> The radial nerve is prone to damage during humeral shaft fractures, leading to symptoms of pain or weakness, especially when bending the wrist back.

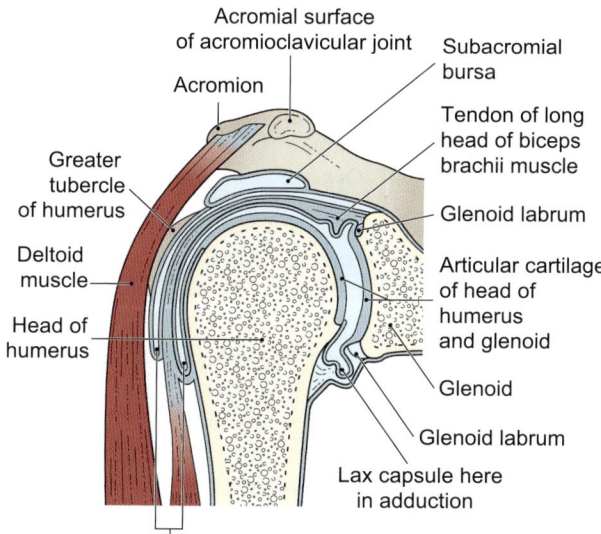

Acromial surface
of acromioclavicular joint
Acromion
Subacromial
bursa
Greater
tubercle
of humerus
Tendon of long
head of biceps
brachii muscle
Deltoid
muscle
Glenoid labrum
Head of
humerus
Articular cartilage
of head of
humerus
and glenoid
Glenoid
Glenoid labrum
Lax capsule here
in adduction
Synovial sheath around long head
of tendon of biceps brachii muscle

Fig. 6.9 A coronal cross section of the glenohumeral joint and related structures.

The glenohumeral joint is a multiaxial ball-and-socket joint (Fig. 6.9). The glenoid cavity is shallow, and a fibrous labrum helps to deepen the joint and provide stability. The joint capsule is reinforced by the superior, middle and interior glenohumeral ligaments, which are actually thickenings of the capsule rather than separate ligaments. The tendons of the rotator cuff muscles (teres minor, supraspinatus, infraspinatus and subscapularis) also support this joint. The muscles that move this joint are shown in Table 6.2.

Elbow and forearm

Elbow

The elbow joint is a synovial hinge joint formed by the distal humerus and the proximal ulna and radius (Fig. 6.10). The articular surfaces of the joint are:

- The capitulum of the humerus, which articulates with the head of the radius.
- The trochlear of the humerus, which articulates with the trochlear notch of the ulna.

In addition to elbow flexion/extension, independent movement of the proximal radioulnar joint can produce pronation and supination.

The elbow joint capsule is generally lax to allow for flexion, but it is supported by three ligaments:

1. Ulnar collateral: On the medial side of the joint between the ulna and medial epicondyle of the humerus.
2. Radial collateral: On the lateral side of the joint between the annular ligament of the radius and the lateral epicondyle of the humerus.

Table 6.2 Movements and muscles of the glenohumeral joint

Movement	Muscles
Flexion	Pectoralis major, anterior fibres of deltoid
Extension	Posterior fibres of deltoid, latissimus dorsi, teres major
Abduction	Deltoid, supraspinatus
Adduction	Pectoralis major, latissimus dorsi
Lateral rotation	Infraspinatus, teres minor, posterior fibres of deltoid
Medial rotation	Pectoralis major, anterior fibres of deltoid, latissimus dorsi, teres major, subscapularis
Circumduction	Varying combinations of flexion, extension, abduction and adduction muscles

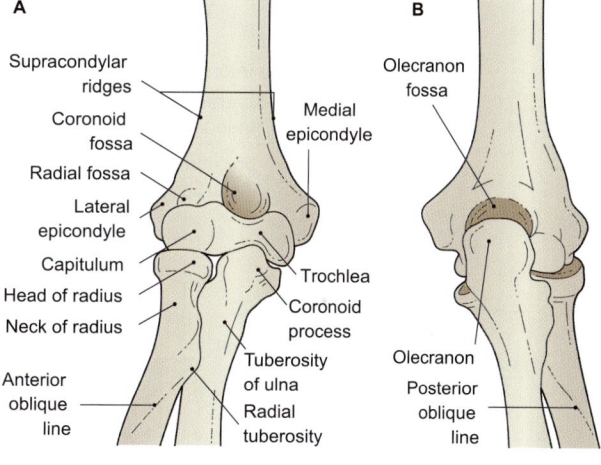

A

Supracondylar
ridges
Coronoid
fossa
Radial fossa
Lateral
epicondyle
Capitulum
Head of radius
Neck of radius
Anterior
oblique
line
Medial
epicondyle
Trochlea
Coronoid
process
Tuberosity
of ulna
Radial
tuberosity

B

Olecranon
fossa
Olecranon
Posterior
oblique
line

Lateral   Medial   Lateral

Fig. 6.10 Anterior (A) and posterior (B) aspects of the humerus and upper ulna and radius.

3. Annular ligament: Runs around the radial head to keep it in position during pronation/supination.

Forearm

The ulna and radius are the bones of the forearm and are joined for most of their length by the interosseous membrane, as shown in Fig. 6.16. Superiorly, this membrane is incomplete to allow the passage of vessels and nerves. The interosseous membrane is the site of muscle attachment. At the distal end is another radioulnar joint, which also moves during pronation/supination.

Wrist and hand

The bones of the wrist and hand are shown in Fig. 6.11.

The radiocarpal (wrist) joint is a synovial joint lying between the distal radius and the scaphoid, lunate and triquetral

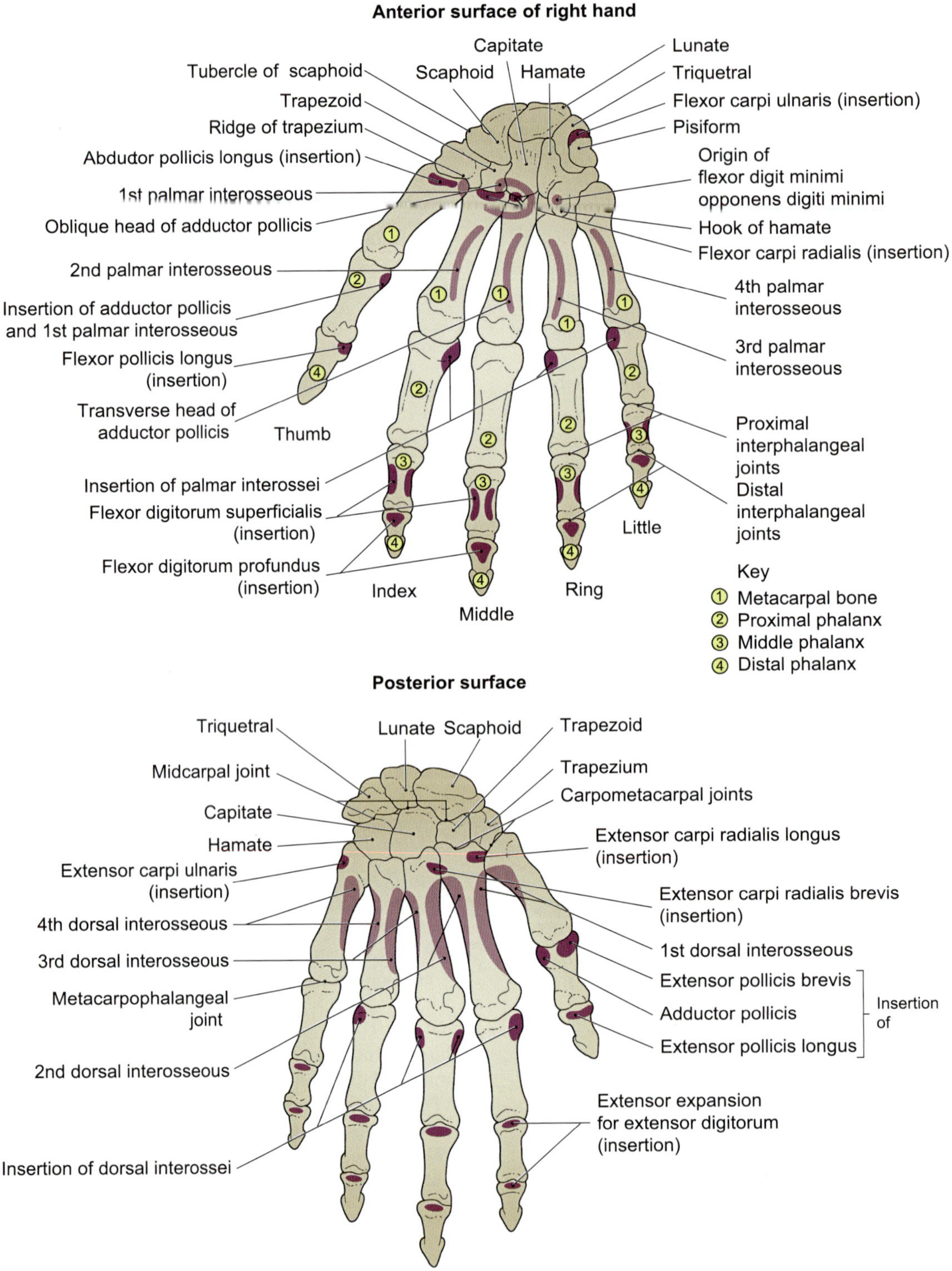

Anterior surface of right hand

Capitate

Tubercle of scaphoid — Scaphoid — Hamate — Lunate

Triquetral

Trapezoid

Ridge of trapezium

Abductor pollicis longus (insertion)

1st palmar interosseous

Oblique head of adductor pollicis

2nd palmar interosseous

Insertion of adductor pollicis and 1st palmar interosseous

Flexor pollicis longus (insertion)

Transverse head of adductor pollicis — Thumb

Insertion of palmar interossei

Flexor digitorum superficialis (insertion)

Flexor digitorum profundus (insertion) — Index

Middle

Flexor carpi ulnaris (insertion)

Pisiform

Origin of flexor digit minimi opponens digiti minimi

Hook of hamate

Flexor carpi radialis (insertion)

4th palmar interosseous

3rd palmar interosseous

Proximal interphalangeal joints

Distal interphalangeal joints

Little

Ring

Key

① Metacarpal bone
② Proximal phalanx
③ Middle phalanx
④ Distal phalanx

Posterior surface

Triquetral — Lunate — Scaphoid — Trapezoid

Midcarpal joint

Capitate

Hamate

Extensor carpi ulnaris (insertion)

4th dorsal interosseous

3rd dorsal interosseous

Metacarpophalangeal joint

2nd dorsal interosseous

Insertion of dorsal interossei

Trapezium

Carpometacarpal joints

Extensor carpi radialis longus (insertion)

Extensor carpi radialis brevis (insertion)

1st dorsal interosseous

Extensor pollicis brevis ⎤
Adductor pollicis   ⎥ Insertion of
Extensor pollicis longus ⎦

Extensor expansion for extensor digitorum (insertion)

Fig. 6.11 Bones of the wrist and hand.

250

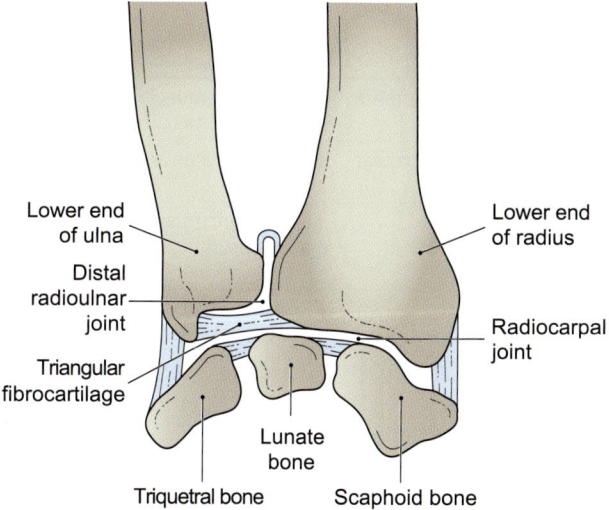

Fig. 6.12 Relationship of the distal radioulnar to the radiocarpal joint.

bones (Fig. 6.12). The joint capsule is reinforced by radiocarpal, ulnocarpal and collateral ligaments. The styloid process of the radius extends further than the ulnar styloid and limits abduction, compared to adduction. The range of flexion/extension is supported by movement at the midcarpal joint. Adduction occurs mainly at the triquetral–radial joint and abduction at the midcarpal joint.

HINTS AND TIPS

The bones in the wrist can be remembered using the mnemonic 'Skeletons Love Telling People That They Can Hiccup'.

MUSCLES OF THE UPPER LIMB

The muscles of the upper limb are shown in Tables 6.3 through 6.7 and Figs 6.11 through 6.16.

Table 6.3 Major muscles of the shoulder region

Name of muscle (nerve supply)	Origin	Insertion	Action
Latissimus dorsi (thoracodorsal nerve)	Iliac crest, lumbar fascia, spinous processes of lower six thoracic vertebrae, lower ribs, scapula	Floor of intertubercular sulcus of humerus	Extends, adducts and medially rotates arm
Levator scapulae (C3 and C4 and dorsal scapular nerve)	Transverse processes of C1–C4	Medial border of scapula	Elevates scapula
Rhomboid minor (dorsal scapular nerve)	Ligamentum nuchae, spines of C7 and T1	Medial border of scapula	Elevates and retracts medial border of scapula
Rhomboid major (dorsal scapular nerve)	Spines of T2–T5	Medial border of scapula	Elevates and retracts medial border of scapula
Trapezius (spinal part of XI nerve and C2 and C3)	Occipital bone, ligamentum nuchae, spinous processes of thoracic vertebrae	Lateral third of clavicle, acromion, spine of scapula	Elevates scapula, retracts scapula and pulls medial border of scapula downwards
Subclavius (nerve to subclavius)	First costal cartilage	Clavicle	Depresses and stabilizes the clavicle
Pectoralis major (medial and lateral pectoral nerves)	Clavicle, sternum, upper six costal cartilages	Lateral lip of intertubercular sulcus of humerus	Adducts arm, rotates it medially and flexes humerus
Pectoralis minor (medial pectoral nerve)	Third, fourth and fifth ribs	Coracoid process of scapula	Depresses point of shoulder Protracts shoulder
Serratus anterior (long thoracic nerve)	Upper eight ribs	Medial border and inferior angle of scapula	Protracts the scapula
Deltoid (axillary nerve)	Clavicle, acromion, spine of scapula	Lateral surface of humerus (deltoid tubercle)	Abducts, flexes and medially rotates, extends and laterally rotates arm
Supraspinatus (suprascapular nerve)	Supraspinous fossa of scapula	Greater tubercle of humerus, capsule of shoulder joint	Rotator cuff muscle Initiates abduction of the arm (first 15 degrees)

(Continued)

Table 6.3 Major muscles of the shoulder region—cont'd

Name of muscle (nerve supply)	Origin	Insertion	Action
Subscapularis (upper and lower subscapular nerves)	Subscapular fossa	Lesser tubercle of humerus	Rotator cuff muscle Medially rotates arm
Teres major (lower subscapular nerve)	Lateral border of scapula	Medial lip of intertubercular sulcus of humerus	Medially rotates and adducts arm
Teres minor (axillary nerve)	Lateral border of scapula	Greater tubercle of humerus, capsule of shoulder joint	Rotator cuff muscle Laterally rotates arm
Infraspinatus (suprascapular nerve)	Infraspinous fossa of scapula	Greater tubercle of humerus, capsule of shoulder joint	Rotator cuff muscle Laterally rotates arm

Table 6.4 Muscles of the arm[a]

Name of muscle (nerve supply)	Origin	Insertion	Action
Flexor compartment			
Biceps brachii—long head (musculocutaneous nerve)	Supraglenoid tubercle of scapula	Tuberosity of radius and bicipital aponeurosis into deep fascia of forearm	Supinator of flexed forearm, flexor of elbow joint, weak flexor of shoulder joint
Biceps brachii—short head (musculocutaneous nerve)	Coracoid process of scapula		
Coracobrachialis (musculocutaneous nerve)	Coracoid process of scapula	Shaft of humerus	Flexes and adducts shoulder joint
Brachialis (musculocutaneous nerve and radial nerve)	Anterior surface of humerus	Ulnar tuberosity and coronoid process	Flexes elbow joint
Extensor compartment			
Triceps—long head (radial nerve) Triceps—lateral head (radial nerve)	Infraglenoid tubercle of scapula Posterior surface of humerus (upper part)	Olecranon process of ulna	Extends elbow joint
Triceps—medial head (radial nerve)	Posterior surface of humerus (lower part)		

[a]Adapted from Snell, R. S. (2000). *Clinical anatomy, an illustrated review with questions and explanations* (2nd ed.). Little Brown & Co.

Table 6.5 Flexor muscles of the forearm

Name of muscle (nerve supply)	Origin	Insertion	Action
Superficial			
Pronator teres—humeral head (median nerve)	Common flexor origin and medial supracondylar ridge	Lateral aspect of shaft of radius	Pronation of forearm and flexion of elbow
Pronator teres—ulnar head (median nerve)	Coronoid process of ulna		
Flexor carpi radialis (median nerve)	Common flexor origin	Second and third metacarpal bones	Flexion and abduction of wrist joint
Flexor carpi ulnaris—humeral head (ulnar nerve)	Common flexor origin	Pisiform, hamate and fifth metacarpal bone	Flexion and abduction of wrist joint
Flexor carpi ulnaris—ulnar head (ulnar nerve)	Olecranon process and posterior border of ulna		
Palmaris longus (median nerve)	Common flexor origin	Palmar aponeurosis	Flexion of wrist joint

Table 6.5 Flexor muscles of the forearm—cont'd

Name of muscle (nerve supply)	Origin	Insertion	Action
Flexor digitorum superficialis—humeroulnar head (median nerve)	Common flexor origin and coronoid process of ulna	Middle phalanges of medial four digits	Flexion of PIP and MCP joints of the medial four digits and wrist joint
Flexor digitorum superficialis—radial head (median nerve)	Anterior oblique line of radius		
Deep			
Pronator quadratus (anterior interosseous nerve)	Anterior surface of ulna	Anterior surface of radius	Pronation of forearm
Flexor pollicis longus (anterior interosseous nerve)	Anterior surface of radius and interosseous membrane	Distal phalanx of thumb	Flexion of interphalangeal and MCP joints
Flexor digitorum profundus (medial half by ulnar nerve and lateral half by anterior interosseous nerve)	Anterior surface of ulna and interosseous membrane	Distal phalanges of medial four digits	Flexion of DIP, PIP, MCP and wrist joint

DIP, *Distal interphalangeal*; MCP, *metacarpophalangeal*; PIP, *proximal interphalangeal*.

Table 6.6 Extensor muscles of the forearm

Name of muscle (nerve supply)	Origin	Insertion	Action
Brachioradialis (radial nerve)	Lateral supracondylar ridge of humerus	Styloid process of radius	Flexes elbow and rotates forearm
Extensor carpi radialis longus (radial nerve)	Common extensor origin	Base of second metacarpal bone	Extends and abducts hand at wrist joint
Extensor carpi radialis brevis (posterior interosseous nerve)		Base of third metacarpal bone	Extends and abducts hand at wrist joint
Extensor digitorum (posterior interosseous nerve)		Extensor expansion of middle and distal phalanges of the medial four digits	Extends the medial four fingers and hand at the wrist joint
Extensor digiti minimi (posterior interosseous nerve)		Extensor expansion of little finger	Extends little finger
Extensor carpi ulnaris (posterior interosseous nerve)		Base of fifth metacarpal bone	Extends and adducts hand at the wrist
Anconeus (radial nerve)		Olecranon process and shaft of ulna	Extends and stabilizes the elbow joint
Supinator (posterior interosseous nerve)	Common extensor origin and supinator crest of ulna	Neck and shaft of radius	Supination of forearm
Abductor pollicis longus (posterior interosseous nerve)	Shafts of radius and ulna and interosseous membrane	Base of first metacarpal bone	Abducts thumb
Extensor pollicis brevis (posterior interosseous nerve)	Shaft of radius and interosseous membrane	Base of proximal phalanx of thumb	Extends metacarpophalangeal joint of thumb
Extensor pollicis longus (posterior interosseous nerve)	Shaft of ulna and interosseous membrane	Base of distal phalanx of thumb	Extends thumb
Extensor indicis (posterior interosseous nerve)		Extensor expansion of index finger	Extends index finger

Table 6.7 Muscles of the hand

Name of muscle (nerve supply)	Origin	Insertion	Action
Thenar eminence muscles			
Abductor pollicis brevis (recurrent branch of median nerve)	Scaphoid, trapezium and flexor retinaculum	Base of proximal phalanx	Abducts thumb at the MCP joint.
Flexor pollicis brevis (recurrent branch of median nerve)	Trapezium and flexor retinaculum	Base of proximal phalanx	Flexes thumb at the MCP joint.
Opponens pollicis (recurrent branch of median nerve)	Trapezium and flexor retinaculum	First metacarpal	Rotates metacarpal at the carpometacarpal joint to oppose the thumb.
Hypothenar eminence muscles			
Abductor digiti minimi (deep branch of ulnar nerve)	Pisiform and flexor retinaculum	Base of proximal phalanx	Abducts little finger at the MCP joint.
Flexor digiti minimi (deep branch of ulnar nerve)	Hook of hamate and flexor retinaculum	Base of proximal phalanx	Abducts little finger at the MCP joint.
Opponens digiti minimi (deep branch of ulnar nerve)	Hook of hamate and flexor retinaculum	Fifth metacarpal	Assists in flexing the carpometacarpal joint, cupping the palm to assist in gripping.
Other intrinsic hand muscles			
Lumbricals (first and second: median nerve; third and fourth: deep branch of ulnar nerve)	Tendons of flexor digitorum profundus	Extensor expansion of the medial four digits	Extends the DIP and PIP joints of medial four digits. Flexes the MCP joint of the medial four digits.
Palmar interossei (deep branch of ulnar nerve)	First, second, fourth and fifth metacarpal bones	Base of proximal phalanx and extensor expansion	Adduct the digits towards the middle finger. Flexes digit at MCP and extends interphalangeal joints.
Dorsal interossei (deep branch of ulnar nerve)	Adjacent sides of the five metacarpal bones	Base of proximal phalanx and extensor expansion	Abduct the digits away from the middle finger. Flexes digit at MCP and extends interphalangeal joints.
Adductor pollicis (deep branch of ulnar nerve)	Oblique head: capitate, trapezoid and second and third metacarpals. Transverse head: distal part of third metacarpal	Base of proximal phalanx	Adducts thumb.
Palmaris brevis (superficial branch of the ulnar nerve)	Palmar aponeurosis and flexor retinaculum	Dermis of the skin on medial border of hand	Wrinkles the skin over the hypothenar eminence and improve the grip of the hand.

DIP, *Distal interphalangeal*; MCP, *metacarpophalangeal*; PIP, *proximal interphalangeal*.

- The muscles of the arm are divided into the anterior and posterior compartments which are separated by medial and lateral intermuscular septae arising from the deep fascia.
- The muscles of the forearm are divided into flexor and extensor compartments.
  - The flexor compartment is further separated into superficial and deep groups. The six superficial muscles all arise from the medial humeral epicondyle (the common flexor origin). The three deep muscles arise from the forearm bones and the interosseous membrane.
  - The extensor compartment is also subdivided into superficial and deep groups. The superficial group has seven muscles that all originate from the lateral epicondyle (the common extensor origin). There are five deep muscles.

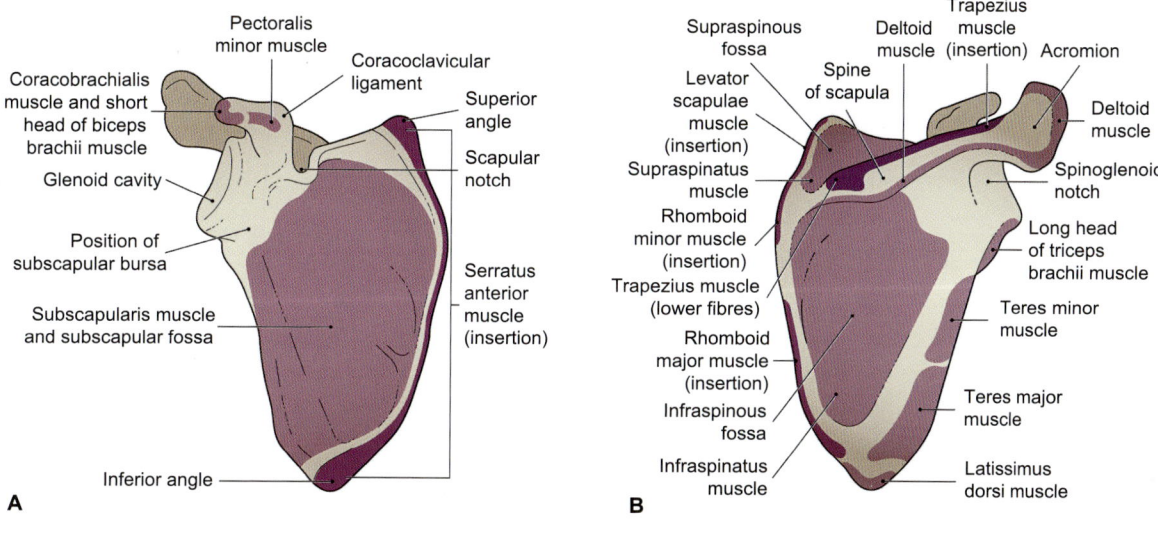

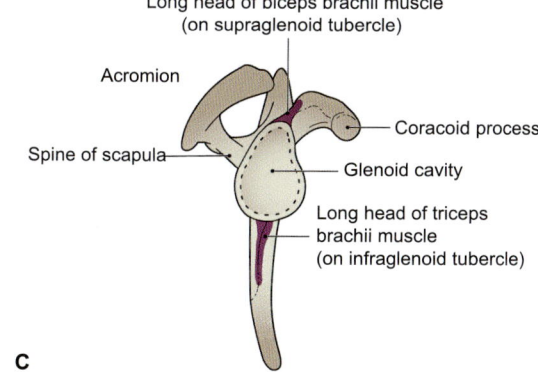

Fig. 6.13 Anterior (A), posterior (B) and lateral (C) aspects of the right scapula and its muscular attachments.

Muscles of the hand

Thenar and hypothenar eminence

The thenar eminence is the prominent muscle mass between the base of the thumb and the wrist. It contains the abductor pollicis brevis, the flexor pollicis brevis and opponens pollicis. These muscles are important for fine movements of the thumb, particularly pinching. The hypothenar eminence is the muscle mass between the base of the little finger and the wrist. Its muscles mirror the thenar eminence. The muscles of the thenar eminence and the lateral two lumbricals are innervated by the median nerve.

Other intrinsic muscles of the hand

The other intrinsic muscles of the hand include the adductor pollicis, interossei muscles and lumbricals. The dorsal and palmar interossei muscles abduct and adduct the fingers, respectively. The first dorsal interosseous muscle can be felt as the muscle mass bulk on the posterior hand at the base of the thumb. The interossei muscles also assist the lumbricals in the flexion of the metacarpophalangeal joints and extension of the interphalangeal joints.

Palmar aponeurosis

The palmar aponeurosis is a thickening of the deep fascia. Proximally, it attaches to the flexor retinaculum and is

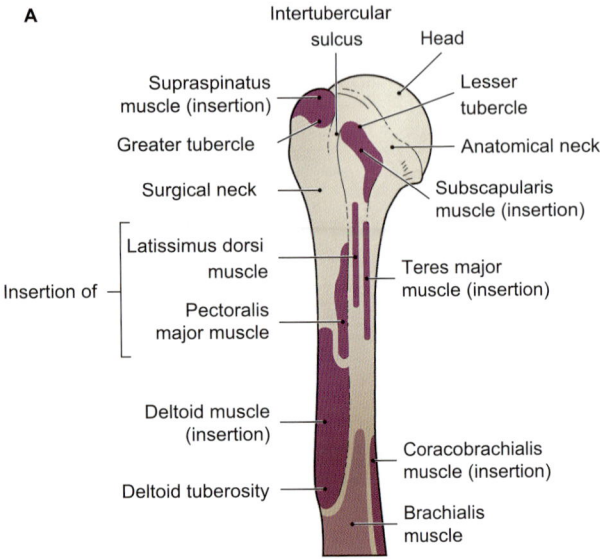

A

Intertubercular
sulcus
Head
Supraspinatus
muscle (insertion)
Lesser
tubercle
Greater tubercle
Anatomical neck
Surgical neck
Subscapularis
muscle (insertion)
Latissimus dorsi
muscle
Teres major
muscle (insertion)
Insertion of
Pectoralis
major muscle
Deltoid muscle
(insertion)
Coracobrachialis
muscle (insertion)
Deltoid tuberosity
Brachialis
muscle

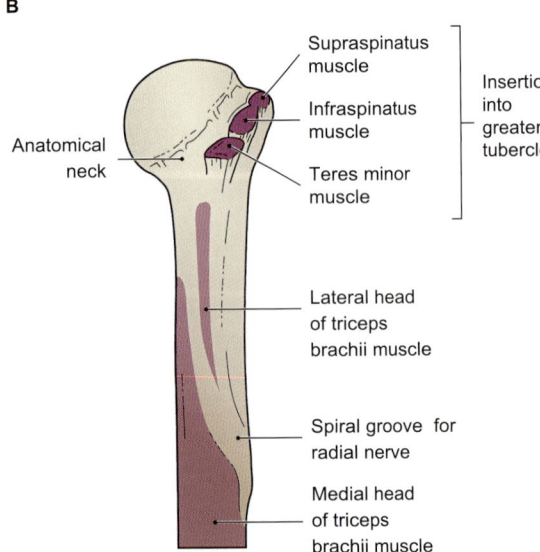

B

Supraspinatus
muscle
Insertions
into
greater
tubercle
Infraspinatus
muscle
Anatomical
neck
Teres minor
muscle
Lateral head
of triceps
brachii muscle
Spiral groove for
radial nerve
Medial head
of triceps
brachii muscle

Fig. 6.14 Anterior (A) and posterior (B) views of the proximal end of the humerus and its muscular attachments.

continuous with the palmaris longus muscle. Distally it divides into four sheaths which cross the metacarpophalangeal joints and insert into the proximal phalanges.

Tendons in the hand
Long flexor tendons in the hand
Flexor digitorum superficialis and flexor digitorum profundus tendons share a common synovial sheath in the hand. This

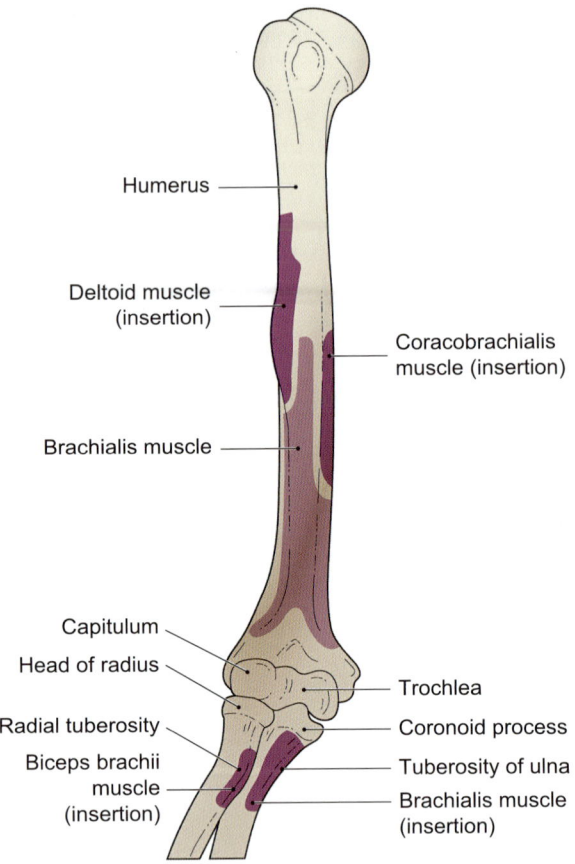

Humerus
Deltoid muscle
(insertion)
Coracobrachialis
muscle (insertion)
Brachialis muscle
Capitulum
Head of radius
Trochlea
Radial tuberosity
Coronoid process
Biceps brachii
muscle
(insertion)
Tuberosity of ulna
Brachialis muscle
(insertion)

Fig. 6.15 Skeleton of the arm and its muscle attachments.

sheath begins just proximal to the flexor retinaculum. The sheath stops briefly in the palm for the attachment of the lumbricals before continuing into the phalanges. The superficialis tendon inserts into the middle phalanx, and the profunda continues to insert into the distal phalanx (Fig. 6.17). The extensor tendon insertion is shown in Fig. 6.18.

NERVE SUPPLY TO THE UPPER LIMB

Brachial plexus

The brachial plexus is formed from the anterior rami of spinal nerves C5 to T1. Fig. 6.19 shows the division of the plexus into roots (behind the scalene), trunks (posterior triangle of the neck), divisions (behind the clavicle), cords (described relative to the axillary artery) and terminal nerves. The axillary nerve

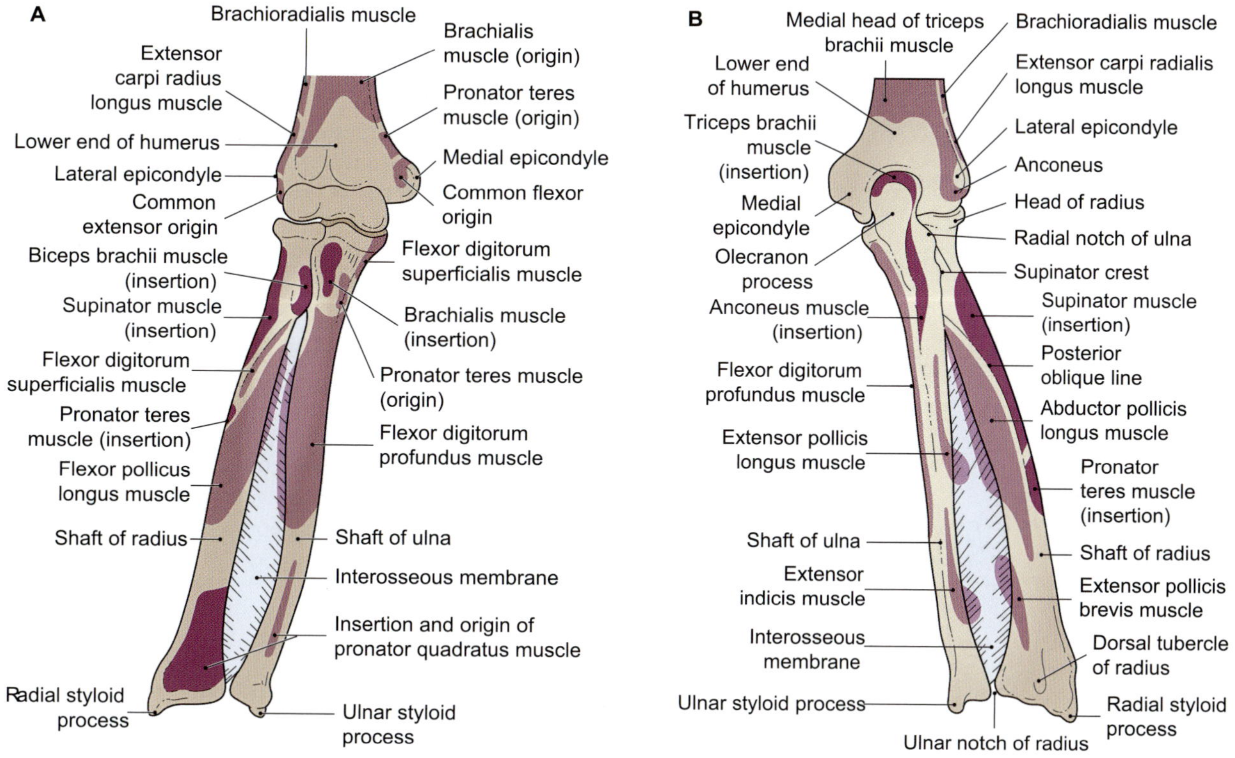

A

- Brachioradialis muscle
- Extensor carpi radius longus muscle
- Lower end of humerus
- Lateral epicondyle
- Common extensor origin
- Biceps brachii muscle (insertion)
- Supinator muscle (insertion)
- Flexor digitorum superficialis muscle
- Pronator teres muscle (insertion)
- Flexor pollicus longus muscle
- Shaft of radius
- Radial styloid process

- Brachialis muscle (origin)
- Pronator teres muscle (origin)
- Medial epicondyle
- Common flexor origin
- Flexor digitorum superficialis muscle
- Brachialis muscle (insertion)
- Pronator teres muscle (origin)
- Flexor digitorum profundus muscle
- Shaft of ulna
- Interosseous membrane
- Insertion and origin of pronator quadratus muscle
- Ulnar styloid process

B

- Medial head of triceps brachii muscle
- Lower end of humerus
- Triceps brachii muscle (insertion)
- Medial epicondyle
- Olecranon process
- Anconeus muscle (insertion)
- Flexor digitorum profundus muscle
- Extensor pollicis longus muscle
- Shaft of ulna
- Extensor indicis muscle
- Interosseous membrane
- Ulnar styloid process

- Brachioradialis muscle
- Extensor carpi radialis longus muscle
- Lateral epicondyle
- Anconeus
- Head of radius
- Radial notch of ulna
- Supinator crest
- Supinator muscle (insertion)
- Posterior oblique line
- Abductor pollicis longus muscle
- Pronator teres muscle (insertion)
- Shaft of radius
- Extensor pollicis brevis muscle
- Dorsal tubercle of radius
- Radial styloid process
- Ulnar notch of radius

Fig. 6.16 Anterior (A) and posterior (B) aspects of the right radius and ulna with their muscle attachments.

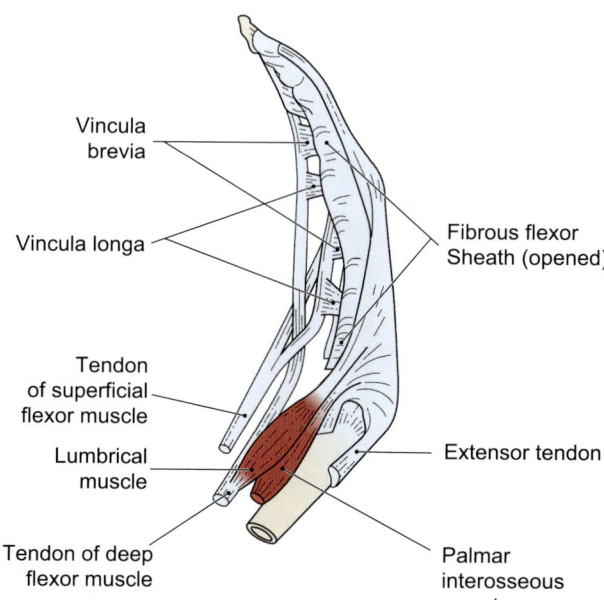

- Vincula brevia
- Vincula longa
- Tendon of superficial flexor muscle
- Lumbrical muscle
- Tendon of deep flexor muscle
- Fibrous flexor Sheath (opened)
- Extensor tendon
- Palmar interosseous muscle

Fig. 6.17 Long flexor tendons in the fingers.

stays in the shoulder and wraps around the neck of the humerus.

Nerves to the arm, forearm and hand

Musculocutaneous nerve

The musculocutaneous nerve is the terminal branch of the lateral cord of the brachial plexus. It pierces the coracobrachialis muscle and then travels between the brachialis and biceps brachii. It supplies the muscles in the flexor compartment of the arm and then pierces the deep fascia to become the lateral cutaneous nerve of the forearm.

Median nerve

The median nerve is formed from the medial and lateral roots of the brachial plexus. In the arm, it initially lies lateral to the brachial artery before crossing anteriorly to run medial to the artery. It enters the cubital fossa between the tendon of biceps brachii and the brachial artery, where it lies deep to the biceps aponeurosis. The median nerve has no branches in the arm; however, the

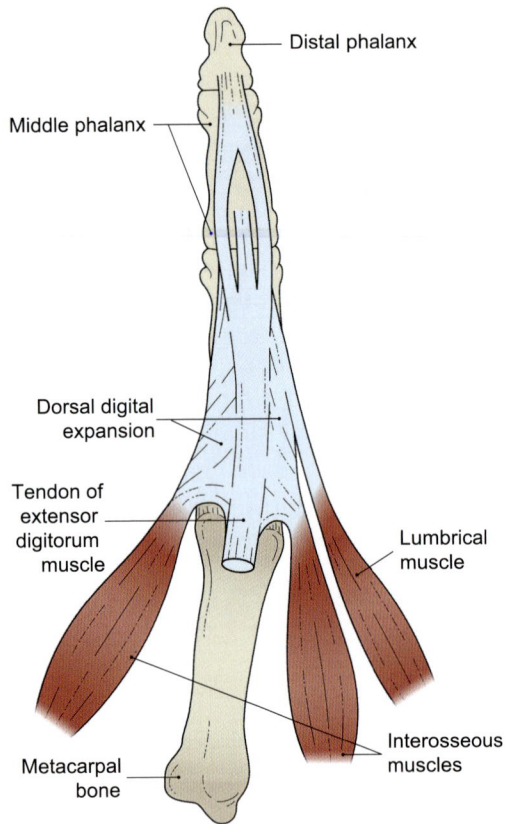

Fig. 6.18 Dorsal digital expansion and extensor tendon.

branch to pronator teres may arise before the elbow. In the forearm, the nerve enters between the two heads of pronator teres and travels between flexor digitorum superficialis and flexor digitorum profundus. It supplies all of the muscles of the flexor compartment except for flexor carpi ulnaris and the medial half of flexor digitorum profundus.

The median nerve passes through the carpal tunnel, and in the hand, it supplies the thenar eminence and lateral two lumbricals. Its cutaneous innervation is shown in Fig. 6.20.

CLINICAL NOTES

CARPAL TUNNEL SYNDROME

The median nerve can be compressed in the carpal tunnel to cause carpal tunnel syndrome. Patients suffer from weakness and pain in the hand with wasting of the thenar eminence. On clinical examination, Tinel and Phalen tests may be used to elicit the symptoms, aiding diagnosis.

Ulnar nerve

After leaving the brachial plexus, the ulnar nerve travels medial to the brachial artery. At the elbow, it passes behind the medial epicondyle and enters the flexor compartment of the forearm between the heads of flexor carpi ulnaris. It then travels between flexor carpi ulnaris and flexor digitorum profundus alongside the ulnar artery. In the distal forearm, the ulnar nerve becomes

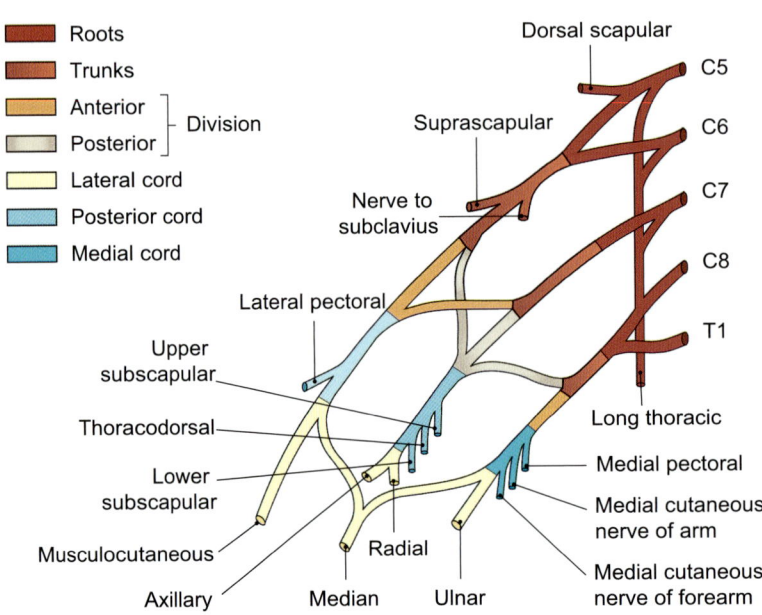

Fig. 6.19 A schematic of the brachial plexus.

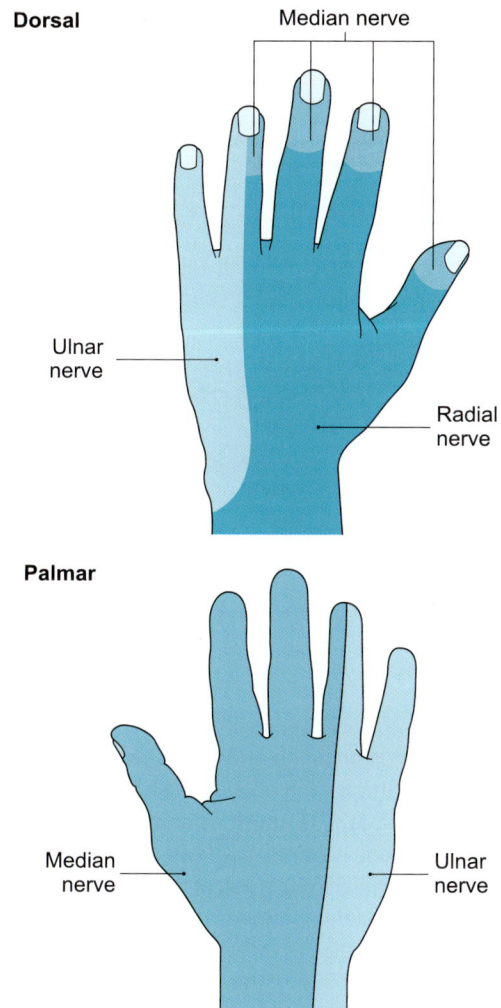

Dorsal

Median nerve

Ulnar nerve

Radial nerve

Palmar

Median nerve

Ulnar nerve

Fig. 6.20 Cutaneous innervations of the dorsal and palmar surfaces of the hand.

superficial and, along with the ulnar artery, lies medial to the tendon of flexor carpi ulnaris.

In the forearm, the ulnar nerve supplies the flexor carpi ulnaris and the medial half of flexor digitorum profundus. It gives two branches: a medial cutaneous branch, which supplies the medial part of the palm, and a dorsal branch, which supplies the medial 1½ digits.

It enters the hand through the ulnar (Guyon) canal superficial to the flexor retinaculum. Its cutaneous innervation is shown in Fig. 6.20.

Radial nerve

The radial nerve is a continuation of the posterior cord of the brachial plexus. In the arm, it runs in the radial groove of the humerus and supplies the muscles of the posterior compartment and anconeus, as well as the posterior cutaneous nerve of the arm and forearm. At the elbow, the radial nerve passes anterior to the lateral epicondyle and deep to brachioradialis. In the forearm, the radial nerve immediately divides into a superficial and deep branch. The deep branch passes between the two heads of the supinator and becomes the posterior interosseous nerve which supplies motor function to the extensor compartment of the forearm. The superficial branch runs with the radial artery into the hand to supply the skin of the dorsum of the hand (see Fig. 6.20).

ARTERIAL SUPPLY TO THE UPPER LIMB

The upper limb is supplied by the subclavian artery which becomes the axillary artery at the lateral border of the first rib. Along with the brachial plexus, the axillary artery is enclosed by the axillary sheath, which is a continuation of the prevertebral fascia.

The axillary artery can be divided into three segments by the pectoralis minor muscle (Fig. 6.21):

1. The first segment lies proximal to the pectoralis minor and has one branch to the superior thoracic artery.
2. The second segment lies posterior to the pectoralis minor and has two branches: the thoracoacromial and lateral thoracic arteries.
3. The third segment lies distal to the pectoralis minor and has three branches: the subscapular, anterior and posterior circumflex humeral arteries.

The axillary artery becomes the brachial artery at the inferior border of teres major. The brachial artery branches into the profunda brachii artery, which passes through the triangular space and then travels in the radial groove of the humerus to supply the extensor compartment. The brachial artery continues through the arm until the cubital fossa, where it divides into the radial and ulnar arteries.

The ulnar artery has a common interosseous branch (which further divides into an anterior and posterior interosseous artery) that supplies the forearm. The radial and ulnar arteries continue through the forearm into the hand to feed the deep and superficial palmar arches, respectively. The radial artery passes through the anatomical snuffbox before becoming the deep arch. Three common digital arteries arise from the arch to supply the metacarpals and eventually the fingers.

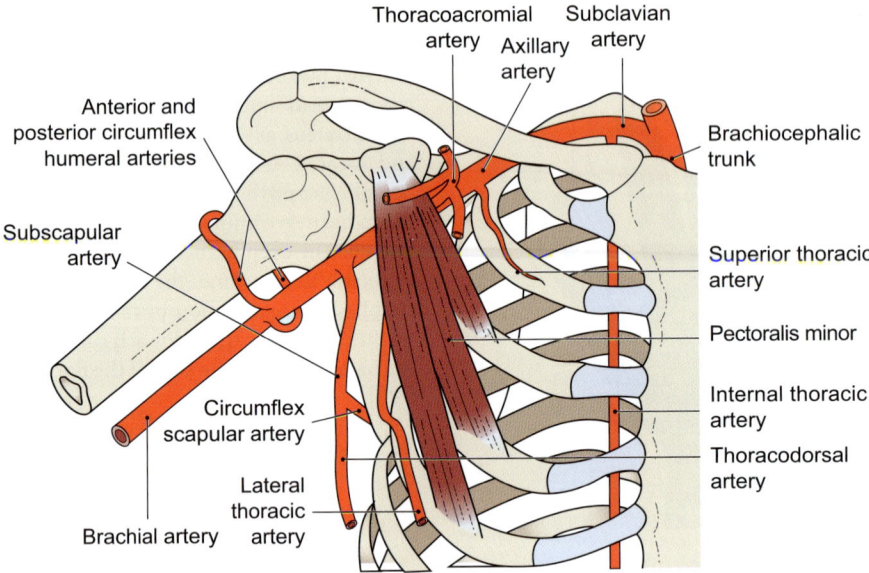

Fig. 6.21 The axillary artery and its branches.

MEASUREMENT OF BLOOD PRESSURE

During manual measurement of blood pressure, the cuff of the sphygmomanometer is wrapped around the arm, and the stethoscope is placed over the brachial artery in the cubital fossa. As the cuff is slowly deflated, Korotkoff sounds (K1–K5) are heard on auscultation. The first sound heard after cuff pressure is released is known as K1—the pressure reading on the sphyg-momanometer at which this is heard represents the systolic blood pressure. The sounds heard on ausculta-tion are owing to turbulent arterial blood flow as a result of a narrowing of the arterial lumen by the cuff. K5 denotes the point at which sounds heard on ausculta-tion disappear. This equates to diastolic blood pressure.

CLINICAL NOTES

ALLEN TEST

Allen test can be performed to assess the patency of the arterial supply to the hand before cannulating the radial artery or before taking an arterial blood gas

sample. These procedures can result in radial artery spasm or occlusion of the artery by a clot; therefore an adequate collateral circulation to the hand is required to prevent ischaemia. The patient is asked to elevate their hand and make a fist for 20 to 30 seconds. The radial and ulnar arteries are occluded at the wrist by applying pressure. If sufficient pressure is applied, the hand will blanch (become pale). Pressure on the ulnar artery is released and the colour of the hand is observed. If the hand refills with blood within 5 to 7 seconds, turning pink, the ulnar artery is patent. This means there is ade-quate collateral circulation, implying it is safe to take an arterial blood sample or cannulate the radial artery.

VENOUS DRAINAGE OF THE UPPER LIMB

Superficial venous drainage

Dorsal and palmar veins in the hand drain into the dorsal venous network (Fig. 6.22); this comprises the basilic and cephalic veins on the medial and lateral sides of the forearm, respectively. In the arm, the basilic vein pierces the deep fascia to become the

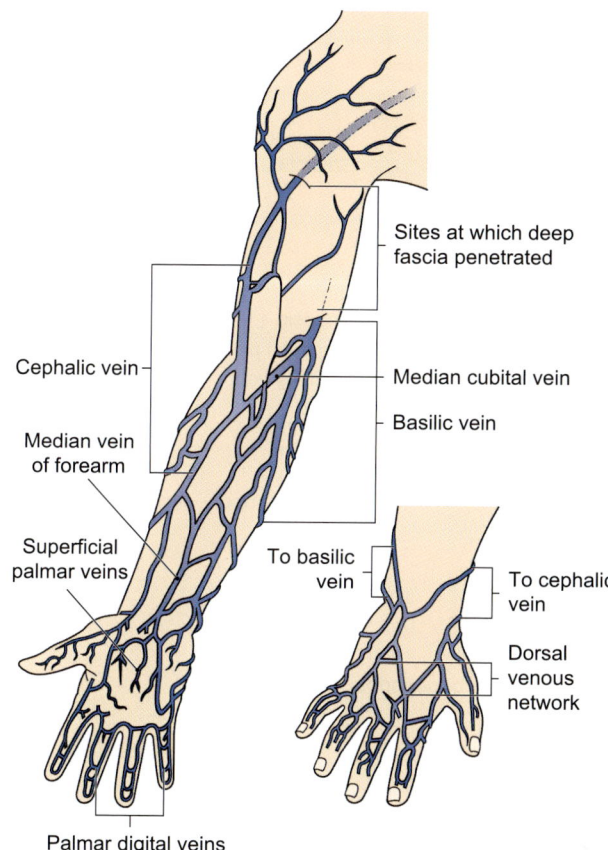

Sites at which deep fascia penetrated

Cephalic vein

Median cubital vein

Basilic vein

Median vein of forearm

Superficial palmar veins

To basilic vein

To cephalic vein

Dorsal venous network

Palmar digital veins

Fig. 6.22 Superficial venous drainage of the upper limb.

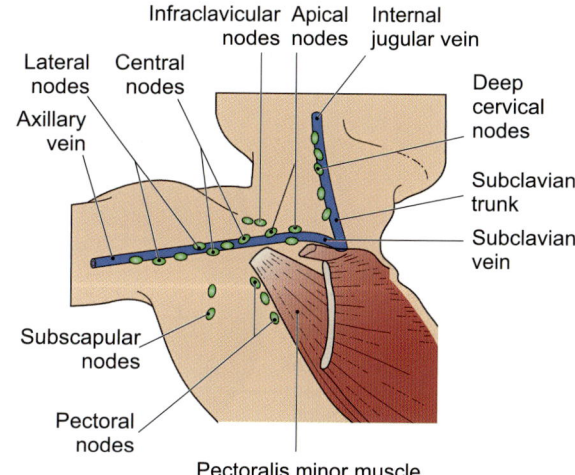

Infraclavicular nodes   Apical nodes   Internal jugular vein

Lateral nodes   Central nodes

Axillary vein

Deep cervical nodes

Subclavian trunk

Subclavian vein

Subscapular nodes

Pectoral nodes

Pectoralis minor muscle

Fig. 6.23 Arrangement of the right axillary lymph nodes.

axillary vein. The cephalic vein pierces the clavipectoral fascia in the deltopectoral triangle to drain into the axillary vein. The cephalic and basilic veins anastomose via the medial cubital vein at the elbow.

CLINICAL NOTES

VENEPUNCTURE

Venepuncture is a procedure that allows blood samples to be taken for a variety of biochemical, microbiological or immunological investigations. The median cubital vein in the median cubital fossa is a commonly used site for venepuncture. A tourniquet is applied to the arm above the cubital fossa to hinder venous return from the forearm, engorging the medial cubital vein and making it more prominent.

Deep venous drainage
The deep veins mirror the arterial system described above.

LYMPHATIC DRAINAGE OF THE UPPER LIMB

Lymphatic drainage follows the venous drainage and ends in the axillary lymph nodes. The basilic system may be interrupted at the elbow by the supratrochlear node. The axillary nodes form several groups (Fig. 6.23):

- Lateral
- Pectoral
- Subscapular
- Central
- Infraclavicular
- Apical

SPECIAL REGIONS OF THE UPPER LIMB

Axilla
The axilla is an anatomical space in the shoulder between the humerus and thoracic wall, through which passes major vessels and nerves (Fig. 6.24). The axilla is formed by four walls, a base and an apex.

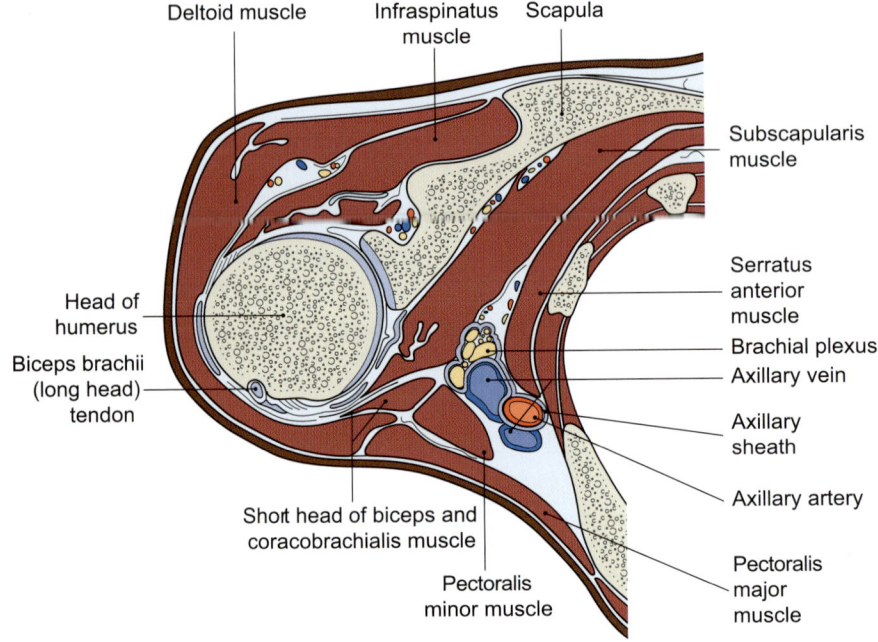

Fig. 6.24 Cross section through the axilla demonstrating its contents and muscular boundaries.

- The apex is continuous with the root of the neck and is formed by the lateral border of the first rib, the clavicle and the scapula.
- Anterior wall: pectoralis major and minor, subclavius and clavipectoral fascia.
- Posterior wall: lateral border of the scapula, latissimus dorsi and teres major.
- Medial wall: ribs 1 to 4 and the serratus anterior muscle.
- Lateral wall: intertubercular sulcus of the humerus.
- Base: skin and fascia.

Quadrangular and triangular spaces

Two spaces are formed by the arrangement of muscles in the shoulder region, forming gateways between the axilla, shoulder and subscapular region (Fig. 6.25).

Triangular space

Boundaries:

- Teres major
- Triceps
- Teres minor

  Contains the scapular circumflex vessels.

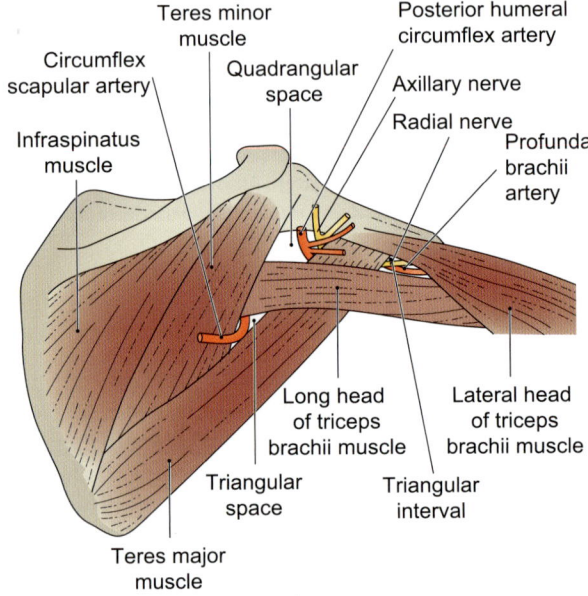

Fig. 6.25 Triangular and quadrangular spaces.

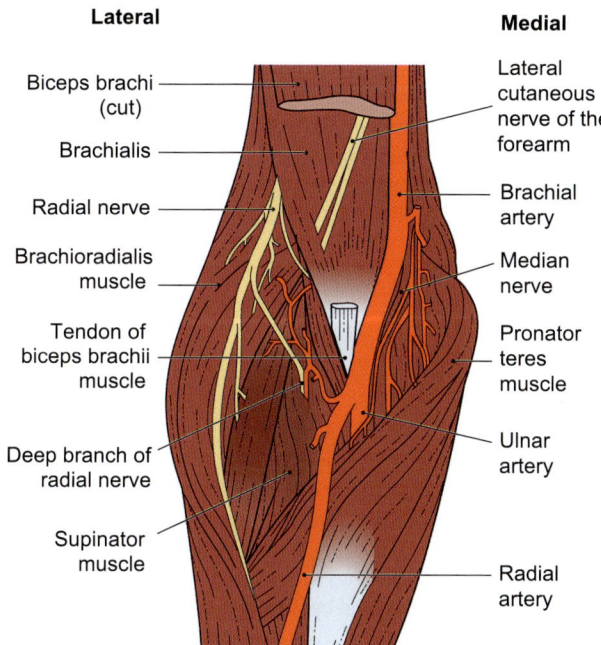

Fig. 6.26 The cubital fossa and its contents.

Lateral

- Biceps brachi (cut)
- Brachialis
- Radial nerve
- Brachioradialis muscle
- Tendon of biceps brachii muscle
- Deep branch of radial nerve
- Supinator muscle

Medial

- Lateral cutaneous nerve of the forearm
- Brachial artery
- Median nerve
- Pronator teres muscle
- Ulnar artery
- Radial artery

Quadrangular space

Boundaries:

- Teres major
- Teres minor
- Surgical neck of the humerus
- Triceps

Contains the axillary nerve and the anterior and posterior circumflex humeral vessels.

Cubital fossa

Boundaries (Fig. 6.26):

- An imaginary line between the medial and lateral epicondyles of the humerus
- Brachioradialis
- Pronator teres
- Floor: brachialis and supinator
- Roof: deep fascia and bicipital aponeurosis

The cubital fossa contains the brachial artery, median nerve and biceps brachii tendon.

Carpal tunnel

The carpal tunnel is formed by the carpal bones and is roofed by the flexor retinaculum (Fig. 6.27). Its contents include:

- Flexor digitorum profundus (four tendons)
- Flexor digitorum superficialis (four tendons)
- Flexor pollicis longus
- Median nerve

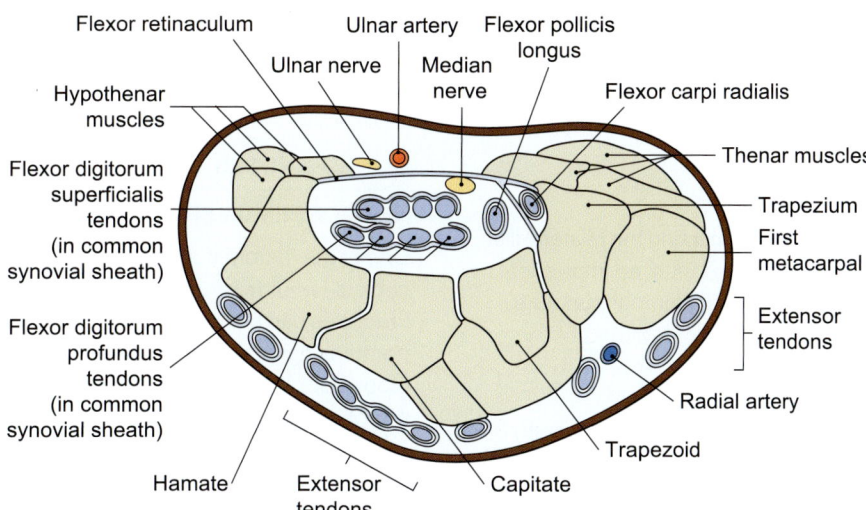

Flexor retinaculum
Ulnar artery
Flexor pollicis longus
Ulnar nerve
Median nerve
Flexor carpi radialis
Hypothenar muscles
Flexor digitorum superficialis tendons (in common synovial sheath)
Flexor digitorum profundus tendons (in common synovial sheath)
Thenar muscles
Trapezium
First metacarpal
Extensor tendons
Radial artery
Hamate
Extensor tendons
Capitate
Trapezoid

Fig. 6.27 Cross section of the carpal tunnel and its contents. (Adapted from Williams, P. (Ed.). (1995). *Gray's anatomy* (38th ed.). Churchill Livingstone.)

REGIONS AND COMPONENTS OF THE LOWER LIMB

The lower limbs are key to locomotion and maintain an upright posture. The line of gravity lies posterior to the hip joint but anterior to the knee and ankle. The hip joint is a ball-and-socket joint formed by the acetabulum and head of the femur. The femur is the bone of the thigh and articulates with the tibia to form the knee joint. The fibula is adjacent to the knee for muscle attachment but is non-weight-bearing. The tibia and fibula are the bones of the leg and articulate with the talus at the ankle joint, where flexion/extension movements occur. Inversion and eversion of the foot occur at the subtalar joint.

The gluteal region is supplied by the superior and inferior gluteal arteries, which are branches of the internal iliac artery. The external iliac artery supplies the lower limb and becomes the femoral artery when it passes under the inguinal ligament. At the popliteal fossa, the femoral artery becomes the popliteal artery.

The gluteal region is supplied by the superior and inferior gluteal nerves. The legs are supplied by the lumbar and sacral plexuses, which form the sciatic, femoral and obturator nerves.

SURFACE ANATOMY OF THE LOWER LIMB

Hip and thigh

In the hip, the pelvis is palpable with its iliac crest, anterior and posterior superior iliac spines. The femur is mostly surrounded by muscles; the greater trochanter can be palpated laterally, and the medial and lateral epicondyles at the knee can be felt.

CLINICAL NOTES

LUMBAR SURFACE ANATOMY

Posteriorly, an imaginary line connecting the bilateral iliac crests (Tuffier line) corresponds to L3/L4, an important landmark appropriate for performing lumbar puncture.

Knee and leg

The circumference of the knee can be palpated, as well as the knee joint line medially and laterally. The patellar ligament attaches inferiorly to the patella and inserts on the tibial tuberosity. Posteriorly, the diamond shape of the popliteal fossa formed by the tendons of the hamstring muscles and the head of the gastrocnemius can be felt.

The anteromedial border of the tibia is felt as the bony shin, and the head of the fibula can be felt lateral to the knee.

Ankle and foot

The two prominences on the sides of the ankle are the medial and lateral malleoli of the tibia and fibula, respectively. In the foot, the metatarsal and phalanx bones are palpable along their length. On the plantar surface, the calcaneum can be felt as the heel. The base of the fifth metatarsal can be palpated laterally, but the remaining metatarsal heads are obscured by the plantar aponeurosis.

BONES AND JOINTS OF THE LOWER LIMB

Hip

The hip joint is a ball-and-socket joint. The C-shaped articular surface of the acetabulum is deepened by the fibrocartilaginous labrum. At the centre of the femoral head is a depression called the fovea, which is the site of attachment of the ligament of the head of the femur.

The joint capsule attaches around the labrum and onto the femoral head. It is supported by three ligaments:

1. Pubofemoral: Prevents excessive abduction and hyperextension.
2. Ischiofemoral: Prevents excessive medial rotation and hyperextension.
3. Iliofemoral: Prevents hyperextension and lateral rotation.

The joint capsule is crucial for the blood supply to the femoral head, which travels in the distal to proximal direction. This supply is from the trochanteric and cruciate anastomoses. The trochanteric anastomosis is composed of the following arteries:

- Medial and lateral circumflex femoral arteries.
- Superior and inferior gluteal arteries.
- Obturator artery.

CLINICAL NOTES

NECK OF FEMUR FRACTURES

One of the factors that influences the management of neck of femur fractures is the fracture location. Fractures can be intra- or extracapsular. Intracapsular fractures have a greater degree of risk of disrupting the blood supply to the femoral head, putting it at a higher risk of avascular necrosis.

Knee joint

The knee joint comprises two articulations: the femur on the tibia and the patella on the femur. It is mostly a flexion/extension joint, but a small degree of rotation is possible. The joint surfaces are lined with hyaline cartilage.

Menisci

Between the femoral and tibial condyles lie the medial and lateral menisci, which are formed from fibrocartilage. They act as shock absorbers and assist in proprioception and joint stability. The menisci are attached peripherally via the coronary ligament to the joint capsule (Fig. 6.28). The menisci are easily injured during twisting movements (medial more commonly than the lateral).

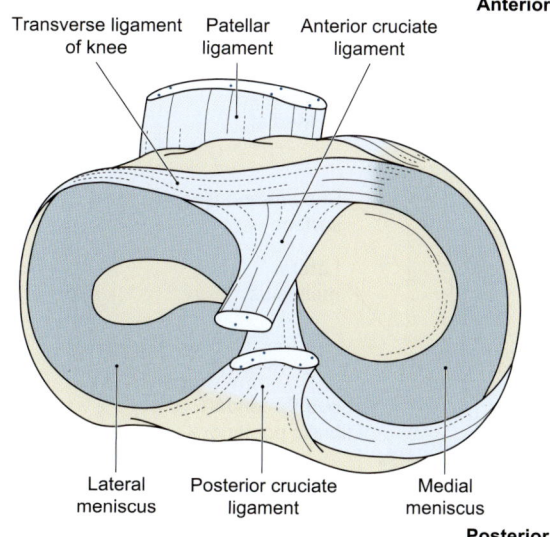

Fig. 6.28 Menisci of the knee viewed from above.

Bursae around the knee joint

The bursae around the knee joint (Fig. 6.29) include:

- Suprapatellar: Between the inferoanterior surface of the femur and the quadriceps tendon.
- Prepatellar: Between the patella and the skin.
- Superficial and deep infrapatellar: Between the patellar ligament and the skin, and the tibia and the patellar ligament.

Ligaments

- The anterior and posterior cruciate ligaments cross over each other to form an X. They keep the articular surfaces opposed and prevent displacement of the femur and tibia. The anterior cruciate ligament (ACL) runs between the medial surface of the lateral femoral condyle and the anterior intercondylar region of the tibia. It prevents anterior displacement of the tibia on the femur. In knee extension, the ACL becomes taut to prevent hyperextension. The posterior cruciate ligament (PCL) runs between the lateral surface of the medial femoral condyle and the posterior intercondylar region of the tibia. The PCL prevents posterior displacement of the tibia on the femur.
- The patellar ligament is a continuation of the quadriceps tendon and attaches at the apex of the patella and inserts on the tibial tuberosity.
- Medial and lateral collateral ligaments stabilize the knee during flexion and extension to prevent abduction and adduction of the knee joint.

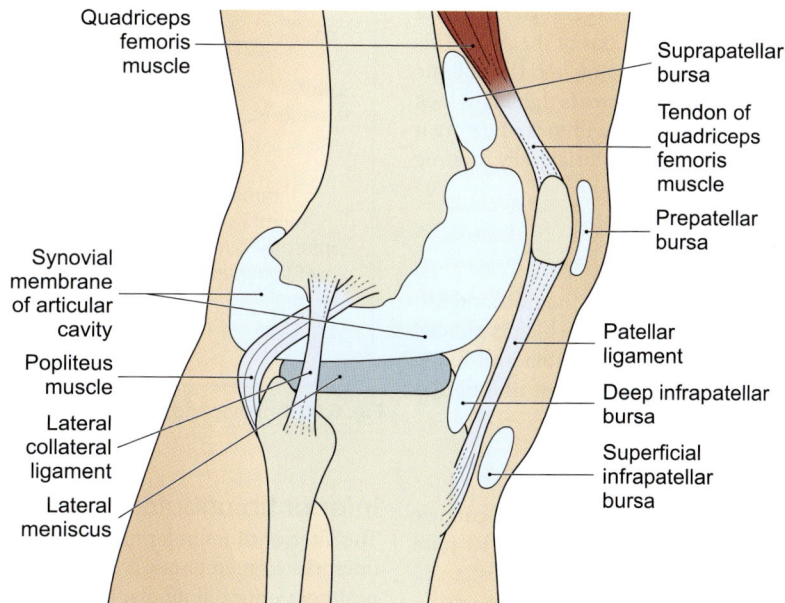

Fig. 6.29 Synovial membrane, bursae and ligaments of the right knee (lateral view).

Table 6.8 Movements of the knee joint

Movement	Muscle
Flexion	Initiated by popliteus hamstrings, gastrocnemius, gracilis and sartorius
Extension	Quadriceps femoris
Medial rotation	Semitendinosus and semimembranosus (when the knee is flexed); popliteus (when the knee is extended)
Lateral rotation	Biceps femoris (when the knee is flexed)
Unlocking of knee	Popliteus
Locking of knee—a passive rotation of the femur on the tibia	Is caused at the end of extension by the anterior cruciate ligament becoming taut and the femoral medial condyle moving around this ligament

- The oblique popliteal ligament is an expansion of the semimembranosus tendon to support the joint capsule posteriorly.

Movements at the knee

The movements of the knee joint are described in Table 6.8. Locking of the knee joint holds it in a slightly hyperextended position. As the knee extends, the ACL becomes taut; however, because the medial condyle of the femur is larger than the lateral condyle, it continues to move around the axis of the ACL. This creates some medial rotation of the knee joint, and the oblique popliteal, medial and lateral collateral ligaments tighten to lock the knee in position. The knee joint must be unlocked before it can flex, which is done by the popliteus muscle laterally rotating the femur.

Bones of the leg

The skeleton of the leg is shown in Fig. 6.30. The tibia and fibula are joined by the interosseous membrane, which is pierced superiorly by the anterior tibial artery. The tibia and fibula articulate at two points: the superior and inferior tibiofibular joints.

Superior tibiofibular joint

The superior tibiofibular joint is formed from the lateral condyle of the tibia and the head of the fibula. It is a synovial joint with limited movement due to the anterosuperior and posterosuperior tibiofibular ligaments.

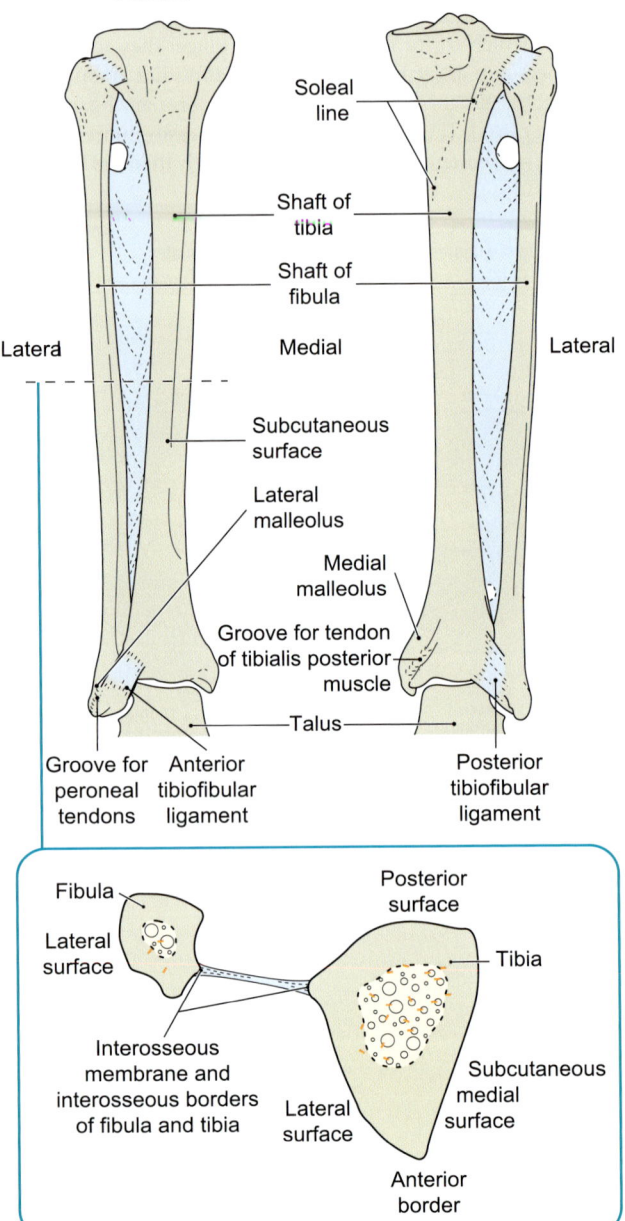

Fig. 6.30 Anterior and posterior views of the tibia and fibula.

Inferior tibiofibular joint

The interior tibiofibular joint is a fibrous joint stabilized by the interosseous membrane. It is stabilized by the anteroinferior and posteroinferior tibiofibular ligaments.

Bones of the ankle and foot

Ankle joint

The ankle joint is a synovial hinge joint between the medial and lateral malleoli of the tibia and fibula and the trochlea of the talus. Plantarflexion is controlled by the muscles in the posterior compartment of the leg, and dorsiflexion is controlled by the anterior compartment (see later). The articular surface of the talus is wider anteriorly so the joint is most stable in full dorsiflexion.

The joint is supported medially by the deltoid ligament and laterally by the anterior talofibular, posterior talofibular and calcaneofibular ligaments.

The bones of the foot (Fig. 6.31) can be divided into the hindfoot (talus and calcaneus), midfoot (navicular, cuboid and cuneiforms) and the forefoot (metatarsals and phalanges). The hallux (great toe) has two phalanges, and the other toes have three.

Intertarsal joints

All of the intertarsal joints are synovial except for the cuboideonavicular joint, which is fibrous. The important intertarsal joints are:

- Subtalar (talocalcaneal) joint: Connects the talus and calcaneum and is strengthened by medial, lateral and posterior talocalcaneal ligaments. Inversion and eversion of the foot occur at this joint.
- Midtarsal (transverse tarsal) joint: Made up of the talocalcaneonavicular joint and the calcaneocuboid joint.

Arches of the foot

The foot has three arches, which act as shock absorbers when walking over uneven ground. These are the medial and lateral longitudinal arches and the transverse arch.

- The medial longitudinal arch is higher than the lateral one and comprises the calcaneus, talus, navicular, cuneiforms and medial three metatarsals with the talus acting as the keystone of the arch. The medial arch is supported by the spring and deltoid ligaments, the long and short plantar ligaments, the plantar aponeurosis as well as several muscles (flexor hallucis longus, flexor digitorum longus, tibialis muscles and peroneus longus).
- The lateral arch consists of the calcaneus, cuboid and lateral two metatarsals. It is supported by ligaments (long and short plantar), the plantar aponeurosis and muscle tendons (flexor digitorum longus and peroneus longus and brevis).

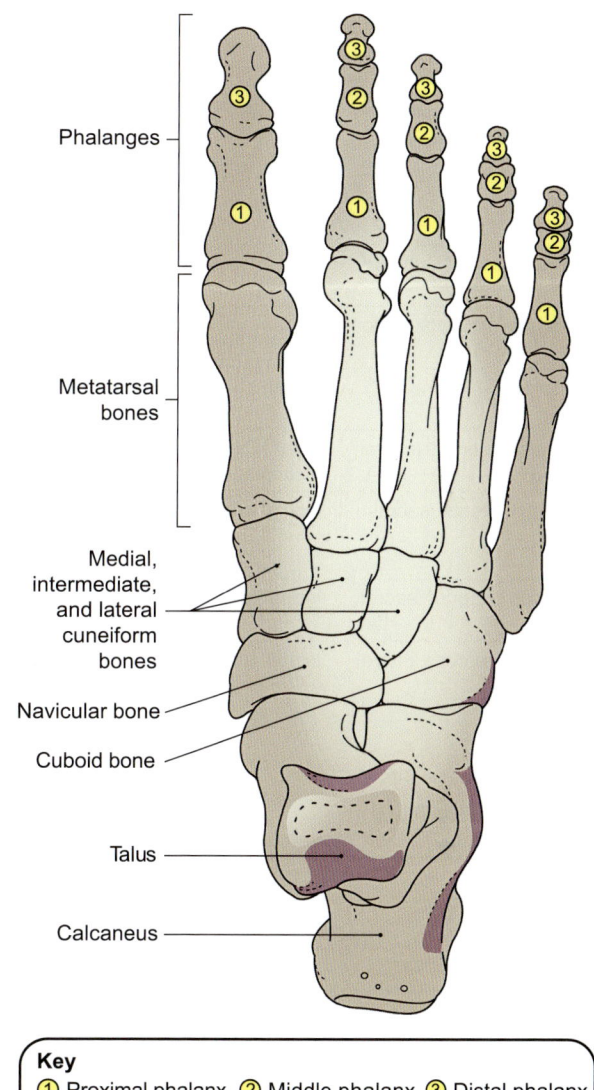

Key
① Proximal phalanx ② Middle phalanx ③ Distal phalanx

Fig. 6.31 Skeleton of the foot.

- The transverse arch consists of the metatarsal bones, cuboid and three cuneiforms. It is maintained by long and short plantar ligaments, deep transverse ligaments and the peroneus longus tendon.

MUSCLES AND TENDONS OF THE LOWER LIMB

The lower limb muscles are shown in Tables 6.9 through 6.15 and Figs 6.32 through 6.38.

Table 6.9 Muscles of the gluteal region

Name of muscle (nerve supply)	Origin	Insertion	Action
Tensor fasciae latae (superior gluteal nerve)	Iliac crest	Iliotibial tract	Extends knee joint Tenses iliotibial tract
Gluteus maximus (inferior gluteal nerve)	Ilium, sacrum, coccyx and sacrotuberous ligament	Iliotibial tract and gluteal tuberosity of femur	Extends and laterally rotates thigh at hip joint Extends knee joint
Gluteus medius (superior gluteal nerve)	Ilium	Greater trochanter of femur	Abducts thigh at hip joint and tilts pelvis when walking
Gluteus minimus (superior gluteal nerve)	Ilium	Greater trochanter of femur	Works with gluteus medius to abduct the thigh and for medial rotation
Piriformis (S1, S2 nerves)	Anterior surface of sacrum	Greater trochanter of femur	
Obturator internus (sacral plexus)	Inner surface of obturator membrane	Greater trochanter of femur	
Gemellus inferior (sacral plexus)	Ischial tuberosity	Greater trochanter of femur	All of these muscles rotate thigh laterally at hip joint and stabilize the hip joint
Gemellus superior (sacral plexus)	Ischial spine	Greater trochanter of femur	
Quadratus femoris (sacral plexus)	Ischial tuberosity	Quadrate tubercle on femur	

Table 6.10 Movements of the hip

Movement of the thigh on the trunk	Movement at the hip joint	Muscles involved	Factors limiting movement
Flexion	Head of the femur moves about a transverse axis passing through both acetabula and causes the shaft to swing anteriorly	Psoas major, iliacus, tensor fasciae latae, pectineus, sartorius	Thigh touching abdomen, hamstring muscle tension if leg is extended
Extension	As flexion but opposite direction	Gluteus maximus, hamstrings	Iliofemoral ligament, pubofemoral ligament
Abduction	Head of the femur moves in the acetabulum about an anteroposterior axis and causes the femoral neck and shaft to swing laterally	Gluteus medius, gluteus minimus	Abductor muscle tension, pubofemoral ligament
Adduction	As abduction but opposite direction	Adductors, gracilis	Gluteus medius, gluteus minimus, other leg
Medial rotation	Rotation of the femoral head in the acetabulum about a vertical axis that passes through the femoral head and medial condyle The neck of the femur swings anteriorly	Tensor fasciae latae, gluteus medius, gluteus minimus, iliopsoas, pectineus, adductor longus	Ischiofemoral ligament
Lateral rotation	As medial rotation but opposite direction	Obturator internus, obturator externus, piriformis, gemelli, quadratus femoris, gluteus maximus	Iliofemoral ligament

Table 6.11 Muscles of the extensor compartment of the thigh

Name of muscle (nerve supply)	Origin	Insertion	Action
Quadriceps femoris—rectus femoris; vastus lateralis, medialis and intermedius (femoral nerve)	Ilium and upper part of femoral shaft	Quadriceps tendon into the patella and via the patellar ligament onto the tibial tuberosity	Extends leg at the knee joint Flexes thigh at hip joint
Sartorius (femoral nerve)	Anterior superior iliac spine	Medial surface of tibial shaft	Flexes, abducts and laterally rotates thigh at the hip joint Flexes and medially rotates leg at the knee joint
Psoas major (lumbar plexus, L1–L3 nerves)	T12 body, transverse processes, bodies and intervertebral discs L1–L5	Lesser trochanter of femur (together with the iliacus muscle)	Flexes thigh on the trunk
Iliacus (femoral nerve)	Iliac fossa of hip bone	Lesser trochanter of femur	Flexes thigh on the trunk
Pectineus (femoral nerve and obturator nerve)	Superior ramus of pubis	Upper shaft of the femur	Flexes and abducts thigh at hip joint

Table 6.12 Flexor muscles of the thigh

Name of muscle (nerve supply)	Origin	Insertion	Action
Biceps femoris: Long head (tibial division of sciatic nerve) Short head (common peroneal division of the sciatic nerve)	Ischial tuberosity	Head of fibula	Flexes leg at knee joint and extends thigh at the hip joint
Semitendinosus (tibial division of the sciatic nerve)	Ischial tuberosity	Proximal tibia (medial to tibial tuberosity)	Flexes leg at the knee joint and extends thigh at the hip joint
Semimembranosus (tibial division of sciatic)	Ischial tuberosity	Medial condyle of the tibia forms the oblique popliteal ligament	Flexes leg at the knee joint and extends thigh at the hip joint

Table 6.13 Adductor muscles of the thigh

Name of muscle (nerve supply)	Origin	Insertion	Action
Gracilis (obturator nerve)	Ischiopubic ramus	Proximal medial surface of tibia	Adducts thigh at hip joint Flexes leg at the knee joint and medially rotates leg when the knee is flexed
Adductor longus (obturator nerve)	Body of pubis	Linea aspera of femur	Adducts and flexes thigh at hip joint
Adductor brevis (obturator nerve)	Inferior ramus of pubis	Linea aspera of femur	Adducts and flexes thigh at hip joint
Adductor magnus (adductor part—obturator nerve; hamstring part—sciatic nerve)	Adductor part—ischiopubic ramus Hamstring part—ischial tuberosity	Adductor part—posterior surface of femur Hamstring part—adductor tubercle of femur	Adductor part—adducts and flexes thigh at hip joint Hamstring part—extends thigh at hip joint
Obturator externus (obturator nerve)	Outer surface of obturator membrane	Greater trochanter of femur	Lateral rotation of thigh at the hip joint

Table 6.14 Muscles of the anterior compartment of the leg

Name of muscle (nerve supply)	Origin	Insertion	Action
Extensor digitorum longus (deep peroneal nerve)	Fibula and interosseous membrane	Phalanges of lateral four digits	Extends toes and dorsiflexes foot at the ankle joint
Extensor hallucis longus (deep peroneal nerve)	Fibula and interosseous membrane	Base of distal phalanx of the great toe	Extends great toe and dorsiflexes foot at the ankle joint
Peroneus tertius (deep peroneal nerve)	Fibula and interosseous membrane	Base of the fifth metatarsal bone	Dorsiflexes at the ankle joint and everts foot
Tibialis anterior (deep peroneal nerve)	Tibia and interosseous membrane	Medial cuneiform and base of first metatarsal bone	Dorsiflexes and inverts foot

Table 6.15 Muscles of the posterior compartment of the leg

Name of muscle (nerve supply)	Origin	Insertion	Action
Superficial group			
Plantaris (tibial nerve)	Lateral supracondylar ridge of femur	Via tendocalcaneus (Achilles tendon) into calcaneus	These muscles plantarflex the foot at the ankle joint
Soleus (tibial nerve)	Tibia and fibula		
Gastrocnemius (tibial nerve)	Medial and lateral condyles of femur		
Deep group			
Flexor digitorum longus (tibial nerve)	Tibia	Distal phalanges of lateral four toes	Flexes lateral four toes Plantarflexes foot
Flexor hallucis longus (tibial nerve)	Fibula	Distal phalanx of great toe	Flexes hallux Plantarflexes foot
Tibialis posterior (tibial nerve)	Tibia and fibula and interosseous membrane	Navicular bone and surrounding bones	Plantarflexes and inverts foot

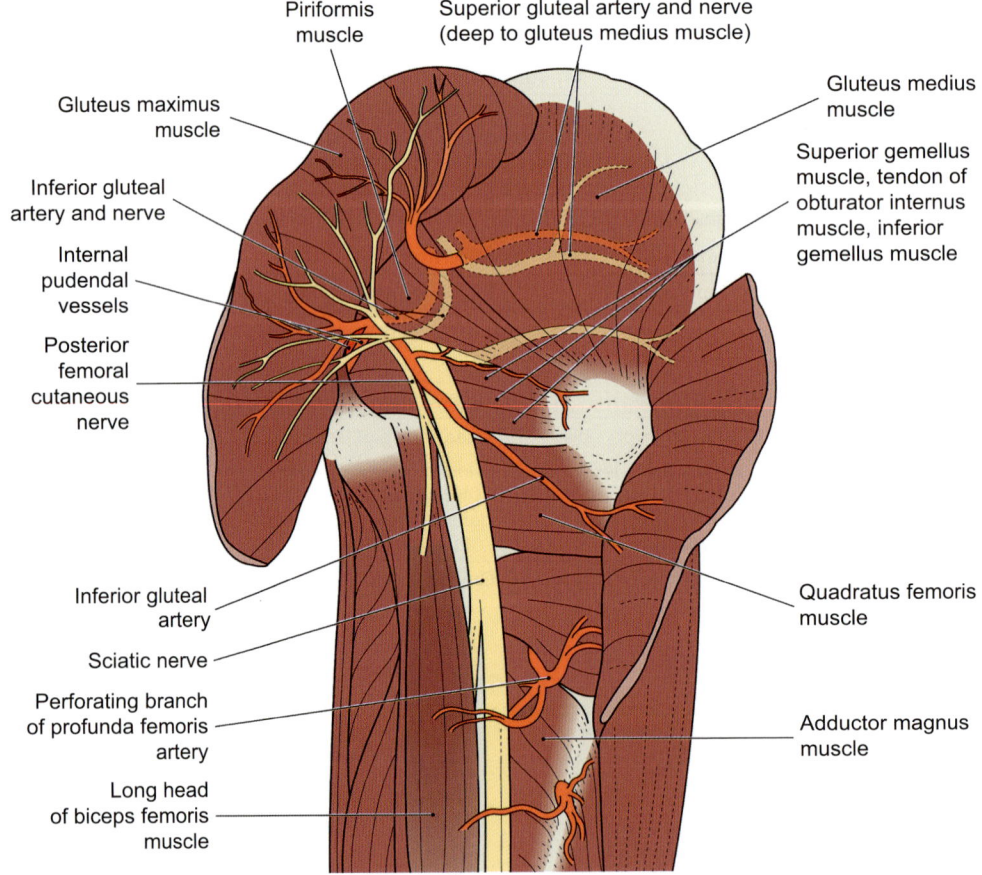

Fig. 6.32 The main muscles, arteries and nerves of the gluteal region.

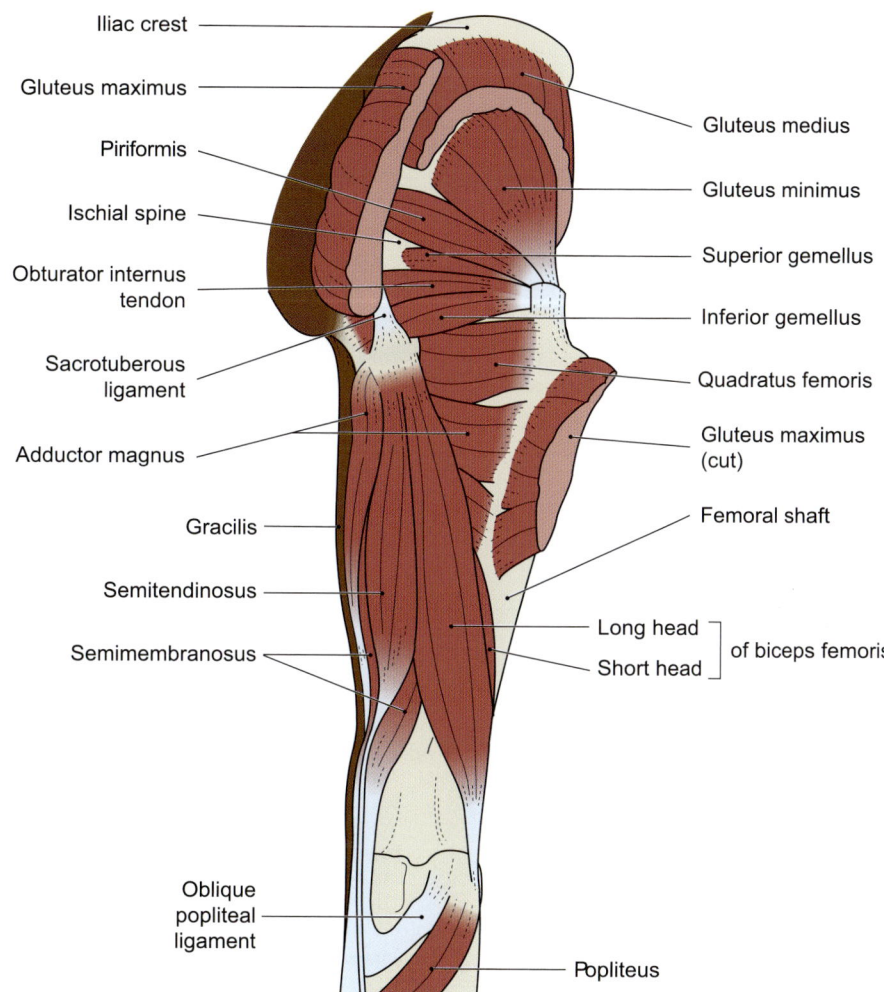

Fig. 6.33 Muscles of the posterior gluteal region and posterior right thigh.

Labels (clockwise from top left): Iliac crest, Gluteus maximus, Piriformis, Ischial spine, Obturator internus tendon, Sacrotuberous ligament, Adductor magnus, Gracilis, Semitendinosus, Semimembranosus, Oblique popliteal ligament, Gluteus medius, Gluteus minimus, Superior gemellus, Inferior gemellus, Quadratus femoris, Gluteus maximus (cut), Femoral shaft, Long head / Short head of biceps femoris, Popliteus.

Muscles of the thigh

The thigh is divided into three muscle compartments (anterior, posterior and medial) by intermuscular septae, which are derived from the fascia lata.

Muscles of the leg

The muscles of the leg are divided into three compartments: anterior, posterior and lateral (see Fig. 6.35). The muscles in the anterior compartment causing dorsiflexion of the ankle are shown in Table 6.14 and Fig. 6.36. The tendons of these muscles enter the foot underneath the extensor retinaculum, which is a thickening of the deep fascia between the anterior tibia and anterior fibula (see Fig. 6.37).

The muscles of the posterior compartment are shown in Table 6.15. The soleus is an important antigravity muscle that maintains posture and initiates walking to overcome the body's weight. The gastrocnemius muscle activates to increase the speed of movement, for example jumping. The muscles also

271

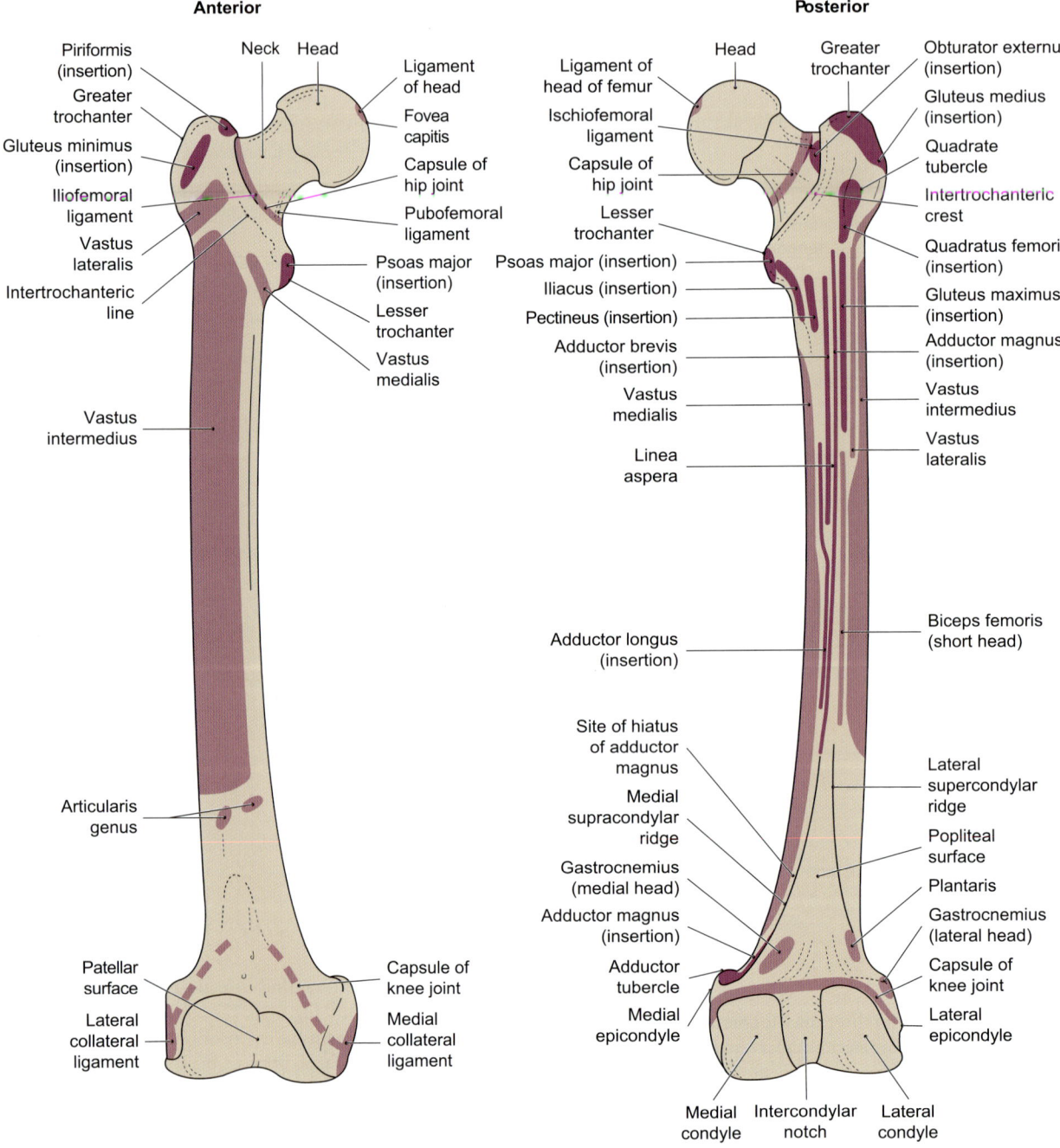

Anterior

Piriformis (insertion)

Greater trochanter

Gluteus minimus (insertion)

Iliofemoral ligament

Vastus lateralis

Intertrochanteric line

Vastus intermedius

Articularis genus

Patellar surface

Lateral collateral ligament

Neck Head

Ligament of head

Fovea capitis

Capsule of hip joint

Pubofemoral ligament

Psoas major (insertion)

Lesser trochanter

Vastus medialis

Capsule of knee joint

Medial collateral ligament

Posterior

Head   Greater trochanter

Ligament of head of femur

Ischiofemoral ligament

Capsule of hip joint

Lesser trochanter

Psoas major (insertion)

Iliacus (insertion)

Pectineus (insertion)

Adductor brevis (insertion)

Vastus medialis

Linea aspera

Adductor longus (insertion)

Site of hiatus of adductor magnus

Medial supracondylar ridge

Gastrocnemius (medial head)

Adductor magnus (insertion)

Adductor tubercle

Medial epicondyle

Obturator externus (insertion)

Gluteus medius (insertion)

Quadrate tubercle

Intertrochanteric crest

Quadratus femoris (insertion)

Gluteus maximus (insertion)

Adductor magnus (insertion)

Vastus intermedius

Vastus lateralis

Biceps femoris (short head)

Lateral supracondylar ridge

Popliteal surface

Plantaris

Gastrocnemius (lateral head)

Capsule of knee joint

Lateral epicondyle

Medial condyle   Intercondylar notch   Lateral condyle

Fig. 6.34 Origins and insertions of muscles on the anterior and posterior femur.

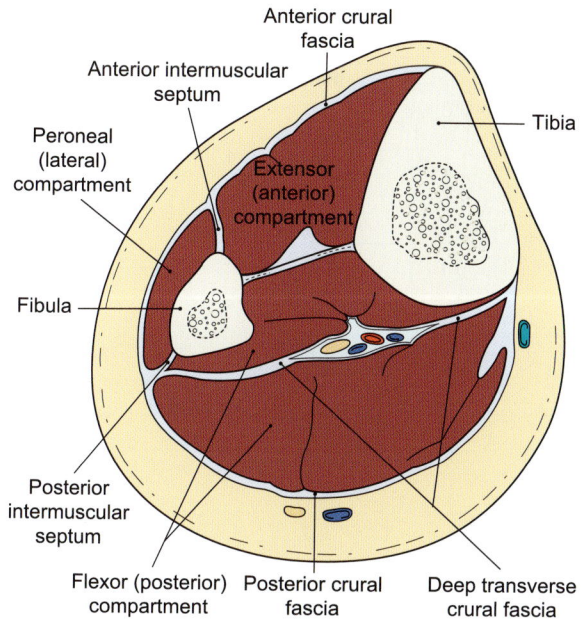

Fig. 6.35 Cross section of the leg.

Anterior crural fascia

Anterior intermuscular septum

Peroneal (lateral) compartment

Extensor (anterior) compartment

Tibia

Fibula

Posterior intermuscular septum

Flexor (posterior) compartment

Posterior crural fascia

Deep transverse crural fascia

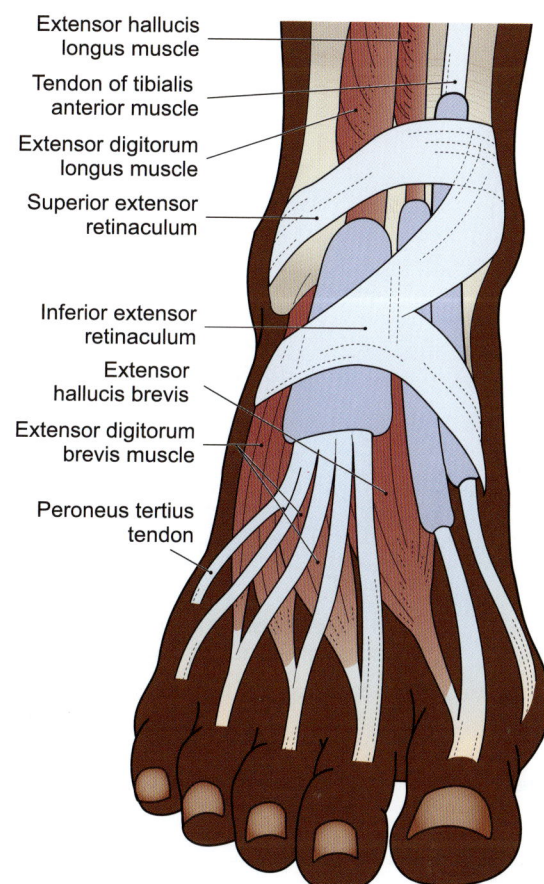

Extensor hallucis longus muscle

Tendon of tibialis anterior muscle

Extensor digitorum longus muscle

Superior extensor retinaculum

Inferior extensor retinaculum

Extensor hallucis brevis

Extensor digitorum brevis muscle

Peroneus tertius tendon

Fig. 6.37 Structure of the extensor retinaculum.

create the calf pump required to move venous blood against gravity back up to the heart. The soleus and gastrocnemius muscles insert into the calcaneum as the Achilles tendon. The remaining muscles pass under the flexor retinaculum to enter the foot (see Fig. 6.38).

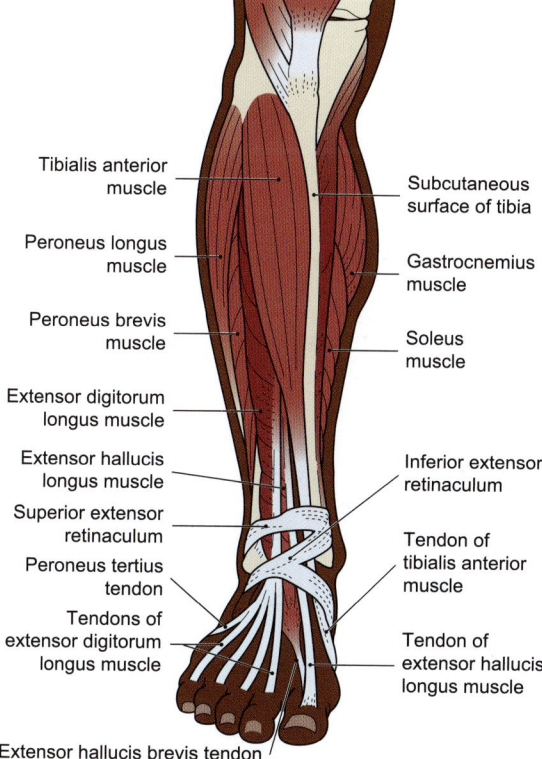

Tibialis anterior muscle

Peroneus longus muscle

Peroneus brevis muscle

Extensor digitorum longus muscle

Extensor hallucis longus muscle

Superior extensor retinaculum

Peroneus tertius tendon

Tendons of extensor digitorum longus muscle

Extensor hallucis brevis tendon of extensor hallucis brevis muscle

Subcutaneous surface of tibia

Gastrocnemius muscle

Soleus muscle

Inferior extensor retinaculum

Tendon of tibialis anterior muscle

Tendon of extensor hallucis longus muscle

Fig. 6.36 Muscles of the anterior compartment of the leg.

> **HINTS AND TIPS**
>
> The contents under the flexor retinaculum (from anterior to posterior) can be remembered with the saying 'Tom, *D*ick and *v*ery *n*aughty *H*arry'—*t*ibialis posterior, flexor *d*igitorum longus, *a*rtery, *v*ein, *n*erve, flexor *h*allucis longus.

The muscles of the lateral compartment are shown in Table 6.16 and Fig. 6.39.

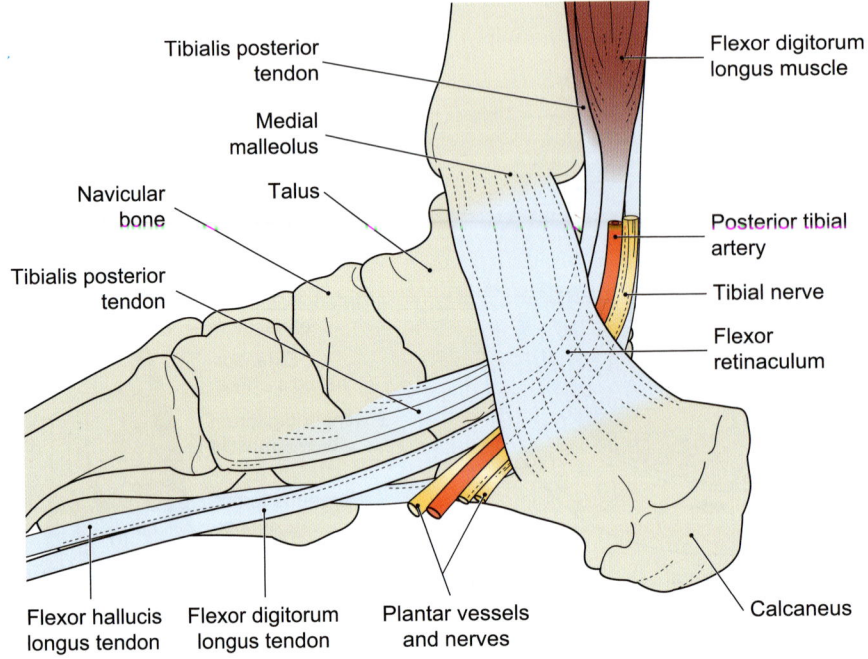

Fig. 6.38 Medial view of the foot and the flexor retinaculum.

Table 6.16 Muscles of the lateral compartment of the leg

Name of muscle (nerve supply)	Origin	Insertion	Action
Peroneus longus (superficial peroneal nerve)	Fibula	First metatarsal and medial cuneiform	Plantarflexes and everts the foot
Peroneus brevis (superficial peroneal nerve)	Fibula	Fifth metatarsal bone	Plantarflexes and everts the foot

Muscles of the foot

The intrinsic muscles of the foot are shown in Table 6.17.

NERVE SUPPLY TO THE LOWER LIMB

The nerves to the lower limb are derived from the lumbosacral plexus. The lumbar plexus is formed from the anterior rami of spinal nerves T12 to L4 and the sacral plexus is from L4 to S4.

The lumbar plexus is shown in Fig. 6.40 and the sacral plexus is shown in Fig. 6.41. The main branches innervating the leg are the sciatic, femoral and obturator nerves.

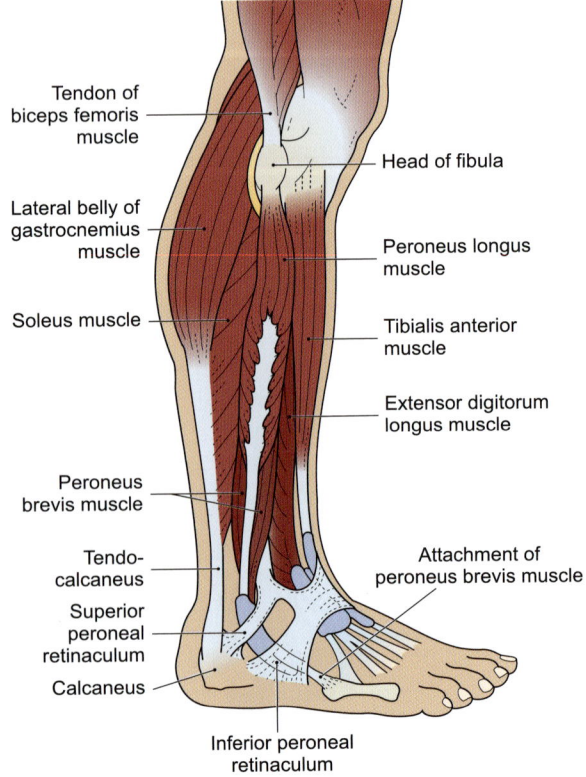

Fig. 6.39 The lateral compartment of the leg.

Table 6.17 Intrinsic muscles of the foot

Muscle (nerve supply)	Origin	Insertion	Action
First layer			
Abductor hallucis (medial plantar nerve)	Calcaneus, flexor retinaculum, plantar aponeurosis	Proximal phalanx of hallux	Abducts great toe
Flexor digitorum brevis (medial plantar nerve)	Calcaneus, plantar aponeurosis	Each tendon bifurcates and inserts into the middle phalanx of the lateral four digits	Flexes lateral four digits
Abductor digiti minimi (lateral plantar nerve)	Calcaneus, plantar aponeurosis	Proximal phalanx of digitus minimus	Abducts digitus minimus (little toe)
Second layer			
Flexor accessorius or quadratus plantae (lateral plantar nerve)	Calcaneus	Tendon of flexor digitorum longus	Pulls on the tendon of flexor digitorum longus and takes up the slack of this tendon when the ankle is plantarflexed This allows the digits to be flexed in this position
Lumbricals (first medial lumbrical—medial plantar nerve; lateral three lumbricals—lateral plantar nerve)	Tendons of flexor digitorum longus	Extensor expansions of lateral four digits	Maintains extension of the digits at DIP and PIP joints while flexor digitorum longus tendons are flexing the lateral four digits at the MTP
Third layer			
Flexor hallucis brevis (medial plantar nerve)	Cuboid and three cuneiforms	Proximal phalanx of hallux	Flexes hallux (great toe)
Adductor hallucis (lateral plantar nerve) Oblique head Transverse head	Second to fourth metatarsal bases and plantar ligament Deep transverse ligament	Both heads insert into the proximal phalanx of the hallux	Adducts hallux towards second toe
Flexor digiti minimi brevis (lateral plantar nerve)	Fifth metatarsal	Proximal phalanx of digitus minimus	Flexes digitus minimus (little toe)
Fourth layer			
Plantar interossei (lateral plantar nerve)	Third, fourth and fifth metatarsals	Proximal phalanx of digits and their extensor expansions	Adduct digits towards second digit
Dorsal interossei (lateral plantar nerve)	First and second; second and third; third and fourth; fourth and fifth metatarsals	Proximal phalanx of digits and their extensor expansions	Abduct digits away from second digit With plantar interossei and lumbricals, they extend the DIP, PIP joints and flex the MTP joint

DIP, *Distal interphalangeal joint*; MTP, *metatarsophalangeal joint*; PIP, *proximal interphalangeal joint*.

Sciatic nerve

The sciatic nerve exits the pelvis through the greater sciatic foramen, beneath the piriformis muscle. In the thigh, it travels through and supplies the muscles of the posterior compartment. At the popliteal fossa, it branches into the tibial and common fibular nerves; the former goes through the fossa and the latter loops around the lateral knee at the femoral head.

In the leg, the tibial nerve runs in the posterior compartment deep to the soleus muscle. It supplies the posterior compartment.

The common fibular nerve has deep and superficial branches; the former supplies muscles of the anterior compartment and the latter supplies the lateral compartment.

Femoral nerve

The femoral nerve is derived from L2 to L4 and enters the leg underneath the inguinal ligament. It innervates the anterior compartment of the thigh and continues as the saphenous cutaneous nerve.

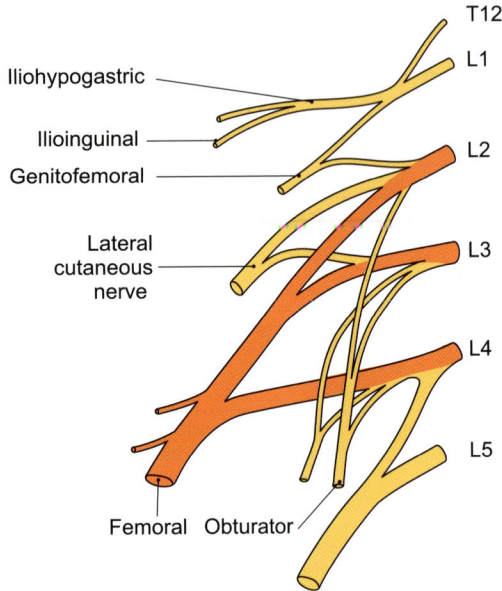

Iliohypogastric

Ilioinguinal

Genitofemoral

Lateral
cutaneous
nerve

Femoral   Obturator

T12
L1
L2
L3
L4
L5

Fig. 6.40 The lumbar plexus.

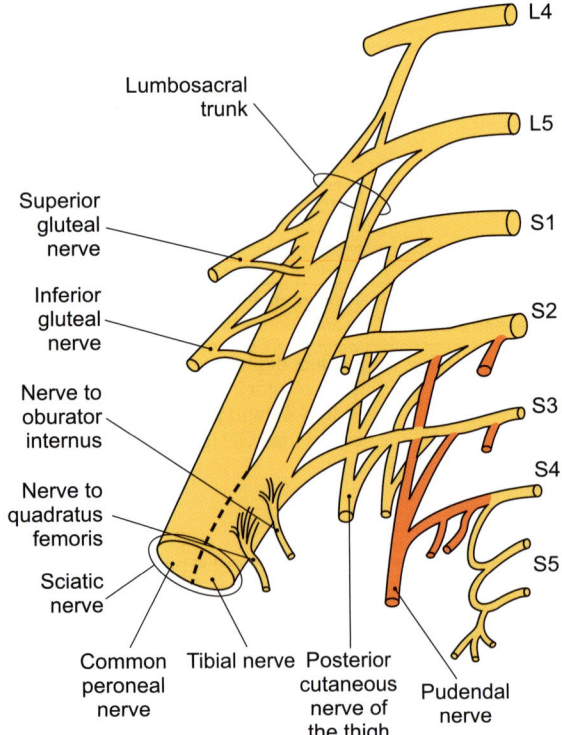

Lumbosacral
trunk

Superior
gluteal
nerve

Inferior
gluteal
nerve

Nerve to
oburator
internus

Nerve to
quadratus
femoris

Sciatic
nerve

Common
peroneal
nerve

Tibial nerve

Posterior
cutaneous
nerve of
the thigh

Pudendal
nerve

L4
L5
S1
S2
S3
S4
S5

Fig. 6.41 The sacral plexus.

Table 6.18 Nerves of the thigh

Nerve (origin)	Course and distribution
Ilioinguinal (lumbar plexus: L1)	Supplies skin over the upper and medial part of the thigh, the skin over the root of the penis and upper part of the scrotum or the skin over the mons pubis and labia majora
Genitofemoral (lumbar plexus: L1–L2)	Descends on the anterior surface of psoas major and divides into genital and femoral branches The femoral branch supplies skin over femoral triangle The genital branch supplies the cremaster muscle and scrotum or the labia majora
Lateral cutaneous nerve of thigh (lumbar plexus: L2–L3)	Passes deep to inguinal ligament, 2–3 cm medial to anterior superior iliac spine Supplies skin on anterior and lateral aspects of thigh
Medial and intermediate femoral cutaneous (femoral nerve)	Arise in femoral triangle and pierce fascia lata of the thigh Supplies skin on the medial and anterior aspects of the thigh
Posterior cutaneous nerve of thigh (sacral plexus: S2–S3)	Passes through greater sciatic foramen inferior to piriformis Supplies skin over the posterior aspect of thigh, buttock and proximal leg
Femoral (lumbar plexus: L2–L4)	Passes deep to inguinal ligament Supplies muscles of the anterior compartment of the thigh, hip and knee joints, and skin on anteromedial side of thigh
Obturator (lumbar plexus: L2–L4)	Enters thigh through obturator foramen and divides The anterior branch supplies adductor longus, adductor brevis, gracilis and pectineus The posterior branch supplies obturator externus and adductor magnus
Sciatic (sacral plexus: L4–S3)	Enters gluteal region through the greater sciatic foramen inferior to or through piriformis, descends along the posterior aspect of thigh and divides proximal to the knee into the tibial and common peroneal nerves The tibial division innervates the hamstrings (except for short head of biceps femoris— innervated by the common peroneal division) and has articular branches to the hip and knee joints

Obturator nerve

The obturator nerve is derived from L2 to L4 and exits the pelvis through the obturator foramen. In the leg, it supplies the adductor compartment.

The nerves of the thigh, leg and foot are shown in Tables 6.18, 6.19 and 6.20, respectively. The cutaneous supply to the foot is shown in Fig. 6.42.

Table 6.19 Nerves of the leg

Nerve (origin)	Course	Distribution
Common peroneal (sciatic nerve)	Arises at the apex of popliteal fossa and follows medial border of biceps femoris and its tendon Passes over the posterior aspect of head of fibula and then winds around the neck of fibula, deep to peroneus longus, where it divides into deep and superficial peroneal nerves	Supplies skin on posterolateral part of leg via its branch—lateral sural cutaneous nerve
Deep peroneal (common peroneal nerve)	Arises between peroneus longus and neck of fibula Descends on interosseous membrane and enters dorsum of the foot	Supplies extensor muscles of leg and skin of the first interdigital cleft
Saphenous (femoral nerve)	Descends with femoral vessels and the great saphenous vein	Supplies skin on the medial side of leg and foot
Superficial peroneal (common peroneal nerve)	Arises between peroneus longus and neck of fibula and descends in the lateral compartment of leg	Supplies peroneus longus and brevis and skin on the anterior surface of leg and dorsum of foot
Sural (usually arises from both tibial and common peroneal nerves)	Descends between heads of gastrocnemius and becomes superficial at the middle of leg	Supplies skin on posterolateral aspects of leg and lateral side of foot
Tibial (sciatic nerve)	Descends through popliteal fossa and lies on popliteus Then runs interiorly with posterior tibial vessels and terminates beneath flexor retinaculum by dividing into medial and lateral plantar nerves	Supplies flexor muscles of leg, knee joint and skin, and muscles of the sole of the foot

Table 6.20 Nerves of the foot

Nerve (origin)	Distribution
Saphenous (femoral nerve)	Supplies skin on the medial side of foot as far anteriorly as head of first metatarsal
Superficial peroneal (common peroneal nerve)	Supplies skin on the dorsum of foot and all digits, except adjoining sides of first and second digits
Deep peroneal (common peroneal nerve)	Supplies extensor digitorum brevis, extensor hallucis brevis and skin on contiguous sides of first and second digits
Medial plantar (larger terminal branch of the tibial nerve)	Supplies skin of medial side of sole of foot and plantar surfaces of first three digits and half of fourth digit Also supplies abductor hallucis, flexor digitorum brevis, flexor hallucis brevis and first lumbrical
Lateral plantar (smaller terminal branch of tibial nerve)	Supplies quadratus plantae, abductor digiti minimi and flexor digiti minimi brevis Deep branch supplies plantar and dorsal interossei, lateral three lumbricals and adductor halluces Supplies skin on sole lateral to a line splitting fourth digit
Sural (tibial and common peroneal nerves)	Lateral aspect of foot
Calcaneal nerves (tibial and sural nerves)	Skin of heel

ARTERIAL SUPPLY TO THE LOWER LIMB

The arterial supply to the lower limb is from the external iliac artery. When the external iliac artery passes under the inguinal ligament, it is renamed as the common femoral artery. In the femoral triangle, the common femoral artery bifurcates into the superficial femoral artery and the profunda femoris. The profunda femoris is the main supply to the muscles of the thigh. The other arteries in the thigh are shown in Table 6.21.

The superficial femoral artery continues through the thigh and enters the posterior compartment through the adductor canal. After passing through the adductor canal, the artery is renamed the popliteal artery. In the popliteal fossa, the artery is the deepest structure in the neurovascular bundle sitting next to the knee joint capsule. Around the knee is an anastomotic network of geniculate arteries (Fig. 6.43). At the lower border of the popliteus muscle, the artery divides into the anterior and posterior tibial arteries. The posterior tibial artery quickly gives off the peroneal branch.

In the leg, the anterior tibial and posterior tibial arteries continue into the foot. In the foot, the anterior tibial becomes the dorsalis pedis which in turn bifurcates into the first metatarsal artery and the deep plantar artery.

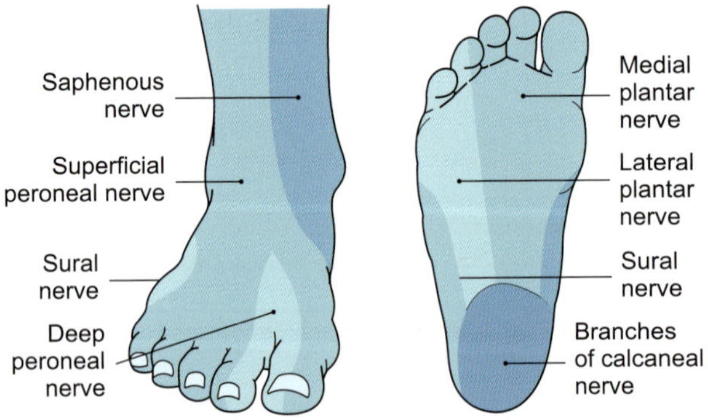

VENOUS DRAINAGE OF THE LEG

The deep venous drainage of the leg follows the arterial branching pattern described above.

Superficial venous drainage

On the dorsum of the foot is the superficial dorsal venous arch, which drains into the great saphenous vein medially and the short saphenous vein laterally (Fig. 6.44). The great saphenous vein lies anterior to the medial malleolus and the short saphenous lies posterior to the lateral malleolus.

Great saphenous vein

At the medial malleolus, the great saphenous vein courses up the medial aspect of the leg in the superficial fascia and then posterior to the medial epicondyle of the femur. In the thigh, it remains medial until it pierces the cribriform fascia (an opening in the fascia lata) so that it can merge with the femoral vein at the saphenofemoral junction.

Small saphenous vein

The Small saphenous vein runs up the posterior leg alongside the sural nerve and pierces the fascia of the popliteal fossa to merge with the popliteal vein.

Fig. 6.42 Distribution of the cutaneous nerves to the foot.

Table 6.21 Arteries of the thigh

Artery	Origin	Course and distribution
Femoral	Continuation of external iliac artery distal to inguinal ligament	Descends through femoral triangle, enters the adductor canal and ends by passing through the adductor hiatus (where it becomes the popliteal artery) Supplies anterior and anteromedial surfaces of the thigh
Profunda femoris	Femoral artery in the femoral triangle	Passes inferiorly, deep to adductor longus Gives off perforating branches to supply posterior and lateral compartments of thigh
Lateral circumflex femoral	Profunda femoris; may arise from femoral artery	Passes laterally deep to sartorius and rectus femoris Supplies the anterior part of gluteal region, the femur and the knee joint
Medial circumflex femoral	Profunda femoris	Passes medially and posteriorly between pectineus and iliopsoas and enters gluteal region Supplies head and neck of femur
Obturator	Internal iliac artery	Passes through obturator foramen and enters medial compartment of thigh Supplies obturator externus, pectineus, adductors of thigh and gracilis—muscles attached to ischial tuberosity and head of femur

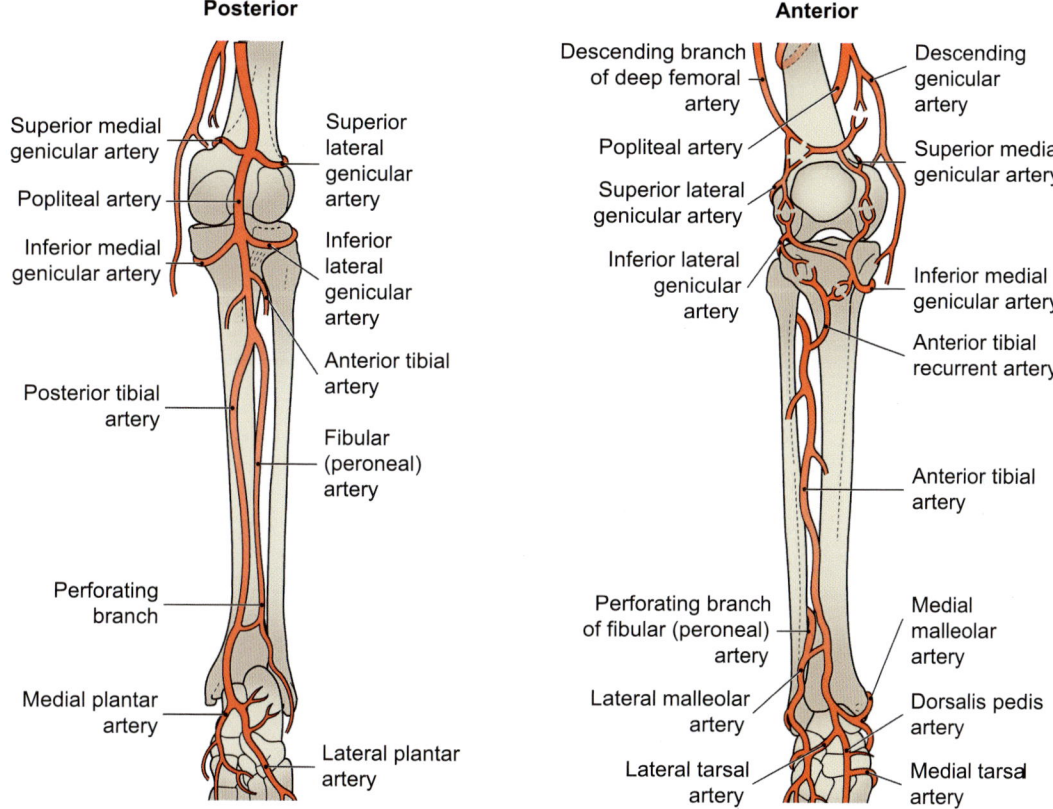

Posterior

Superior medial
genicular artery

Popliteal artery

Inferior medial
genicular artery

Posterior tibial
artery

Perforating
branch

Medial plantar
artery

Superior
lateral
genicular
artery

Inferior
lateral
genicular
artery

Anterior tibial
artery

Fibular
(peroneal)
artery

Lateral plantar
artery

Anterior

Descending branch
of deep femoral
artery

Popliteal artery

Superior lateral
genicular artery

Inferior lateral
genicular
artery

Perforating branch
of fibular (peroneal)
artery

Lateral malleolar
artery

Lateral tarsal
artery

Descending
genicular
artery

Superior medial
genicular artery

Inferior medial
genicular artery

Anterior tibial
recurrent artery

Anterior tibial
artery

Medial
malleolar
artery

Dorsalis pedis
artery

Medial tarsal
artery

Fig. 6.43 Arterial supply of the lower leg: posterior and anterior views.

LYMPHATIC DRAINAGE OF THE LOWER LIMB

The lymphatic drainage of the superficial tissues in the leg is into the superficial inguinal lymph nodes around the termination of the great saphenous vein. The deep tissues drain into the deep nodes around the femoral veins (Fig. 6.45).

SPECIAL REGIONS OF THE LOWER LIMB

Femoral triangle
Boundaries:

- Inguinal ligament
- Adductor longus

- Sartorius
- Floor: pectineus and adductor longus
- Roof: fascia lata

It contains the femoral nerve, arteries, veins and deep lymph nodes.

Popliteal fossa
Boundaries:

- Semimembranosus and semitendinosus tendons
- Biceps femoris tendon
- Medial and lateral heads of gastrocnemius
- Floor: capsule of the knee joint and popliteus muscle
- Roof: superficial and deep fascia

It contains the tibial nerve, popliteal artery and vein, termination of the short saphenous vein and common fibular nerve.

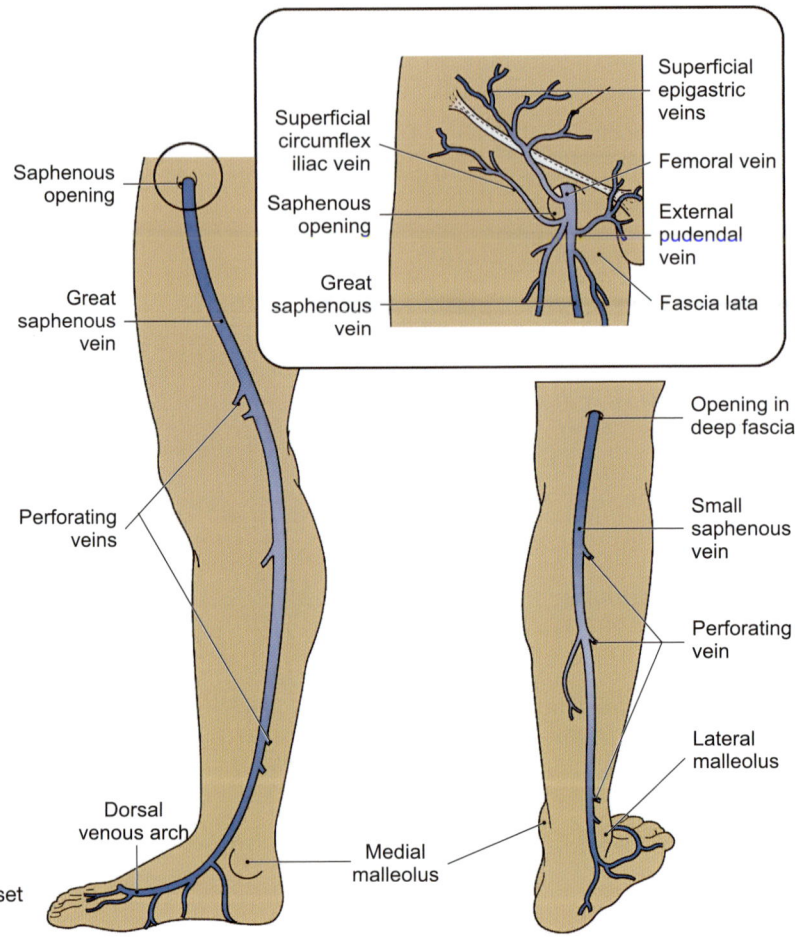

Fig. 6.44 Great and small saphenous veins. Inset shows saphenofemoral junction.

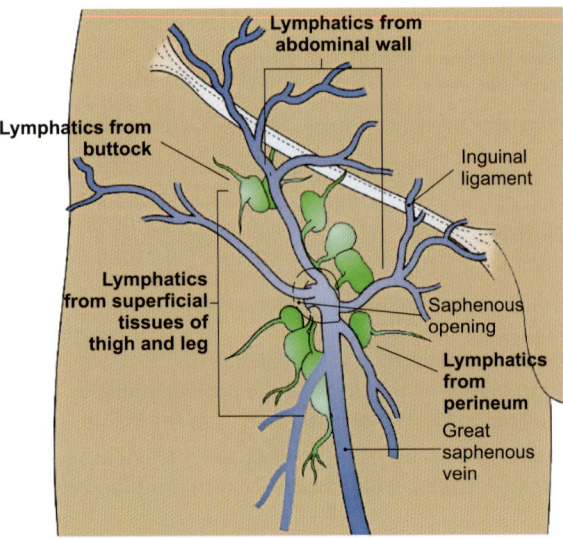

Fig. 6.45 Superficial inguinal lymph node.

VERTEBRAL COLUMN

The key surface landmarks of the vertebral column are shown in Fig. 6.46.

Osteology of the cerebral column

The vertebral column consists of 33 vertebrae arranged in five distinct regions (5 cervical, 12 thoracic, 5 lumbar, 5 sacral and 4 coccygeal). The sacral and coccygeal vertebrae fuse into one unit. The vertebrae articulate with each other through the intervertebral discs and the facet joints.

There are four curvatures of the spine (Fig. 6.47).

Features of a vertebra

The features of a typical vertebra are shown in Fig. 6.48. The vertebral body is responsible for 80% of the weight-bearing capability of the spine, and the vertebral bodies get larger progressively

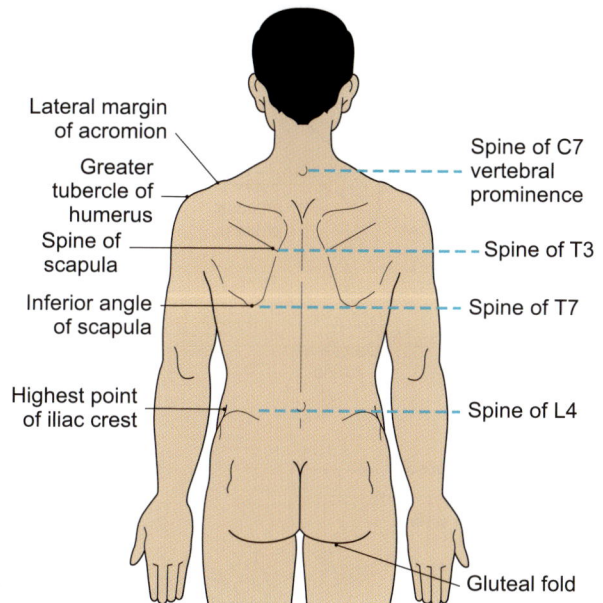

Lateral margin of acromion

Greater tubercle of humerus

Spine of scapula

Inferior angle of scapula

Highest point of iliac crest

Spine of C7 vertebral prominence

Spine of T3

Spine of T7

Spine of L4

Gluteal fold

Fig. 6.46 Surface anatomy of the back.

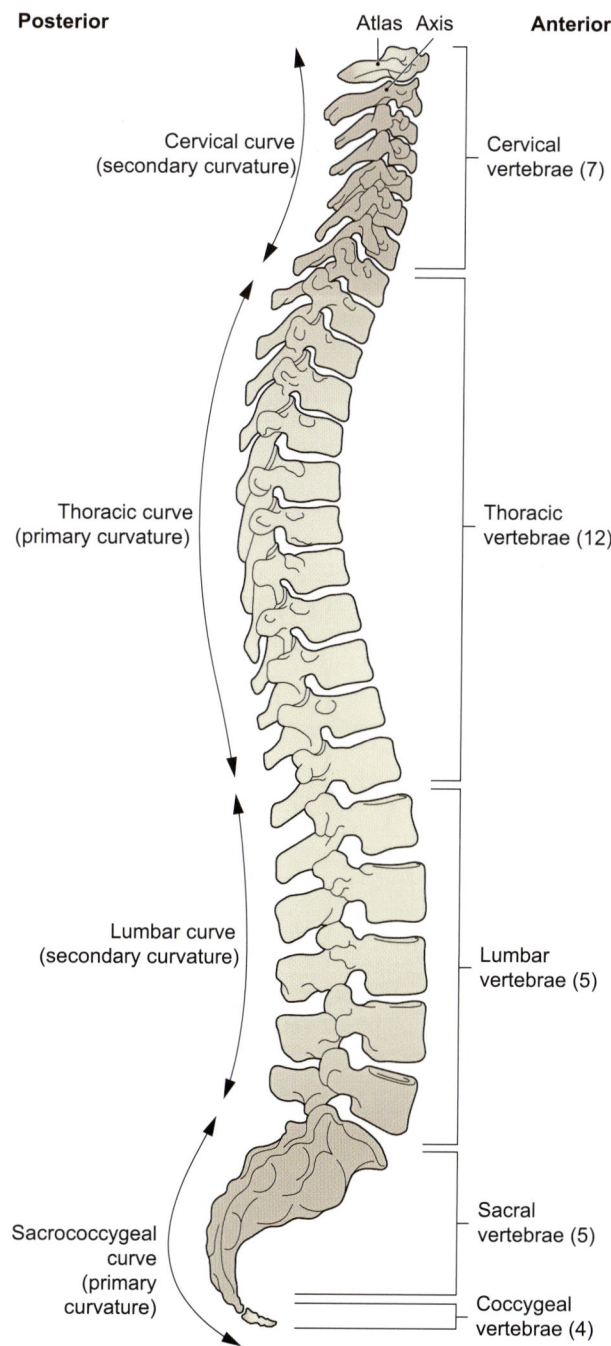

Posterior   Atlas Axis   Anterior

Cervical curve (secondary curvature)

Cervical vertebrae (7)

Thoracic curve (primary curvature)

Thoracic vertebrae (12)

Lumbar curve (secondary curvature)

Lumbar vertebrae (5)

Sacrococcygeal curve (primary curvature)

Sacral vertebrae (5)

Coccygeal vertebrae (4)

Fig. 6.47 Lateral view of the vertebral column.

down the spine. The vertebral foramen is formed by the posterior arch, and the vertebral canal is formed when the vertebral foramen is put together along the length of the spine.

Each region of the spine has some atypical features that are unique to that region. These are listed in Table 6.22. The C1 (atlas) and C2 (axis) vertebrae are highly specialized to allow rotation of the head at the C1 to C2 joint (see Fig. 6.48).

Joints of the vertebral column

Atlantooccipital joint

The atlantooccipital joint is formed by the articular surface of the lateral mass of C1 and the occipital condyles. It is a synovial joint and allows a total of 30 degrees of flexion/extension.

Atlantoaxial joints

The atlantoaxial joints are formed by articulations between the lateral masses of the atlas (C1) and axis (C2) vertebrae and between the odontoid process and anterior arch. The odontoid is held in position by the transverse ligament across the anterior atlas arch and alar ligaments to the occipital bone. The main motion is rotation, which covers 50 degrees and represents 50% of the total rotation of the cervical spine.

Facet joints

Facet joints (zygapophysial) are synovial joints between the superior and inferior articular processes. Their orientation, and thus the movements they allow, change in different regions of the

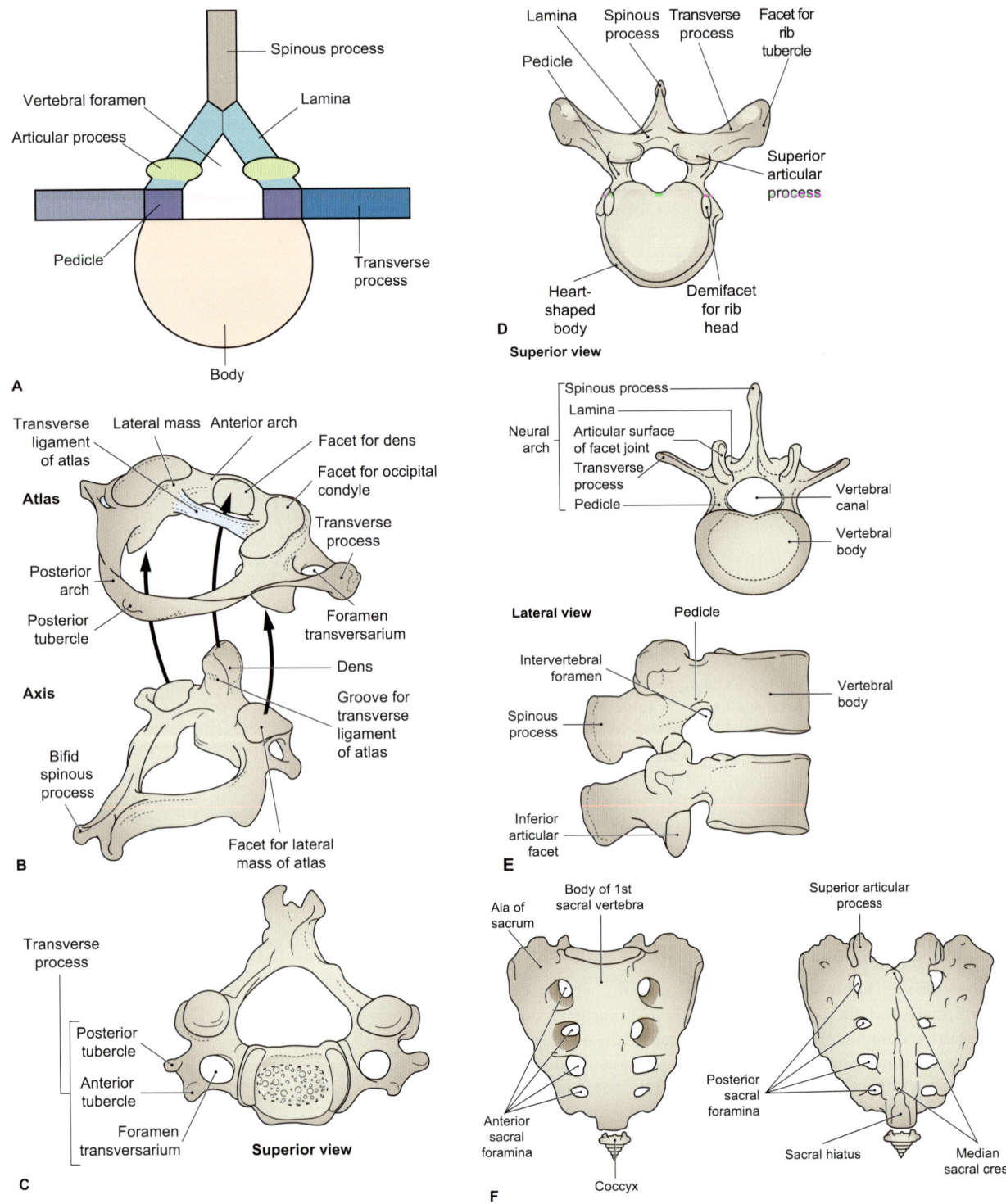

Fig. 6.48 Features of a typical vertebrae (A), atlas and axis (B), cervical vertebrae (C), thoracic vertebrae (D), lumbar vertebrae (E) and the sacrum viewed from anterior and posterior (F).

Table 6.22 Features of atypical vertebrae

Vertebral region	Differentiating characteristics
Cervical	• Small vertebral bodies—transverse diameter greater than anteroposterior diameter. Concave superior surface, convex inferior surface • Large triangular vertebral foramina • Short and bifid spinous processes (except C6 and particularly C7) • Foramina transversaria for the passage of the vertebral arteries
Thoracic	• Heart-shaped vertebral bodies with costal facets for articulation with the ribs • Small circular vertebral foramina • Long transverse processes (T1–T10 have facets for articulation with the ribs) • Long spinous processes
Lumbar	• Large, kidney-shaped vertebral bodies • Triangular vertebral foramina • Long, thin transverse processes • Bulky, square spinous processes
Sacral	• Fused vertebral bodies • Sacral foramina

Table 6.23 Ligaments of the vertebral column

Ligament	Action
Anterior longitudinal	Extends from the anterior tubercle of C1 vertebra (the atlas) to the sacrum. Is attached to the anterior surfaces of the vertebral bodies and intervertebral discs. Prevents hyperextension of the vertebral column and maintains the stability of the intervertebral discs.
Posterior longitudinal	Extends from C2 vertebra to the sacrum. Is attached to the posterior aspect of the vertebral bodies and intervertebral discs (therefore lines the anterior surface of the vertebral canal). Prevents hyperflexion of the vertebral column and posterior protrusion of the intervertebral discs.
Supraspinous	Crosses and unites the tips of the spinous processes from C7 to the sacrum (between the skull and C7 this ligament is known as the ligamentum nuchae).
Interspinous	Ligaments uniting adjacent spinous processes.
Ligamentum flavum	Unites adjacent laminae, limits flexion of the vertebral column, assists in extending the spine after flexion and helps to preserve the curvatures of the vertebral column.

spine. In the lumbar region they are orientated in the sagittal plane and so only allow flexion/extension and no rotation or lateral flexion. Further up the spine, they become more coronally aligned and so allow more rotation and lateral flexion.

Intervertebral discs

Intervertebral discs lie between the vertebral bodies. They act as shock absorbers in the spine. There are two components to the disc:

1. Anulus fibrosus: outer rings of fibrocartilage.
2. Nucleus pulposus: gelatinous core.

Ligaments of the vertebral column

The ligaments of the spine are shown in Table 6.23. The nuchal ligament is only found in the cervical spine and is a continuation of the supraspinal ligament to attach to the spinous processes and the external occipital protuberance.

Muscles of the vertebral column

The majority of a person's weight is anterior to the vertebral column, so strong back muscles are required to maintain posture. There are two main groups of back muscles (Fig. 6.49):

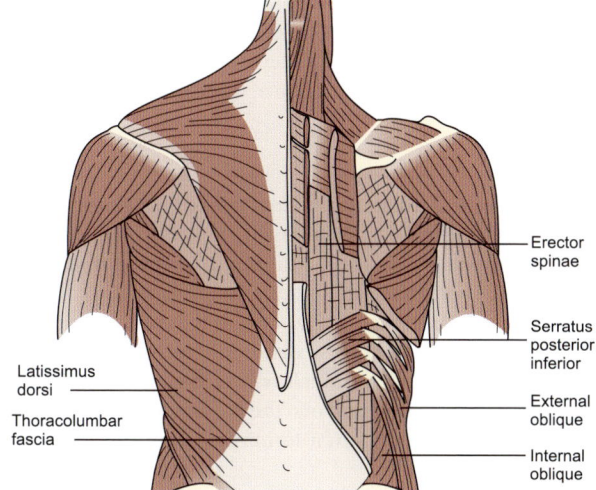

Fig. 6.49 Muscles of the back.

1. Superficial: trapezius, latissimus dorsi, levator scapulae and rhomboid major and minor.
2. Deep: erector spinae muscles (multifidus, longissimus and iliocostalis).

283

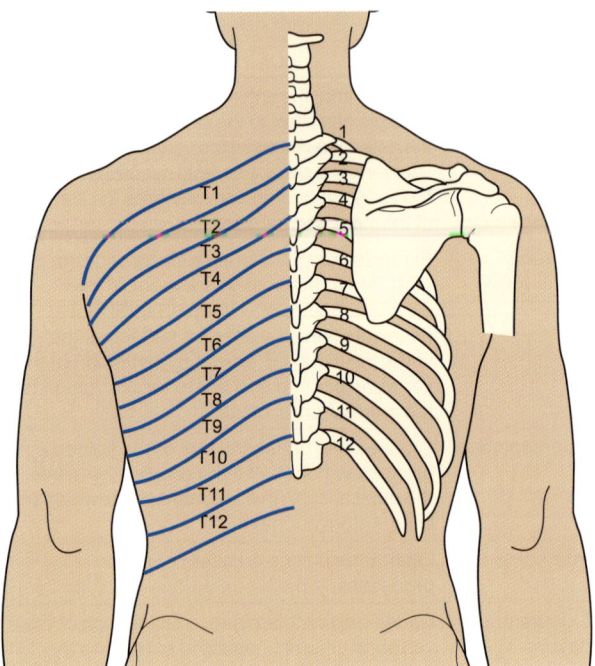

Fig. 6.50 Dermatomes of the back.

Cutaneous innervation of the back

The cutaneous innervation of the back follows a dermatomal pattern from the posterior rami of the spinal nerves. The distribution is shown in Fig. 6.50. Key levels are at the spine of the scapula at T2 and the inferior angle of the scapula at T7.

Spinal cord

The spinal cord is a slightly flattered cylindrical structure that extends from the foramen magnum of the skull (it is a continuation of the medulla oblongata of the brain) to approximately the level of the L2 vertebra in adults (L3 vertebra in infants). The terminal end of the spinal cord is known as the conus medullaris. The pia mater of the meninges extends inferiorly from the conus medullaris, as the filum terminale which attaches to the coccyx. Inferior to the conus medullaris, the lumbosacral spinal nerve roots, together with the filum terminale, comprise the cauda equina.

There are two regions of enlargement within the spinal cord, which give rise to the upper and lower limb plexuses. A nervous plexus is an interconnected network of branching nerves. The cervical enlargement (C5–T1 segments of the spinal cord) gives rise to the nerves of the brachial plexus, while the lumbosacral enlargement (L2–S3) gives rise to the nerves of the lumbosacral plexus (Fig. 6.51).

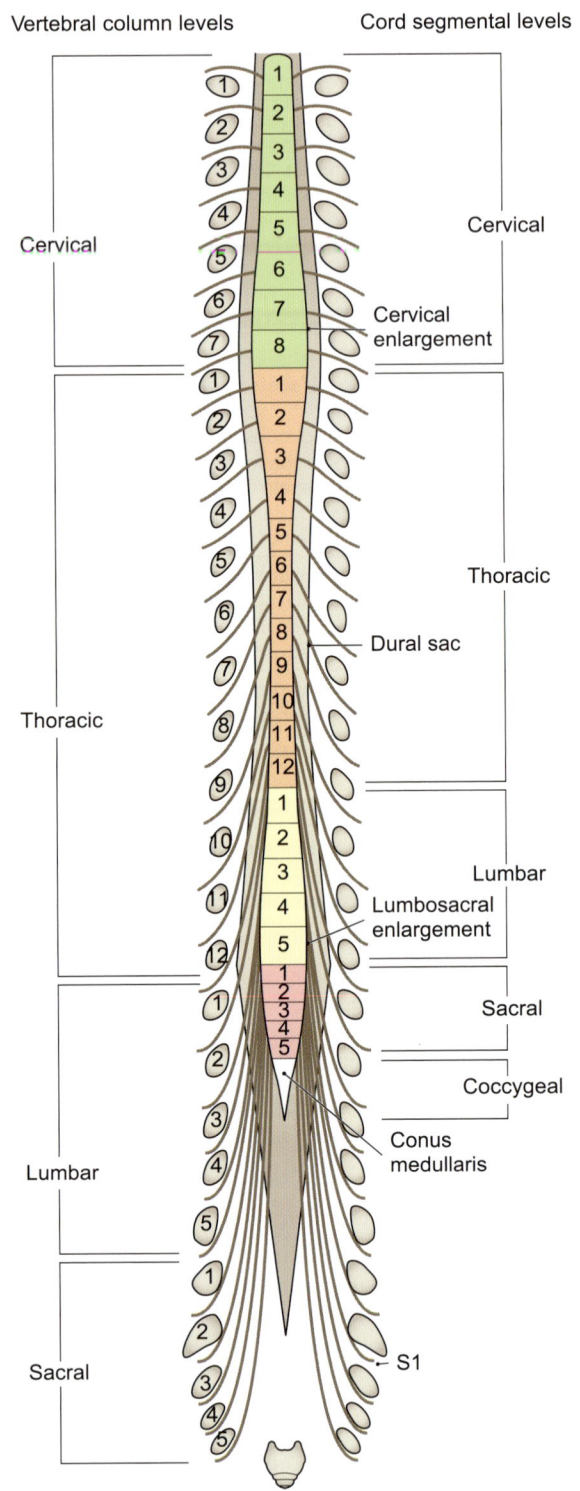

Fig. 6.51 Spinal cord showing vertebral and segmental levels.

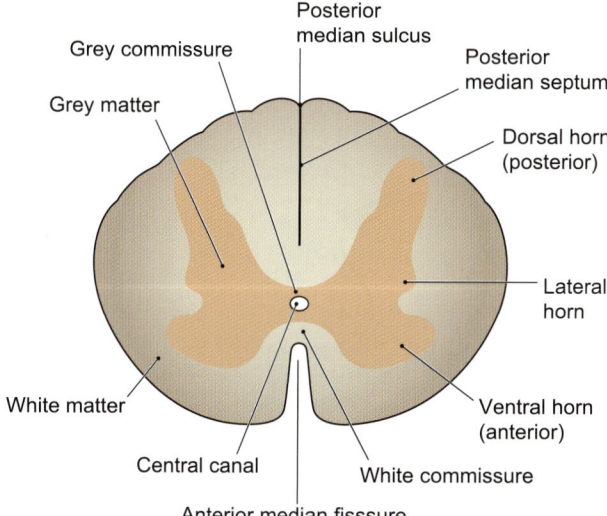

Fig. 6.52 labels:
- Posterior median sulcus
- Grey commissure
- Posterior median septum
- Grey matter
- Dorsal horn (posterior)
- Lateral horn
- White matter
- Ventral horn (anterior)
- Central canal
- White commissure
- Anterior median fisssure

Fig. 6.52 Transverse section of the spinal cord illustrating the major features.

On the anterior surface of the cord lies the anterior median fissure, while on the posterior surface lies the posterior median sulcus, which continues internally as the posterior median septum. A cross section of the spinal cord reveals a central H-shaped structure, composed of grey matter (cell bodies of neurones), surrounded by white matter (axons of neurones). The grey matter is composed of two lateral horns connected by a grey commissure. Within the grey commissure lies the central canal, filled with cerebrospinal fluid. The grey matter is divided into anterior (ventral), lateral and posterior (dorsal) horns, and the white matter is divided into anterior, lateral and posterior columns (Fig. 6.52).

The cell bodies of motor neurones are in the ventral (anterior) horn of the spinal cord (Fig. 6.53). The axons of these neurones synapse with the sarcolemma (plasma membrane) of muscle cells at the neuromuscular junction. Depolarization of a motor neurone results in the release of neurotransmitters into the synaptic cleft, causing depolarization of the sarcolemma and initiation of muscle contraction.

The receptors of sensory neurones in skin, muscle or viscera respond to specific stimuli, for example mechanical, chemical or thermal. The axons of these neurones (known as first-order neurones) carry impulses from the receptor to the dorsal (posterior) horn of the spinal cord. First-order neurones synapse with second-order neurones either at the same level or at a higher level within the spinal cord. The second-order neurones carry impulses to higher centres in the brain, where they synapse with third-order neurones. Sensory neurones can also synapse directly with motor neurones at the same spinal level or via an interneurone. This is the structural and physiological basis of a reflex arc (see Fig. 6.53).

CLINICAL NOTES

EXAMINING REFLEXES

When testing reflexes, the reflex arc is assessed at a spinal cord level. For example, on striking the patellar tendon, the quadriceps muscle is stretched. This triggers an action potential within a muscle spindle (receptors within the muscle which monitor muscle length). The action potential travels to the spinal cord via an afferent neurone, where it synapses with an efferent neurone, leading to contraction of the muscle and a knee jerk. The common limb reflexes tested, with their spinal cord levels are:

Biceps brachii (C5–C6)
Triceps brachii (C7–C8)
Brachioradialis (C6–C7)
Quadriceps femoris (L3–L4)
Gastrocnemius (S1–S2)

Although reflexes occur at the level of the spinal cord, they can be influenced by higher centres. For example, after a stroke, inhibitory input from higher centres, which would normally dampen reflex activity, may be lost and hyperreflexia (exaggerated limb reflexes) can occur.

Blood supply to the spinal cord

The anterior portion of the spinal cord is supplied by the anterior spinal artery that arises from branches of the vertebral arteries and is reinforced by several contributory arteries, especially the artery of Adamkiewicz. The posterior portion of the spinal cord is supplied by two posterior spinal arteries. In roughly 75% of humans, these arrive from the posterior inferior cerebellar artery. In the remaining 25% of humans, they arise from the vertebral arteries.

Spinal Tracts

Several white matter tracts exist within the spinal cord to conduct information from the brain to the spinal cord and subsequently the peripheries and vice versa. These are termed the spinal tracts and are broadly split between ascending tracts (sensory) and descending tracts (motor).

Ascending (sensory) tracts
Spinothalamic tract

The spinothalamic tract conveys the sensation of crude touch, pressure, pain and temperature to the brain. It is a three-neurone system. The first-order neurone synapses in the dorsal root ganglion in the spinal cord at its representative level. The

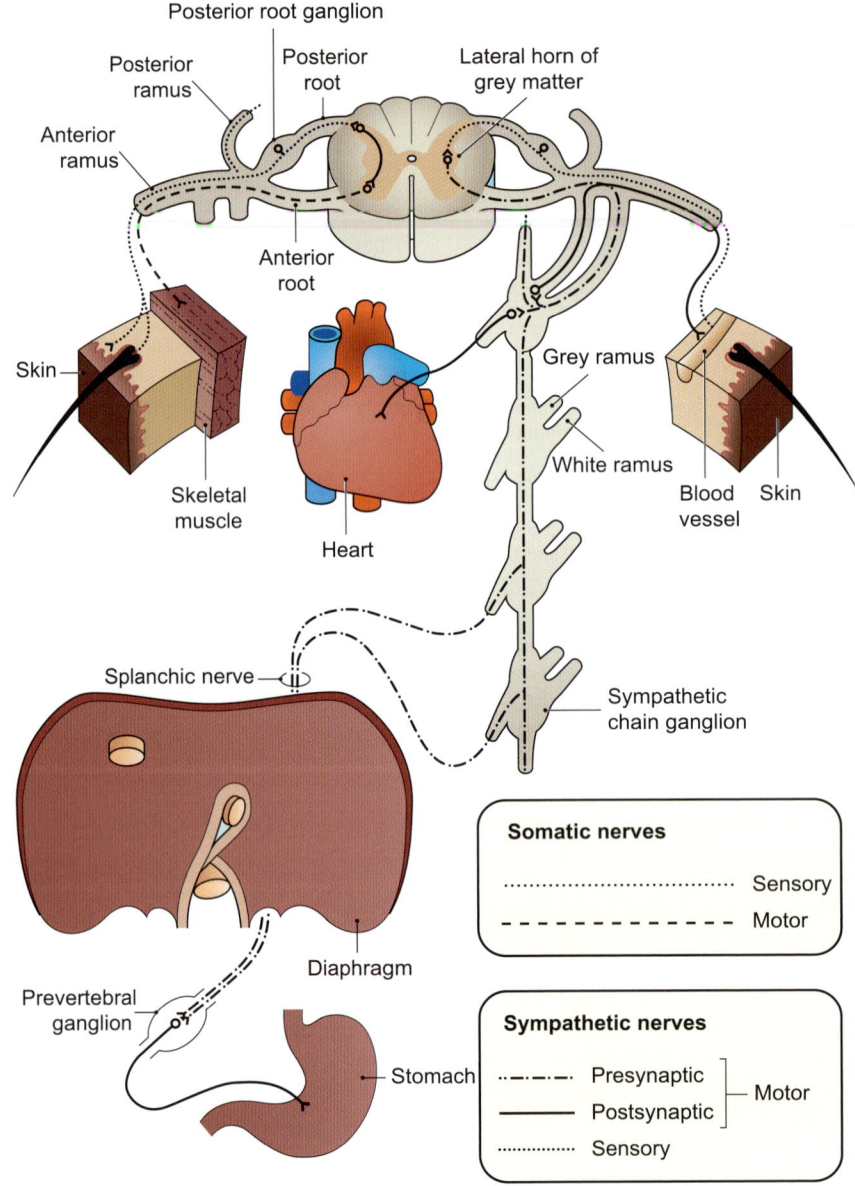

Fig. 6.53 Components of a typical spinal nerve and the sympathetic nervous system.

second-order neurone then decussates at that level and ascends contralaterally to terminate in the thalamus. From the thalamus, the third-order neurone projects to the sensory cortex (Fig. 6.54).

Dorsal column/medial-lemniscal pathway

The second major sensory pathway is the dorsal column, or medial-lemniscal pathway, which conveys fine touch, conscious proprioception and vibration sensation. The first-order neurone

enters the spinal cord via the dorsal root ganglion and ascends ipsilaterally within the dorsal columns of the spinal cord. The dorsal columns are formed of two bundles of fibres: the fasciculus gracile and fasciculus cuneate. The fasciculus gracile carries information from the lower half of the body (approximately midthoracic level), and the fasciculus cuneate, which lies more laterally within the spinal cord, carries information from the upper half of the body (see Fig. 6.54).

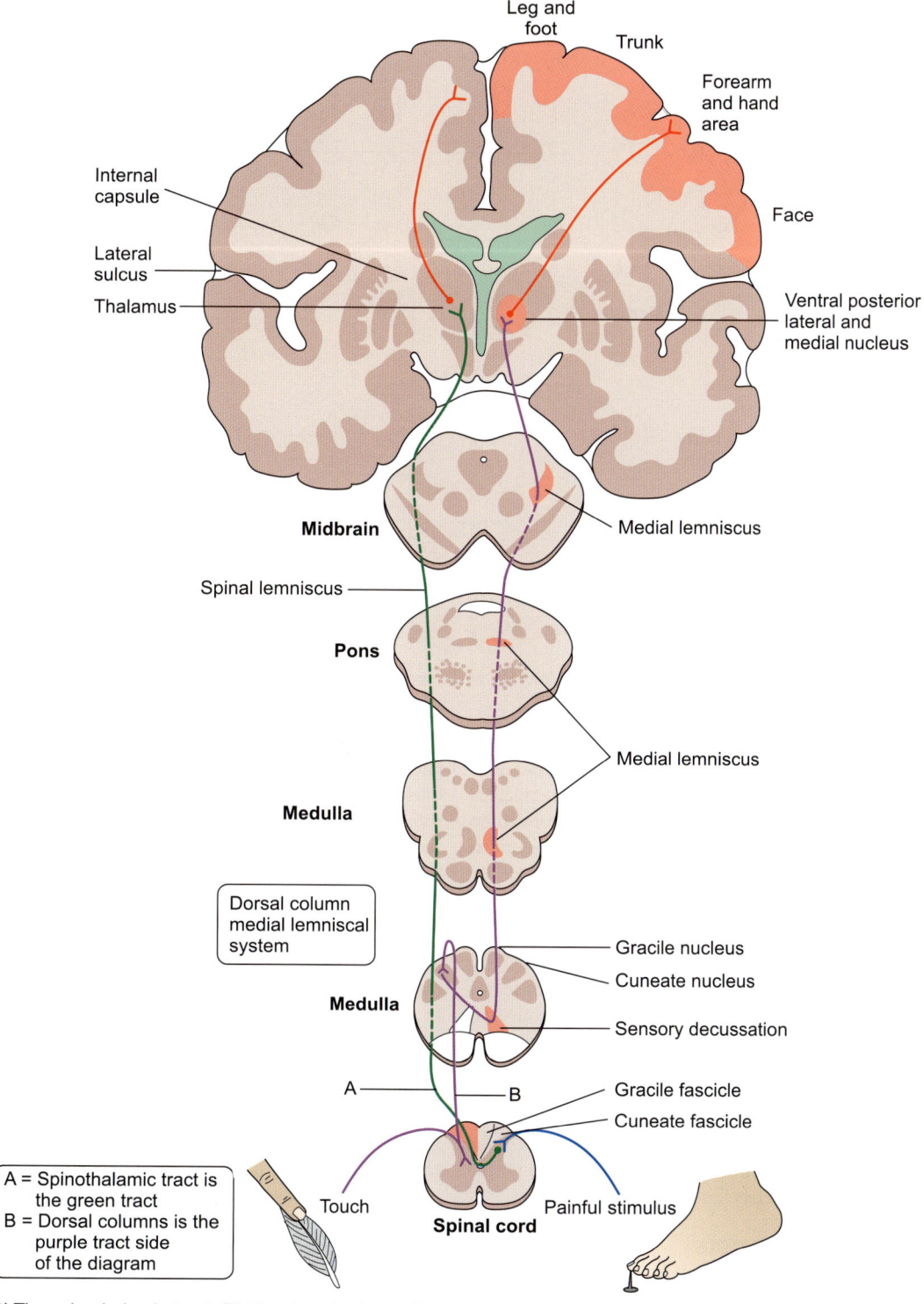

Fig. 6.54 (A) The spinothalamic tract. (B) The dorsal columns/medial-lemniscal pathway.

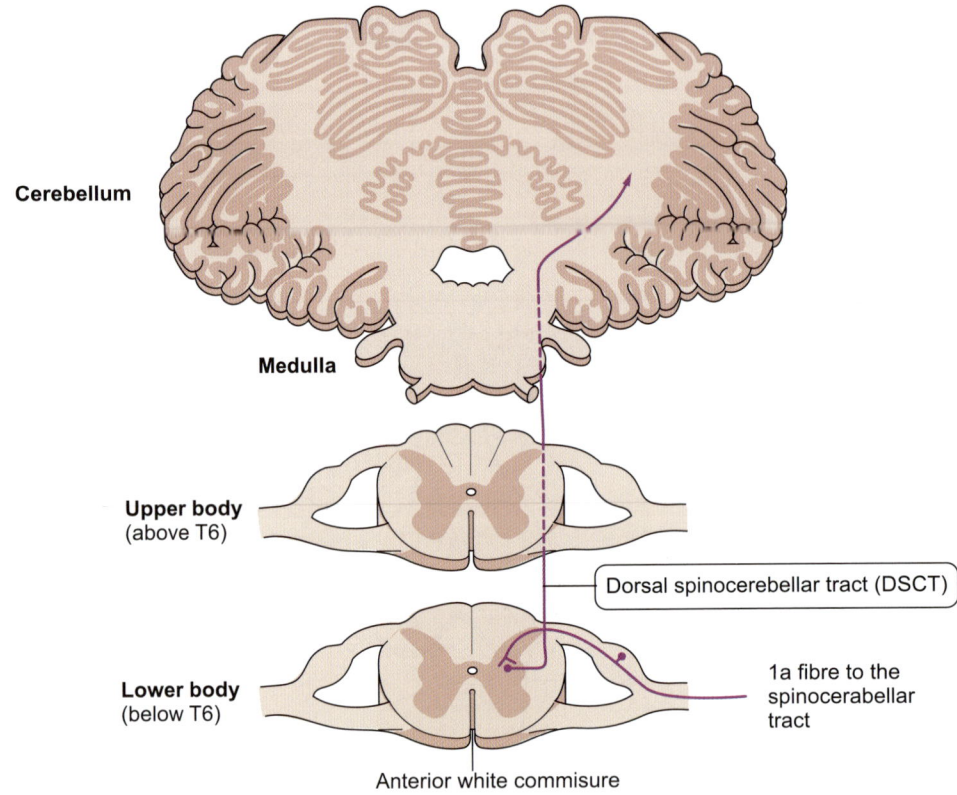

Cerebellum

Medulla

Upper body (above T6)

Dorsal spinocerebellar tract (DSCT)

Lower body (below T6)

1a fibre to the spinocerabellar tract

Anterior white commisure

Fig. 6.55 The spinocerebellar tract.

The first-order neurone synapses with the second-order neurone at its respective nuclei in the medulla—either the nucleus gracile or nucleus cuneate. The second-order neurone then decussates the midline within the medial lemniscus of the brainstem (hence the name 'medial-lemniscal pathway') to enter the thalamus, where it synapses to become a third-order neurone which then projects to the cortex.

Spinocerebellar tract

To maintain smooth motor control, information on unconscious sensations of joint position and muscle tension must be conveyed from the limbs to the brain. The spinocerebellar tract acts to relay information from the muscle spindles and Golgi tendon organs to the cerebellum for this purpose. Sensory information enters the spinal cord via the dorsal root ganglion as first-order neurones. These neurones then synapse with the spinocerebellar fibres in the grey matter of the spinal cord to ascend ipsilaterally to enter the cerebellum via the inferior cerebellar peduncle (Fig. 6.55).

Descending (motor) tracts

The control of movement is a combination of both voluntary and involuntary inputs. Voluntary control of skeletal muscle is conducted in the corticospinal and corticobulbar tracts, also known as the 'pyramidal' pathways. Modifications of these skeletal muscle contractions are made via the 'extrapyramidal pathways': rubrospinal, tectospinal, vestibulospinal and reticulospinal tracts. Anatomically, the distinction between these pathways is whether their course involves the pyramids, the two 'humps' at the anterior aspect of the medulla formed by bundles of motor axons.

Corticospinal tract

The main pathway for voluntary movement control, the corticospinal tract, contains two neurones. It begins with its nucleus in the primary motor cortex and premotor area. It then descends through the internal capsule and cerebral crus before forming the pyramids of the medulla. At this point, roughly 85% of fibres decussate (i.e. crossover) to become contralateral fibres and enter the spinal cord to become the lateral corticospinal tracts. The remaining 15% of fibres continue ipsilaterally (i.e. on the same side) within the smaller anterior corticospinal tract, decussating at the spinal level they innervate. This decussation of fibres explains why the left side of the brain controls the skeletal movements of the right side of the body and vice versa. At the spinal level, each fibre innervates, synapsing with the respective lower motor neurone in the ventral horn of the spinal cord (Fig. 6.56).

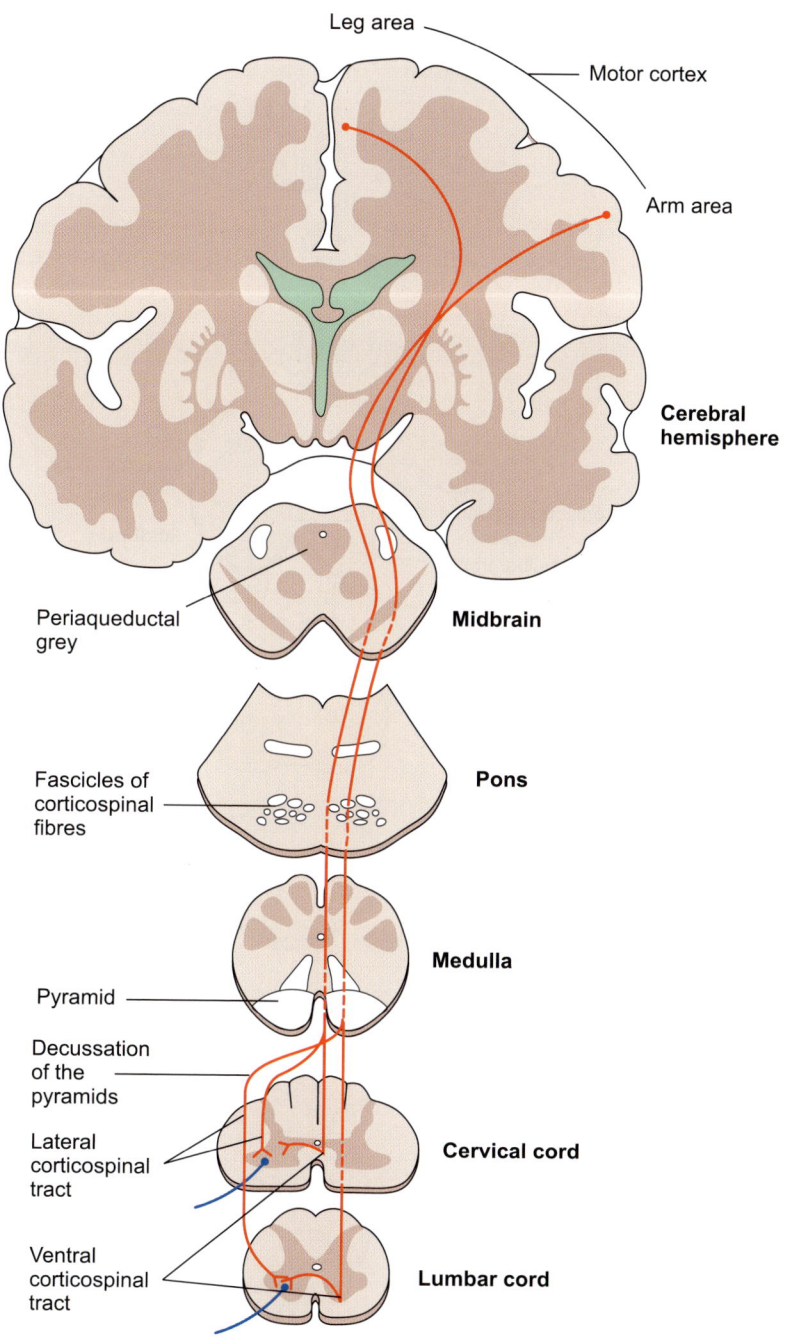

Fig. 6.56 The corticospinal tract.

Corticobulbar tract

The corticobulbar tract is the primary motor pathway connecting the motor cortex and the cranial nerve (CN) nuclei. Again a two-neurone tract originates in the primary motor cortex before descending through the internal capsule into the brainstem to travel within the cerebral crus. The corticobulbar fibres then exit at the appropriate level of the brainstem to synapse with the lower motor neurone of the respective cranial nerve. Except for the lower facial nuclei (CN 7) and hypoglossal nuclei (CN 12), the corticobulbar tract innervates each motor nucleus bilaterally (Fig. 6.57).

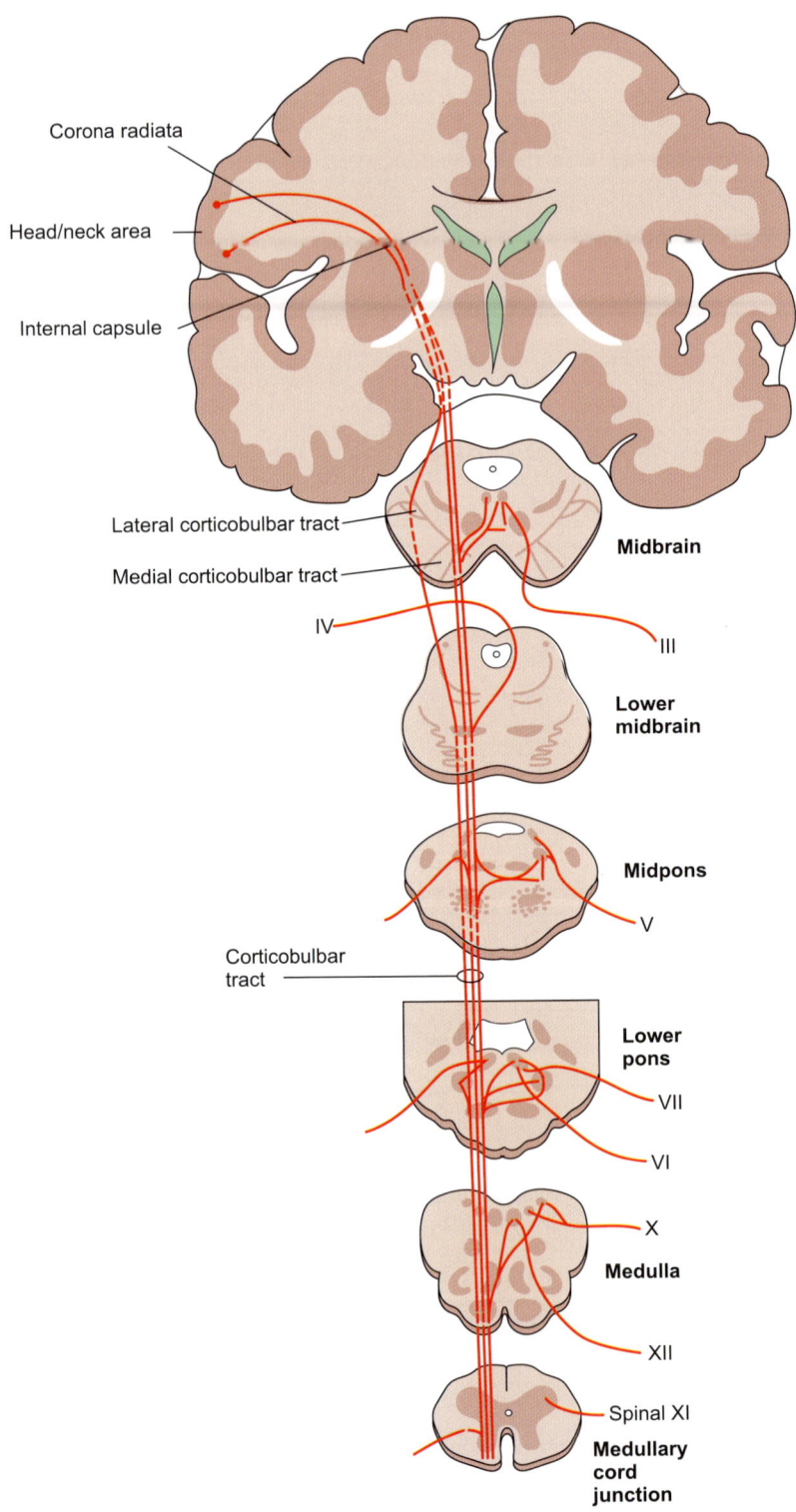

Corona radiata

Head/neck area

Internal capsule

Lateral corticobulbar tract

Medial corticobulbar tract

IV

Midbrain

III

Lower midbrain

Midpons

V

Corticobulbar tract

Lower pons

VII

VI

X

Medulla

XII

Spinal XI

Medullary cord junction

Fig. 6.57 The corticobulbar tract.

Rubrospinal tract

The purpose of the rubrospinal tract is to mediate large voluntary movements and fine motor control. It originates in the red nucleus of the midbrain and primarily facilitates flexion of the upper limb extremities.

Tectospinal tract

The tectospinal tract is involved in the mediation of reflexes of the head in response to visual and auditory information, that is to bright lights and loud noises. The tract originates from the superior and inferior colliculi of the midbrain which processes visual and auditory information, respectively. It then descends through several brainstem nuclei before terminating in the cervical spinal cord.

Vestibulospinal tract

The vestibulospinal tract receives information from the vestibular section of the vestibulospinal nerve (CN 8). The primary purpose of the tract is to maintain upright balance, conscious realization of spatial orientation and head–eye coordination in response to head position.

Reticulospinal tract

The reticulospinal tract is divided into two tracts, the medial and lateral reticulospinal tracts. It is involved in locomotion and posture control by supplying the flexors and extensors of the trunk and proximal limbs. Clinically, the reticulospinal tract is mainly inhibited by the corticospinal tract. Damage to the reticulospinal tract at the level of or below the red nucleus can cause decerebrate rigidity and upset extension of the head and limbs.

Spinal nerves

Spinal nerves are mixed nerves, carrying motor, sensory and autonomic information between the spinal cord and the peripheral nervous system. There are 31 pairs of spinal nerves: 8 cervical, 12 thoracic, 5 lumbar, 5 sacral and 1 coccygeal nerve. In the intervertebral foramina, the anterior and posterior roots of each segment of the spinal cord join to form a spinal nerve (see Fig. 6.53):

- The anterior root contains motor neurons supplying skeletal muscle. The anterior roots of T1 to L2 also contain preganglionic sympathetic fibres, while S2 to S4 contain preganglionic parasympathetic fibres.
- The posterior root contains sensory neurons, the cell bodies of which are located in the dorsal root ganglion.

Immediately after formation, the spinal nerve divides into ventral and dorsal rami. The ventral rami supplies the limbs and the trunk. The dorsal rami supply the erector spinae muscles of the back along with the overlying skin.

Each spinal nerve provides sensory innervation to an area of skin known as a dermatome (except for the skin of the face, which is supplied by the trigeminal nerve (CN 5)). There is a degree of overlap in sensory innervation between adjacent dermatomes. Testing for loss of sensation over a dermatome helps to identify the level of a lesion within the spinal cord.

MLA Single Best Answer (SBA) questions

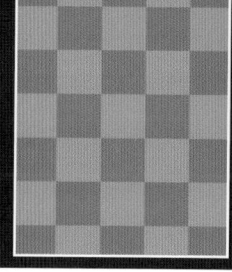

Chapter 1 Introduction

1. A 50-year-old male builder comes to your clinic. He has noticed an enlarging mole on his right shoulder. You refer him to the dermatology department of his local hospital, where he is diagnosed with a malignant melanoma. He is required to undergo further tests to stage his disease (determine the extent of any spread). To which of the following regions of the body are metastases from melanoma likely to spread?
   A. Colon, liver, bones, brain
   B. Colon, liver, bones, kidney
   C. Kidneys, liver, bones, lung
   D. Liver, bones, lung, brain
   E. Liver, bones, lung, colon

2. A 70-year-old male presents to his general practitioner (GP) with generalized weakness. The GP tests his muscle power as part of his examination. He decides that the patient is able to contract his muscles against resistance. According to the Medical Research Council (MRC) muscle scale, what level of power does the patient have?
   A. Grade 1
   B. Grade 2
   C. Grade 3
   D. Grade 4
   E. Grade 5

3. The anatomical position is the standard reference for describing the position of the body. What is the position of the hands in the anatomical position?
   A. The hands are adducted at the wrist.
   B. The little fingers lie lateral to the thumbs.
   C. The palms face anteriorly.
   D. The palms lie in the lateral plane.
   E. The thumbs point medially.

4. A 35-year-old male is diagnosed with leukaemia. He is found to have pancytopaenia (a deficiency of all types of blood cells) due to the infiltration of his bone marrow by leukaemic cells. In adults, which of the following sites contain red marrow?
   A. Fibula
   B. Phalanges
   C. Radius
   D. Sternum
   E. Tibia

5. A 25-year-old female patient comes to see you with pain in the left shoulder. You examine the shoulder and while examining ask them to abduct their shoulder at the glenohumeral joint. Which of the following best describes abduction?
   A. Movement away from the median sagittal plane.
   B. Movement in the coronal plane where there is a reduction in the angle between two parts of the body.
   C. Movement in the sagittal plane where there is an increase in the angle between two parts of the body.
   D. Movement in the sagittal plane where there is a reduction in the angle between two parts of the body.
   E. Movement towards the median sagittal plane.

6. A 15-year-old boy is admitted to the hospital after having a torrential nosebleed after minor sports trauma. The ENT surgeons have found it difficult to control. He reports that his father had similar problems on a number of occasions while a teenager. After investigations, the haematologist informs him that he has haemophilia A, a genetic deficiency of which clotting factor?
   A. Factor VIII
   B. Factor IX
   C. Fibrinogen
   D. Prothrombin
   E. Von Willebrand factor

Chapter 2 Head and neck

1. A 28-year-old amateur cook is making brunch for his friends. While removing the stone from an avocado, the knife slips and strikes the palm of his hand giving him a deep laceration. He immediately feels pain caused by the knife. The painful stimulus will be carried along which type of fibre?
   A. Myelinated A α fibres
   B. Myelinated A δ fibres
   C. Myelinated C fibres
   D. Myelinated γ fibres
   E. Unmyelinated C fibres

2. In response to a stressful situation, a large dose of adrenaline is released into the circulation of a 14-year-old girl. Adrenaline is a neurotransmitter that can act to do what?
   A. Cause pupillary constriction
   B. Dilate bronchial smooth muscle
   C. Dilate peripheral blood vessels
   D. Increase blood flow to the gastrointestinal tract
   E. Reduce the strength of myocardium contraction

3. A 25-year-old male presents to the accident and emergency department with a temperature, headache, vomiting and photophobia. He undergoes a lumbar

puncture for suspected meningitis. Cerebrospinal fluid (CSF) is removed and sent for microscopy and culture. CSF drains via arachnoid granulations into which structure?

A. Cavernous sinus
B. Choroid plexus
C. Jugular vein
D. Petrosal sinus
E. Superior sagittal sinus

4. A 38-year-old female attends her optician as she has been experiencing problems with her vision. The results of her eye test concern her optician and so he refers her to the local hospital for further investigation. She undergoes a computed tomography (CT) scan which reveals a pituitary adenoma, compressing the optic chiasma. This will result in which of the following?

A. Complete blindness
B. Loss of left and right temporal (outer) fields of vision
C. Loss of left inferior fields of vision
D. Loss of vision in the left eye
E. Loss of vision in the right eye

5. A 20-year-old male presents to the accident and emergency department with a reduced level of consciousness (Glasgow Coma Scale of 13: E3, V4, M6) and confusion. His girlfriend tells you that he fell over earlier that day and hit the side of his head on some steps. He briefly lost consciousness but recovered quickly and did not appear to have any injuries as a result of the fall.
A CT scan shows that the patient has suffered a skull fracture and an extradural haemorrhage. In which region of the skull is the fracture most likely to have occurred?

A. Bregma
B. Lambda
C. Occiput
D. Orbit
E. Pterion

6. Given the location of the patient's fracture (see the question above), which vessel has been ruptured?

A. Middle cerebral artery
B. Middle meningeal artery
C. Occipital artery
D. Supraorbital artery
E. Superficial temporal artery

7. You are asked to examine a 77-year-old female who has been admitted to hospital with left-sided weakness. As part of your assessment, you perform a cranial nerve examination. In which part of the brain do the nuclei of the cranial nerves originate?

A. Brainstem
B. Cerebellar cortex
C. Cerebral cortex
D. Corpus callosum
E. Diencephalon

8. A patient is concerned about their general health. The main complaint is that she is frequently 'tripping' over her own feet for no apparent reason. You perform a full neurological examination and find she has a loss of distal joint position sense in both feet. Which spinal tract has been affected?

A. Corticobulbar tract
B. Corticospinal tract
C. Dorsal columns/medial-lemniscal pathway
D. Spinocerebellar tract
E. Spinothalamic tract

9. Which of the following is not supplied by the facial nerve?

A. Posterior belly of digastric
B. Stapedius
C. Anterior belly of digastric
D. Buccinator
E. Frontalis

10. Which nerve in the orbit controls the medial rectus muscle?

A. Oculomotor
B. Trochlear
C. Trigeminal V_1
D. Abducens
E. Optic

11. Which cranial nerve supplies the parasympathetic component to the vidian nerve?

A. Oculomotor
B. Facial
C. Vestibulocochlear
D. Glossopharyngeal
E. Vagus

12. Which cranial nerve supplies general somatic sensation to the anterior two-thirds of the tongue?

A. Trigeminal
B. Facial
C. Glossopharyngeal
D. Vagus
E. Hypoglossal

13. What is the main method by which thyroid hormones are carried in the blood?

A. Dissolved free in plasma
B. Bound to plasma proteins
C. Bound to calcitonin
D. Bound to thyroid-stimulating hormone
E. Bound to colloid matrix

14. Which nerve innervates the platysma muscle?

A. Trochlear
B. Trigeminal
C. Abducens
D. Facial
E. Vestibulocochlear

15. Which cranial nerve provides parasympathetic supply to the lacrimal gland?
    A. Facial
    B. Glossopharyngeal
    C. Lacrimal
    D. Vidian
    E. Pterygopalatine

16. Which parasympathetic ganglion controls pupil size?
    A. Oculomotor
    B. Facial
    C. Glossopharyngeal
    D. Ciliary
    E. Lacrimal

17. What is the anterior border of the posterior triangle of the neck?
    A. Digastric
    B. Omohyoid
    C. Sternocleidomastoid
    D. Submandibular
    E. Trapezius

18. The anterior midline of the neck is a boundary of which triangle?
    A. Carotid
    B. Posterior
    C. Muscular
    D. Submental
    E. Submandibular

19. Which muscle forms a boundary of the submandibular triangle?
    A. Digastric
    B. Omohyoid
    C. Genioglossus
    D. Sternothyroid
    E. Sternohyoid

20. Which bone forms the posterior part of the nasal septum?
    A. Vomer
    B. Palatine
    C. Sphenoid
    D. Zygoma
    E. Nasal

21. The superior orbital fissure is bounded by which bone?
    A. Vomer
    B. Palatine
    C. Sphenoid
    D. Zygoma
    E. Frontal

22. Which artery passes through the foramen spinosum?
    A. Superficial temporal
    B. Middle meningeal
    C. Ascending pharyngeal

    D. Occipital
    E. Retroauricular

23. Which artery supplies the contents of the temporal fossa?
    A. Maxillary
    B. Superficial temporal
    C. Ascending pharyngeal
    D. Deep temporal
    E. Sphenopalatine

Chapter 3 Thorax

1. A 25-year-old female undergoes an exploratory laparoscopy for abdominal pain. Postoperatively, she has pain around the shoulder which the surgeon explains is due to CO_2 used in the laparoscopy accumulating under the diaphragm and irritating it. Which nerve is responsible for the sensation of pain in this situation?
    A. Accessory
    B. Axillary
    C. Phrenic
    D. Sympathetic trunk
    E. Vagus

2. A 68-year-old male smoker presents with a 3-month history of cough and weight loss. He is investigated with a CT scan, which shows a left-sided bronchial carcinoma. The physician notices that he has a hoarse voice. Compression of which structure is responsible for the voice changes?
    A. Left main bronchus
    B. Left phrenic nerve
    C. Left recurrent laryngeal nerve
    D. Left sympathetic trunk
    E. Left vagus nerve

3. A 55-year-old female undergoes a routine mammogram which shows an abnormality in the right breast consistent with breast cancer. Which of the following statements about the anatomy of the breast is true?
    A. The breast lies in the deep fascia.
    B. The breast lies deep to the pectoralis major and serratus anterior muscles.
    C. The base of the breast lies between the first and eighth ribs.
    D. The breast is composed of 15 to 20 lobules.
    E. The majority of lymph from the breast drains into the parasternal nodes.

4. The patient discussed in the previous question undergoes a right-sided mastectomy. During a follow-up appointment in the clinic, she was noted to have winging on the scapula. Which nerve has been injured?
    A. Right accessory nerve
    B. Right long thoracic nerve
    C. Right supraclavicular nerve

D. Right suprascapular nerve
E. Right thoracodorsal nerve

5. An 8-year-old girl chokes on a peanut. Where is the peanut most likely to lodge?
   A. Left lower lobar bronchus
   B. Left main bronchus
   C. Left superior segmental bronchus
   D. Right upper lobe bronchus
   E. Right main bronchus

6. A 68-year-old female presents to the accident and emergency unit with shortness of breath and chest pain. She has a CT pulmonary angiogram, which shows a pulmonary embolism. Which of the following statements regarding ventilation–perfusion of the lungs is correct?
   A. Perfusion is greatest at the lung apex.
   B. Individuals with shunts have higher PaO_2.
   C. Lower V/Q values result in higher PaO_2.
   D. Inspired $PO_2 = 100$ mm Hg.
   E. Lower V/Q values result in higher $PaCO_2$.

7. A 72-year-old male has a carotid endarterectomy to treat stenosis of the carotid artery. This results in the destruction of the carotid body. Which of the following statements about the carotid body is correct?
   A. Peripheral chemoreceptors are most sensitive to carbon dioxide.
   B. Peripheral chemoreceptors monitor arterial values only.
   C. Carotid bodies have the least significant respiratory effect.
   D. Peripheral chemoreceptors are stimulated by anaemia.
   E. Type 2 cells of the carotid bodies are believed to monitor PaO_2.

8. A 45-year-old female suffers from chronic pain and is taking opiate analgesia. Opiates reduce the central control over ventilation. Which of the following statements regarding the central chemoreceptors is correct?
   A. Central chemoreceptors form part of the dorsal respiratory group.
   B. Central chemoreceptors provide 50% of the ventilator drive.
   C. Central chemoreceptors are most sensitive to acidaemia.
   D. Central chemoreceptors primarily respond to hypoxia.
   E. Central chemoreceptors are located on the floor of the fourth ventricle.

9. A 60-year-old male with a 30-pack-year history of smoking presents to his general practitioner (GP) with increasing shortness of breath and a chronic cough. The GP diagnoses chronic obstructive pulmonary disease (COPD) and arranges for the patient to have spirometry testing. Which of the results below is consistent with COPD?
   A. Forced expiratory volume in 1 second (FEV1) 60% predicted and normal forced vital capacity (FVC)

B. FEV1 and FVC 60% of predicted
C. FEV1 normal and FVC 60% of predicted
D. FEV1 and FVC normal
E. FEV1 80% predicted and normal FVC

10. A 65-year-old male presents to the accident and emergency unit with chest pain. The pain is crushing, radiates to his left arm and jaw, and is associated with nausea and sweating. An electrocardiogram (ECG) shows he is having a myocardial infarction with ST elevation in leads II and V_2 to V_4. He undergoes primary percutaneous coronary intervention (primary PCI) and is found to have occlusions of his coronary arteries, secondary to atheroma. Which coronary artery is most likely to be affected by this atheroma?
    A. Anterior interventricular artery (left anterior descending artery)
    B. Circumflex artery
    C. Left marginal artery
    D. Posterior interventricular artery
    E. Right marginal artery

11. Several months later, the patient discussed in the previous question is readmitted to the hospital suffering from a new myocardial infarction. He is bradycardic, with a heart rate of 52 beats per minute. It is thought that the infarction has affected his sinoatrial (SA) node. Which artery most commonly supplies the SA node?
    A. Anterior interventricular artery
    B. Circumflex artery
    C. Left coronary artery
    D. Posterior interventricular artery
    E. Right coronary artery

12. The same patient discussed in the previous two questions continues to suffer from angina and eventually undergoes a coronary artery bypass. During surgery, the anterior interventricular artery is located. Which vein lies adjacent to the anterior interventricular artery?
    A. Anterior cardiac vein
    B. Coronary sinus
    C. Great cardiac vein
    D. Middle cardiac vein
    E. Small cardiac vein

13. The veins of the heart drain into the coronary sinus. Into which structure does the coronary sinus drain?
    A. Inferior vena cava (IVC)
    B. Left atrium
    C. Right atrium
    D. Right auricular appendage
    E. Superior vena cava (SVC)

14. A 55-year-old male presents to his general practitioner with headaches and fatigue. A set of observations shows his blood pressure (BP) to be 204/105 mm Hg. His mean arterial blood pressure (MAP) is:

A. 133 mm Hg
B. 138 mm Hg
C. 139 mm Hg
D. 141 mm Hg
E. 142 mm Hg

15. A 45-year-old intravenous drug user is admitted to hospital critically unwell. He has developed septic shock secondary to bacterial infective endocarditis (IE). The source of infected tissue is most likely to be the:
    A. Aortic valve
    B. Combined mitral and aortic valve
    C. Mitral valve
    D. Pulmonary valve
    E. Tricuspid valve

16. A 6-month-old female presenting with increased work of breathing and failure to thrive is diagnosed with patent ductus arteriosus (PDA). This pathological patency lies between which two vessels?
    A. Pulmonary artery and descending aorta
    B. Pulmonary artery and superior vena cava
    C. Pulmonary artery and pulmonary vein
    D. Pulmonary vein and ascending aorta
    E. Superior vena cava and ascending aorta

17. Salbutamol is a drug used in asthma and chronic obstructive pulmonary disease. Salbutamol is an agonist of which receptor type to cause bronchodilation?
    A. Leukotrienes
    B. β1-receptors
    C. β2-receptors
    D. α1-receptors
    E. α2-receptors

18. Which of the following is primarily secreted from the adrenal medulla?
    A. Adrenaline
    B. Adrenocorticotrophic hormone (ACTH)
    C. Aldosterone
    D. Atrial natriuretic peptide
    E. Renin

19. Which of the following structures attaches the papillary muscles to the cusps of the atrioventricular valve?
    A. Moderator band
    B. Sinoatrial node
    C. Chordae tendineae
    D. Bundle of His
    E. Interventricular groove

Chapter 4 Abdomen

1. An 18-year-old presents with pain in the right iliac fossa, pyrexia and vomiting. They are diagnosed with appendicitis and undergo appendicectomy. The base of the appendix lies deep to the McBurney point. Which of the following best describes the location of McBurney point?
   A. It lies one-third of the way between the anterior superior iliac spine (ASIS) and the umbilicus.
   B. It lies one-third of the way between the posterior superior iliac spine (PSIS) and the umbilicus.
   C. It lies one-third of the way between the umbilicus and ASIS.
   D. It lies 2 cm above the midpoint of the inguinal ligament (half of the way between ASIS and pubic tubercle).
   E. It lies at the mid-inguinal point (halfway between ASIS and pubic symphysis).

2. When the surgeon makes an incision to reach the appendix, what is the correct order of the layers of the abdominal wall through which the scalpel must pass to reach the appendix?
   A. External oblique, internal oblique, peritoneum, transversus abdominis
   B. External oblique, internal oblique, transversus abdominis, peritoneum
   C. Internal oblique, external oblique, peritoneum, transversus abdominis
   D. Internal oblique, peritoneum, external oblique, transversus abdominis
   E. Rectus abdominis, external oblique, internal oblique, peritoneum

3. The appendicular artery supplies the appendix. It is a branch of which of the following arteries?
   A. Anterior caecal artery
   B. Ileal artery
   C. Ileocolic artery
   D. Inferior mesenteric artery (IMA)
   E. Right colic artery

4. A 75-year-old male presents to his general practitioner (GP) complaining of a swelling in his groin. On examination, the GP observes a visible bulge in his right groin, which has a cough impulse and can be reduced by gentle pressure. He suspects it is a direct inguinal hernia. Which of the following is true about direct inguinal hernias?
   A. They arise medial to the inferior epigastric artery.
   B. They occur only in young males.
   C. They occur secondary to a patent processus vaginalis.
   D. They may pass into the scrotum.
   E. They pass through the deep inguinal ring.

5. Inguinal hernias may exit the superficial inguinal ring. The spermatic cord also exits through the superficial inguinal ring. The external spermatic fascia is one of the coverings of the spermatic cord. From which of the following layers does it arise?
   A. Aponeurosis of the external oblique
   B. Aponeurosis of the internal oblique
   C. Internal oblique muscle

D. Transversalis fascia

E. Tunica vaginalis

6. Direct inguinal hernias pass through the Hesselbach triangle in the posterior wall of the inguinal canal. What are the boundaries of the Hesselbach triangle?
   A. Conjoint tendon, inferior epigastric vessels, inguinal ligament
   B. Conjoint tendon, inferior epigastric vessels, rectus sheath
   C. Conjoint tendon, superior epigastric vessels, inguinal ligament
   D. Rectus sheath, inferior epigastric vessels, inguinal ligament
   E. Rectus sheath, superior epigastric vessels, inguinal ligament

7. During embryonic development of the peritoneal cavity, there is a greater and lesser sac. How do these two compartments communicate?
   A. Epiploic foramen
   B. Foramen ovale
   C. Paracolic gutters
   D. Transverse mesocolon
   E. Sac foramen

8. A 50-year-old female who was admitted with worsening jaundice, dark urine, pale stools and pain in the right upper quadrant is diagnosed with gallstones. The common bile duct drains into which of the following?
   A. First part of the duodenum
   B. Second part of the duodenum
   C. Third part of the duodenum
   D. Fourth part of the duodenum
   E. Junction of the second and third parts of the duodenum

9. The above patient undergoes cholecystectomy. The fundus of the gallbladder lies posterior to which costal cartilage, at the intersection of the transpyloric plane with the costal margin?
   A. Sixth costal cartilage
   B. Seventh costal cartilage
   C. Eighth costal cartilage
   D. Ninth costal cartilage
   E. 10th costal cartilage

10. An 80-year-old male presents with severe abdominal pain. He undergoes a CT scan which shows an ischaemic bowel. At laparotomy, he has a region of ischaemic gut extending from approximately two-thirds of the way along his transverse colon to the distal part of his sigmoid colon. Which blood vessel has become occluded, causing this pattern of ischaemia?
    A. Coeliac trunk
    B. Inferior mesenteric artery (IMA)
    C. Middle rectal artery
    D. Sigmoid artery
    E. Superior mesenteric artery

11. A 34-year-old patient undergoes an erect chest x-ray that reveals air under the right hemidiaphragm. What is the diagnosis?
    A. No pathology—this is a normal finding
    B. Perforated abdominal viscus
    C. Pneumonia
    D. Right-sided pneumothorax
    E. Small bowel obstruction

12. Which one of these organs is not retroperitoneal?
    A. Second part of the duodenum
    B. Adrenal glands
    C. Sigmoid colon
    D. Rectum
    E. Ureters

13. A 15-year-old girl presents with abdominal pain. Her history reveals that her pain is around the umbilical region. Which part of the gastrointestinal tract is likely to be the cause of her pain?
    A. Ascending colon
    B. Duodenum
    C. Ileum
    D. Jejunum
    E. Stomach

14. With regard to the liver, which of the following is true?
    A. Deoxygenated blood exits the liver via the porta hepatis.
    B. It is completely covered by the peritoneum except over its anterior surface.
    C. The bare area of the liver lies in direct contact with the stomach.
    D. The division into left, quadrate and caudate lobes is based on function.
    E. The falciform ligament attaches the liver to the anterior abdominal wall.

15. Which parasympathetic nerves innervate the hindgut?
    A. Pelvic splanchnic
    B. Phrenic
    C. Vagus
    D. Pudendal
    E. Lumbar splanchnic

16. Which hormone is secreted by the zona fasciculata?
    A. Adrenaline
    B. Aldosterone
    C. Cortisol
    D. DHEA (dehydroepiandrosterone)
    E. Noradrenaline

17. What is the action of prostaglandins on the renal vasculature?
    A. Afferent arteriole dilatation
    B. Afferent arteriole constriction
    C. Efferent arteriole dilatation

D. Efferent arteriole constriction

E. Both afferent and efferent arteriole constriction

18. Which hormone is a mineralocorticoid?
    A. Aldosterone
    B. Angiotensin I
    C. Angiotensin II
    D. Cortisol
    E. Antidiuretic hormone (ADH)

19. A patient with Guillain–Barré syndrome with acute respiratory involvement will have which pattern on her arterial blood gas?
    A. Low PCO_2, low pH, normal HCO_3^-
    B. High PCO_2, low pH, normal HCO_3^-
    C. High PCO_2, high pH, normal HCO_3^-
    D. High PCO_2, low pH, high HCO_3^-
    E. High PCO_2, low pH, low HCO_3^-

20. Through which receptors does antidiuretic hormone cause increased water absorption in the collecting ducts?
    A. V_1
    B. V_2
    C. V_3
    D. V_4
    E. V_5

Chapter 5 Pelvis

1. A 36-year-old female is a pedestrian in a road traffic collision. She sustains a fracture of her pelvis.
   Which of the following is true about the pelvis?
   A. The greater or false pelvis lies below the pelvic brim.
   B. The male pubic arch is wider than the female pubic arch.
   C. The sacrum is attached to the hip bones via two synovial joints.
   D. The pubic tubercle lies in the midline.
   E. When standing upright, the anterior inferior iliac spines and pubic symphysis lie in the same vertical plane.

2. A 30-year-old male who presented with a lump in his left testicle was diagnosed with a malignant tumour. To which lymph nodes do testicular tumours most commonly metastasize?
   A. Deep inguinal
   B. Femoral nodes
   C. Popliteal nodes
   D. Para-aortic nodes
   E. Superficial inguinal nodes

3. Inguinal hernias may extend into the scrotum. Which of the following lists the correct order of the layers within the wall of the scrotum?
   A. Skin, cremasteric fascia, superficial fascia, internal spermatic fascia, external spermatic fascia, parietal layer of the tunica vaginalis

B. Skin, superficial fascia, cremasteric fascia, external spermatic fascia, internal spermatic fascia, parietal layer of the tunica vaginalis

C. Skin, superficial fascia, external spermatic fascia, cremasteric fascia, internal spermatic fascia, parietal layer of the tunica vaginalis

D. Skin, superficial fascia, external spermatic fascia, internal spermatic fascia, cremasteric fascia, parietal layer of the tunica vaginalis

E. Skin, superficial fascia, internal spermatic fascia, cremasteric fascia, external spermatic fascia, visceral layer of the tunica vaginalis

4. Following the birth of her second child, a 40-year-old female presents to her general practitioner with faecal incontinence. She attends the gynaecology department of her local hospital where the investigation reveals that she sustained damage to the muscles of her pelvic floor during the delivery of her baby. Injury to which structure is responsible for her faecal incontinence?
   A. Deep transverse perineal muscle
   B. External anal sphincter
   C. Iliococcygeus
   D. Internal anal sphincter
   E. Puborectalis

5. Which nerve supplies the muscle responsible for the above patient's incontinence?
   A. Inferior rectal nerve
   B. Nerve to obturator internus
   C. Obturator nerve
   D. Pudendal nerve
   E. Superior rectal nerve

6. Which of the following is true about the rectum?
   A. It commences where the sigmoid mesocolon ends.
   B. The middle third of the rectum is covered laterally by the peritoneum.
   C. The rectovesical pouch in females separates the rectum from the bladder.
   D. The rectum is supplied by branches of the superior mesenteric artery.
   E. The rectum has taeniae coli.

7. A 75-year-old male presents to his general practitioner with difficulty passing urine. He describes frequency, urgency, nocturia and terminal dribbling. He is diagnosed with benign prostatic hyperplasia (BPH). Which region of the prostate is most likely to be affected by BPH?
   A. Anterior lobe
   B. Lateral lobes
   C. Middle lobe
   D. Peripheral zone
   E. Posterior lobe

8. An 80-year-old male who presented with weight loss, back pain, nocturia, frequency and urgency is diagnosed with prostate cancer. Which lobe of the prostate is most likely to be affected by prostate cancer?
   A. Anterior
   B. Left lateral
   C. Middle
   D. Posterior
   E. Right lateral

9. A 25-year-old female presents to her general practitioner (GP) with pelvic pain. She undergoes an examination, including a bimanual vaginal examination. In which position is the GP most likely to find her uterus?
   A. Anteflexed and anteverted
   B. Anteflexed and inverted
   C. Anteflexed and retroverted
   D. Retroflexed and anteverted
   E. Retroflexed and retroverted

10. A 65-year-old female presents to her general practitioner having noticed blood in her urine. For the past few weeks she has also experienced urinary frequency and urgency. She undergoes a cystoscopy and biopsy and is diagnosed with a malignant tumour of the bladder. What type of epithelium lines the internal surface of the bladder?
    A. Columnar epithelium
    B. Cuboidal epithelium
    C. Keratinized stratified squamous epithelium
    D. Stratified squamous epithelium
    E. Transitional epithelium

11. Which section of the urethra runs the length of the penis?
    A. Preprostatic
    B. Prostatic
    C. Membranous
    D. Spongy
    E. Postspongy

12. A 51-year-old female presents to her GP with low mood among many other symptoms. After taking a history, the GP suspects that the patient is suffering from menopause. Which of the following is not a typical symptom of menopause?
    A. Reduced ability to concentrate
    B. Hot flushes
    C. Insomnia
    D. Decreased libido
    E. Diarrhoea

13. Which of the following is not one of the key factors that contribute to the mechanism of labour?
    A. Passage
    B. Passenger
    C. Psyche
    D. Potential
    E. Power

14. The placenta develops from the blastocyst following implantation within the uterus. How many weeks into the pregnancy does this occur?
    A. 2 weeks
    B. 4 weeks
    C. 6 weeks
    D. 8 weeks
    E. 10 weeks

15. A 68-year-old patient presents to A+E with pelvic pain. The patient is a transgender female and has previously had male-to-female vaginoplasty surgery. Which of the following structures is most likely to have been surgically removed during the procedure?
    A. Prostate
    B. Testes
    C. Urethra
    D. Seminal vesicle
    E. Perineal body

16. Which of the following hormones is primarily responsible for the decrease in bone mineral density in postmenopausal females?
    A. Oestrogen
    B. Progesterone
    C. Testosterone
    D. Follicle-stimulating hormone (FSH)
    E. Luteinizing hormone (LH)

Chapter 6 Musculoskeletal system

1. What is the definition of isometric contraction?
   A. The muscle shortens during contraction.
   B. The muscle contracts but does not change length.
   C. Controlled relaxation where the muscle gradually lengthens.
   D. A single action potential that is insufficient in causing movement.
   E. The changes in muscle relative to its functional requirement.

2. In the clinic, you examine a 65-year-old who has injured their biceps brachii muscle while playing sport. Which nerve supplies the biceps brachii muscle?
   A. Axillary
   B. Musculocutaneous
   C. Median
   D. Radial
   E. Ulnar

3. Which muscle in the hand is supplied by the median nerve?
   A. Abductor pollicis brevis
   B. Adductor pollicis
   C. Medial two lumbricals
   D. Flexor digiti minimi
   E. Interosseous

4. Which one of these structures is not found in the carpal tunnel?
   A. Flexor digitorum profundus
   B. Flexor digitorum superficialis
   C. Flexor pollicis longus
   D. Flexor pollicis brevis
   E. Median nerve

5. Which of these muscles is not considered a rotator cuff muscle?
   A. Supraspinatus
   B. Infraspinatus
   C. Subscapularis
   D. Teres minor
   E. Teres major

6. A person comes into the out-of-hours clinic complaining of hand pain following a fall onto their outstretched hand. On examination, you note they have tenderness when the anatomical snuffbox is palpated. Which bone is most likely affected?
   A. Hamate
   B. Lunate
   C. Capitate
   D. Scaphoid
   E. Trapezoid

7. Which muscle forms the lateral boundary of the femoral triangle?
   A. Sartorius
   B. Rectus femoris
   C. Vastus intermedius
   D. Adductor longus
   E. Pectineus

8. An 18-year-old has a superficial injury to their first and second toe. The sensation of the skin between the first and second toe ('the sandal gap') is supplied by which nerve?
   A. Superficial peroneal
   B. Saphenous
   C. Sural
   D. Deep peroneal
   E. Femoral

9. The common peroneal nerve runs very close to the skin over which bony landmark?
   A. Medial epicondyle of the femur
   B. Lateral epicondyle of the femur
   C. Patella
   D. Head of the fibula
   E. Tibial tuberosity

10. A 21-year-old female presents to the accident and emergency department complaining of a severe headache and photophobia. She has been vomiting over the past few hours and is becoming increasingly drowsy. The doctors are concerned that she may have meningitis and so after a CT scan, decide to perform a lumbar puncture. Below which of the following vertebral levels is a lumbar puncture safe to perform in an adult?
    A. T10 to T11
    B. T11 to T12
    C. T12 to L1
    D. L1 to L2
    E. L2 to L3

11. The lumbar region is an ideal site of access to the subarachnoid space where a sample of cerebrospinal fluid (CSF) may be obtained without damage to the spinal cord. What feature is used as a surface landmark when preparing to undertake a lumbar puncture?
    A. The disc between L1 and L2
    B. The disc between L3 and L4
    C. The line between the iliac crests
    D. The lower border of the L5 vertebra
    E. The lower border of the S2 vertebra

12. What is the sensory information carried by the tibial nerve?
    A. Plantar surface of the foot
    B. Dorsal surface of the foot
    C. Posterior compartment of the foot
    D. Anterior compartment of the leg
    E. Lateral compartment of the leg

13. Which of these muscles attaches to both the radius and ulna?
    A. Flexor digitorum profundus
    B. Flexor digitorum superficialis
    C. Pronator quadratus
    D. Extensor indicis
    E. Extensor digitorum

14. Which term best describes the part of the spine where the tubercle of the rib articulates in the thoracic spine?
    A. Transverse process
    B. Spinous process
    C. Superior articulating facet
    D. Pedicle
    E. Lamina

15. A 45-year-old experiences severe pain in their lower back. An MRI scan shows an L4/L5 intervertebral disc prolapse that is putting pressure on a spinal nerve. A disc prolapse involves:
    A. The nuchal ligament of the spine tearing.
    B. Spread of the nucleus pulposus through the annulus fibrosus.
    C. Twisting of the facet joint to put pressure on a spinal nerve.
    D. Bulging of the erector spinae muscles into the spinal canal.
    E. An intervertebral disc pushing through the foramen transversarium.

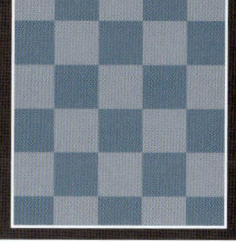

MLA SBA answers

Chapter 1 Introduction

1. **D**—Liver, bones, lung, brain. The common sites to which malignant melanoma metastasizes are the liver, bones, lung and brain. The likelihood of metastasis can be related to the 'Breslow depth' of the primary cutaneous lesion. The Breslow depth describes the thickness of a tumour at the deepest point of dermal invasion. The deeper the depth, the more likely the melanoma is to metastasize, which is also linked with a poorer prognosis. A depth of 4mm or greater appears to be a critical depth, beyond which prognosis is poorer with a higher likelihood of metastasis.

2. **D**—Grade 4. The MRC scale is a universally accepted scale to quantitatively assess a patient's muscle power throughout different muscles. It acts as an internationally accepted and reproducible scale to monitor a patient's improvement to treatment or physical decline. Grade 4 describes the active movement of a muscle or group of muscles against gravity and resistance. The full MRC scale is:
   A—Grade 1: A flicker or trace of contraction.
   B—Grade 2: Active movement, with gravity eliminated.
   C—Grade 3: Active movement against gravity.
   E—Grade 5: Normal power.

3. **C**—The palms face anteriorly. Remember, the anatomical position can be described as a patient standing upright with their head to the front, legs together and feet facing forwards, arms by the side with the palms also facing forwards; the clitoris or penis is in the erect position.
   The following answers are all incorrect as in the anatomical position:
   A—The hands are neither adducted nor abducted and lie in a neutral position, facing anteriorly.
   B—The little fingers lie medial to the thumbs.
   D—The palms lie in the coronal plane, facing anteriorly.
   E—The thumbs face laterally.

4. **D**—Sternum. The majority of red bone marrow is found in the flat bones, such as the pelvis, sternum and cranium vertebrae, and in the cancellous material of the epiphyseal ends of long bones, for example femur or humerus. In contrast, yellow marrow is found in the middle portion of short bones, specifically in the medullary cavity, the hollow interior of such bones.

5. **A**—Movement away from the median sagittal plane. To abduct is to take something away. In this scenario,

abduction of the arm means to take the arm away from the median sagittal plane and therefore away from the body and the median sagittal plane.
   B—Movement in the coronal plane to reduce the angle between two body parts describes adduction.
   C—Movement in the sagittal plane that increases the angle between two body parts describes extension. An example is the extension at the elbow joint increases the angle between the humerus and the radius and ulnar of the forearm.
   D—Movement in the sagittal plane that decreases the angle between two body parts describes flexion. An example is flexion at the hip which decreases the angle between the leg and the torso.
   E—Movement towards the median sagittal plane describes adduction. Remember: ADDuction, is like adding the limb back towards the body.

6. **A**—Factor VIII. Haemophilia A is caused by an X-linked inherited disorder leading to the absence of Factor VIII. Clinically, it is characterized by spontaneous or traumatic bleeding despite minimal trauma. Intraarticular, subcutaneous or intramuscular bleeding can also occur.
   B—A genetic deficiency in factor IX is called haemophilia B (or Christmas disease). Like haemophilia A, it is inherited in an X-linked recessive manner; however, it is rarer.
   C—Fibrinogen is the name given to factor I. When activated, thrombin and ionized Ca^{2+} cause fibrinogen (soluble) to become fibrin (insoluble). This fibrin can then be activated to form a cross-linked fibrin mesh to stabilize blood clots.
   D—Prothrombin is the name given to factor II. Prothrombin is activated by prothrombinase and ionized Ca^{2+} to form thrombin. In turn, thrombin causes the activation of fibrinogen to become fibrin (see previous).
   E—Von Willebrand factor is required for platelet adhesion. A deficiency in the quality or quantity of this factor can be caused by von Willebrand disease, the most common hereditary blood clotting disorder. It presents with a tendency for bleeding, including bruising easily, bleeding gums, recurrent nosebleeds and heavy menstrual blood loss.

Chapter 2 Head and neck

1. **B**—Myelinated A δ fibres. This scenario portrays a fast pain response that involved the medium-diameter myelinated A δ fibres. Myelinated A α fibres are primarily involved in the conduction of sensation from

proprioceptive muscle spindles. Myelinated γ fibres are indeed motor fibres and therefore are not involved in sensation. Unmyelinated C fibres are sensory fibres but are involved in slow pain conduction, with pain being perceived 1 to 2 seconds after the stimulus. The pain can persist and is typically less localized than fast pain perception. An example of pain transmitted via unmyelinated C fibres would be biliary colic.

2. **B**—Dilate bronchial smooth muscle. Adrenaline will cause bronchial dilation. It can be administered in medical emergencies such as an acute exacerbation of asthma or an allergic reaction. In these situations, bronchial constriction can create a life-threatening situation; therefore adrenaline can be administered to reverse this and cause bronchodilation.

Adrenaline will also cause the opposite of all the remaining answers—it will cause pupillary dilation, constriction of peripheral blood vessels, reduced blood flow to the gastrointestinal tract and an increased strength of myocardium contraction.

3. **E**—Superior sagittal sinus. CSF is absorbed via the arachnoid granulations and drains into the superior sagittal sinus. The superior sagittal sinus is a large sinus that runs in the midline in an anteroposterior direction. It produces the confluence of sinuses at the internal occipital protuberance which then drains into the transverse sinus.

The cavernous sinus is a pair of two true venous sinuses (a left and a right) that communicate via the anterior and posterior intercavernous sinuses. It is the only anatomical location in the body where an artery (the internal carotid artery) travels completely through a venous structure.

The choroid plexus is located throughout the ventricular system. It is a collection of ependymal cells that *produce* CSF.

On each side of the body, there are two sets of jugular veins—an external jugular vein and an internal jugular vein. Their function is to deliver deoxygenated blood from the head and neck back into the heart via the superior vena cava.

4. **B**—Loss of left and right temporal (outer) fields of vision. A lesion compressing the optic chiasm can typically lead to loss of vision in the temporal (outer) fields of both eyes—this is also known as bitemporal hemianopia.

The loss of vision in the left inferior fields may be caused by a lesion (e.g. a stroke, tumour) in the lower right optic radiation.

Complete blindness in either eye can be caused by direct damage to the eye from trauma, a lesion to the respective optic nerve, retinal injury or a vitreous haemorrhage.

5. **E**—Pterion. The pterion is the point on the skull, in the temple region, where the frontal, parietal, temporal and sphenoid bones join together. Fracture at this point puts a patient at high risk of extradural haemorrhage.

The bregma describes the point on the skull where the coronal suture is intersected by the sagittal suture. The lambda is the point in the occiput where the sagittal and lambdoid sutures meet. An extradural haemorrhage in the midline directly underneath the bregma or lambda is rare.

The occiput describes the lower back part of the skull and again it is rare to find an extradural haemorrhage in the posterior fossa.

The orbit is the bony cavity in the face that contains the eyes and their surrounding structures. All four walls of the orbit (inferior, superior, lateral and medial) are prone to fracture in trauma. The orbit provides protection to the globe. The orbital roof provides the floor to the anterior cranial fossa, but fracture typically does not cause significant intracranial haemorrhage. This type of fracture is known as a skull base fracture and can lead to an increased risk of meningitis or abscess formation.

6. **B**—Middle meningeal artery. The middle meningeal artery is a branch of the maxillary artery which itself arises from the external carotid artery. The middle meningeal artery enters the skull through the foramen spinosum. Along with the anterior and posterior meningeal arteries, it supplies the meninges and the calvarium. The anterior branch of the middle meningeal artery runs beneath the pterion and at this point the artery is vulnerable to injury that can lead to an extradural haematoma.

The middle cerebral artery is an extension of the internal carotid artery from both the left and right sides of the brain. The middle cerebral artery is a major artery that supplies the lateral cerebral cortex, anterior temporal lobes and insular cortex. Insufficiency of blood flow in this artery (e.g. caused by a stroke) can lead to significant neurological dysfunction which may or may not be reversible.

The occipital artery is a branch of the external carotid artery, which supplies blood to the back of the scalp, deep muscles of the back and neck and the sternomastoid muscles.

The supraorbital artery is a branch of the ophthalmic artery and is absent in 10% to 20% of people.

When the external carotid artery bifurcates, it creates the superficial temporal artery and maxillary artery. The superficial temporal artery is palpable anterior and superior to the tragus, just above the zygomatic arch.

7. **A**—Brainstem. The brainstem is the location of the cranial nerve nuclei. The nuclei lie at various levels throughout the brainstem. All but one of the cranial nerve rootlets leave the brainstem from its anterior or lateral aspect, on both the left and right sides. The only nerve that exits the brainstem posteriorly is the trochlear nerve

(cranial nerve IV). At the level of the inferior colliculus, the trochlear nerve exits the brainstem and wraps around the brainstem on both sides before appearing at its anterior aspect at the junction between the midbrain and the pons.

The cerebral cortex is the origin of the corticobulbar tract—a motor pathway that connects the motor cortex to the cranial nerve nuclei.

The corpus callosum is a long flat commissure in the midline, about 10 cm in length, that connects the right and left sides of the brain.

The diencephalon is a region of the embryonic neural tube that gives rise to the posterior forebrain structures, including the hypothalamus, thalamus, epithalamus (including the pineal gland) and the subthalamus.

8. **C**—Dorsal columns/medial-lemniscal pathway. The dorsal columns/medial-lemniscal pathway relay sensory information about vibration, conscious proprioception, fine touch and two-point discrimination. The joint position sense test involves asking the patient to close their eyes and moving the distal phalanx of their large toe or finger either upwards or downwards. The patient's awareness of which way their toe or finger is moving is a test of the function of conscious proprioception. A lesion of the dorsal columns/medial-lemniscal pathway can lead to the loss of this sense.

The corticobulbar tract is the motor pathway that connects the cerebral cortices to the cranial nerve nuclei.

The corticospinal tract is the primary motor pathway relaying motor information from the cortex to the limbs and trunk. A lesion in this tract will cause paralysis of the respective muscles.

The spinocerebellar tract is the sensory pathway that conveys information from the peripheries to the cerebellum.

The spinothalamic tract is also sensory in nature and transmits pain and temperature sensations from the peripheries to the thalamus.

9. **C**—Anterior belly of digastric. The anterior belly of the digastric muscle is supplied by the trigeminal nerve.

10. **A**—Oculomotor. The oculomotor nerve controls four of the six extraocular muscles (medial rectus, superior rectus, inferior rectus and inferior oblique). The trochlear nerve innervates the superior oblique, and the abducens nerve innervates the lateral rectus.

11. **B**—Facial. The parasympathetic fibres of the Vidian nerve come from the nervus intermedius component of the facial nerve. These fibres branch from the facial nerve as the greater superficial petrosal nerve, which combines with the deep petrosal nerve (sympathetic) to form the Vidian nerve.

12. **A**—Trigeminal. The general somatic sensation of the anterior two-thirds of the tongue is supplied by the lingual branch of the trigeminal nerve and taste to the anterior two-thirds is supplied by the facial nerve via the chorda tympani.

13. **B**—Bound to plasma proteins. The majority of the thyroid hormones are bound to plasma proteins, in particular thyroid-binding globulin.

14. **D**—The cervical branch of the facial nerve provides motor innervation to the platysma muscle.

15. **A**—The facial nerve supplies the lacrimal gland via the greater superficial petrosal nerve and the pterygopalatine ganglion.

16. **D**—The ciliary ganglion receives parasympathetic input from the oculomotor nerve to control pupil size.

17. **C**—Sternocleidomastoid. The borders of the posterior triangle of the neck are the sternocleidomastoid (anterior), trapezius (posterior) and the middle third of the clavicle (inferior).

18. **C**—The muscular triangle is bound by the omohyoid, sternocleidomastoid and hyoid bone as well as the midline.

19. **A**—Digastric. The submandibular triangle is formed by the mandible superiorly and the digastric muscle inferiorly.

20. **A**—The vomer bone attaches to the hard palate and forms the bony part of the nasal septum.

21. **C**—The superior orbital fissure is an opening bounded by the greater and lesser wings of the sphenoid bone.

22. **B**—The middle meningeal artery branches from the maxillary artery and enters the skull through the foramen spinosum to supply the dura mater.

23. **D**—The deep temporal arteries are branches from the maxillary artery to supply the temporalis muscle and other contents of the temporal fossa.

Chapter 3 Thorax

1. **C**—Phrenic. The correct answer is the phrenic nerve that supplies motor function to the diaphragm. Abdominal pathology irritating the diaphragm to cause shoulder pain is called Kerr sign.

2. **C**—Left recurrent laryngeal nerve. The correct answer is the left recurrent laryngeal nerve, which branches from the vagus nerve at the level of the aortic arch, passes underneath it and then traverses back up into the neck in a groove between the oesophagus and trachea. In the larynx, the recurrent laryngeal nerve supplies all the intrinsic muscles (except for the cricothyroid muscle). The hoarse voice implies that the tumour has invaded

the nerve. Invasion of the sympathetic trunk would cause Horner syndrome.

3. **D**—The breast is composed of 15 to 20 lobules which are responsible for milk production. The breast lies superficial to the deep fascia and the muscles. The base of the breast lies between the first and sixth ribs. Eighty per cent of the lymph drainage is to the axillary nodes, with the remainder to the parasternal and subclavicular nodes.

4. **B**—Right long thoracic nerve. The long thoracic nerve supplies the serratus anterior muscle and, when paralyzed, causes winging of the scapula. Damage to the right accessory nerve would present with trapezius and sternocleidomastoid dysfunction. The supraclavicular nerve is a cutaneous nerve supplying the shoulder and upper chest. The suprascapular nerve supplies the supraspinatus and infraspinatus, and damage would present with weakness in the first 15 degrees of shoulder abduction and shoulder external rotation. The thoraco-dorsal nerve supplies the latissimus dorsi muscle, and damage would cause weakness in adduction and extension of the shoulder.

5. **E**—Right main bronchus. The right main bronchus is shorter and straighter than the left, so foreign objects are more likely to lodge there than the left side.

6. **E**—Lower V/Q values result in higher $PaCO_2$. A V/Q = 0 means no ventilation; thus if the V/Q values are lower, the lungs are underventilated and CO_2 accumulates in the blood, giving a higher $PaCO_2$.

7. **E**—Type 2 cells of the carotid bodies are believed to monitor PaO_2. Peripheral chemoreceptors measure arterial values and are most sensitive to hypoxia. They are also stimulated by hypercapnia, pH and rate of blood flow but not anaemia.

8. **C**—Central chemoreceptors are most sensitive to acidaemia. Central chemoreceptors provide 80% of the respiratory drive and are most sensitive to acidosis. They are on the ventral surface of the medulla (the floor of the fourth ventricle is on the dorsal surface) and are not part of either the dorsal or ventral respiratory groups.

9. **A**—Forced expiratory volume in 1 second (FEV1) 60% predicted and normal forced vital capacity (FVC). An obstructive pattern is a reduction in FEV1 with preserved FVC.

10. **A**—Anterior interventricular artery (left anterior descending artery). This man has had an anterior ST-elevation myocardial infarction. The anterior interventricular artery supplies the anterolateral myocardium, apex and interventricular septum. This artery has been termed

'the widow maker'. Typically, this artery supplies 45% to 55% of the left ventricle and therefore severe occlusion of the artery can often lead to sudden death. Infarction of the circumflex artery (B) would lead to a posterior infarction. Given that the ECG leads V_1 to V_3 are directed towards the internal surface of the posterior myocardium, the typical injury pattern of ST elevation becomes ST depression. The left marginal artery is a branch of the circumflex artery. A branch of the right coronary artery, the posterior interventricular artery anastomoses with the anterior interventricular artery, close to the apex. It supplies posterior sections of the myocardium. Occlusion of the right marginal artery usually leads to the infarction of the right ventricle. Presence of ST elevation in lead V_1 would occur, the only standard ECG looking directly at the right ventricle.

11. **E**—Right coronary artery. The SA node, the natural pacemaker of the heart, is supplied by the sinoatrial artery, a branch of the right coronary artery in 60% to 70% of patients. The circumflex artery also supplies the SA node; however, only in 20% to 30% of patients.

12. **C**—Great cardiac vein. The great cardiac vein begins near the apex of the heart in the anterior interventricular groove where the interventricular artery lies. It then passes superiorly within the groove, alongside the artery, to merge with the left end of the coronary sinus. It drains the territories supplied by the left coronary artery, for example the left atrium and ventricle.
    The anterior cardiac vein comprises two to five small veins. The anterior cardiac veins return blood from the anterior portion of the right ventricle. They run across the anterior surface of the right ventricle and drain into the right atrium. The coronary sinus is the main drainage channel of the myocardium. It is situated between the left atrium and left ventricle on the posterior surface of the heart. It receives deoxygenated blood from multiple smaller veins, typically, from right to left, the small cardiac veins, middle cardiac vein, posterior vein of the left ventricle, oblique vein of the left atrium and the great cardiac vein. The middle cardiac vein runs alongside the posterior interventricular artery in the posterior interventricular groove. The small cardiac vein drains the anterior wall of the right ventricle, bridging the right coronary artery from the superior side.

13. **C**—Right atrium. The coronary sinus drains through the Thebesian valve into the right atrium. It lies on the posterior, inferior surface of the heart.
    The inferior vena cava (IVC) is formed by joining the left and right common iliac veins approximately at the L5 level. It then runs along the posterior abdominal cavity receiving multiple tributaries including the lumbar, right gonadal, right suprarenal, renal, hepatic and inferior phrenic veins. It delivers deoxygenated blood into the right atrium. The IVC is a retroperitoneal structure.

The left atrium receives oxygenated blood from the pulmonary veins. Blood then flows through the mitral valve to the left ventricle during diastole.

The right auricular appendage is a small pouch–shaped structure attached to the right atrium. It is an extension of the pectinate muscles.

The SVC is formed by the union of the right and left brachiocephalic veins. It is joined by the azygos vein before entering the right atrium.

14. **B**—138 mm Hg. Remember MAP = diastolic BP + 1/3 (systolic BP – diastolic BP). Therefore MAP = 105 + 1/3(99) = 138 mm Hg.

15. **E**—Tricuspid valve. Fifty per cent of IE in intravenous drug users involves the tricuspid valve, with the most common causative organism being *Staphylococcus aureus*. Factors influencing the high incidence of IE of the tricuspid valve include the relatively low flow rates through the valve as well it being the first in contact with the systemic circulation before renal/hepatic filtration if the injection site is on the upper limb.

With respect to the aortic valve, calcific aortic stenosis in the elderly remains the most common underlying condition for patients with IE involving this valve.

The third most common site for IE to develop is a combination of the mitral and aortic valves.

Underlying rheumatic heart disease or mitral valve prolapse significantly increases the incidence of subacute IE involving the mitral valve.

The pulmonary valve is the least common site for IE to develop.

16. **A**—Pulmonary artery and descending aorta. Patency between the pulmonary artery and descending aorta is pathological in humans after birth, a condition termed patent ductus arteriosus (PDA). The PDA existing in the developing foetus allows blood from the right ventricle to bypass the nonfunctioning, fluid-filled lungs and enter the systemic circulation. Typically it closes at birth to form the ligamentum arteriosum. Failure of closure is termed a PDA, which can lead to congestive heart failure if left untreated. Handy tip: PDA = *P*ulmonary artery and *D*escending *A*orta.

17. **C**—β2-Adrenoreceptors are G protein–coupled receptors that cause bronchodilation by relaxing the smooth muscles in the bronchial walls.

18. **A**—Adrenaline is produced and released from the adrenal medulla in response to stresses imparted to the body (e.g. excitement, threat). Production and release are stimulated by ACTH and directly via the sympathetic nervous system. Adrenaline acts on both α- and β-receptors and plays a vital role in the 'fight or flight' response.

19. **C**—Chordae tendineae are predominantly made up of collagen (80%) and connect the papillary muscles to the atrioventricular valves. They ensure the atrioventricular valves remain closed during ventricular contraction.

Chapter 4 Abdomen

1. **A**—McBurney point is a surface-marking point that lies one-third of the way between anterior superior iliac spine (ASIS) and the umbilicus. It corresponds with the location of where the base of the appendix connects with the caecum.

D—Two centimetres above the midpoint of the inguinal ligament is considered to correspond with the deep inguinal ring beneath it. The deep inguinal ring transmits the round ligament in females and the spermatic cord in males.

E—It describes the surface marking for the femoral artery. Clinically, this point can be useful in assessing the femoral pulse volume in an acutely unwell patient where the radial and brachial pulse may be lost due to hypotension. Femoral artery venepuncture can also be performed at this point.

2. **B**—External oblique, internal oblique, transversus abdominis, peritoneum is the correct order from superficial to deep.

3. **C**—Ileocolic artery. The ileocolic artery is the lowest branch of the superior mesenteric artery that supplies the ileum, caecum and appendix. The ileocolic artery divides into superior and inferior branches which subsequently anastomose with the right colic artery and the end of the superior mesenteric artery, respectively. The ileocolic artery has multiple arteries that branch from it to supply specific sections of the gastrointestinal tract.

A—The anterior caecal artery, a branch of the ileocaecal artery, supplies the anterior portion of the caecum.

B—The ileal artery, again a branch of the ileocolic artery, supplies the ileum.

D—The IMA branches off the anterior aspect of the aorta at the level of L3. It branches into the left colic artery, sigmoid arteries and the superior rectal artery, which all have further divisions. The proximal branches of the IMA anastomose with branches of the middle colic artery of the superior mesenteric artery. The IMA supplies the structures of the hindgut which include the distal third of the transverse colon, descending colon, sigmoid colon and proximal part of the rectum.

E—The right colic artery is a major branch of the superior mesenteric artery that supplies the ascending colon. It can be divided into an ascending branch that anastomoses with the middle colic artery and a descending branch that anastomoses with the ileocolic artery.

4. **A**—They arise medially to the inferior epigastric artery. An inguinal hernia occurs where part of the abdominal contents (usually fatty tissue or bowel) protrudes into the inguinal canal; an inguinal hernia is either described as direct or indirect depending on the location of the hernia and its underlying pathology. Direct hernias occur as a result of a weakness in the posterior abdominal wall, formed by the transversalis fascia. They arise medial to the inferior epigastric artery and may pass through the superficial inguinal ring. Risk factors for developing a direct inguinal hernia include any cause for an increased intra-abdominal pressure (chronic cough, constipation) or a weakness in the abdominal muscles (obesity, advanced age). For these reasons, direct inguinal hernias are far more common in middle-aged and elderly patients. The inguinal ring is larger in males than in females to transmit the spermatic cord and its contents; therefore males are at significantly higher risk of an inguinal hernia than females.

   B—For the reasons described above, direct inguinal hernias are most common in middle-aged and elderly males.

   C—*Indirect* inguinal hernias occur as a result of a patent processus vaginalis, which remains patent following the failure of embryonic closure. This gives a path for abdominal contents to protrude through the deep inguinal ring into the inguinal canal and ultimately through the superficial ring.

   D—Indirect inguinal hernias may pass into the scrotum. In healthy individuals, the processus vaginalis closes after the testicle has descended from the abdominal cavity and into the scrotum. When the processus vaginalis fails to close, this tract essentially remains open, giving a path for abdominal contents to pass from the abdominal cavity through the inguinal canal and into the scrotum.

   E—Indirect inguinal hernias pass through the deep inguinal ring, whereas direct inguinal hernias do not.

5. **A**—Aponeurosis of the external oblique. There are three layers of the sheath surrounding the spermatic cord, each of which is formed by the extension of a layer of the abdominal wall. The external spermatic fascia is an extension of the aponeurosis of the external oblique.

   C—The cremasteric muscle is an extension of the internal oblique muscle.

   D—The internal spermatic fascia is a continuation of the transversalis fascia.

6. **D**—Rectus sheath, inferior epigastric vessels, inguinal ligament. Hesselbach triangle is the eponymous name given to the inguinal triangle through which direct inguinal hernias pass. Its boundaries are:

- Medial border: lateral margin of the rectus sheath.
- Superolateral border: inferior epigastric vessels.
- Inferior border: inguinal ligament.

7. **A**—The epiploic foramen.

   B—Foramen ovale is found in the skull. The paracolic gutter separates the supracolic and infracolic compartment. The transverse mesocolon divides the supracolic and infracolic compartments.

8. **B**—Second part of the duodenum. The biliary system drains its contents into the duodenum at the major duodenal papilla (also known as papilla of Vater) which lies roughly 8 cm distal to the pylorus of the stomach, in the second part of the duodenum (descending duodenum). The release of bile and pancreatic fluid into the duodenum is controlled by the sphincter of Oddi.

   E—Some patients may have an anatomical variant in the location of the major duodenal papilla. The junction between parts two and three of the duodenum is the most common site of this variant.

9. **D**—Ninth costal cartilage. The fundus of the gallbladder is the rounded end of the gallbladder that faces forwards. The fundus comes into contact with the anterior abdominal wall at the costal margin of the ninth costal cartilage. This corresponds with the lateral border of the rectus abdominis at the level of the transpyloric plane.

10. **B**—Inferior mesenteric artery (IMA). The IMA supplies the structures of the hindgut, which begin approximately two-thirds of the way along his transverse colon to the proximal part of the rectum.

    A—The coeliac trunk branches from the anterior aspect of the aorta at the level of T12. After approximately 1 cm, it divides into three major branches: the left gastric, splenic and common hepatic arteries. These branches further divide to supply the structures of the embryological foregut, including the abdominal oesophagus, stomach, proximal half of the duodenum, liver, pancreas and spleen. Several anastomoses of arteries exist within this region, including major anastomoses around the stomach and the head of the pancreas.

    C—The middle rectal artery is a branch of the internal iliac artery that supplies blood to the rectum. It has anastomoses with the inferior vesicle artery as well as the superior and inferior rectal arteries. Branches from the middle rectal artery supply the vagina in females and the seminal vesicles and prostate in males.

    D—As the name suggests, the sigmoid artery supplies the sigmoid colon. It is a branch of the IMA.

    E—The superior mesenteric artery arises from the anterior aspect of the aorta at the lower border L1. Its main branches are inferior pancreaticoduodenal artery, intestinal arteries, ileocolic artery, right colic artery and middle colic artery. These supply the structures of the embryological midgut including distal duodenum, jejunum, ileum, caecum, appendix, ascending colon and approximately the proximal two-thirds of the transverse colon.

11. **B**—Perforated abdominal viscus. The rupture of an intra-abdominal viscus will produce air under the diaphragm visible on an erect chest x-ray. This is because free air rises. The presence of a gastric air bubble below the diaphragm is a normal finding on the *left* side of a chest x-ray. If free air is seen under the right diaphragm, this must be considered as an emergency with the underlying cause investigated and treated appropriately. Perforated abdominal viscus is a surgical emergency, and an urgent surgical review must be arranged. Further imaging such as a CT scan of the abdomen may provide more information on the underlying cause or site of the perforated viscus.

   A—It is worth noting that free intra-abdominal air may be considered a normal finding only in a postoperative patient where the abdomen has been opened or laparoscopic abdominal surgery performed. However, if the clinical picture is of concern, perforated abdominal viscus must be the main differential until proven otherwise, even in a postoperative patient.

   C—Pneumonia will appear as an increased opacification (the x-ray appearance of an underlying consolidation of the lung) in a lung field/multiple lung fields. Therefore the pathology will be seen above the diaphragm.

   D—A pneumothorax describes the pathological presence of air in the pleural space—between the lung and chest wall. On a chest x-ray, a pneumothorax appears as a rim of air (appears black) between the lung and the chest wall. Again, this would be seen above the diaphragm in the thorax.

   E—A small bowel obstruction is best seen on an abdominal x-ray. Typical features of small bowel obstruction on an x-ray include centrally located, distended gas-filled bowel loops. A hallmark feature of the small bowel is the presence of valvulae conniventes, which appear as thin white lines that pass across the full width of the bowel. Small bowel obstruction may lead to perforation of the small bowel if not treated in a timely and effective manner.

12. **C**—Sigmoid colon is not retroperitoneal.

13. **A**—Ascending colon. The ascending colon is formed from the foetal midgut. Pain from structures formed from the foetal midgut is felt around the umbilical region.

   B, C, D and E—These structures are all part of the foetal foregut and therefore pain is felt in the epigastric region.

14. **E**—The falciform ligament, which separates the left and right lobes of the liver, attaches the anterior surface of the liver to the anterior abdominal wall. Within the free edge of the ligament is the ligamentum teres, a remnant of the umbilical vein.

A—The porta hepatis describes the short and deep fissure beneath the right lobe of the liver that transmits the common hepatic duct (bile), hepatic artery (oxygenated blood) and hepatic portal vein (deoxygenated blood from the gastrointestinal tract). It therefore transmits both oxygenated and deoxygenated blood. Sympathetic nerves, the hepatic branch of the vagus nerve and lymphatics are also transmitted in the porta hepatis.

B—The liver is covered entirely by the peritoneum apart from an area on the diaphragmatic section of the liver known as the bare area.

C—The bare area of the liver is in contact with the diaphragm via the coronary ligaments.

D—When viewing the liver from an anterior perspective, the liver can be divided into the left and right lobes, with the falciform ligament creating this divide. Viewed from the underside, there are two further lobes, the quadrate and caudate lobes, which are part of the right lobe. These divisions are created on an anatomical basis and not on a functional basis.

15. **A**—Pelvic splanchnic nerves. The vagus nerve innerves the foregut and midgut, while the lumbar splanchnic nerve supplies sympathetic innervation to the hindgut.

16. **C**—Cortisol. The correct answer is cortisol which is secreted under the control of adrenocorticotrophic hormone (ACTH) produced by the pituitary gland.

17. **A**—Afferent arteriole dilatation. Prostaglandins cause vasodilatation of the afferent arteriole to increase glomerular perfusion and thus increase glomerular filtration.

18. **A**—Aldosterone is a mineralocorticoid hormone, whereas cortisol is a glucocorticoid.

19. **B**—High PCO_2, low pH, normal HCO_3^-. Guillain–Barré syndrome is a neurological disease that causes muscle weakness. The lungs are not able to ventilate properly so the PCO_2 rises. CO_2 drives the formation of carbonic acid and thus the pH falls. Chronic acidosis will result in a compensatory high in bicarbonate, but Guillain–Barré syndrome is an acute disorder so bicarbonate will be normal in this case.

20. **B**—V_2. The V_2 receptor promotes the fusing of aquaporin water channels to the luminal membrane of the collecting ducts.

Chapter 5 Pelvis

1. **C**—The sacrum is attached to the hip bones via two modified synovial joints—the sacroiliac joints. Each hip bone develops from three bones, the ilium, ischium and pubis, which fuse at the acetabulum. They also

form a joint with each other at the pubis symphysis, a secondary cartilaginous joint. This forms the pelvic ring.

A—The greater pelvis lies above the pelvic brim with the lesser pelvis below.

B—Females have a wider pelvic arch than males. This is to accommodate the passage of the foetus during childbirth.

D—There are two pubic tubercles, both of which are part of the superior ramus of the pubis. It is the most anterior point of the pubis and is palpable. Each pubic tubercle, either the left or right pubic tubercle, lies off the midline of the body. Instead, the pubic symphysis, the secondary cartilaginous joint that joins the left and right hip bones, lies in the midline.

E—When standing upright, the anterior superior iliac spine and superior border of the pubic symphysis lie in the same vertical plane—not the inferior border of the pubic symphysis.

2. **D**—Para-aortic nodes. The testes originate on the posterior abdominal wall, close to the kidney, and descend into the scrotum during foetal development. Lymphatic drainage is, therefore, to the para-aortic nodes in the abdomen and not to the inguinal nodes.

A—The deep inguinal lymph nodes lie medial to the femoral vein within the femoral triangle. Normally up to 2 cm in size, they may swell during infections such as orchitis or malignancies of the vulvar or anus.

C—The popliteal lymph nodes are a group of small lymph nodes located in the fat of the popliteal fossa (i.e. behind the knee). They drain the territories of the lower leg and knee with efferents along the femoral vessels to the deep inguinal lymph nodes.

E—The superficial inguinal lymph nodes lie in a chain directly beneath the inguinal ligament. They receive a number of afferents throughout the genital region, lower abdominal wall, buttocks and anus. The superficial inguinal nodes drain into the deep inguinal nodes, which subsequently drain superiorly via the external iliac nodes, pelvic nodes and onto the para-aortic lymph nodes.

3. **C**—Skin, superficial fascia, external spermatic fascia, cremasteric fascia, internal spermatic fascia, parietal layer of the tunica vaginalis. This correctly describes the layers within the scrotum from superficial to deep.

4. **E**—Puborectalis. Puborectalis is one of three muscle components of the levator ani muscle, situated on either side of the pelvis. The other two components are pubococcygeus and iliococcygeus. The puborectalis muscles from either side of the body meet to form a sling around the rectum. Relaxation of the puborectalis muscle increases the angle between the rectum and anus, thus assisting with defaecation if the internal and external anal sphincters also relax.

A—A component of the pelvic floor, the deep transverse perineal muscle acts to fix the perineal body and aid the expulsion of semen in males, as well as the last few drops of urine in males and females.

B—The external anal sphincter is adherent to the skin at the margin of the anus. To keep the anal orifice closed, it remains in tonic contraction. However, under voluntary control, relaxation assists in defaecation. Damage to this structure may cause incontinence but it is not a pelvic floor muscle.

C—Iliococcygeus, part of the levator ani, supports the pelvic cavity viscera. As a group, the levator ani muscle group rhythmically contracts during orgasm.

D—The internal anal sphincter is also part of the control mechanism of defaecation. Under complete involuntary control, it remains under continuous contraction to prevent the escape of fluid, liquid or solid matter. On distension of the rectal ampulla secondary to voluntary contraction of the puborectalis and external anal sphincter, the internal anal sphincter will relax to allow defaecation. It is not a pelvic floor muscle.

5. **D**—Pudendal nerve. The pudendal nerve has both a sensory and motor function. Damage to the nerve, such as in childbirth, can lead to faecal incontinence as it can lead to the disruption of the innervation to the levator ani muscles.

A—The inferior rectal nerve is the first branch of the pudendal nerve as it enters the pudendal canal. It conveys sensory information of the skin to the pectinate line and the external anal sphincter.

B—Originating from the ventral aspects of L5 to S1 nerve roots, the nerve to obturator internus supplies this muscle, as well as the gemellus superior. They both act to stabilize the femoral head in the acetabulum.

C—Arising from L2 to L4, the obturator nerve has sensory and motor components. Although the name may suggest otherwise, the obturator nerve does not supply the obturator internus muscle. It does, however, innervate the adductor muscles of the leg and sensory components of the skin over the medial thigh.

6. **A**—The rectum begins where the mesocolon ends, approximately at the level of the S3 vertebra. It continues for approximately 12 cm until terminating at the anorectal junction.

B—The middle third of the rectum is only covered by the peritoneum on its anterior surface, which subsequently reflects onto the posterior surface of the bladder in males and posterior surface of the vagina in females. The upper third of the rectum has perineum covering the anterior and lateral surfaces, whereas the lower portion of the rectum has no peritoneal coverage.

C—The rectovesical pouch is only present in males, where it is formed by the peritoneum of the middle third of the rectum reflecting onto the posterior surface of the bladder. In females, this peritoneal reflection from the rectum adheres to the superior aspect of the uterus and upper vagina to form the rectouterine pouch—the pouch of Douglas.

D—The rectum has no blood supply from the superior mesenteric artery. Instead, its arterial supply is from the superior, middle and inferior rectal arteries. The superior rectal artery is a continuation of the inferior mesenteric artery, and the middle and inferior rectal arteries are branches of the internal iliac artery via the inferior vesicle artery and inferior pudendal artery, respectively.

E—A defining feature of the rectum that allows it to be distinguished from the colon is the lack of taeniae coli, haustra and appendices epiploicae.

7. **B**—Lateral lobes. The lateral lobes of the prostate have a high glandular composition and are therefore the most common site for BPH. BPH is the noncancerous enlargement of the prostate caused by hyperplasia of stroma and epithelial cells. As the prostate enlarges, it can compress the prostatic urethra causing symptoms of lower urinary tract obstruction (LUTS), including urinary hesitancy, poor flow, straining to urinate, terminal dribbling, frequency, nocturia and urgency. Given the proximity of the affected lobe to the urethra, LUTS can occur in the early stages of enlargement. On digital rectal examination, a patient with BPH will have a symmetrically enlarged prostate that feels smooth. Importantly, the size of the prostate enlargement does not correspond to symptom severity.

8. **D**—Posterior. Adenocarcinoma of the prostate typically occurs in the posterior lobe. Given this fact, compression of the urethra and subsequent lower urinary tract obstruction may occur later in the clinical course compared to benign prostatic hyperplasia. On digital rectal examination (DRE), the prostate may feel enlarged, asymmetrical and hard. The loss of sulci between lobes may also be noted. However, malignancy of the prostate may not be detected on DRE.

9. **A**—Anteflexed and anteverted. The normal position of the uterus is described as anteflexed and anteverted. This means the body of the uterus is flexed forwards, and the cervix is angled to the front of the body. Some patients may have a uterus that lies in an abnormal position, that is retroflexed or retroverted. This does not pose any inherent medical problem but may increase a female's risk of uterine prolapse into the vagina.

10. **E**—Transitional epithelium. Transitional epithelium is found only in the urothelium, which is in the renal pelvis, bladder, ureters, superior urethra and the prostatic and ejaculatory ducts of the prostate. These specialized epithelial cells exist in multiple layers and have the ability to contract and expand depending on the varying degrees of distension placed on them, that is when the bladder becomes full. Carcinoma of these epithelial cells, a transitional cell carcinoma, is by far the most common cause (approximately 90%) of bladder cancer.

A—Columnar epithelium has a cell height greater than its width and can be found at many sites throughout the body but most abundantly throughout the gastrointestinal tract. With variability in structure depending on function, the majority of columnar epithelium lies at sites where both secretion and absorption are required.

B—Cuboidal epithelium is also specialized and able to secrete and absorb. As suggested by the name, the cells are cuboid in shape with a height and width of similar size. Cuboidal epithelium is found in the ovaries, nephrons, renal tubules, eyes and thyroid gland.

C—Found in the skin and masticatory mucosa, keratinized, stratified squamous epithelium consists of multiple layers of squamous epithelial cells. To be able to withstand insults/trauma, this type of epithelium contains the fibrous protein, keratin.

D—Stratified squamous epithelium is found in areas that require a high turnover of epithelium, owing to cells being frequently lost as a result of repeated trauma. Its location includes the vagina and oesophagus. Containing multiple layers of cells, not all cells within the epithelium will necessarily be flattened squamous cells; however, those cells at the surface will be squamous.

11. **D**—Spongy. The spongy urethra runs the length of the penis in the spongy cavernosum. There is no postspongy urethra!

12. **E**—Diarrhoea. There are multiple and varied symptoms that are associated with menopause and perimenopause, but diarrhoea is not typical. Mental health symptoms can include anxiety, low mood, mood swings and problems with memory and concentration. There are a myriad of potential physical symptoms including hot flushes, insomnia, night sweats, palpitations, headaches, vaginal dryness, dyspareunia, recurrent urinary tract infections, myalgia, arthralgia, weight gain, skin changes and decreased libido.

13. **D**—Potential. The interaction of passage, passenger and power determine the progress of labour, and psyche takes into account the emotional state of the mother.

14. **B**—4 weeks. The blastocyst implants into the wall of the uterus at 4 weeks.

15. **B**—Testes. In a typical male-to-female vaginoplasty, the testes are removed via orchidectomy while the prostate, perineal body and seminal vesicles remain in situ. The urethra is shortened via penectomy with much of the spongy urethra amputated; however, the proximal urethra remains.

16. **A**—Oestrogen. The hormone primarily responsible for the decrease in bone mineral density in postmenopausal females is oestrogen.

Chapter 6 Musculoskeletal system

1. **B**—The muscle contracts but does not change length. This is important for maintaining body posture as it requires holding a steady position. Isotonic contraction refers to the shortening of a muscle during contraction, and eccentric contraction is a controlled relaxation where the muscle gradually lengthens while lowering an object.

2. **B**—Musculocutaneous. The musculocutaneous nerve supplies the anterior compartment of the arm, which includes the coracobrachialis, biceps brachii and brachialis muscles.

3. **A**—Abductor pollicis brevis. The median nerve controls the thenar eminence muscles (abductor pollicis brevis, pollicis opponens and flexor pollicis brevis) and the lateral two lumbricals.

4. **D**—Flexor pollicis brevis. The carpal tunnel is formed by the carpal bones and is roofed by the flexor retinaculum. Flexor pollicis brevis originates at the trapezoid and capitate bones and travels on the radial side of flexor pollicis longus.

5. **E**—Teres major. The rotator cuff muscles stabilize the shoulder joint and include all four options except teres major, which inserts onto the shaft of the humerus rather than on the head.

6. **D**—Scaphoid. Anatomical snuffbox tenderness is indicative of a scaphoid fracture. This type of fracture is prone to avascular necrosis as the scaphoid has a retrospective blood supply.

7. **A**—Sartorius. The boundaries of the femoral triangle are the sartorius (laterally), adductors longus and pectineus (medially) and the inguinal ligament (superiorly).

8. **D**—Deep peroneal. The deep peroneal nerve has a cutaneous supply to a very specific area in the 'sandal gap'.

9. **D**—Head of the fibula. The common peroneal nerve wraps around the head of the femur where it is prone to damage, for example owing to bad positioning in an operating theatre.

10. **D**—L1 to L2. The level of L1 to L2 is where the spinal cord terminates at the conus medullaris. To avoid the spinal cord during lumbar puncture, the procedure is performed below the level of L1 to L2. Below this level extends the lumbar cistern which terminates around the level of S2. The lumbar cistern contains some nerve roots of the cauda equina, as well as cerebrospinal fluid (CSF). This is where CSF is drawn from in a lumbar puncture.

11. **C**—The line between the iliac crests. The iliac crest is a reliable landmark that is both visible and palpable as a surface marking. From here an 'imaginary line' can be made between both iliac crests and the point on this line that crosses the midline corresponding to the L3 to L4 level. You can then palpate the vertebral body above (L3) and below (L4) to find the L3 to L4 disc space. This is where a lumbar puncture is performed.
    The L3 to L4 disc itself is not palpable and therefore an alternate landmark is required.
    The lumbar cistern terminates around S2 and therefore attempting to access CSF below this level would be futile. Furthermore, the sacral vertebrae are fused, with a slim fibrocartilage between each vertebral connection. This means that you would not be able to readily access the space anterior to the vertebral column with a transcutaneous needle.

12. **C**—The tibial nerve originates from L4 to S3 and supplies sensory innervation to most of the posterior surface of the leg and foot. C to E are compartments, which would be muscle groups and come under motor control, not sensory.

13. **C**—The pronator quadrates attach to both bones in the deep layer of the flexor compartment of the distal forearm.

14. **A**—In the thoracic spine, the transverse processes are longer to allow articulation with the ribs.

15. **B**—A disc prolapse involves the spread of the nucleus pulposus through a tear in the annulus fibrosus which can compress surrounding structures including nerve roots. This can happen acutely due to trauma or gradually as a chronic process. Depending on the location of the tear, this may be in a posterior or lateral direction which may then place pressure on a spinal nerve or the spinal cord.

Glossary

Anatomy and Physiology

A- Absence of, lacking, e.g., avascular—absence of a blood supply.

Abscess A localized collection of pus.

Adenosine triphosphate (ATP) A general source of energy for all intracellular metabolic reactions.

Afferent Carrying towards a given point. Afferent nerve impulses (i.e., sensory) are carried towards the brain and spinal cord.

Agonist A muscle that, when it contracts, causes a specific movement (prime mover), e.g., biceps brachii causes flexion of the elbow. Contraction of the agonist usually requires the relaxation of the antagonist. See Antagonist.

Anaesthesia Loss of feeling owing to nerve damage, resulting from disease or trauma.

Anastomosis Network of communicating arteries, veins or nerves (plural—anastomoses).

Aneurysm A dilatation of an arterial wall.

Antagonist A muscle that has the opposite action of the agonist muscle. It returns limbs to their original position.

Antigen-presenting cell A cell that displays foreign material (antigen) to immune cells (lymphocytes). Antigen-presenting cells may be macrophages, dendritic cells, or B cells.

Apex Pointed end of a cone-shaped structure, e.g., apex of the axilla.

Aponeurosis Strong, flattened tendon with a wide area of attachment, e.g., external oblique aponeurosis.

Appendicular Relating to the appendages (the limbs), e.g., appendicular skeleton.

Arteriogram Digital image or film produced as a result of arteriography.

Arteriography The use of contrast medium and X-rays, to visualize the lumina of arteries, or of the chambers of the heart.

Arterioles Blood vessels that are smaller than arteries and that branch from arteries with variable amounts of elastic and smooth tissue.

Arthro- Relates to joints, e.g., arthrodesis, arthritis, arthroscope.

Atrophy Wasting of a tissue or organ owing to cell loss, e.g., muscle atrophy after prolonged bedrest.

Autonomic nervous system (ANS) The ANS regulates bodily functions not under conscious control. It is divided into sympathetic and parasympathetic divisions.

Autoregulation Process by which tissue perfusion remains relatively constant despite blood pressure changes.

Axial Relating to the axis of the body, as in axial skeleton, which consists of the skull, vertebral column and thoracic cage.

Axilla Region where the upper limb joins the trunk (commonly known as the armpit).

Axon A neuron consists of a nerve cell body and an axon, which conducts impulses away from the cell body.

Barium sulphate An insoluble compound which is used as a contrast medium in imaging the gastrointestinal tract.

Baroreceptors Sensitive to pressure and located in the aorta, internal carotid arteries and other large arteries in the neck and chest.

Bifurcation The point at which an anatomical structure, e.g., trachea, divides into two parts, i.e., primary bronchi.

Bipennate Usually a term that describes the structure of a muscle. A bipennate muscle is one in which the tendon lies in the centre of the muscle and the muscle fibres pass to it from either side (e.g., rectus femoris). See Unipennate and Multipennate.

Brachial Relates to the arm (between the shoulder and elbow)—hence brachial artery.

Branchial At the cranial end of the embryonic digestive system there are a series of branchial arches (primitive gill arches) which give rise to specific structures of the head and neck.

Bronchiole A microscopic branch of the bronchi.

Bronchus First branches of the trachea (plural—bronchi; adjective—bronchial).

Buccal Relating to the mouth.

Bursa Small sac lined by synovial membrane that ensures free movement of tendons close to joints, e.g., infrapatellar bursa.

Bursitis Inflammation of a bursa.

Canal A tubular passage, e.g., adductor canal of the thigh.

Capillaries Join arterioles and venules and are present in almost every tissue in the body.

Carcinoma Cancer of epithelial origin.

Cardia Heart (adjective—cardiac).

Cardiac output (CO) The volume of blood ejected by one ventricle into its respective artery each minute. Calculated as the heart rate multiplied by the stroke volume.

Cerebellum Part of the brain that controls coordinated movement, balance and muscle tone (adjective—cerebellar).

Cerebrum Largest part of the brain, composed of the two cerebral hemispheres (adjective—cerebral).

Cerebrospinal fluid Fluid surrounding the central nervous system and filling the ventricles of the brain.

Cerebrovascular accident (CVA) See Stroke.

Cervix Literally means 'the neck'. Also used to refer to the narrow part or 'neck' of an organ. In anatomy 'cervix' usually refers to the neck of the uterus (adjective—cervical).

Chemoreceptors Located in the carotid sinus and aortic arches in small structures known as carotid and aortic bodies.

Chondro- Relates to cartilage, e.g., chondrocytes—cartilage cells.

Collateral Accessory or secondary, e.g., collateral circulation is an accessory route of blood flow to an organ.

Condyle Literally means 'knuckle'. A rounded articular surface, e.g., femoral condyles.

Connective tissue A tissue composed of cells, fibres and extracellular matrix, which supports and separates more specialized tissues and organs.

Contrast studies A procedure involving the use of contrast medium, allowing improved visualization of structures on plain X-rays, computed tomography (CT) or magnetic resonance imaging (MRI) scans.

Coronary Encircling like a crown, e.g., coronary arteries, arteries which encircle and supply the heart.

Cortex Outer part of a structure, e.g., cortex of the kidney (adjective—cortical); see also Medulla.

Costa Literally means 'rib' (adjective—costal), e.g., intercostal muscles lie between the ribs.

Cranial nerves Twelve pairs of nerves that emerge from the brain (the majority from the brainstem)—unlike spinal nerves, which emerge from the spinal cord.

Cranium The section of the skull containing the brain.

Cruciate Structures arranged like a cross, e.g., the cruciate ligaments.

Cusp Leaflet of a heart valve. Hence bicuspid valve means a valve comprising two leaflets.

Cutaneous Relating to the skin.

Dendrite A short branch of the neuron cell body which forms synapses with other neurons.

Dental Related to teeth (the dens is a tooth-shaped structure).

Depolarization A change in the membrane potential of a cell, usually resulting in an action potential.

Dermatome An area of skin supplied by a single spinal segment.

Diastole Relaxation phase of the cardiac cycle (adjective—diastolic).

Diffusion The passive, simple movement of a substance down a concentration gradient.

Discharge The release of fluid or pus from its site of production, e.g., an infected wound.

Dislocate Joint displacement where the contact between the articular surface of bones is lost.

Dural venous sinuses Venous spaces lying between the endosteal and meningeal layers of the dura, within the cranium, e.g., superior sagittal sinus.

Dyspnoea Difficulty in breathing.

Electrocardiogram (ECG) Records the electrical activity of the heart.

Efferent Carrying away from. Efferent (i.e., motor) nerve impulses are carried away from the central nervous system.

Endo Within, or inner part of a structure, e.g., endocardium—the innermost layer of the heart.

Endocardium Consists of three layers and is continuous with the endothelial lining of the large blood vessels attached to the heart.

Endoplasmic reticulum Forms a network of membranes within the cell.

Epi- Above or on the surface of a structure, e.g., epidermis—outermost layer of the skin.

Epithelium One of the four basic tissue types. It forms glands, covers all surfaces and lines the body cavities (adjective—epithelial).

Erythema Reddening of the skin owing to dilatation of dermal capillaries.

Eversion Turning the sole of the foot outwards (laterally).

Ex-, Extra- Out, e.g., expiration—to breathe out; extracapsular—outside a joint capsule.

Facet A flat articular surface of a bone, e.g., facet joints of the vertebra.

Facilitated diffusion This process is faster than simple diffusion, with the passage of substances down their concentration gradients requiring a transporter.

Fissure A groove or cleft, e.g., the oblique fissure of the left lung separates upper and lower lobes.

Foramen Opening or passage through a bone, e.g., foramen magnum through which the spinal cord passes (plural—foramina).

Fossa Literally means 'a ditch'; therefore, a depression, hollow or pit (antecubital fossa of the elbow).

Fracture A break in the continuity of a bone.

Fundus Base of a hollow organ, or the part furthest from the opening (stomach, uterus).

Ganglion A swelling. In the nervous system, it is a collection of nerve cell bodies outside the central nervous system (CNS), e.g., a sensory ganglion (without synapses), or an autonomic ganglion (with synapses). See Nucleus.

Gastro- Relates to the stomach, e.g., gastric artery, gastrointestinal (GI) tract, gastroscopy.

Genicular Relates to the knee joint, e.g., genicular arteries, which supply the knee.

Glosso- Relates to the tongue. The hypoglossal nerve lies below the tongue.

Glottis Gap between the vocal folds (adjective—glottal).

Golgi apparatus Membranous sacs that sort and modify proteins arriving from the granular endoplasmic reticulum, packing them into vesicles before sending them to other organelles or secreting them.

Golgi tendon organs Bundles of collagen fibres encapsulated by a connective tissue layer present at the muscle–tendon junction.

Gonads Sex organs—ovaries and testes (adjective—gonadal).

Greater sac General peritoneal cavity.

Gyrus Raised area of the cerebral cortex (pleural—gyri). See Sulcus.

Haemo- Relates to blood, e.g., haematology is the study of blood, haematoma (bruising) is the swelling caused by bleeding into the tissues.

Haemopoiesis The formation of red blood cells in the bone marrow.

Haemoptysis Coughing up blood, commonly a sign of infection or malignancy.

Haemostasis Control of bleeding.

Heart rate (HR) Number of ventricular contractions in one minute.

Hemi- Denotes one half of the body or a structure, e.g., hemidiaphragm, hemiplegia.

Hepato Relates to the liver, e.g., hepatic artery, hepatitis—inflammation of the liver.

Hernia Protrusion of an organ or tissue through the wall of a cavity that normally encloses it, e.g., femoral and inguinal hernias.

Hiatus An opening, e.g., adductor hiatus of adductor canal.

Hilum Place where vessels and nerves enter or leave an organ, e.g., hilum of the lung (plural—hila, adjective—hilar).

Homeostasis The maintenance of constant conditions within the body.

Hyper Literally 'above', or 'excessive', e.g., hyperextension—forced extension of a joint beyond normal limits, hypertrophy—increase in size.

Hypo- Literally 'below' or 'depressed', e.g., hypochondrium—below the costal cartilages, hypoglossal—below the tongue.

Hyperplasia An increase in tissue/organ size owing to an increase in cell numbers.

Hypertrophy An increase in tissue/organ size owing to an increase in cell size.

Ilium Part of the hip bone, along with the pubis and ischium (adjective—iliac).

Infra- Below or lower, e.g., infraorbital, below the orbit of the skull, infrahyoid below the hyoid bone.

Infundibulum A funnel-shaped passage.

Inguinal Relates to the groin where the lower limb meets the trunk, e.g., inguinal hernia, inguinal ligament.

Inotropes Substances that affect the force of cardiac contractility.

Insertion Relates to the more distal attachment of a muscle, which moves on contraction of the muscle.

Inter Between, e.g., interosseous membrane lies between the bones, intercostal between the ribs.

Intra- Inside, e.g., an intracapsular tendon lies inside the capsule of the joint (see Extra-).

Intraperitoneal A viscus suspended from the posterior abdominal wall by a mesentery, e.g., the ileum and jejunum.

Intervertebral discs Secondary cartilaginous joints between the vertebrae.

Ischaemia Reduction of blood flow to a tissue or organ, often resulting in damage to the tissue or organ.

Isthmus Narrow region connecting two parts, e.g., isthmus of the thyroid gland.

-itis Inflammation, e.g., gastritis—inflammation of the stomach, arthritis—inflammation of joints.

Labium Lip (pleural—labia, adjective—labial).

Labrum Lip or a lip-like structure, e.g., glenoid labrum of the glenoid fossa of the shoulder joint.

Larynx The part of the airway between the pharynx and trachea containing the vocal cords (adjective—laryngeal).

Lesser sac Diverticulum of peritoneum posterior to the stomach.

Ligament Tough connective tissue bands connecting two or more structures, most commonly bones. (adjective—ligamentous).

Lingula Tongue (adjective—lingual).

Loculus A small, enclosed cavity or space (plural—loculi, adjective—loculated).

Lumen Central cavity of a tube, e.g., artery, vein, intestine, etc. (adjective—luminal).

Lysosome Single-membraned oval organelle containing highly acidic digestive enzymes that break down bacteria, cell debris and dead organelles.

Macro- Indicates the large size of a structure (macroscopic—visible with the naked eye).

Mast- Relating to the breast, e.g., mastectomy—removal of the breast, mastitis—inflammation of the breast.

Mediastinum The space within the thorax, between the two pleural cavities.

Medulla Inner part of a solid organ (adjective—medullary), e.g., medulla of the kidney. See Cortex.

Mesentery Double layer of peritoneum attaching viscera to the posterior abdominal wall (adjective—mesenteric).

Messenger RNA (mRNA) Carries the genetic code from the nucleus to the cytoplasm.

Metastasis The spread of a malignant tumour to distant sites, e.g., breast carcinoma to axillary lymph nodes.

Mitral Describes the valve between the left atrium and left ventricle (also known as the atrioventricular valve).

Mitochondria Double-membraned, elongated, ovoid structures that function to make energy available to cells in the form of adenosine triphosphate.

Motor Relates to structures or activities involving transmission of nerve impulses away from the central nervous system. See Efferent.

Motor endplate The enlarged end of a motor neuron that forms a synapse with part of the muscle membrane.

Motor units Each skeletal muscle fibre is innervated by a single motor neurone, which comprises a motor neurone and all the muscle fibres it innervates.

Mucus A thick glycoprotein secretion produced by glands (adjective—mucous).

Multipennate A term describing the structure of a muscle. A multipennate muscle may be arranged as a series of bipennate muscles lying alongside one another (e.g., the acromial fibres of the deltoid) or may have the tendon lying within its centre and the muscle fibres passing to it from all sides, converging as they go (e.g., tibialis anterior).

Muscle spindles These organs lie parallel to the skeletal muscle fibres and measure the extent of muscle stretch.

Myo Relating to muscle, e.g., myocardium—muscle of the heart, myometrium—uterine muscle, myalgia—muscle pain.

Myocardium Consists of cardiac muscle cells (myocytes), which are responsible for cardiac contractility.

Myocytes Muscle cells.

Myofibrils Filamentous bundles on the individual muscle fibre that run along the entire length of the fibre.

Necrosis Death of a tissue, e.g., cardiac muscle, resulting from a myocardial infarction.

Nerve A term that may be used rather loosely. Strictly, it should refer to a large collection of nerve fibres that can be seen with the naked eye, e.g., the ulnar nerve. However, it may be used when referring to a single neurone, or its axon.

Neuro- Relates to nerves, e.g., neurology—study of the nervous system.

Neuromuscular junction (NMJ) NMJ is the synapse between a neurone and the muscle cell membrane.

Noxious Harmful, e.g., a substance that causes damage to cells.

Nucleus In terms of the CNS, a nucleus describes a collection of nerve cell bodies that share a similar function. See Ganglion.

Nuclear membrane/envelope Two membranes surrounding the nucleus containing pores that regulate the entry and exit of molecules.

Nucleoli Highly coiled structures not enveloped by a nuclear membrane and containing RNA and protein components.

-oma Denotes a tumour, e.g., lymphoma (of the lymph nodes), carcinoma (of an epithelium), melanoma (of the skin).

Omental bursa See Lesser sac.

Omentum Folds of peritoneum linking the stomach to other viscera, e.g., lesser omentum connects the stomach to the liver.

Orifice An opening to a cavity.

Oss-, Osteo- Relates to bones, e.g., ossification—process of bone formation, osteoporosis—abnormal loss of bone density.

Ossification The conversion of fibrous tissue or cartilage into bone; can either be intramembranous or endochondral.

-ostomy Making a permanent opening, e.g., colostomy—opening of the colon onto the surface of the abdomen, ileostomy—opening of the ileum onto the surface of the abdomen.

-otomy Making a small, temporary opening, e.g., laparotomy—emergency opening of the abdomen.

Palpebral Relates to the eyelids (palpebrae), e.g., the muscle that lifts the eyelids is levator palpebrae superioris.

Papilloedema Swelling of the optic disc, seen on fundoscopy. Often a sign of raised intracranial pressure.

Para- By the side of, e.g., paravertebral muscles, alongside the vertebral column, paraaortic, beside the aorta, paranasal air sinuses.

Paraesthesia Abnormal sensation in the distribution of a peripheral nerve, e.g., pins and needles along the medial border of the forearm and medial one-and-a-half digits, in ulnar nerve damage.

Paralysis Loss of muscle function.

Parietal Relates to the surface of the inner walls of a body cavity, e.g., parietal pleura. Also relates to the parietal bone of the skull.

Pectoral Relating to the chest (adjective).

Perforation The formation of a hole in an organ or tissue, usually through a disease process.

Peri- Around or near, e.g., periosteum—membrane covering the surface of bone, pericardium—sac surrounding the heart.

Pericardium Fibrous sac covering the whole heart.

Perineum The region between the anus and external genitalia, inferior to the pelvic diaphragm and bounded by the pelvic outlet.

Peristalsis Motion by which intestinal contents are moved through the alimentary tract.

Peritoneum Membrane lining the abdominal cavity.

Peroxisomes Single-membraned, oval organelles that destroy the highly toxic hydrogen peroxide (H_2O_2) that is produced by certain cell reactions.

Phrenic Relating to the diaphragm.

Pia Innermost, vascular layer of the meninges.

Pleura The epithelial covering of the lungs.

Plexus Network, e.g., brachial plexus is the network of nerves that supply the upper limb.

Portal system Venous system carrying blood through a second capillary bed before returning blood to the heart, e.g., hepatic portal vein delivers blood from the gastrointestinal tract to the capillaries of the liver before it is returned to the right atrium via the hepatic vein and the inferior vena cava.

Post- After or following, e.g., postganglionic describes a neurone that leaves a ganglion and terminates in an effector (muscle or gland).

Pre- Preceding or before, e.g., preganglionic describes a neuron that leaves the spinal cord and terminates in a ganglion.

Process A thin prominence or protuberance, e.g., spinous process of vertebrae.

Prominence A projection of bone.

Prone Lying face down.

Proprioception Ability to sense the position of the body in space. Proprioceptors are present in muscles and tendons and register mechanical changes in position.

Protuberance A rounded projection of bone.

Pulmonary circulation Vessels that carry blood from the right side of the heart to the alveolar capillaries of the lungs and back to the left side of the heart. In the process, gaseous exchange occurs, with oxygen entering the blood and carbon dioxide leaving it.

Radiolucent A structure that does not absorb X-rays and appears dark on an X-ray film.

Radiopaque A structure which absorbs X-rays and appears white on an X-ray film.

Raphe Literally 'a seam'. A line of union between two muscles such as is found in the pharyngeal constrictors.

Recess A depression or hollow cavity of an organ.

Reflex An unconscious, autonomic and involuntary action, e.g., muscle contraction through a neuronal circuit.

Regurgitation The backflow of a liquid against its normal direction, e.g., blood flows from the left ventricle to left atrium through a defective mitral valve.

Renal Relating to the kidneys, e.g., renal artery.

Retinaculum A thickened connective tissue band holding other tissues in position, e.g., extensor tendons held by the extensor retinaculum in the forearm.

Retro- At the back or behind a structure, e.g., retroperitoneal.

Retroperitoneal A viscus lying against the posterior abdominal wall and covered by peritoneum on its anterior surface only, e.g., pancreas, kidneys, etc.

Ribosomes Large particles composed of about 70 proteins and several RNA molecules. There are two subunits of different sizes, 30s and 50s, with the former being smaller.

Ribosomal RNA (rRNA) Where the protein molecules are actually assembled.

Sarcoma Cancer of connective tissue origin.

Sarcomere Fundamental contractile unit within the muscle, from one Z-line to the next.

Sarcoplasm Muscle fibre matrix where the myofibrils are suspended.

Sarcoplasmic reticulum (SR) An endoplasmic reticulum equivalent in the muscle fibre. Runs longitudinally along the myofibrils and wraps around groups of myofibrils.

Sclerosis Hardening of a tissue.

Sensory Relates to structures or activities that involve transmitting nerve impulses towards the CNS from the periphery. See Afferent.

Septum A partition which divides an anatomical structure, e.g., interventricular septum—between the ventricles.

Serous Thin, watery secretions, secreted by a serous membrane such as the pleura. See Mucus.

Sesamoid An oval or round-shaped bone within a tendon that slides over another bone, e.g., the patella within the patellar tendon, which slides over the patellar surface of the femur.

Sheath A connective tissue envelope that surrounding anatomical structures, e.g., nerve, muscle or tendon.

Sinoatrial (SA) node Part of the heart that causes the pacemaker potential.

Sinus Cavity or channel; has many meanings, e.g., paranasal sinus, hepatic sinus, dural venous sinus.

Somatic Relating to the structures that make up the body wall, or its primitive divisions, known as somites.

Sphincter Muscular valve which controls the diameter of a tube, e.g., the pyloric sphincter lies between the stomach and duodenum.

Splanchnic Equivalent to visceral—splanchnic is derived from Greek, visceral from Latin.

Squamous Flattened, scale-like cells, e.g., squamous epithelium consists of very flattened cells.

Stroke Sudden onset of weakness due to interruption of blood flow to the brain.

Stroke volume (SV) Volume of blood ejected in one ventricular contraction.

Sub- Below or underlying, e.g., subcostal—below the ribs.

Sulcus Gutter or depression, particularly used in relation to the surface of the cerebrum where sulci lie between the gyri, e.g., central sulcus of the cerebral cortex (plural—sulci).

Supine Lying on the back, face up.

Supra Above, e.g., supraorbital nerve, suprarenal gland.

Synapse- Junction between two neurones or between a nerve and an effector e.g., a muscle.

Synovial Synovial means 'like an egg'. Describes joints that are freely movable. Synovial fluid secreted by synovial membrane has the consistency of egg white and lubricates and nourishes the joint surfaces.

Systemic circulation Vessels carrying blood from the left side of the heart, to the capillary beds of the entire body (except the lungs), and returning blood to the right side of the heart. In the process gaseous exchange occurs with oxygen leaving the blood to enter the tissues, and carbon dioxide exiting the tissues and entering the blood.

Systole Contraction phase of the cardiac cycle (adjective—systolic). See Diastole.

Tachycardia An increased heart rate.

Tachypnoea An increased respiratory rate.

Tamponade An abnormal pressure on a part of the body, e.g., the presence of fluid within the pericardial cavity, compressing the heart.

Tendon The tough extension of the connective tissue associated with muscles, which forms the attachment of muscle to bone.

Thermoregulation Regulation of body temperature through shivering or peripheral capillary dilatation and sweating.

Thoraco- Relating to the thorax.

Thrombus A blood clot.

Tissue A collection of similar cells that perform specialized functions. There are four basic tissue types epithelia, muscle, nerve and connective tissues.

Total peripheral resistance Resistance to blood flow in the circulatory system.

Transcription mRNA synthesis.

Transfer RNA (tRNA) Transfers amino acids to the ribosomes to manufacture proteins.

Translation Formation of proteins from the mRNA.

Transmural pressure The pressure across the wall of the vessel; can be affected by external and internal pressures.

Transverse A plane dividing a structure into superior and inferior parts.

Tubercle A small rounded bony protuberance, e.g., lesser tubercle of the humerus.

Tuberosity A large rounded bony protuberance, e.g., the greater tuberosity of the femur.

Tunica A layer of an anatomical structure, e.g., tunica media—the smooth muscle layer of an artery.

Umbilicus Abdominal site of attachment of the umbilical cord.

Unipennate Relates usually to muscle. Describes a muscle in which the tendon lies along one side of the muscle and the muscle fibres pass oblique to it. See Bipennate and Multipennate.

Ureter Muscular tube that carries urine between the kidney and bladder.

Urethra Muscular tube that carries urine from the bladder to the exterior.

Varicose Enlarged and twisted superficial veins, especially in the lower limb.

Vaso Relating to vessels, e.g., vasoconstriction—physiological narrowing of blood vessels (plural—vasa).

Venae comitantes Veins that closely accompany arteries, e.g., the deep veins of the limbs.

Venules Collect the blood from the capillaries and transport it to the veins.

Venepuncture The puncture of a vein to obtain a sample of blood or administer medication, e.g., antibiotics.

Ventricle Chamber, e.g., chambers of the heart. There are also four ventricles in the brain.

Vinculae A band of synovial tissue connecting the flexor tendons to the phalanges.

Visceral Relates to internal organs. Visceral nerves tend to be under involuntary control, and sensation tends to be vague, imprecisely perceptible or even imperceptible. See Somatic.

Viscus Internal organ, e.g. heart, spleen, etc. (plural—viscera).

Index

Note: Page numbers followed by *f* indicate figures, *t* indicate tables and *b* indicate boxes.